Evaluation of Advanced Semiconductor Materials by Electron Microscopy

NATO ASI Series

Advanced Science Institutes Series

A series presenting the results of activities sponsored by the NATO Science Committee, which aims at the dissemination of advanced scientific and technological knowledge, with a view to strengthening links between scientific communities.

The series is published by an international board of publishers in conjunction with the NATO Scientific Affairs Division

A	**Life Sciences**	Plenum Publishing Corporation
B	**Physics**	New York and London
C	**Mathematical and Physical Sciences**	Kluwer Academic Publishers
		Dordrecht, Boston, and London
D	**Behavioral and Social Sciences**	
E	**Applied Sciences**	
F	**Computer and Systems Sciences**	Springer-Verlag
G	**Ecological Sciences**	Berlin, Heidelberg, New York, London,
H	**Cell Biology**	Paris, and Tokyo

Recent Volumes in this Series

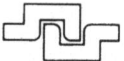

Series B: Physics

Evaluation of Advanced Semiconductor Materials by Electron Microscopy

Edited by

David Cherns

University of Bristol
Bristol, United Kingdom

Plenum Press
New York and London
Published in cooperation with NATO Scientific Affairs Division

Proceedings of a NATO Advanced Research Workshop on
the Evaluation of Advanced Semiconductor Materials
by Electron Microscopy,
held September 12–17, 1988,
in Bristol, United Kingdom

Library of Congress Cataloging in Publication Data

NATO Advanced Research Workshop on the Evaluation of Advanced Semiconductor Materials by Electron Microscopy (1988: Bristol, England)
    Evaluation of advanced semiconductor materials by electron microscopy /
edited by David Cherns.
        p.   cm.—(NATO ASI series. Series B, Physics; vol. 203)
    "Proceedings of a NATO Advanced Research Workshop on the Evaluation of
Advanced Semiconductor Materials by Electron Microscopy, held September
12–17, 1988, in Bristol, United Kingdom"—Verso t.p.
    "Held within the program of activities of the NATO Special Program on Con-
densed Systems of Low Dimensionality, running from 1983 to 1988 as part of the
activities of the NATO Science Committee".
    "Published in cooperation with NATO Scientific Affairs Division."
    Includes bibliographical references.
    ISBN-13: 978-1-4612-7850-4   e-ISBN-13: 978-1-4613-0527-9
    DOI: 10.1001/13: 978-1-4613-0527-9
    1. Semiconductors—Surfaces—Congresses. 2. Electron microscopy—Tech-
nique—Congresses. 3. Electrons—Diffraction—Congresses. I. Cherns, David. II.
North Atlantic Treaty Organization. Scientific Affairs Division. III. Special Program on Condensed Systems of Low Dimensionality (NATO) IV. Title. V. Series:
NATO ASI series. Series B, Physics; v. 203.
QC611.6.S9N36   1988   89-16354
530.4'1—dc20   CIP

© 1989 Plenum Press, New York
Softcover reprint of the hardcover 1st edition 1989
A Division of Plenum Publishing Corporation
233 Spring Street, New York, N.Y. 10013

SPECIAL PROGRAM ON CONDENSED SYSTEMS OF LOW DIMENSIONALITY

This book contains the proceedings of a NATO Advanced Research Workshop held within the program of activities of the NATO Special Program on Condensed Systems of Low Dimensionality, running from 1983 to 1988 as part of the activities of the NATO Science Committee.

Other books previously published as a result of the activities of the Special Program are:

SPECIAL PROGRAM ON CONDENSED SYSTEMS OF LOW DIMENSIONALITY

PREFACE

The last few years have seen rapid improvements in semiconductor growth techniques which have produced an expanding range of high quality heterostructures for new semiconductor devises. As the dimensions of such structures approach the nanometer level, it becomes increasingly important to characterise materials properties such as composition uniformity, strain, interface sharpness and roughness and the nature of defects, as well as their influence on electrical and optical properties. Much of this information is being obtained by electron microscopy and this is also an area of rapid progress. There have been advances for thin film studies across a wide range of techniques, including, for example, convergent beam electron diffraction, X-ray and electron energy loss microanalysis and high spatial resolution cathodoluminescence as well as by conventional and high resolution methods. Important developments have also occurred in the study of surfaces and film growth phenomena by both microscopy and diffraction techniques.

With these developments in mind, an application was made to the NATO Science Committee in late summer 1987 to fund an Advanced Research Workshop to review the electron microscopy of advanced semiconductors. This was subsequently accepted for the 1988 programme and became the "NATO Advanced Research Workshop on the Evaluation of Advanced Semiconductor Materials by Electron Microscopy". The Workshop took place in the pleasant and intimate surroundings of Wills Hall, Bristol, UK, during the week 11-17 September 1988 and was attended by fifty-five participants from fourteen countries.

The scientific programme was mostly divided into morning and evening sessions, each session comprising between one and four invited lectures followed by a general discussion. Sessions were almost equally divided between those reviewing progress in techniques and those concerned more with applications, or "hot" topics as viewed by the Organising Committee. The papers of the invited speakers are included in these Proceedings, and have been assembled mostly in the order of presentation and under the actual session headings. A Study Group, chaired by Dr. J.M. Gibson, met in three sessions towards the end of the week to discuss future scientific and instrumental developments. The report of the Study Group is included as an appendix to the Proceedings.

It was generally agreed that the Workshop was both very useful and stimulating, as may indeed be judged by the quality of the submitted papers. A key factor in organising the meeting was, of course, the availability of sufficient funds to assist with travel expenses of invited speakers. The NATO Science Committee has already been mentioned as the principal source of funds for the Workshop. However, the Organising Committee also gratefully acknowledges grants from JEOL (UK) Ltd and Philips (Eindhoven) which provided valuable additional support and flexibility in planning the programme.

Several members of the Physics Department, Bristol University helped with the organisation and running of the Workshop, and particular thanks go to Dr. R. Vincent and P. Spellward. Miss A. Carton and Mrs. F.A. Hanley provided secretarial support both prior to the meeting and in preparation of these Proceedings.

D. Cherns
20th March, 1989

CONTENTS

High Resolution Electron Microscopy

Convergent Beam Electron Diffraction

X-ray and Electron Energy Loss Microanalysis

Defects in Heteroepitaxy

Appendix

HREM OF EDGE-ON INTERFACES AND DEFECTS

Rob W. Glaisher, J.C. Barry and David J. Smith*

Center for Solid State Science
Arizona State University
Tempe, Arizona 85287, U.S.A.

INTRODUCTION

The latest generation of intermediate-voltage high-resolution electron microscopes (HREMs) offer the exciting prospect of resolution limits of 2Å or better [1,2]. Moreover, under certain well-defined conditions, it is even possible to deduce useful structural details down to small fractions of this limit [3-5], and some limited chemical information can also be extracted. In this paper, the potentialities and limitations of the high-resolution technique will be considered, with particular reference to edge-on interfaces and defects in various elemental and compound semiconductors. Specific examples described include: i the identification of crystal polarity in <110>-orientated sphalerite materials; ii intensity variations across <100> GaAs/Ga$_{1-x}$Al$_x$As interfaces; iii stacking fault symmetry and dislocations; iv refinement of the diamond <100> platelet defect; v distinguishing shuffle and glide models for the Si 30° partial dislocation. Prospects and practical problems associated with the HREM technique, as it applies to imaging semiconductors, are briefly discussed.

CRYSTALLOGRAPHY

The crystal orientations of most interest when imaging elemental or sphalerite compound semiconductors are <100> or <110>. Schematic drawings for the binary sphalerite structure are shown in Fig. 1, together with corresponding diffraction patterns. The sphalerite structure has space group F43m (No. 216). Several relationships between the kinematical structure factors (F_{hkl}) have important consequences for imaging these materials. For example, c^*-axis related reflections have equal equivalent structure factors due to mirror symmetry, eg. $F_{\overline{1}11}=F_{1\overline{1}1}$. For specific structure factors the following hold:

   i h+k+l=4n (n=0,1,2....) (for example, 220, 400) contain sum terms (f_A+f_B) only, and therefore provide no chemical information;

   ii h+k+l=4n+2 (for example, 200) contain difference terms (f_A-f_B) only. These beams can provide chemical information;

   iii h+k+l=4n+1, 4n+3 (for example, 111, 311) contain both sum and difference terms and give information about polarity. The degree of polarity (i.e. non-centrosymmetry) is given by the ratio of (f_A+f_B) to (f_A-f_B).

---

*Also at Department of Physics

iv Bijvoet-related reflections, i.e. (hkl), ($\bar{h}k\bar{l}$), are non-equivalent, as a consequence of the crystal's non-centrosymmetry, eg. $F_{\bar{1}11} \neq F_{1\bar{1}\bar{1}}$;

v The {002} and {020} reflections differ in structure phase by 180°; these relationships are retained under dynamical scattering conditions when the related reflections have equivalent excitation errors; they are utilized later for deriving expressions for image intensity under zone axis imaging conditions. In the <110> orientation, information from {111} reflections will be used to determine polarity, whereas in the <100> orientation information from {200} reflections will be used to investigate chemical changes at interfaces.

The <110> orientation is preferred for the investigation of dislocations in diamond/sphalerite crystals by HREM since the dominant slip system is <110> {111}. A <110> orientation aligns the core of the dislocation parallel to the electron beam and thus provides the most useful projected view of the core. For multilayer structures such as GaAs/Ga$_x$Al$_{1-x}$As, which are grown on <100>, the extent of structural and chemical abruptness at the interface is of critical importance. In order to assess the structural flatness of the interface by HREM, either <100> or <110> projections are suitable. However, <100> is preferred for the determination of chemical information due to the contributions of four chemically-sensitive {002} reflections to the diffraction pattern [6], whereas the two {002} reflections in the <110> orientation also derive considerable intensity from {111} reflections by double diffraction.

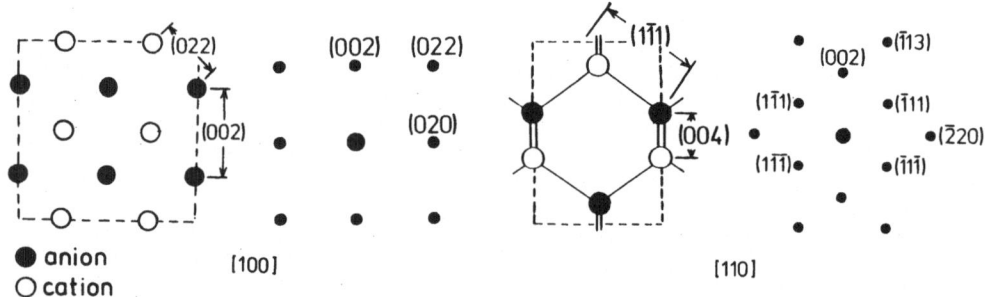

● anion
○ cation

[100]   [110]

Fig.1. Schematic of sphalerite structure drawn in [100] and [110] projections, together with corresponding electron diffraction patterns. Open, closed circles represent cation, anion species respectively.

The wurtzite structure, as shown in Fig. 2, has space group P6$_3$mc (No. 186). It consists of two interpenetrating hexagonal-close-packed lattices separated along the c-axis by u, which is a distance ideally equal to 3/8 in fractional coordinates. Atoms of one atomic species are located on one sublattice at (000)(1/3, 2/3, 1/2), those of the other species are located on the other sublattice at (00u), (1/3, 2/3, 1/2 + u). The close-packed (0001) planes have a stacking sequence ...AaBbAaBb... compared with the 3-layer sequence ...AaBbCcAaBbCc... of diamond and sphalerite crystals. The structure does not possess a center of symmetry and the <0001> axis is polar. Important relationships between the structure factors, which again depend upon the choice of origin (see Fig. 2), include the following:

i systematic absences of kinematic reflections occur for h+k=3n, l=odd, e.g. (0001), ($\bar{3}$301);

ii the {0004} reflections of wurtzite are chemically sensitive, with structure factors of the form $F_{0004}=i4\Delta$ and $F_{000\bar{4}}=-i4\Delta$, where Δ is the difference in electron scattering factors of the two species; and

iii there is a phase difference of 180° between c*-axis mirror-related reflections, due to c-axis glide plane symmetry, which results in structure

2

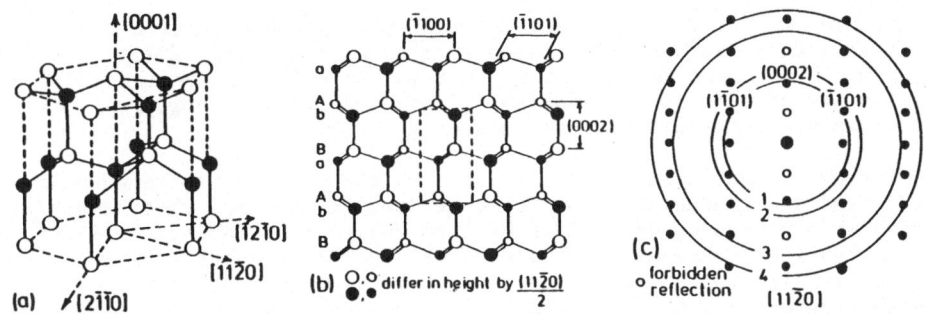

Fig.2. Schematic of the hexagonal wurtzite structure (a) in perspective, and (b) in [11$\bar{2}$0] projection, together with (c) corresponding electron diffraction pattern showing schematic objective lens apertures.

factors of the form $F_{hkil}=A+iB$ and $F_{\bar{h}\bar{k}il}=-A-iB$. This symmetry element ensures the continued extinction of kinematically-forbidden reflections under dynamical scattering conditions, in accord with the Gjønnes-Moodie rules[7].

The $\langle 11\bar{2}0\rangle$ projections, i.e. [11$\bar{2}$0], [2$\bar{1}\bar{1}$0], [$\bar{1}$2$\bar{1}$0], are preferred for the investigation of defects in wurtzite materials by HREM since the dominant slip system in the wurtzite structure is $\langle 11\bar{2}0\rangle$ {0001}, and dislocation cores can thus be viewed 'end-on', i.e. imaged along the line of the dislocation. This particular projection is shown in Fig. 2b, with the open and closed circles indicating atomic columns of different species, and its corresponding electron diffraction pattern is shown in Fig. 2c. (Circles of dissimilar size correspond to atoms separated by half the (11$\bar{2}$0) repeat distance in the beam direction).

THEORETICAL ANALYSIS

The contrast of high-resolution images of small-unit-cell materials can be readily assessed in a quantitative manner. The image intensity at a point $\underline{r}$ within the unit cell, under conditions of coherent axial illumination and unit magnification, has the general form [8]:

$$I(\underline{r}) = U_0^2 + 2\sum_{\underline{g}}{}' U_{\underline{g}} U_0 \cos\left[2\pi \underline{g}\cdot\underline{r} - (\theta_{\underline{g}} - \theta_0 + \chi_{\underline{g}})\right]$$
$$+ \sum_{\underline{g}}{}' \sum_{\underline{g}'}{}' U_{\underline{g}} U_{\underline{g}'} \exp\left[-i(2\pi\underline{g}\cdot\underline{r} - 2\pi\underline{g}'\cdot\underline{r} - (\theta_{\underline{g}} - \theta_{\underline{g}'} + \chi_{\underline{g}} - \chi_{\underline{g}'}))\right] \tag{1}$$

where $\underline{g}$ is the scattering vector, U_o, $U_{\underline{g}}$ are the amplitudes of the transmitted and scattered beams and θ_o, $\theta_{\underline{g}}$, are their respective dynamical phases. The effect of the transfer function of the objective lens is incorporated in the phase change caused by $\chi_{\underline{g}}$ (where $\chi_{\underline{g}} = \pi C_s \lambda^3 g^4/2 + \pi\lambda g^2 \Delta f$, with C_s= spherical aberration coefficient, λ=electron wavelength and Δf=defocus). The summation, as indicated by ', is only for those reflections within the objective aperture. Equation (1) emphasizes that intensity contributions to a point $\underline{r}$ are received from two different interference processes, namely linear and non-linear interactions which correspond to $\underline{g}\rightarrow\underline{0}$ and $\underline{g}\rightarrow\underline{g}'$ processes respectively. For centrosymmetric materials, such as the elemental semiconductors, it can be useful to rearrange Equation (1) to emphasize the contributions to image intensity which result from linear and non-linear interactions [8,9]. Cosine fringes with a spatial periodicity $2\pi\underline{g}.\underline{r}$ result from linear interference and have a maximum possible peak intensity of $2U_{\underline{g}}U_o$. The smallest linear fringe periodicity is equal to $2\pi\underline{g}_{max}.\underline{r}$ where

3

g_{max} is the maximum scattering vector admitted by the objective aperture. Fringe periodicities and peak intensities are respectively $2\pi(g.\underline{r}-g'.\underline{r})$ and $2U_gU_g$, for non-linear interference. The smallest fringe spacing could be half the periodicity of the smallest linear fringe, i.e. $4\pi g_{max}.\underline{r}$, resulting from cross-aperture interference between g_{max} and $\bar{g}_{max}$.

For small-unit-cell materials, such as the compound tetrahedrally-coordinated semiconductors, the low-order reflections and their associated interference processes determine the chemically- or polarity-sensitive contrast morphology, whereas the higher-order reflections basically only modulate the low-resolution image detail to produce high frequency detail. In general, these contributions cannot, however, cause any contrast reversals. Thus, a useful characterization of the image contrast can be accomplished by deliberately restricting analysis to low-resolution conditions as carried out below. It will also prove convenient later, for the purposes of classifying the contrast behaviour, to restrict $\underline{r}$ to specific strategic points within the unit cell.

POLARITY DETERMINATION

High-resolution images of <110> sphalerite crystals have variable asymmetrical contrast as a direct consequence of the breakdown of Friedel's Law, i.e. the Bijvoet-related reflections (e.g. (hkl), ($\bar{h}k\bar{l}$)) have significantly different amplitudes and phases as a result of dynamical scattering in thicker crystals [10]. This asymmetry, which is present in 5-beam and many-beam images, can be utilized for an absolute determination of crystal polarity, including the polarity of exposed surfaces [11].

Weak-Phase-Object Images

For later reference, kinematic or weak-phase-object (WPO) [8,12] images of [110] InP are shown in Fig. 3. These particular images have been simulated as a function of resolution, with 5-, 7-, 13- and 35-beams included within the objective aperture, which corresponds to {111}, {002}, {113} and {333} beams respectively contributing to the image formation process. A close study of these WPO images reveals several interesting features. Imaging with only five beams results in crossed {111} fringes with the pairs of In-P columns located by black spot contrast. The asymmetry of the crystal structure first becomes apparent with contributions from the chemically-sensitive {002} reflections. Individual atomic columns start to become resolved under 13-beam conditions, with the orientation of the In-P atomic columns clearly distinguishable by the asymmetry of the dumbbell-shaped contrast motif. Finally, in order for the atomic columns to be imaged individually, contributions from the {333} reflections are required.

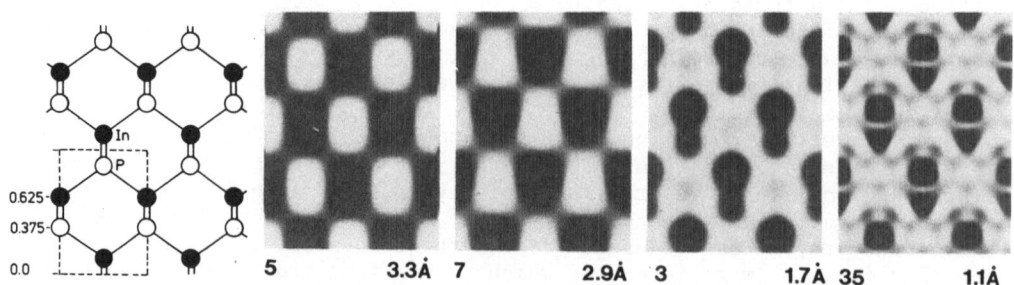

Fig.3. Series of Weak-Phase-Object images of [110] InP. The number of contributing beams and effective image resolution are indicated.

4

5-Beam Images

It appears from Fig. 3 that the asymmetry of the crystal is first revealed under 7-beam conditions. In fact, the 5-beam image contrast is also asymmetric relative to the origin. Intensity measurements indicate that the minima within the black spots are not located symmetrically between the two atomic columns but rather shifted towards the higher atomic number In atomic column. A kinematic analysis shows that the intensity minimum is shifted away from the centrosymmetric position in an <001> direction by

$$\alpha = \frac{a_0}{4\pi}(\theta_1 - \theta_{\bar{1}}) \tag{2}$$

where a_0 is the unit cell length and θ_1, $\theta_{\bar{1}}$ are the structure factor phase values of {111} Bijvoet-related reflections. For InP, with atomic columns orientated as shown in the schematic structural drawing (Fig. 3), the value of $(\theta_1 - \theta_{\bar{1}})$ is +0.597 rad (or +34.2°), which results in a displacement of the intensity minimum towards the In atom by $\alpha = 0.05a_0$, i.e. relative to the unit cell origin, the minimum occurs at $r = 0.55a_0$. Furthermore, note that a phase value for $(\theta_1 - \theta_{\bar{1}})$ of |90°| produces a displacement of $0.125a_0$ which would locate the intensity minimum either above the atomic site at $r = 0.625a_0$ or above $r = 0.375a_0$.

Since the dynamical phase difference $\theta_D = (\theta_1 - \theta_{\bar{1}})$ continually changes from the structure factor value as the crystal thickness increases, there is a continuous relative shift in the spot contrast (black or white) of the image. The amount of fringe movement can be calculated from Equation 1 as shown, for example, in the case of [110] InAs in Fig. 4, for thicknesses up to 200Å, at defocus values of -400Å (black-spot contrast above atom sites) and -1100Å (white spot contrast above atom sites). This contrast movement may initially appear to complicate the process of image interpretation but it actually has the very positive benefit of enabling the crystal polarity to be identified. This identification relies on the fact that, irrespective of defocus, the initial fringe movement is usually towards the lighter atomic species [13]. Thus a single 5-beam image of an approximately wedge-shaped specimen enables the cation-anion orientation to be revealed unambiguously.

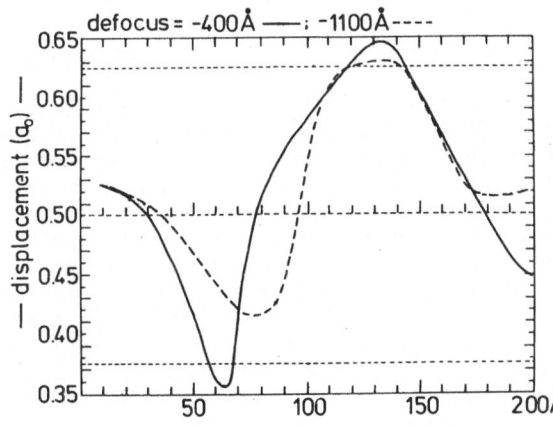

Fig.4. Relative fringe movement, as a function of thickness for [110] InAs at 400kV. Defocus values of -400Å (solid line) and -1100Å (dashed line).

Many-Beam Images

The changes in image symmetry associated with a breakdown in Friedel's Law are easily recognized at higher resolution. For example, a through-thickness series of 15-beam images of [110] InAs, simulated at a defocus of

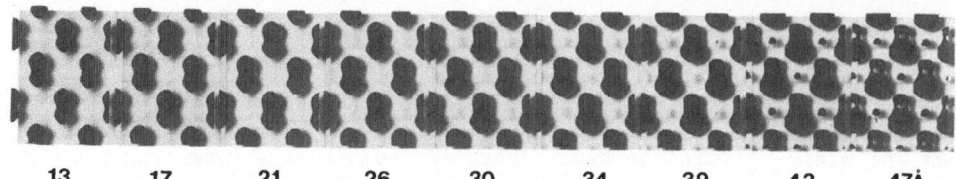

13   17   21   26   30   34   39   43   47Å

Fig.5. Through-thickness series of image simulations for [110] InAs, at an accelerating voltage of 400kV and a defocus of −400Å, under coherent illumination conditions (thickness indicated in Å).

−400Å for coherent illumination conditions, is presented in Fig. 5. A survey of these images shows a continual change from the expected contrast asymmetry which is exhibited by the black dumbbell-shaped motifs located above atomic columns at 13Å thickness. More centrosymmetric contrast is visible from 26 to 32Å and the symmetry is inverted at 47Å thickness. This sequence of changing symmetry closely mimics that for InAs imaged under 5-beam diffraction conditions at the same defocus (see the solid-line curve of Fig. 4), thus confirming the dominant role of {111} reflections and their associated linear and non-linear interference processes in determining contrast morphology. Conversely, it should also be obvious that a small isolated region of a single micrograph, where the thickness is unknown, cannot be reliably used for polarity determination.

Experimental images

Several characteristic image features can be utilized to determine the crystal polarity in <110>-orientated compound semiconductors[11], including:

(a) the sideways shift of 5-beam lattice fringes as the crystal thickness is increased;

(b) the asymmetrical spot contrast which is visible in high-resolution images;

(c) the occurrence and distribution of white-spot contrast within black "dumbbell-shaped" motifs;

(d) the location of <u>white</u> dumbbells at tunnel-anion/cation sites.

However, because of the extreme sensitivity of the image contrast to changes in crystal thickness and objective lens defocus, it should be far more reliable in practice to identify the crystal polarity on the basis of several images and more than one method. For example, application of the fringe shift method confirmed [11] the previous determination of crystal polarity from GaSb images which was based on asymmetrical spot contrast [14]. Figure 6 shows a 400kV high-resolution image of InP recorded at close to the optimum objective lens defocus. Close scrutiny of this image indicates that the progressive changes in its appearance with thickness conform closely with those visible in image simulations (not shown here but see Fig. 5) although, of course, the calculations are not affected by any experimental factors such as the signal-to-noise ratio of the micrograph and the presence of any amorphous surface overlayers on the specimen. A further serious experimental problem for materials with the wurtzite structure is the extreme sensitivity of the electron micrographs to beam and crystal misalignment due to the occurrence of dynamically-forbidden reflections [15]. Experience indicates that only images from the thinnest crystal regions will stand a close comparison with image simulations.

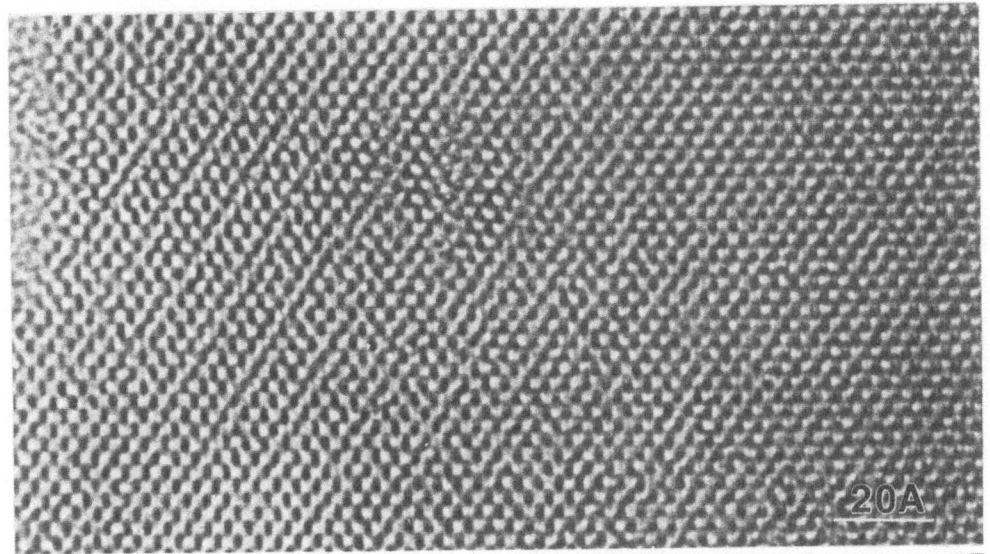

Fig.6. Experimental micrograph of <110> InP recorded at 400kV. Note the
changes in image contrast with increasing thickness from left to right

INTERFACES

The image contrast for <100>-orientated sphalerite materials under 5- and
9-beam imaging conditions can be conveniently characterized in such a way
that the investigation of interfaces is greatly simplified. Furthermore,
under certain conditions, it proves to be possible to interpret the variations in contrast at an interface in terms of compositional changes for
materials of well-matched unit cell size.

5-Beam Images

By starting from Equation (1), and taking account of the scattering
symmetries for sphalerite materials outlined above, then the image intensity
at strategic points within the [100] projected unit cell can be calculated,
as follows:

$$I(B) = I(D) = I(E) = U_0^2 \tag{3}$$

$$I\binom{C}{A} = U_0^2 + 16U_{002}^2 \begin{cases} +8U_{002}U_0T(002) & \tag{4} \\ -8U_{002}U_0T(002) & \tag{5} \end{cases}$$

where $T(002)=\cos(\theta_{002}-\theta_0+\chi_{002})$ is the generalized transfer function [9] and
A...E refer to the positions indicated in Fig. 8.

Analysis of these equations reveals several significant imaging features. The intensity of tunnel sites (eg. points B and E) is independent of
defocus and equal to U_0^2. Conversely, the intensity at C and A is defocus-
dependent due to the influence of T(002). The intensity differences between
these sites depends on the sign, (+) or (−), of T(002). For example, a (+)
value produces enhancement/suppression of the intensity at C/A sites respectively. Furthermore, at thickness/defocus values where T(002) is zero, the
two sublattices are imaged with identical intensity (equal to $U_0^2+16U_{002}^2$).

By providing a graphical representation of T(002), it is straightforward to characterize contrast over extended regions of the thickness-defocus plane. Typical thickness-defocus plots are shown in Figure 7 for (a) [100]AlAs, and (b) [100]GaAs, where, in both cases, the cation is located at site C. A (+) value for T(002) (unshaded regions in Fig. 7) will thus result in C-contrast (for enhanced cation intensity, i.e. white at cation site), a (-) value for A-contrast (i.e. anion enhancement within shaded regions of Fig. 7) and AC-contrast where both sublattices have equal intensity (dashed lines in Fig. 7). 5-beam images of AlAs, simulated at the thickness and defocus values denoted by points 1, 2 and 3 in Fig. 7(a), are presented in Fig. 8. A comparison of the image simulations with the schematic drawing of the projected structure, confirms that the respective simulations (b), (c) and (d) exhibit the expected C, AC and A contrast.

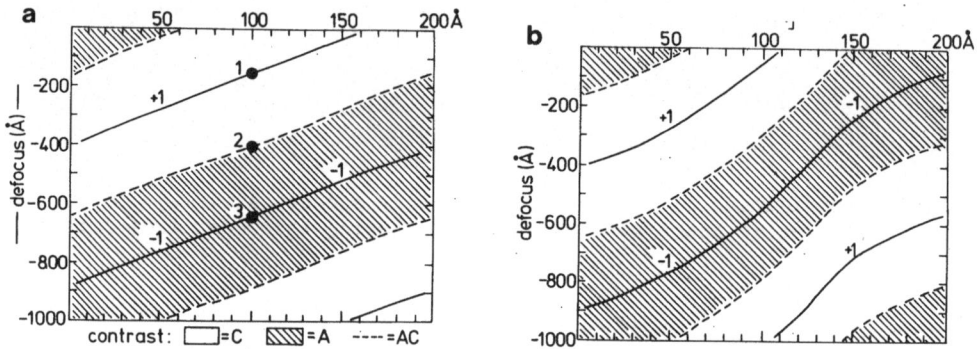

Fig.7. Graphical representation of generalized transfer function, T(002), for (a) [100] AlAs, and (b) [100] GaAs. Unshaded/shaded regions correspond to C (cation) and A (anion) contrast respectively. Accelerating voltage = 400kV and C_s=1.0mm.

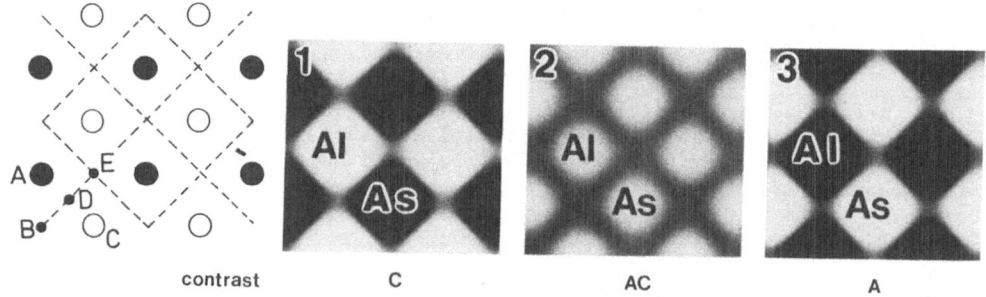

Fig.8. Five-beam simulated images of AlAs at thickness-defocus values denoted by 1,2,3 in Fig. 7(a).

By the simple process of overlaying the separate T(002) curves, it becomes immediately obvious what values of thickness and defocus will be optimum for maximizing contrast differences at an interface between two similar materials. This process is demonstrated in Figs. 9(a) and (b) which correspond, respectively, to GaAs/Ga$_{0.7}$Al$_{0.3}$As and GaAs/AlAs. In the former case, the close similarity in dynamical scattering behaviour of the two materials result in large regions of common sign. As a consequence, both materials should exhibit similar contrast morphology, although different absolute intensities, under most imaging conditions, making it difficult in practice to locate accurately the exact position of any interface and to assess its atomic configuration. The simulated images shown in Fig. 10(a), which correspond to the points 1, 2 and 3 in Fig. 9(a), do however confirm

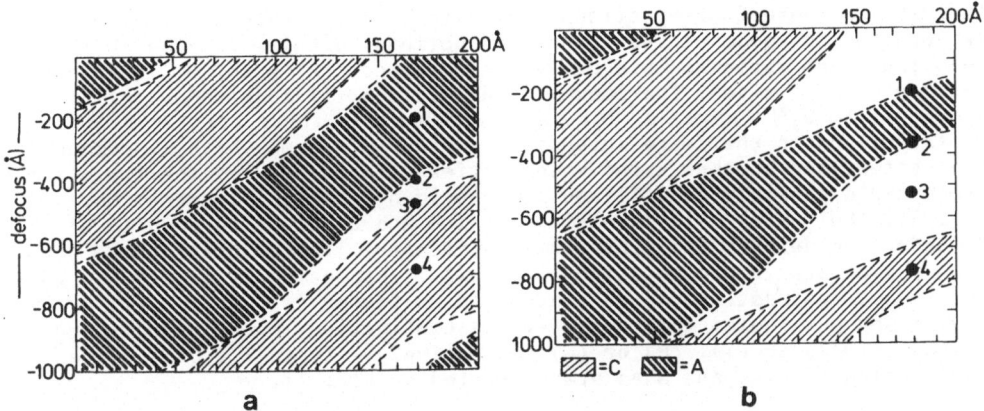

Fig.9. Composite figures resulting from overlay of separate T(002) curves. (a) GaAs/Ga$_{0.7}$Al$_{0.3}$As and (b) GaAs/AlAs. Shaded regions correspond to common sign for both materials.

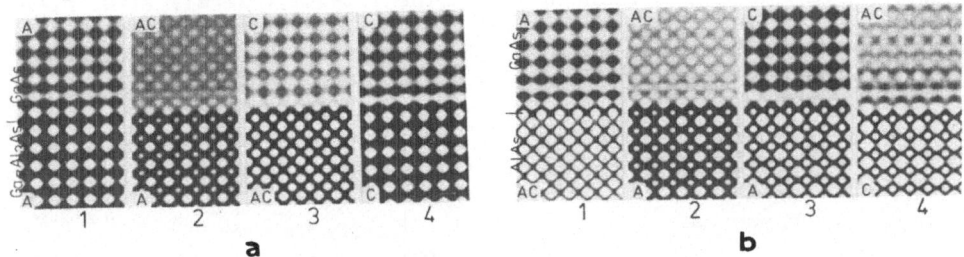

Fig.10 (a) Five-beam simulated images of GaAs/Ga$_{0.7}$ Al$_{0.3}$As at thickness-defocus values denoted in Fig. 9(a). (b) Corresponding to GaAs/AlAs – see Fig. 9(b). A, AC and C indicate contrast type.

the predictions about image appearance based on Fig. 9(a). For the case of GaAs/AlAs, the composite plot in Fig. 9(b) reveals extensive (unshaded) regions where the combination of thickness and defocus values should permit the differences in image contrast between the two materials to be accentuated. The simulated images shown in Fig. 10(b) confirm these predictions.

9-Beam Images

The inclusion of four {022} reflections within the objective aperture makes the imaging process considerably more complicated. Under 9-beam imaging conditions, the image intensity expressions become as follows:

$$I(B) = I(E) = U_0^2 + 16U_{022}^2 + 8U_{022}U_0T(022) \tag{6}$$

$$I(D) = U_0^2 \tag{7}$$

$$+8U_{002}U_0T(002)-32U_{022}U_{002}T(022,002) \tag{8}$$

$$I(^C_A) = U_0^2+16U_{002}^2+16U_{022}^2-8U_{022}U_0T(022)$$

$$-8U_{002}U_0T(002)+32U_{022}U_{002}T(022,002) \tag{9}$$

where $T(022) = \cos(\theta_{022} - \theta_0 + \chi_{022})$

and $T(022,002) = \cos(\theta_{022} - \theta_{002} + \chi_{022} - \chi_{002})$

Analysis of these four equations, and reference to graphical representations for the generalized transfer functions, enables considerable insight into the image formation process to be obtained. At point D, located midway between C and A sites, the image intensity is still independent of defocus and equal to U_0^2. However, for the C and A sites there are two distinct contributions to the image intensity: a group of terms which is <u>common</u> to both sites, and another group which differentiates between the two sites and hence could possibly be utilized for providing chemical information. Finally, the tunnel site intensities (at B and E) are also seen to be dependent on defocus via contributions from the linear interference term. From a graphical representation of T(022) it can actually be deduced whether the tunnel contrast should be classified as strong (s), medium (m) or weak (w) at any particular thickness-defocus combination, i.e. depending on whether T(022) is (+), (0) or (-) respectively. Typical T(022) curves for [100]-oriented AlAs and GaAs are presented in Fig. 11.

The combined effect of these various interference processes, together with modulations by the generalized transfer functions, result in several distinctive contrast morphologies. As illustrated by the image simulations shown in Fig. 12, which correspond to [100] AlAs, these contrast types can be conveniently labelled on the basis of the intensity levels (i.e. s, m, or w) at Al, As and tunnel sites. Similar contrast variations can be anticipated for other <100>-oriented sphalerite crystals, though with obvious differences depending on the behaviour of the corresponding T(022).

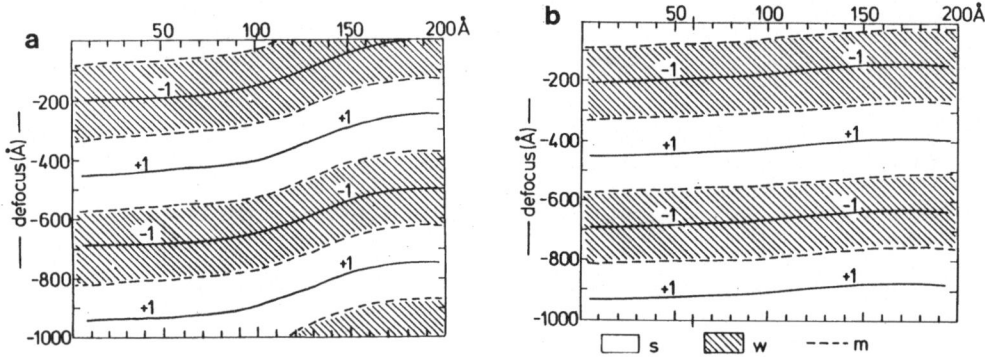

Fig.11. Graphical representation of generalized transfer function T(022) at 400kV and C_s=1.0mm for (a) [100] GaAs and (b) [100] AlAs. Contrast is strong (s) medium (m) or weak (w) for T(022) values of +1, 0 and -1, respectively.

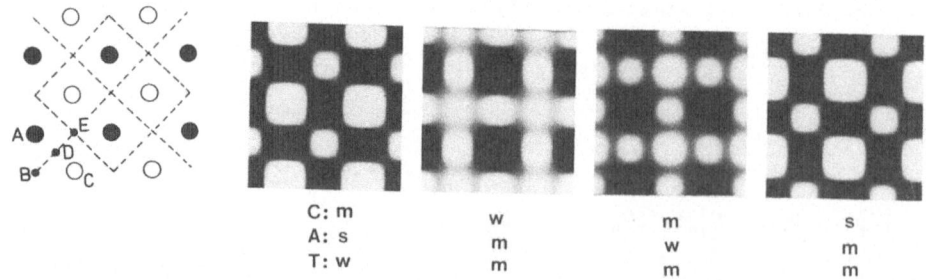

C: m	w	m	s
A: s	m	w	m
T: w	m	w	m

Fig.12. Nine-beam simulated images of [100] AlAs at 60Å thickness and defocus values (from 1. to r.) of -700, -550, -350, -200Å. For comparison, cation (C), anion (A) and tunnel (T) site contrast is classified as being strong (s), medium (m) or weak (w).

Interfacial Chemistry

The essential point of the preceding analyses was to establish the optimum imaging conditions for extracting information about the location and chemical composition of an interface between two compound semiconductors of sphalerite structure. Clearly, 9-beam images will be further complicated by the interaction between the T(002) and T(022,002) functions as summarized in Equations (8) and (9), and considered in more detail elsewhere [16]. Our conclusion was that 5-beam imaging would be expected to provide the best operating conditions for this purpose. As an example, Figs. 13(a) and (b) compare 5-beam image simulations at a defocus of -700Å of an interface between GaAs and Ga$_7$Al$_3$As which include a single buffer layer with composition Ga$_5$Al$_5$ and an ideal abrupt interface. The effect of the buffer layer can be assessed in Fig. 13(c) which shows the intensity difference between the two images, with contrast levels enhanced. It is difficult to be sure whether the contrast difference is solely related to structure or whether it is also influenced by Fresnel fringe contrast.

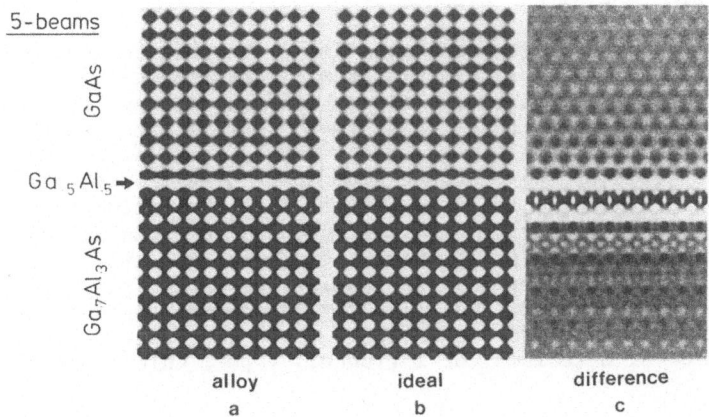

Fig.13. Five-beam simulated images of [100] GaAs/Ga$_7$Al$_3$As (a) with interfacial (buffer) layer of Ga$_5$Al$_5$ composition and b) an ideal abrupt interface. Effect of buffer is shown in (c), which is a difference image, (a)-(b), simulated with enhanced contrast to reveal spatial detail. Accelerating voltage is 400kV and C$_s$=1.0mm.

A further interesting possibility for quantification of local variations in chemistry stems from the fact that, under 5-beam imaging conditions, the combined intensity sum for cation-anion sites is defocus-independent and equal to

$$I(C) + I(A) = 2U_0{}^2 + 32\ U_{002}{}^2 \qquad (10)$$

As an example, Fig. 14(a) shows the summed intensities as a function of thickness for five different materials, namely AlAs, Ga$_x$Al$_{1-x}$As(x=0.3, 0.5 and 0.7) and GaAs. The same results are also displayed in Fig. 14(b) but instead normalized against the GaAs intensity. A similar normalization process could be performed experimentally using an electron micrograph from a wedge-shaped multilayer material.

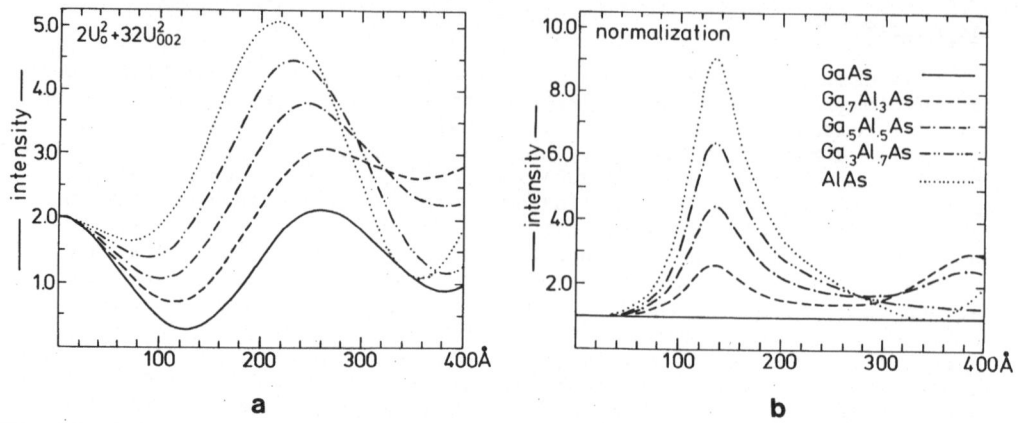

Fig.14. (a) Summed cation-anion site intensities plotted as a function of thickness for ⟨100⟩-oriented sphalerite materials at 400kV (b) Normalized against the GaAs intensity. Solid curve is for GaAs, others are (from top to bottom) for $Ga_xAl_{1-x}As$ (x=0, 0.3, 0.5 and 0.7).

STACKING FAULT SYMMETRY AND DISLOCATIONS

The variations of high-resolution image contrast for small-unit-cell materials, as a function of crystal thickness and objective lens defocus, depend upon complex interactions between diffracted beams which are also modulated by the transfer function of the objective lens. Although the fine detail visible in the final image cannot easily be related back to the projected atomic structure of the specimen, it is usually possible to understand the overall general features of the image by considering the behaviour of the first-order reflections as influenced by the generalized transfer function. As examples, Fig. 15 shows the result of overlaying the generalized transfer functions for (a) the sphalerite InAs in [110] at 100kV, and (b) the wurtzite CdSe in [11$\bar{2}$0] at 400kV. The shaded regions of these graphs indicate thickness-defocus values where the image contrast is predicted to be of C (column) or T (tunnel) type*, which corresponds to T being (−) or

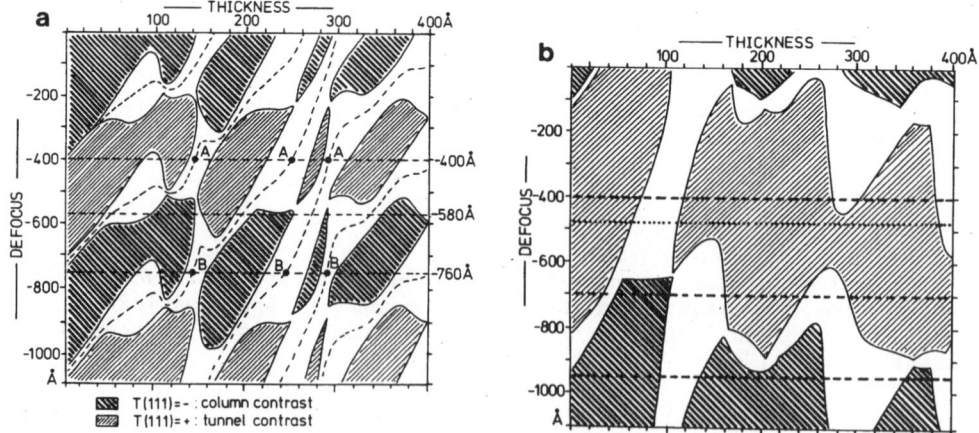

Fig.15. Graphical representation of generalized transfer functions for (a) InAs at 100kV and $C_s=0.7$mm: T($\bar{1}$11) and T(1$\bar{1}\bar{1}$); (b) CdSe at 400kV and $C_s=0.1$mm: T(0002), T(000$\bar{2}$) and T($\bar{1}$100).

---

*C-type contrast refers to white contrast at atomic column positions, whereas T-type corresponds to white contrast at the intermediate tunnel positions.

(+) respectively. Image simulations (not shown here) for several sphalerite and wurtzite compound semiconductors confirm these expectations, thereby emphasizing the general usefulness of these plots for tying down the conditions under which experimental images should be recorded.

For centrosymmetric crystals, the symmetries of the projected structure are reproduced faithfully in the image, at least for thin crystals, provided that the crystal and the incident beam have been well-aligned [17]. For example, the known symmetry of an intrinsic stacking fault was utilized for interpretation of image detail from a dissociated 30° partial dislocation in <110>Si [18]. For non-centrosymmetric crystals, correlation between the perceived image symmetry and the actual projected crystal structure is much more difficult to obtain.

The likelihood of erroneous image interpretation for the particular cases of stacking faults and dislocations is demonstrated in Figs. 16 and 17. For example, Fig. 16(a) shows a schematic for an extrinsic stacking fault in a <110> sphalerite structure. If the differences in chemical species are ignored, then this structure could be considered as containing a two-fold axis located along the tunnel row labelled T. The accompanying through-thickness series of 5-beam image simulations are for [110] InAs at an accelerating voltage of 100kV, spherical aberration of 1.0mm and a defocus of -700Å. Despite the fact that all images exhibit black contrast above tunnel sites, the two-fold axis, as identified by the arrows, apparently changes location and reverses contrast.

Image simulations for 30° shuffle and glide partial dislocations in [110] InAs are shown in Fig. 17, together with a schematic of the projected potential of the defect (at left). These simulations are for an accelerating voltage of 400kV, an objective lens defocus of -500Å, and crystal thicknesses of (b) 20Å, (c) 40Å and (d) 150Å. By reference to the inset at the top left of each simulation, it can be seen that the initial asymmetrical image contrast at a thickness of 20Å corresponds to that which might be expected intuitively given the atomic numbers of the two species whereas, at a thickness of 40Å, the contrast symmetry is reversed in polarity. At a thickness of 150Å, however, the elongated white contrast is not directly related to the locations of the two species, even though it would still be possible, for example, to deduce the atomic configurations and identities at the glide dislocation by reference to the adjacent perfect crystal.

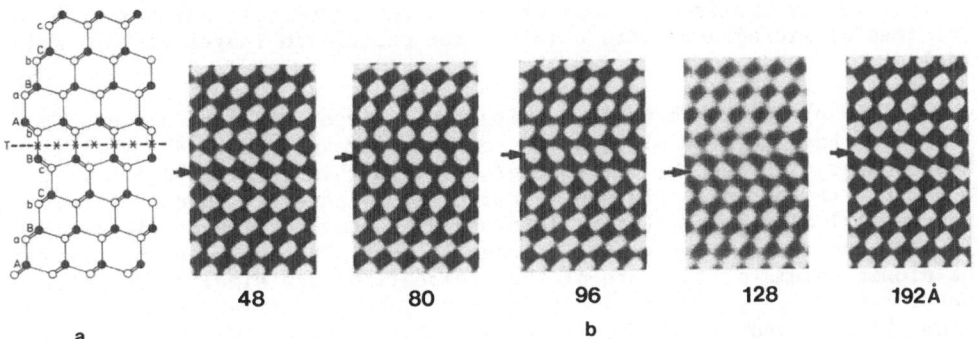

Fig.16. (a) Schematic of extrinsic stacking fault in [110] InAs with location of 'two-fold' axes identified along line T. (b) 15-beam images of (a) simulated at 100kV for -700Å defocus and indicated thicknesses. Arrows identify image fringe on which the 'two-fold' axes appear to reside.

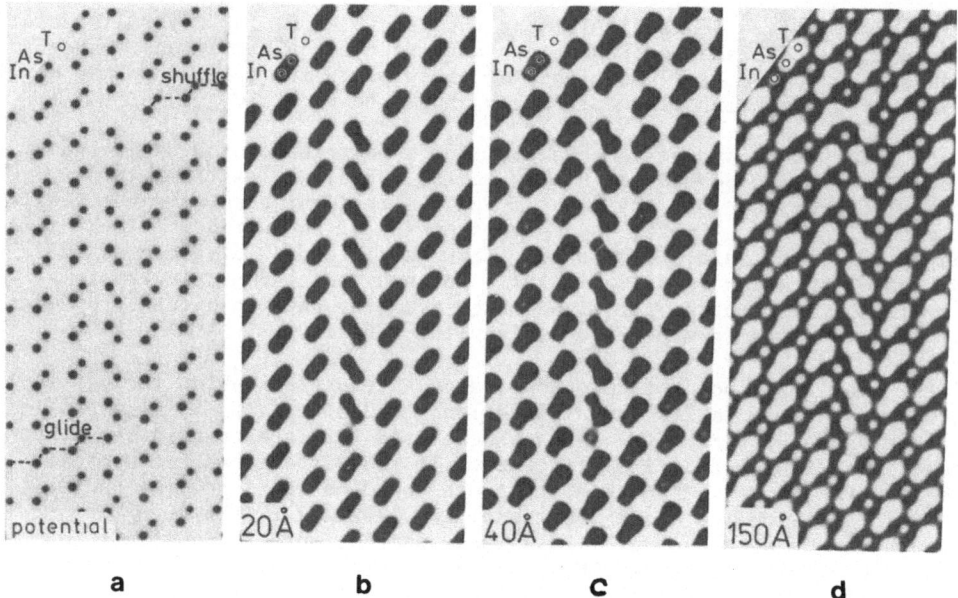

Fig.17. Simulations of 30° glide and shuffle partial dislocations in [110] InAs. (a) Projected potential. (b), (c) and (d) corresponding images for -500Å defocus and indicated thicknesses. Note the change in contrast symmetry between images and in particular, the white dumbbell motif in (c) located above As-tunnel sites.

THE Si 30° PARTIAL DISLOCATION

Dislocations in silicon, for example produced by plastic deformation, are usually dissociated into partials. 60° dislocations, of Burgers vector B=1/2[101], are dissociated into 30° (B=1/6[211]) and 90° (B=1/6[1$\bar{1}$2]) dislocations. The 30° partials may be of either "glide" or "shuffle" type [19]. Lattice images of the 30° partial at 100kV [18] and at 200kV [20,21] have been previously published. Reasonable, though imperfect, matches with the experimental micrographs were obtained for calculated images of the "glide" model.

In the present observations, direct structure images of 30° dislocation cores have been obtained at an accelerating voltage of 400kV [22]. From these images, recorded at optimum defocus from thin crystal regions, it seems that the 30° partials are of glide type. However, in comparisons of experimental micrographs (Figs. 18(a,b)) with computed images (Figs. 18(c-f)), it appears that there are two equally feasible positions for placing the atomic column at the core of the dislocation. The simulations correspond, respectively, to (c) glide (unkinked), (d) shuffle (unkinked), (e) glide (kinked) and (f) shuffle (kinked). The shuffle (unkinked) clearly does not match with the experimental micrographs but both the glide (kinked) and the shuffle (kinked) seem to give good matches. By comparison of the calculated and experimental images, it appears that the 30° partials are kinked such that the dislocation core moves sideways by 3.33Å along the [1$\bar{1}$2] direction within the thin Si foil but it is not possible to tell whether the dislocations are of kinked shuffle or kinked glide type.

14

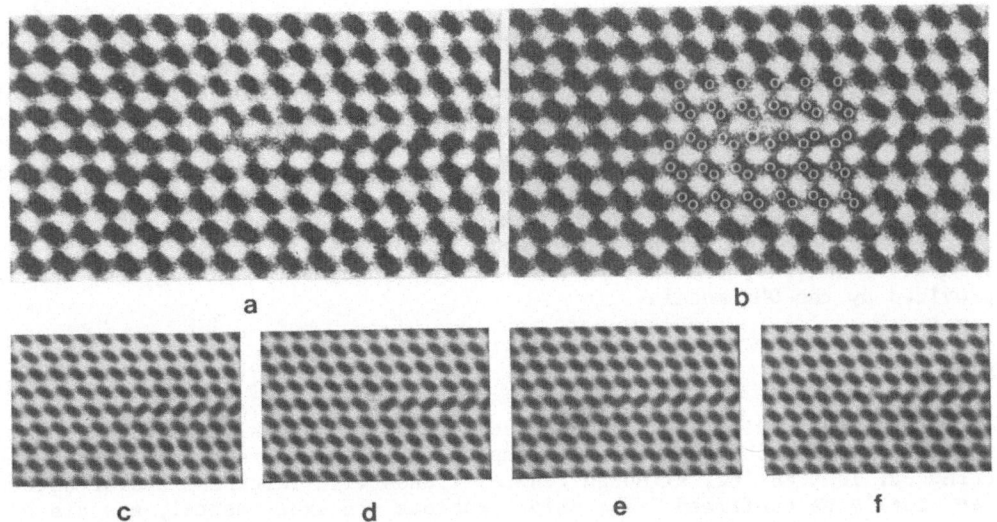

Fig.18. 30° partial dislocation in silicon. a) Experimental image.
b) Experimental image with atomic positions for glide model
overlaid. (c)-(f) Calculated images. c) Glide model. d) Shuffle
model. e) Kinked glide model. f) Kinked shuffle model.

DIAMOND PLATELETS

The majority of naturally-occurring gem-quality diamonds contain {100}
platelet defects, the presence of which was first detected by X-ray diffraction [23]. The debate over the structure and chemical composition of these
platelets has been longstanding and controversial, and centers on the question of whether or not the platelets contain nitrogen. A comprehensive
comparison between high-resolution lattice images (2.5Å structural resolution, 1.7Å information limit) of platelets with computed images for a number
of platelet models found that the double nitrogen layer zig-zag model gave
the best match with the experimental micrographs [24]. Another comparison
between lattice images (also at 2.5Å structural resolution) and computed
platelet images found that the alternative Humble-nitrogen-carbon (HNC)
platelet model gave the best match with the experimental images [25]. In
both studies, a major difficulty was that the largest diamond lattice spacing was only 2.06Å (corresponding to (111) fringes) but the structural
resolution of the available microscopes was limited to 2.5Å.

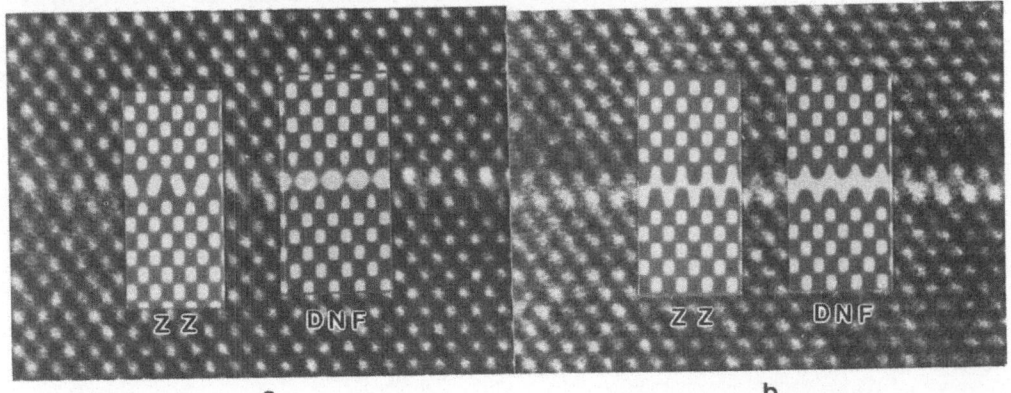

Fig.19. Experimental micrographs of platelet defects in diamond in a) [110]
orientation; b) [1̄10] orientation, with calculated images for zig-
zag model (ZZ) and disordered nitrogen fretwork model (DNF) inset.

15

A detailed reevaluation has since been made using lattice images of diamond platelets for <110> and <100> orientations recorded at 400kV with ~1.7Å structural resolution. Images simulated for five different platelet models indicated that the different models should be clearly distinguishable in thin crystal regions for images recorded close to optimum defocus. Indeed, it was necessary to derive yet another model for the diamond platelets in order to match the latest experimental micrographs [26]. Figure 19 shows experimental platelet images for (a) [110] and (b) [1$\bar{1}$0] orientations, together with simulations for the disordered-nitrogen-fretwork (DNF) and zigzag (zz) model in the same projections. Of the six different models simulated, the only acceptable match to the experimental micrographs was provided by the DNF model.

DISCUSSION

Detailed predictions, based on computer simulations, about the appearance of high-resolution images of compound semiconductors are not yet fully borne out in practice, although general trends with thickness and/or defocus can usually be confirmed. The major problems are experimental, associated mainly with preparation of the sample for observation and with setting up the optimum conditions of the microscope. For example, irrespective of the method used for thinning the specimen, whether it be ion-milling, crushing or polishing techniques, there are invariably amorphous overlayers covering the entire surface. The resulting local variations in contrast will obscure the clarity of the crystalline image [27], particularly in the vicinity of defects where image-averaging techniques will generally be inapplicable. More effort into minimizing this overlayer thickness has been recommended, for example by establishing ultra-high-vacuum conditions at the sample region and by providing in situ cleaning facilities [28,29]. Electron-beam-stimulated desorption of the constituent atoms from the near-surface regions is, however, then likely to become more prevalent [30]. Moreover, the specific defects of interest are not always conveniently located in the thinnest specimen regions where the demands on crystal alignment are less exacting, and dynamical and inelastic electron scattering have less effect on the final image. A further problem stems from the inescapable radiation damage which occurs when the electrons of the incident beam have sufficient energy to cause "knock-on" displacement of one or the other of the separate atomic species. Operation below the threshold voltage for this type of damage is therefore strongly recommended. However, in regard to accelerating voltage, it should also be realized that the optimum imaging conditions implied by the analyses above do not correspond to the highest attainable resolution of the microscope so, in many cases, it will not be necessary to operate at the highest available voltage.

Despite these experimental difficulties, it is nevertheless possible to state that the image formation process for compound semiconductors within the high-resolution electron microscope is well-understood. Because the imaging is dominated by the mutual interaction of the transmitted beam with the low-order diffracted beams, characteristic images can be anticipated which will provide fiducial markers of crystal thickness and objective lens defocus. Consequently, it then becomes feasible to extract quantitative information about atomic locations, and even chemical species, at defects and interfaces.

ACKNOWLEDGEMENTS

Much of the work described here was supported by National Science Foundation Grant DMR-8514583.

REFERENCES

[1] Cowley, J.M. and Smith, D.J., 1987, Acta Cryst., A43:737.
[2] Smith, D.J., 1988, J. Electr. Micro. Techn., in press.
[3] Wood, G.J., Stobbs, W.M. and Smith, D.J., 1984, Phil. Mag. A50:375.
[4] Stobbs, W.M., Wood, G.J. and Smith, D.J., 1984, Ultramicroscopy 14:145.
[5] Saxton, W.O. and Smith, D.J., 1985, Ultramicroscopy 18:39.
[6] Hetherington, C.J.D., Barry, J.C., Bi, J.M., Humphreys, C.J., Grange, J., Wood, C., 1985, Mater. Res. Soc. Symp. Proc. 37:41.
[7] Gjonnes, J. and Moodie, A.F., 1965, Acta Cryst. 19:65.
[8] Glaisher, R.W., Spargo, A.E. and Smith, D.J., 1989, Ultramicroscopy, in press.
[9] Bourret, A., Desseaux, J. and Renault, A., 1975, Acta Cryst. A31:746.
[10] Glaisher, R.W., Spargo, A.E. and Smith, D.J., 1989, Ultramicroscopy, in press.
[11] Smith, D.J., Glaisher, R.W. and Lu, P., 1989, Phil. Mag. Letts., in press.
[12] O'Keefe, M.A. and Pitt, A.J., 1980, in Electron Microscopy 1980 (ed. P. Brederoo and G. Boom) Vol. 1:122.
[13] Glaisher, R.W. and Spargo, A.E.C., 1985, Ultramicroscopy, 18: 323.
[14] Wright, A.C., Ng, T.L. and Williams, J.O., 1988, Phil. Mag. Letts. 57:107.
[15] Smith, D.J., Bursill, L.A. and Wood, G.J., 1984, Ultramicroscopy, 16:19.
[16] Glaisher, R.W., to be published.
[17] Smith, D.J., Saxton, W.O., O'Keefe, M.A., Wood, G.J. and Stobbs, W.M., 1983, Ultramicroscopy, 11:263.
[18] Olsen, A. and Spence, J.C.H., 1981, Phil. Mag. A43:945.
[19] Hornstra, J., 1958, Phys. Chem. Solids, 5:129.
[20] Bourret, A., Desseaux, J. and D'Anterroches, C., 1981, Inst. Phys. Conf. Ser., 60:9.
[21] Anstis, G.R., Hirsch, P.B., Humphreys, C.J., Hutchison, J.L. and Ourmazd, A., 1981, Inst. Phys. Conf. Ser., 60:23.
[22] Barry, J.C. and Alexander, H., 1987, in Proc. 45th Ann. Meet. EMSA (ed. G.W. Bailey, San Francisco Press, San Francisco) pp. 242-243.
[23] Raman, C.V. and Nilakantan, P., 1940, Proc. Indian Acad. Sci.,A11:389.
[24] Barry, J.C., Bursill, L.A. and Hutchison, J.L., 1985, Phil.Mag., A51:15.
[25] Humble, P., Lynch, D.F. and Olsen, A., 1985, Phil. Mag., A52:623.
[26] Barry, J.C., 1986, in Proc. XIth Int. Cong. on Electron Microscopy, Kyoto, pp. 799-800.
[27] Kilaas, R. and Gronsky, R., 1985, Ultramicroscopy 16:193.
[28] Gibson, J.M. and McDonald, M.L., 1987, Mater. Res. Soc. Symp. Proc.82:109.
[29] Ponce, F.A., Suzuki, Kobayashi, H., Ishibashi, Y., Ishida, Y. and Eto, T., 1986, in Proc. 44th Ann. Meet. EMSA (ed. G.W. Bailey, San Francisco) pp. 606-609.
[30] Petford-Long, A.K. and Smith, D.J., 1986, Phil. Mag. A54:837.

IMAGE PROCESSING APPLIED TO HRTEM IMAGES OF INTERFACES

A.F. de Jong

Philips Research Laboratories WY2
P.O. Box 80000
5600 JA Eindhoven, The Netherlands

1. INTRODUCTION

High resolution transmission electron microscopy (HRTEM) images contain a large amount of information. Digital image processing techniques offer opportunities to extract the relevant part of the information, thus simplifying the interpretation of the image. Several textbooks have appeared [1,2] which give an introduction into the subject of image processing in electron microscopy, with main applications in biology and organic materials. For these samples the need for image processing follows mainly from the extreme sensitivity of the specimens to the electron beam. The very bad signal-to-noise ratio (S/N) at high resolution is often improved by spatial averaging or Fourier filtering techniques. An image with a large number of identical contrast units is then needed, preferentially arranged on a periodic lattice.

A whole area of image processing is directed towards obtaining a "restored" image where amplitude- and phase-contrast are separated, and the effects of electron-optical distortions and noise are suppressed. The ultimate aim of these methods is to calculate the projected structure of the object from the restored images (structure retrieval). For very thin, weakly scattering objects (organic molecules, complex metal oxides) this seems to be feasible up to a certain resolution [3,4]. Recently, more general image restoration methods have been proposed [5].

In the fields of metals and semiconductor research, image processing is not nearly as widespread, although some pioneering work has been done by Krakow [6]. Three reasons for this discrepancy may be distinguished. In the first place, radiation damage and the resulting poor S/N is not a serious problem with these materials. In the second place, the materials consist of medium or heavy scattering objects making image restoration, and certainly structure retrieval, extremely difficult. At present, the actual structure of an object is to be determined by careful comparison of experimental and simulated images [7]. In the third place, the structure of the bulk of these materials is often well known. Subsequently, most HRTEM investigations are aimed at resolving non-periodic structural details (from e.g. defects, interfaces, grain boundaries or surfaces). Therefore, image processing techniques to be applied in materials science have to focus more on non-periodic image features.

Application of image processing will be advantageous to separate relevant (but sometimes weak) features from noise. Recently some work has been published where image processing is used to enhance the S/N of HRTEM images in materials science. Tomita et al.[8] and Coene et al.[9] used Fourier transform patterns and filters to analyse HRTEM images of various materials. Moreover, there may be future methods where structure retrieval will become feasible even for heavy scattering, non-periodic objects[10]. Noise filtering, if applied in such a way that all relevant information is preserved, might be a first step.

The techniques designed to enhance the contrast of periodic images might not be valid when applied to non-periodic objects. The main problem is that reduction of noise (which is also non-periodic) conflicts with the preservation of the non-periodic image detail we want to emphasize. A compromise between noise reduction and resolution (of the non-periodic feature) must be found. To find an optimal filter procedure for a particular problem, an analysis of the image to be processed is necessary. Then, promising filter procedures have to be investigated in a systematical way to find the restrictions with which they are to be used. In this paper a general analysis of HRTEM images and filter procedures is presented. Then several Fourier-space filters are investigated and tested on model images. Subsequently they are applied to experimental HRTEM images of (semi-conductor) interfaces.

2. THEORY

2.1. Description of the Signal

An HRTEM image (or "signal") can be thought to consist of three contributions: a known signal, an unknown signal and noise. The "known" signal may be a periodic signal representing the bulk of the material. The "unknown" signal is the more interesting, often non-periodic part of the image. It may also describe the edges of a periodic (known) signal. The objective of a filter procedure is to suppress the noise, and enhance the unknown signal at the same time. To design an optimal filter procedure, a-priori information about the signal is necessary. The success of the procedure depends on how well the available a-priori information in the image can be used for designing the filter.

Some information is available about the noise $n(\mathbf{r})$, which is generated either at the object (by preparation or radiation damage) or during recording of the image (camera noise, counting statistics). The recording noise can be assumed to have a white power spectrum. The object noise, on the other hand, has a power spectrum which is affected by the image formation in the microscope. Coherent and incoherent effects of image formation can be described by the transmission cross coefficient (TCC)[11]. The TCC damps higher spatial frequencies because of instrumental instabilities, chromatic aberrations and a finite source size. Therefore the power spectrum of the object noise has a radial symmetric bell shape around the origin.

Some information may be available about how the known signal $p(\mathbf{r})$ and the unknown signal $x(\mathbf{r})$ are related. They might be additive, multiplicative or convoluted as shown in eqs. (1a-c):

$$s(\mathbf{r}) = n(\mathbf{r}) + p(\mathbf{r}) + x(\mathbf{r}) \ , \tag{1a}$$

$$s(\mathbf{r}) = n(\mathbf{r}) + p(\mathbf{r}) \ x(\mathbf{r}) \ , \tag{1b}$$

$$s(\mathbf{r}) = n(\mathbf{r}) + p(\mathbf{r}) * x(\mathbf{r}) \ . \tag{1c}$$

An appropriate schematic description of the signal may lead to a particular filter procedure. This is illustrated for a signal which consists of a known, periodic part multiplied by an unknown part describing e.g. an interface as the (unknown) edge of the periodic signal (see Fig. 1). In this case areas in reciprocal space can be found where most of the unknown signal is concentrated. The Fourier transform of eq. (1b) reads:

$$S(\mathbf{g}) = N(\mathbf{g}) + P(\mathbf{g}) * X(\mathbf{g}) \ . \tag{2}$$

Theoretically the Fourier tranform of the interface function is non-vanishing over the entire reciprocal space. However, in practice it drops below the noise level quite rapidly. Because $X(\mathbf{g})$ is convoluted with the sharp intensity maxima related to the periodic signal ("Bragg spots"), the unknown signal is concentrated closely around the Bragg positions in reciprocal space (Fig. 1). A Fourier space filter transmitting only these regions (Bragg filter, see Fig. 2a,b) then seems an appropriate filter procedure.

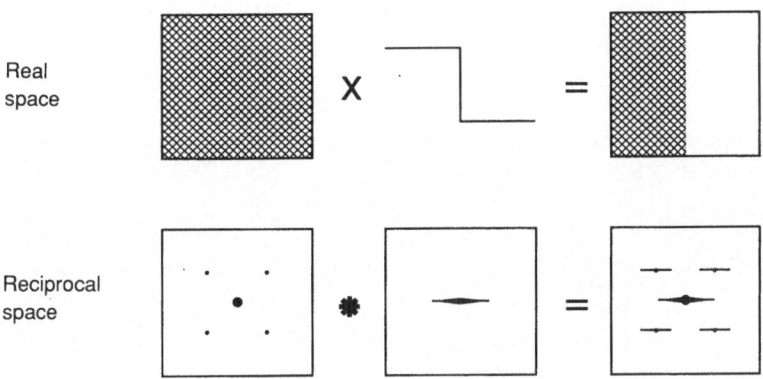

Fig. 1. Schematic picture showing how the HRTEM image of an interface can be described, and where the information about the interface is located in reciprocal space.

Another filter procedure is needed when the known and the unknown signal are convoluted, as in eq. (1c). We can rewrite this equation as:

$$s(\mathbf{r}) = n(\mathbf{r}) + m(\mathbf{r}) * \{ q(\mathbf{r}) + x(\mathbf{r}) \} \ . \tag{3a}$$

Fourier transformation gives:

$$S(\mathbf{g}) = N(\mathbf{g}) + M(\mathbf{g}) \, Q(\mathbf{g}) + M(\mathbf{g}) \, X(\mathbf{g}) \ . \tag{3b}$$

The perfect signal is described by a motive $m(\mathbf{r})$ convoluted by a function $q(\mathbf{r})$ determining where the motive is placed. A disturbance of the perfect signal can be described by the motive convoluted with an (unknown) function $x(\mathbf{r})$. Note that $q(\mathbf{r})$ and $x(\mathbf{r})$ are in fact only a set of weighted delta functions. In this way a dislocation or an interface can be described. A logical filter procedure to extract the unknown signal would be to divide $S(\mathbf{g})$ by $M(\mathbf{g})$ (the Fourier transform of the motive), and then subtract $Q(\mathbf{g})$. However, this deconvolution scheme is not practical because of noise amplification. A correlation procedure turns out to be a better alternative, as will be demonstrated in section 4.

2.2. Analysis of Fourier Filters

In this section a schematic analysis is presented of filters in Fourier space, which can be used to process signals described by eq. (1b). A more detailed analysis is presented elsewhere [12]. In Fourier space and in real space the filtering process is described by, respectively,

$$S_p(\mathbf{g}) = S(\mathbf{g}) \, F(\mathbf{g}) \quad \text{and} \quad s_p(\mathbf{r}) = s(\mathbf{r}) * f(\mathbf{r}) \ , \tag{4}$$

where $F(\mathbf{g})$ is the filter function. The (inverse) Fourier transform of the filter, $f(\mathbf{r})$, is a spread function which disperses the intensity of each image pixel to its environment. The information about the non-periodic feature is spread out in real space, decreasing the resolution. Several Fourier filters, with their corresponding spread functions, are shown in Fig. 2. Obviously the resolution of the non-periodic feature after filtering is proportional to the width of the spread function, and inversely proportional to the width w of the filter itself.

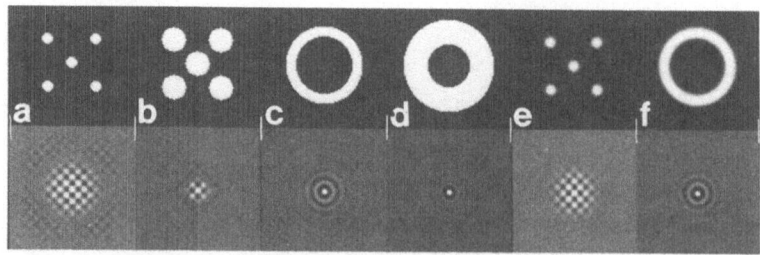

Fig. 2. Filters in Fourier space (top row) and their real-space spread functions (bottom row). (a) Bragg filter with "hole" diameter w = 6.4. (b) Same, w = 16. (c) Ring filter with mean radius A = 22.6 and width w = 6.4. (d) Same, w = 16. (e) Bragg filter with cosine-shaped intensity, w = 6.4. (f) Ring filter with cosine-shaped intensity, A = 22.6 and w = 6.4. (All variables in pixel units.)

This means that filters with a large width are needed to preserve the non-periodic feature with sufficient resolution. On the other hand, the noise left in the processed image is roughly proportional to the size of the filter $(= \int F(\mathbf{g}) \, d\mathbf{g})$, and filters with a small size are needed to suppress the noise. We have to determine the minimum size (width) of the filter which ensures a "sufficient" resolution of the non-periodic feature.

All filters shown in Fig. 2 can be described as a profile function convoluted by a function determining the position of the filter in reciprocal space. The Bragg filters shown in Fig. 2a,b have the same position function (i.e. the Bragg positions), but their profile functions (i.e. the shape of the "holes") have a different width w. For the Ring filters (Fig. 2c,d) the position function is circular symmetric, with radius A. In Fig. 2e and 2f filters are shown having a profile function with cosine-shaped ("soft") edges. The widths of the profiles are then defined as the full width at half maximum. The position functions of Figs. 2e and 2f are the same as for the Bragg filters (2a,b) and Ring filters (2c,d) respectively.

In real space, the spread function can be described as an envelope (the Fourier transform of the profile) multiplied by a fine structure (the Fourier transform of the position function). Figs. 2a, 2b and 2e show the same fine structure, but a different envelope. The spread functions of the soft-edge filters have quickly vanishing tails. Note that the width of the envelopes (at half maximum) is not much smaller than those of the spread functions of corresponding filters with sharp edges.

The resolution of the non-periodic feature in the filtered image is determined by the envelope of the spread function. Therefore, we can define the preserved resolution as the distance ρ where the envelope drops below $1/e$ of its value at the origin. The main parameter influencing the resolution is the width w of the profile of the filter. Computer calculations of a large number of spread functions have shown[12] that to preserve a resolution of ρ, a Bragg filter with $w > 0.8/\rho$ is required; or a Ring filter with $w > 0.5/\rho$. If cosine-shaped profiles are used these numbers hardly change. Of course these theoretical predictions have to be tested. However, it illustrates how a simple analysis can result in quantitative restrictions on the filters.

3. TESTING FOURIER FILTERS

3.1. Test on a Model Image

To test the resolution preserved by the Fourier filters described in the previous section we will apply them to a model image (Fig. 3). The intensity of the left-hand side of the original image can be described by a two-dimensional sine function with period p = 8 pixels in both the x and the y direction. The Fourier spectrum consists of four peaks at positions $(u,v) = (\pm \frac{1}{p} \pm \frac{1}{p})$. In the middle of the picture an abrupt interface between crystalline and amorphous material is modelled. Gaussian noise is added (with mean $= 0$ and $\sigma = 0.5$), and the image with noise is processed using Bragg filters (Fig. 3a) or Ring filters (Fig. 3b), with either "sharp" or "soft" (cosine) edges.

An important feature in Fig. 3a is the pattern of crossed fringes appearing in the amorphous parts of all images, obscuring the interface. This is a result of the fine structure present in all spread functions of Bragg filters (see Fig. 2), irrespective of hole width and edge profile. Even for a filter with $w = 1.0/p$ careful observation is needed. Thus the theoretical predictions ($w > 0.8/p$) are somewhat too optimistic in this case, although this is not a result of the envelope of the spread functions. The fine structure in their spread function makes Bragg-type filters unsuitable for crystalline-to-amorphous interfaces.

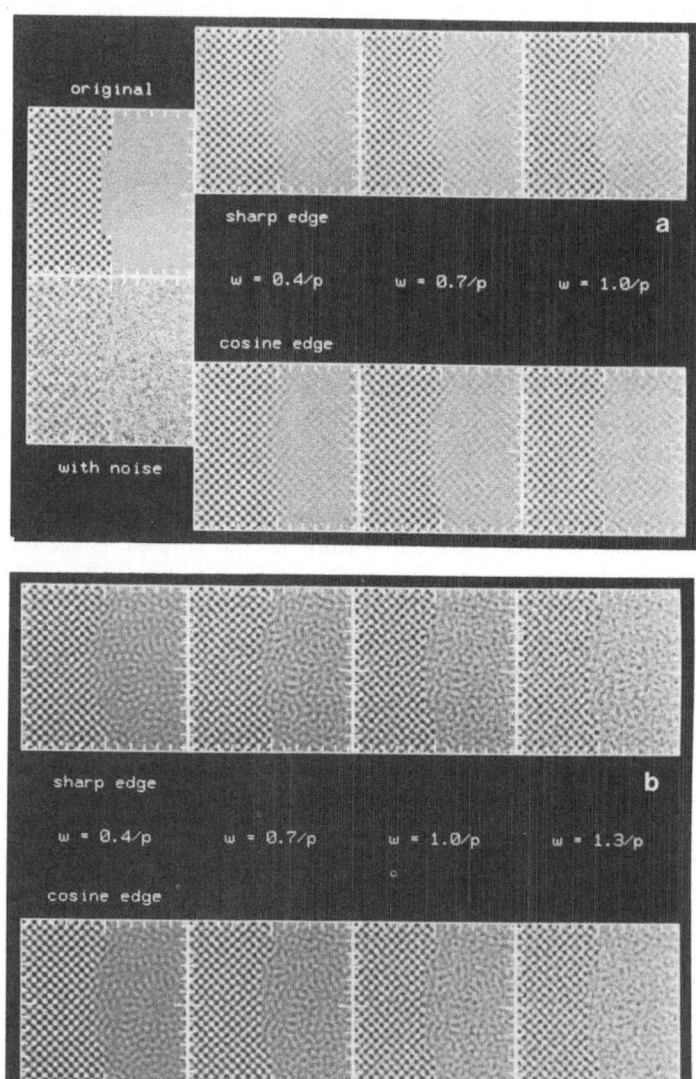

Fig. 3. (a) Model image ("original", note the two steps at the interface), with noise added and subsequently filtered by Bragg filters with either sharp or cosine edges. The diameters w of the holes are given in units of the inverse fringe spacing (1/p) of the left-hand side of the model. (b) The model image filtered by Ring filters with a width w as indicated.

When Ring-filters are used, the fringes imposed on the amorphous part of the image are circular in shape (Fig. 3b). The Ring filter acts in a similar way as the envelope of the TCC, with finer contrast features in the image when the filter (or TCC) extends further into reciprocal space. The resolution preserved at the interface is completely determined by the envelope of the spread function. It seems that at the value of $w = 0.4/p$ the exact shape of the interface is somewhat obscured, but $w = 0.7/p$ is certainly a safe value. This agrees with the theoretical prediction made in section 2.2. Application of "soft" edges has hardly any influence on the resolution preserved (Fig. 3).

A more quantitative comparison of the different Fourier filters can be obtained by processing the original model (without noise) and calculating the deviation between original and filtered image. More details of this comparison are presented elsewhere[12]. The main conclusion is that Bragg filters are in general to be preferred over Ring filters, because for a given resolution their size is smaller and more noise is suppressed.

3.2. Filtering an Experimental Image: APB in a Cu-Pd Alloy

Fourier filtering was also tested on an HRTEM micrograph of a Cu_3Pd alloy containing a quasi-periodic arrangement of anti-phase boundaries (APBs)[13], being an example of a "crystalline-to-crystalline" interface. In perfect parts of the structure the minority (Pd) atom columns are imaged as white dots (Fig. 4a), with fringe distance $p = 0.38$ nm. The APBs display a wavy profile and in addition may have a certain width, caused by mixed Cu-Pd columns.

The "unknown" part of the signal is the exact place and shape of the APBs. An APB is situated where the vertical fringes shift one half lattice spacing. In Fourier space the unknown information is located around the Bragg positions corresponding to these vertical fringes (arrowed in Fig. 4b). A suitable filter procedure then is a Bragg filter around these spots alone. The results (Fig. 4c1-4c5) clearly illustrate the improving resolution at the APB with increasing filter width. The apparently straight APBs in Figs. 4c1 and 4c2 are artificial; a result of the large width of the envelope of the spread functions. The fine structure of the spread function does not influence the resolution, because it coincides with the fine structure in the image at both sides of the APB. An important observation is that the fringe positions in the Cu_3Pd layers, away from the APBs, are not affected by the filter and still coincide with the positions in the original image.

To determine the minimum width necessary to ensure that all relevant information about the APB is preserved, we can compare filtered images of successive widths. The series converges at Fig. 4c4 ($w = 0.67/p$): while there is some more detail (but not much) in Fig. 4c4 compared to Fig. 4c3, Fig. 4c5 does not add any additional information. This indicates that a filter width of $0.7/p$ is sufficient, in agreement with the theoretical predictions.

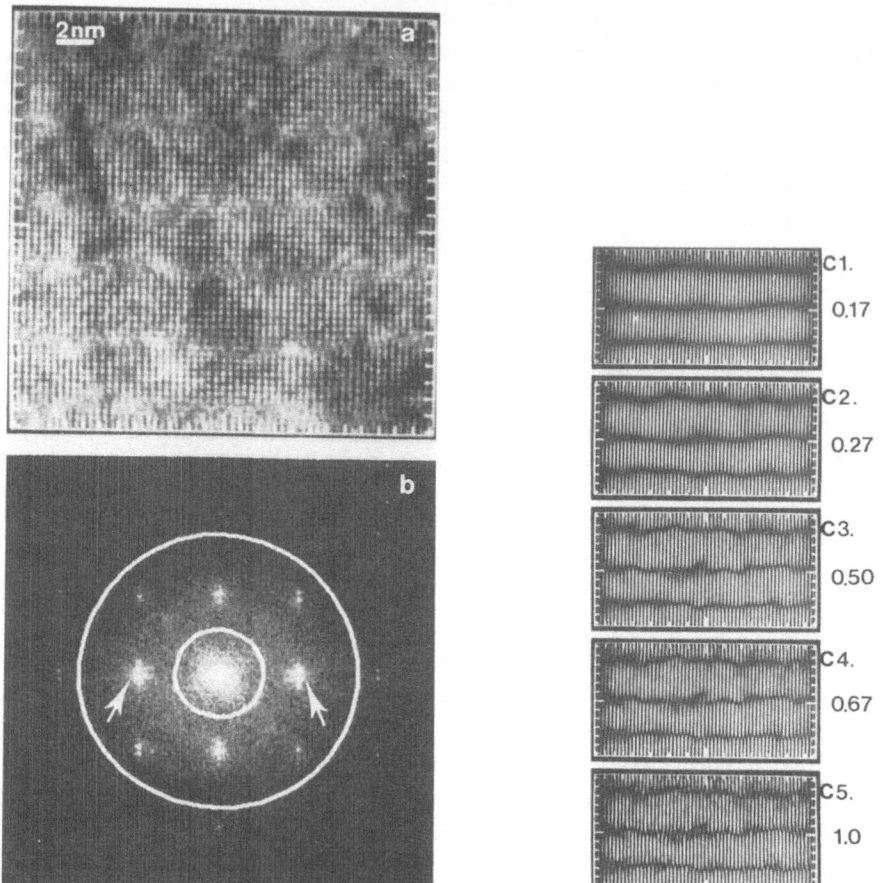

Fig. 4. (a) (100) Lattice image of APBs in Cu_3Pd. (b) Fourier spectrum; spots transmitted by the Bragg filter are arrowed. (c1-c5) Filtered image; the width of the Bragg filter is given in units of the inverse fringe spacing (1/p) of the original image (p = 3.8 nm).

4. CORRELATION PROCEDURE APPLIED TO A GaAs / AlAs INTERFACE

As indicated in section 2.1., an interface may be described by a convolution of a (known) motive with an (unknown) signal determining where the motive is placed (eq. 3). Instead of deconvoluting this signal, the unknown signal may be enhanced by correlation of the image with the motive. Multiplying the Fourier transform of the signal (eq. 3b) by $M^{\cdot}(g)$, the processed signal becomes in reciprocal and real space :

$$S_p(\mathbf{g}) = M^*(\mathbf{g})\, N(\mathbf{g}) + |M(\mathbf{g})|^2\, Q(\mathbf{g}) + |M(\mathbf{g})|^2\, X(\mathbf{g}) \quad, \tag{5a}$$

$$s_p(\mathbf{r}) = m(\mathbf{r}) * n(\mathbf{r}) + c_m(\mathbf{r}) * \{\, q(\mathbf{r}) + x(\mathbf{r}) \,\} \quad. \tag{5b}$$

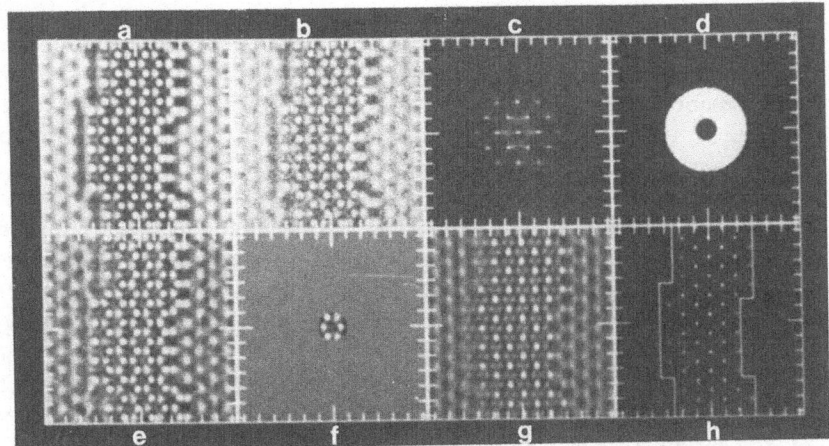

Fig. 5. (a) Simulated image of a GaAs/AlAs interface, thickness = 22 nm and defocus = -90 nm. (b) Noise added. (c) Square root of Fourier spectrum. (d) Ring filter. (e) Filtered image. (f) Small contrast feature from AlAs layer. (g) Correlation of (e) with (f). (h) Threshold applied to (g); the drawn line indicates the exact place of the interface in the model.

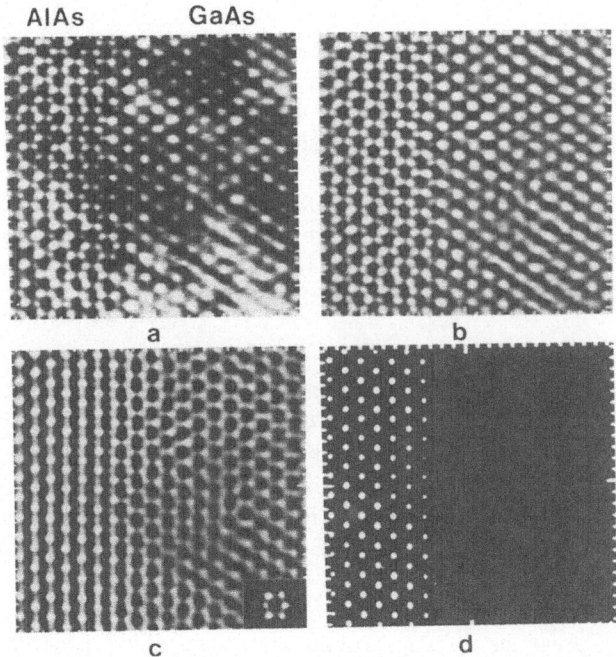

Fig. 6. (a) (110) Lattice image of a GaAs/AlAs interface. (b) Original filtered with Ring filter. (c) Correlation of image (b) with typical feature (inset) from AlAs layer. (d) Correlated image with threshold applied.

Here $c_m(\mathbf{r})$ is the autocorrelation function of the motive itself, which is strongly peaked at the origin. The processed image will have sharp intensity maxima at points having a good correspondence between the original image and the motive. The functions describing the place of the motive, $q(\mathbf{r}) + x(\mathbf{r})$, are enhanced. Noise is reduced because it contributes randomly to $s_p(\mathbf{r})$. Of course, the resolution is reduced to the repeat distance of the motive.

This correlation scheme is first tested on a simulated image of a GaAs/AlAs interface [12] (Fig. 5a), where the AlAs layer exhibits a typical contrast feature (Fig. 5f) because of second order interference effects during image formation. Before the correlation is performed, a Ring filter (Figs. 5d,e) is used to remove long-range intensity fluctuations. The processed image Fig. 5g indeed shows sharp intensity maxima. A threshold (just above the intensity level in the GaAs layer) enhances the visibility of the interface (Fig. 5h). The interface itself is characterized by a series of somewhat weaker spots because of the partial fit there.

Subsequently this procedure is applied to a corresponding experimental image of a GaAs/AlAs interface [14] (Fig. 6a). A Ring filter is applied and the resulting image (Fig. 6b) is correlated with a typical contrast feature or motive from the AlAs layer (Fig. 6c and inset). After thresholding just above the intensity level in the GaAs layer, the interface can clearly be identified as the row of somewhat weaker spots in Fig. 6d.

5. APPLICATION TO AN HRTEM IMAGE OF A $CoSi_2/Si$ (111) INTERFACE

Other "unknown" non-periodic structures which can be analysed by filtering an HRTEM image are crystal defects. Here an example is given of a dislocation associated with a step at the $CoSi_2/Si$ (111) interface. $CoSi_2$ grown epitaxially on (111) Si usually has a twin relationship with the substrate [15, 16], which means that the epilayer is rotated 180° around the [111] surface normal (B-type). This is indicated in the $(1\bar{1}0)$ lattice image of Fig. 7a (from Bulle-Lieuwma et al. [17]). In plan view samples an hexagonal network of dislocations can be observed with Burgers vectors $\mathbf{b} = a/6 <112>$ running in $<110>$ directions. These dislocations can be associated with steps at the interface [16-18].

By image simulation (of Si and $CoSi_2$ separately) it was first established that in Fig. 7a pairs of Si atoms are imaged as white dots. In the $CoSi_2$ this gives rise to pronounced (002) fringes. The Co atoms are at the black dot positions. Subsequently the rigid body shift of the $CoSi_2$ lattice with respect to the Si substrate could be measured. Comparing with simulated images of several interface models, we found in accordance with Gibson et al. [18] that the model with 5-fold coordination of the interfacial Co is the most likely one.

In order to analyse the dislocation associated with the step (of height d_{111}) a Burgers circuit must be drawn around the step. This procedure is facilitated by processing the image using several Bragg filters. The location of the interface is determined from Fig. 7a. In Figs. 7b and 7c only two sets of Bragg spots are transmitted by the filter (insets), clearly revealing the "extra" fringes in the $CoSi_2$ layer. From these images a schematic model is composed (Fig. 7d) of the lattice fringes around the step. Of course in the real lattice the planes will be curved because of relaxation of strain around the dislocation. A Burgers circuit can easily be drawn in this model, connecting equivalent points. The circuit has a closure failure (at the interface) giving a Burgers vector of $\mathbf{b} = a/6\,[11\bar{2}]$, indicating that the dislocation is of edge type. This is in agreement with models describing the association between steps, dislocations, and the coordination of interfacial Co published earlier [17, 18]. The two "extra" fringes in Fig. 7a make up one extra $(11\bar{2})$ plane in the $CoSi_2$ layer. This extra plane relieves some of the strain induced by the mismatch between Si and $CoSi_2$, as the $CoSi_2$ lattice is 1.4% smaller than the Si lattice.

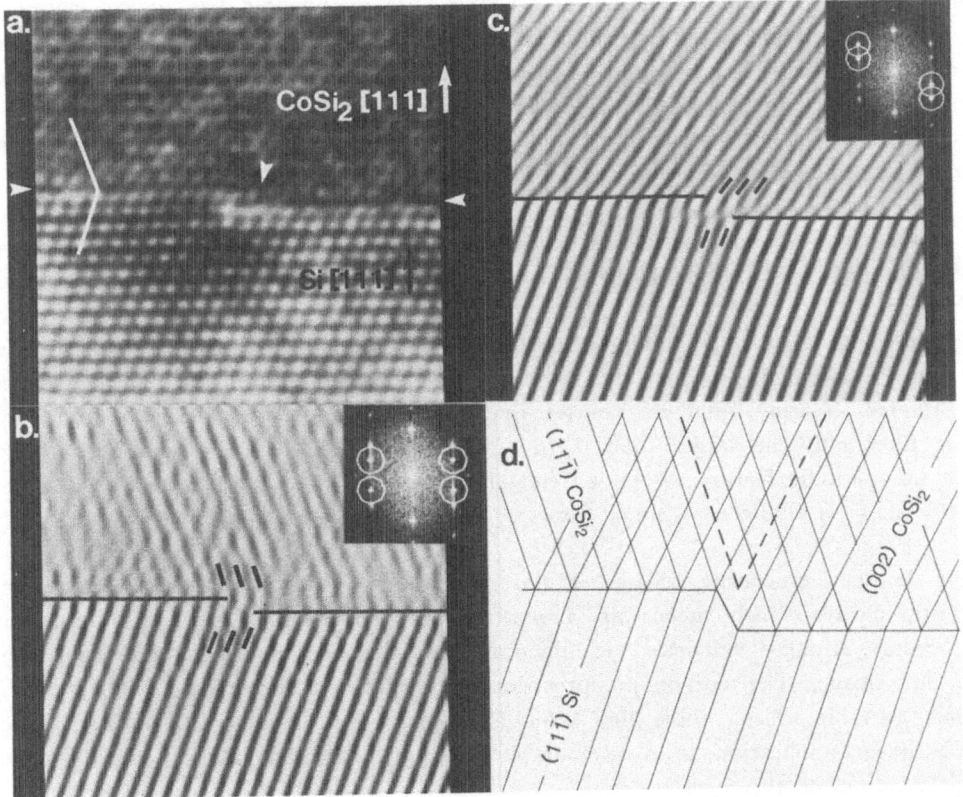

Fig. 7. (a) $(1\bar{1}0)$ Lattice image of a $CoSi_2(B)$ / Si (111) interface, with a monolayer step (arrow). The image was taken at 200 kV with a defocus of -70 nm; sample thickness was between 13 and 19 nm. (b) Image filtered by a Bragg filter on the Si and the $CoSi_2$ $(11\bar{1})$ spots (indicated on the inserted Fourier spectrum). (c) Same, with a Bragg filter on the Si $(11\bar{1})$ spots and the $CoSi_2$ (002) spots. (d) Schematic model of the lattice planes around the interface step, with the "extra" fringes indicated by the dashed lines.

The width of the filters chosen is 0.65/p, with $p = d_{111} = 0.31$ nm . This width is sufficient to ensure a resolution of 0.31 nm around the interfacial step. This resolution would not be sufficient to verify atomistic models of the step itself[17], including possible local relaxation effects. However, the test described in section 3.2. (see Fig. 4.) proves that at a short distance from the interface the fringe positions are not shifted by the filter at all. Thus for Burgers circuit analyses (or even rigid body displacement measurements) Bragg filters with even smaller widths can be used without introducing errors.

6. CONCLUSIONS

As in materials science HRTEM investigations are often aimed at resolving structural defects, interfaces etc. (instead of bulk material), image processing has to focus more on images with non-periodic features. To enhance these features of interest and suppress the noise, as much use as possible has to be made of a-priori information about the different components in the image. Indeed, a careful description of the known and (non-periodic) unknown parts in the image, and their relation, often leads to a particular processing scheme. For instance, if the known and the unknown signal are multiplicative, filtering in Fourier space is an appropriate way of noise reduction.

Once a processing scheme is chosen, it has to be tested. The main objective of this test is to find a good compromise between noise reduction and the preservation of resolution. In this paper several Fourier space filters are tested by applying them to a model image and to an experimental image of APBs in a Cu_3Pd alloy. It appears that when a "crystalline-to-amorphous" type interface is filtered, a Ring filter in Fourier space is most appropriate. The width w of this filter must be larger than $0.5/\rho$, where ρ is the desired resolution around the non-periodic. feature. When a "crystalline-to-crystalline" interface (or dislocation, APB etc.) is filtered, a Bragg filter is better, with $w > 0.7/\rho$.

Another processing scheme is the correlation of an image with the characteristic motive which makes up a part of the image. This "pattern recognition" procedure strongly enhances the function describing where the motive is located in the image. The correlation procedure is tested on a simulated image of a GaAs/AlAs interface, where the AlAs layer displays a characteristic fine-structure. Subsequent application · to a comparable experimental image allows one to locate the position of the interface.

Application of a Bragg-type Fourier space filter to a dislocation associated with a step at the $CoSi_2(B) / Si (111)$ interface illustrates how filtering can help determining the Burgers vector of the dislocation. A schematic model of the dislocation can be constructed after enhancing particular sets of fringes in subsequently processed images. This approach simplifies the Burgers circuit analysis, or the measurement of a rigid body shift.

ACKNOWLEDGEMENTS

It is a pleasure to acknowledge the fruitful cooperation of W. Coene and D. Van Dyck on image processing in general, and of C. Bulle-Lieuwma on the $CoSi_2/Si$ work.

REFERENCES

1. W.O. Saxton, Computer Techniques for Image Processing in Electron Microscopy, in: Adv. in Electr. and El. Phys. suppl. 10, L. Marton and C. Marton, eds., Academic Press, New York (1978).

2. D.L. Misell, Image Analysis, Enhancement and Interpretation, in : "Practical Methods in Electron Microscopy" Vol. 7, A.M. Glauert, ed., North-Holland, Amsterdam (1978).

3. D.N. Wang, S. Hovmoller, L. Kihlborg and M. Sundberg, Ultramicroscopy 25:303 (1988).

4. F.H. Li and D. Tang, Acta Cryst. A41:376 (1985);
   F.S. Han, H.F. Fan and F.H. Li, Acta Cryst. A42:353 (1986).

5. E.J. Kirkland, Ultramicroscopy 15:151 (1984);
   W. Coene and D. Van Dyck, in: Proc. VIth Pfefferkorn Conf., Scanning Microscopy Suppl. 2:117 (1988).

6. W. Krakow, Mat. Res. Soc. Symp. Proc. 31:39 (1984).

7. J.C.H. Spence, "Experimental High-Resolution Electron Microscopy", Clarendon press, Oxford (1981).

8. M. Tomita, H. Hashimoto, T. Ikuta, H. Endoh and Y. Yokota, Ultramicroscopy 16:9 (1985).

9. W. Coene, A.F. de Jong, D. Van Dyck, G. Van Tendeloo and J. Van Landuyt, Phys. Stat. Sol. (a)107:521 (1988).

10. D. Van Dyck and W. Coene, in: Proc. VIth Pfefferkorn Conf., Scanning Microscopy Suppl. 2:131 (1988).

11. J. Frank, Optik 38:519 (1973);
    K. Ishizuka, Ultramicroscopy 5:55 (1980);
    W. Coene, D. Van Dyck and J. Van Landuyt, Optik 73:13 (1986).

12. A.F. de Jong, W. Coene and D. Van Dyck, Ultramicroscopy (1989 in press).

13. D. Broddin, G. Van Tendeloo, J. Van Landuyt, S. Amelinckx and A. Loiseau, Phil. Mag. B 57:31 (1988).

14. A.F. de Jong, W. Coene and H. Bender, Inst. Phys. Conf. Series 87:9 (1987).

15. J.M. Gibson, J.C. Bean, J.M. Poate, and R.T. Tung, Thin Solid Films 93:99 (1982).

16. C.W.T. Bulle-Lieuwma, A.H. van Ommen and J. Hornstra, Inst. Phys. Conf. Series 87:541 (1987).

17. C.W.T. Bulle-Lieuwma, A.H. van Ommen and J. Hornstra, Mat. Res. Soc. Symp. Proc. 102:377 (1988).

18. J.M. Gibson, J.C. Bean, J.M. Poate and R.T. Tung, Appl. Phys. Lett. 41:818 (1982).

II-VI SEMICONDUCTOR INTERFACES

G. ·Feuillet

Commissariat à l'Energie Atomique, C.E.N./Grenoble
Département de Recherche Fondamentale, Service de Physique
Groupe Physique des Semiconducteurs
85 X - 38041 Grenoble, Cedex, France

ABSTRACT

We shall review recent T.E.M. results on II-VI semiconductor Molecular Beam Epitaxial growth. The emphasis will be put on the structure of interfaces in both high misfit systems such as (001)ZnTe, (001) CdTe and (111)CdTe on (001)GaAs substrates, and low misfit ones such as (001)CdTe on (001) $Cd_{0.96}Zn_{0.04}$Te. Quantum wells and superlattices such as CdTe/ZnTe and HgTe/CdTe will also be investigated.

INTRODUCTION

Growing high-quality II-VI semiconductor epitaxial layers such as CdTe, ZnTe or Cd_xHg_{1-x}Te has recently received much attention because of the potential interest of these materials in the fields of solar energy conversion, gamma-ray and infrared detection and of optoelectronics (Panish, 1987).

However, II-VI epitaxial growth is not as well controlled as in the case of III-V compounds and there remain many problems that need much structural characterization (Ponce et Al, 1987). One of the main difficulties lies in the fact that available II-VI substrates are still imperfect with a dislocation density in the range $10^5/cm^2$: these dislocations can thread into the epitaxial layer and may limit the epitaxial film quality. This has led epitaxy teams to resort to alternative substrates such as InSb (Chew et Al, 1984) and GaAs (Otsuka et Al, 1985).

All the layers studied hereafter were grown by Molecular-Beam Epitaxy (M.B.E.) in RIBER 2300 and 1000 systems and T.E.M. observations were carried out in JEOL 200 CX (C_s=1.05 mm) or 4000 EX (C_s = 1.0 mm) microscopes.

$Cd_{0.96}Zn_{0.04}$Te substrates were used rather than CdTe because Zn incorporation tends to reduce the density of dislocations and because these substrates are perfectly lattice matched to HgTe.CdTe growth on these substrates implies a small misfit of the order of 2.3%. As for heteroepitaxy, GaAs or GaAs : In were chosen as much for their good crystallinity and low cost, as for further possible integration of optoelectronic devices. In this case, lattice mismatch is 14.6 % for CdTe and 8 % for ZnTe and structural characterization of these systems yields valuable information of how heteroepitaxy proceeds. We shall report here on our T.E.M. observations of both low and high misfit II-VI epitaxial systems with a particular emphasis on interfaces. Structural analysis of a few typical heterostructures (such as quantum wells and superlattices) will also be detailed.

II-VI EPITAXIAL GROWTH ON (001) GaAs

(001) ZnTe

The lattice mismatch is $\frac{\Delta a}{a}$ = 8% (a_{ZnTe} = 0.610 nm ; a_{GaAs} = 0.565 nm).

Three types of interface dislocations can be found from the <110> lattice images (Fig. 1a) : mainly Lomer type edge dislocations with their $\frac{a}{2}$ <110> Burgers vector in the interface plane, lying at a distance of approximately 5 nm from each other (accounting well for the 8 % misfit), occasional 60° dislocations with their $\frac{a}{2}$ <110> Burgers vector inclined at 45° to the interface (thus twice less efficient for lattice matching), and finally partial dislocations with inclined $\frac{a}{6}$ <112> Burgers vectors bounding intrinsic or extrinsic stacking-faults. We have observed that 60° dislocations are predominant on inclined parts of the interface with their extra {111} and {001} lattice fringes within the substrate on the GaAs side of the surface step (Feuillet et Al. 1987). The partials lying at the ZnTe/GaAs interface were found to be the 30° partial of 60° dissociated dislocations when the stacking fault was of intrinsic nature or 90° partials if of extrinsic nature, which would be coherent with the dissociation sense of 60° misfit dislocations coming over from the surface of the layer upon relaxation of the compressive stress ($a_{ZnTe} > a_{GaAs}$) (Marée et Al. 1987).

The stacking-faults were very often found to intersect each other (Fig. 1b) in the close vicinity of the interfaces, leading to the formation of stair-rod type dislocations. Frank dislocations, resulting from the interaction of partials with 60° undissociated dislocations either at the interface or within the layer, were also detected. Because of these possible reactions, the extent of the highly defective zone in the layer is limited to approximately 50 nm. These reactions will inhibit 60° dislocation glide from the interface towards the top of layer, that might have occurred during specimen cooling from the deposition temperature to room temperature under the effect of the tensile stress due to the different thermal expansion coefficients of ZnTe and GaAs ($\alpha_{ZnTe} > \alpha_{GaAs}$). However, stacking-fault extension was found greater than normal (Lu and Cockayne, 1986), up to 50 nm instead of 9 to 13 nm for dissociated 60° at equilibrium and might be the consequence of the thermal contraction tensile stress that would send the 90° partials up in the layer, while the 30° partials would stay pinned at the interface (this for intrinsic stacking-faults, the other way around for extrinsic ones).

Determination of the stacking sequence at epitaxial interfaces is of much interest if one wants to understand how epitaxy proceeds. Furthermore, it is one of the aims of atomic resolution microscopy to assess the interface atomic roughness, particularly in the case of quantum wells and superlattices. This can be achieved by observation of lattice images obtained under <100> illumination, where the four chemically sensitive <002> reflections contribute to the image (Ourmazd et Al, 1987 ; Bourret et Al, 1988). Such a lattice image obtained at 400 KeV is given in Fig. 1c in the case of (001)ZnTe on (001)GaAs, where it appears feasible to differentiate between Zn and Te because of their very different atomic scattering factors. Image simulations as a function of defocussing distance and sample thickness are presently carried out and will allow us to have these indispensable informations.

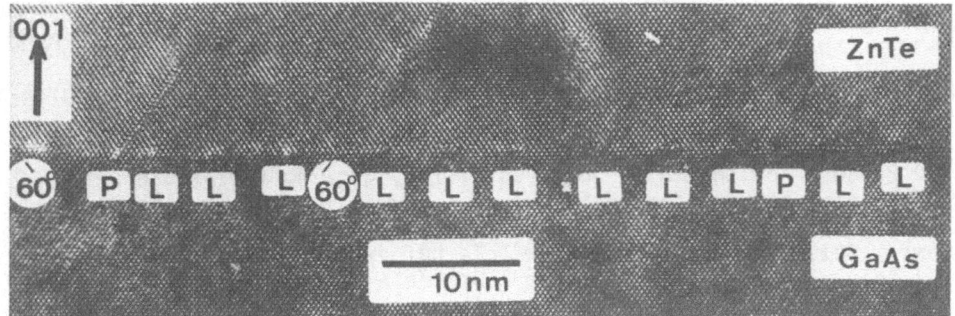

Fig. 1a. (001)ZnTe/(001)GaAs interface ; L=Lomer, 60°, and P=partial dislocations.

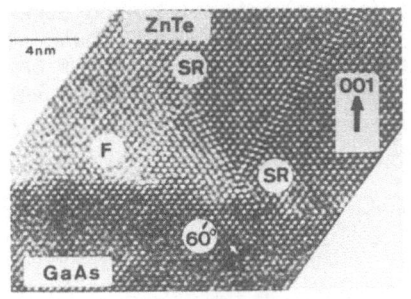

Fig. 1b. Intersection of stacking faults and formation of sessile dislocations.

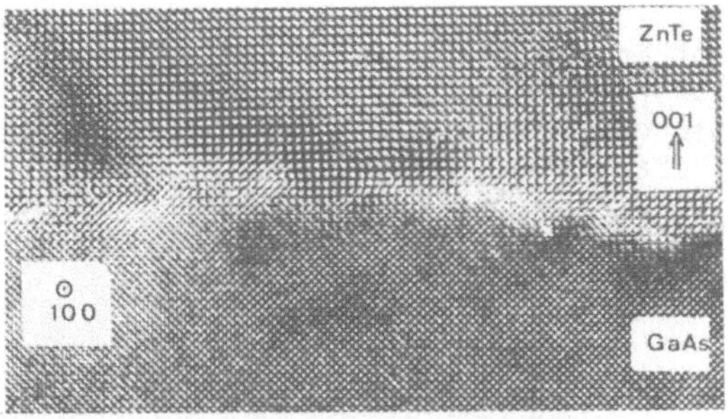

Fig. 1c. (100) lattice image of the (001)ZnTe/GaAs interface

(001) CdTe

The lattice mismatch is $\frac{\Delta a}{a}$ = 14.6 %. (a_{CdTe}=0.6481 nm, a_{GaAs} =0.565 nm).

As for (001)ZnTe, mainly Lomer type edge dislocations with their $\frac{a}{2}$ <110> Burgers vector in the interface plane can be detected (Fig. 2a). Their mean distance, ≈ 2.5 nm, agrees well with the lattice mismatch between CdTe and GaAs. Very many stacking-faults and microtwins exist at the interface that extend into the layer over a maximum distance of approximately 20 nm.

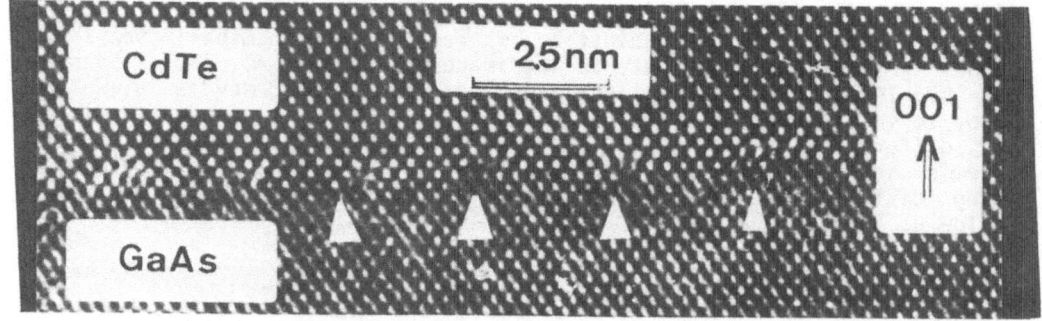

Fig. 2a. Lomer type misfit dislocations at the (001)CdTe/(001)GaAs interface.

Because of the high involved misfit, growing (001) CdTe onto (001) GaAs happens to be rather difficult and anyway leads to a high density of grown-in dislocations. This difficulty can be partly overcome if one grows (001)CdTe on top of a thin ZnTe buffer layer. Fig. 2b represents a (001)CdTe layer grown on a 25 nm thick ZnTe layer : most stacking-faults originating from the ZnTe/GaAs interface stop at the ZnTe/CdTe interface. The partials at this latter interface are utilized to absorb part of the misfit and the stacking-faults cannot extend further. The density of microtwins and stacking-faults in CdTe is greatly reduced. For thicker ZnTe buffers, the quality of the top CdTe layer is not as good which was confirmed by double crystal X-ray diffraction and Rutherford Back Scattering : in this case, all stacking-faults intersect each other within the ZnTe buffer and their bounding partials do not contribute to absorbing part of the CdTe/ZnTe mismatch. Other stacking-faults and microtwins are thus generated again at this interface degrading the overall structural quality of the CdTe layer.

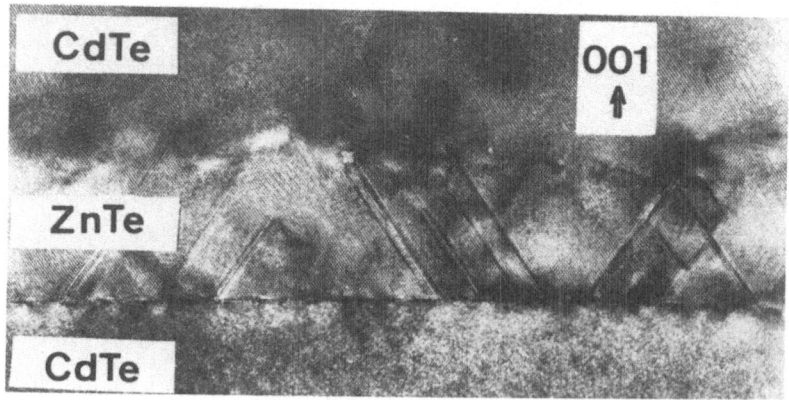

Fig. 2b.   (001)CdTe grown on top of a 25 nm thick ZnTe buffer layer.

Despite this drastic reduction in stacking-fault density, there remain many grown-in dislocations in the layers, the density of which can be highly reduced by depositing, on top of the ZnTe buffer layer, multi-layers of the type $Cd_x Zn_{1-x} Te$ with stepped x values (Million et Al, 1988). Fig. 2c is a low magnification image of such a structure where the thickness of each of the layers is below the critical thickness (70 nm for a 20 % x increase). In this case, it is believed that all the dislocations (other than the partials) bend over at the $Cd_{0.2}Zn_{0.8}Te/ZnTe$ interface under the action of the compressive mismatch stress. These bent threading dislocations might annihilate at the interface or form dislocation nodes. In any case, the density of threading dislocations will decrease on crossing each of the successive interfaces and will allow growth of a "clean" final CdTe epilayer.

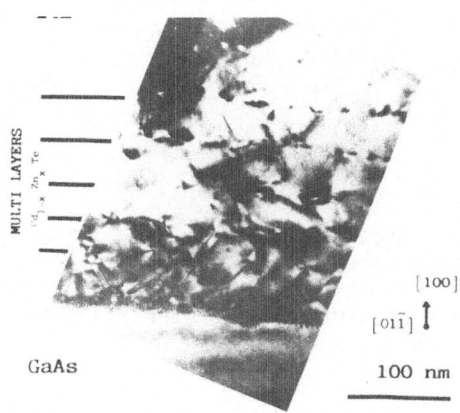

Fig. 2c. (001)CdTe grown on top of a multilayer buffer.

(111) CdTe

We have already mentioned that (001) CdTe growth is not that easy to carry out. Instead CdTe has a natural tendency to grow (111) onto (001) GaAs.

Fig. 3a helps understanding the situation : represented are the atomic positions of the (111) CdTe and (001) GaAs planes when the $[11\bar{2}]$ CdTe direction is aligned with the [110] GaAs one and the $[\bar{1}10]$ GaAs direction is parallel to the $[\bar{1}10]$ CdTe one. Then, one finds out that $(11\bar{2})$ CdTe interreticular distance ($d = \dfrac{a\sqrt{6}}{4} = 0.397$ nm) matches quite perfectly that of the (110) GaAs planes ($d = \dfrac{a}{\sqrt{2}} = 0.40$ nm) the remaining lattice mismatch is 0.7%. In the perpendicular direction, $[\bar{1}10]$ CdTe$\not\!/$$[\bar{1}10]$GaAs, one is left with the total 14.6 % misfit.

Fig. 3b is a lattice image of this interface when viewing it along the [110] GaAs and $[11\bar{2}]$ CdTe directions : lattice match is almost perfect. Misfit dislocations could be detected with their extra half plane on the CdTe side of the interface to relax the tensile 0.7 % misfit.

In the orientation at 90° from the previous one, Fig. 3c, i.e. when viewing the interface along the $[\bar{1}10]$ direction, one finds lattice coïncidences, as expected from Fig. 3a , which are indicated by arrows and which account for the 14.6 % misfit.

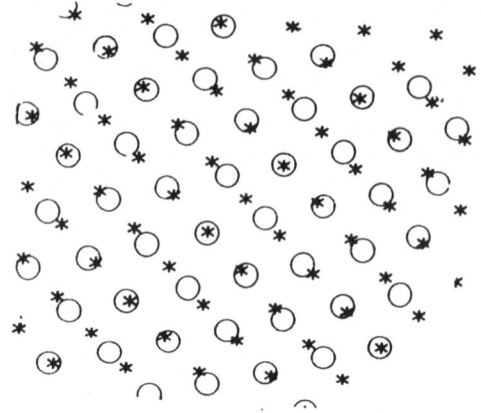

Fig. 3a. Schematic representing the positions of the atoms in the (111)CdTe plane (o) superimposing those in the (001) GaAs plane (x) when [11$\bar{2}$] CdTe is parallel to [110] GaAs.

Image analysis and simulations of these interfaces are under way and should prove very efficient to discuss a growth model that was recently proposed by Cohen-Solal and Coworkers (1986) and that was confirmed by R.B.S. measurements of the relative polarities of GaAs and CdTe (Chami et Al, 1988).

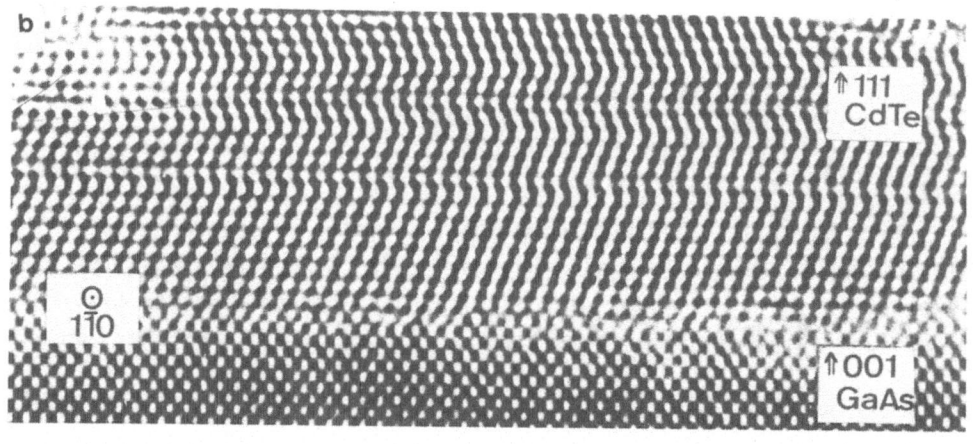

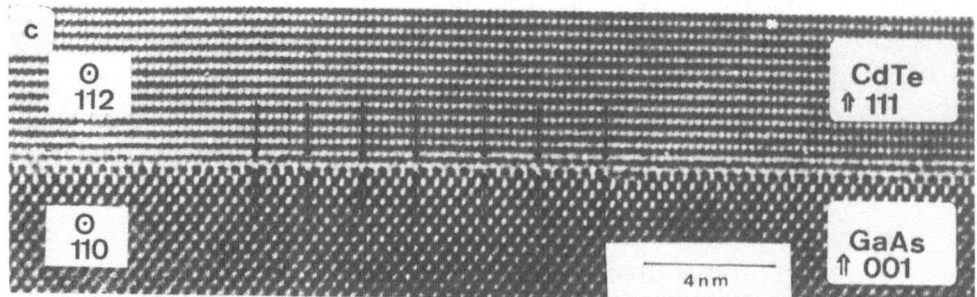

Fig. 3. (111)CdTe/(001)GaAs interface observed in
b. the common [1$\bar{1}$0] azimuth
c. the [112] CdTe∥[110]GaAs azimuth.

Close inspection of the lattice images obtained at this interface revealed monomolecular steps on the (001) GaAs surface aligned along the <110> directions. This is clearly evidenced in Fig. 3d where steps are arrowed and is of much interest to assess the morphology of high-vacuum prepared GaAs surfaces on a fairly large scale and at an atomic level.

As to what concerns growth nucleation, we have studied the early stages of growth by depositing very thin layers and encapsulating them with amorphous Te in order to avoid layer oxidation and degradation during preparation. We could check (Fig. 3e) that, contrary to what R.H.E.E.D. suggests, (111) CdTe growth an (001) GaAs is rather a 3-D process but that islands are somehow extended in the <110> directions. The CdTe lattice parameter has been found to have reached its equilibrium value in all studied thin layers and twinning had occurred right from the beginning of the deposition.

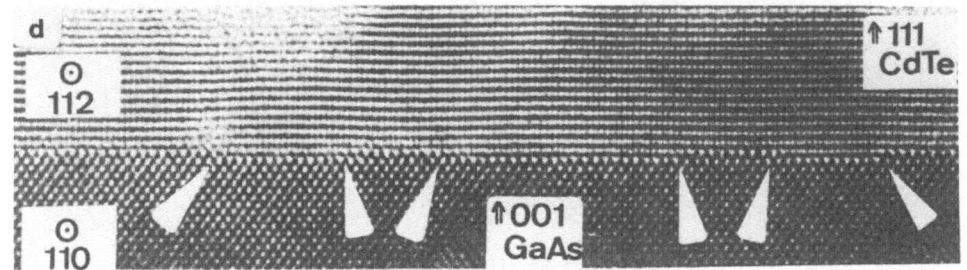

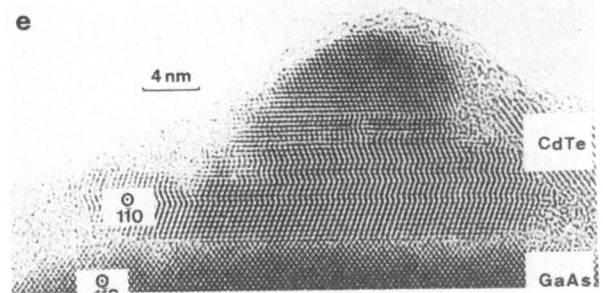

Fig. 3d.   monomolecular steps on the GaAs surface.
    e.   (111)CdTe island on (001)GaAs.

II-VI EPITAXIAL GROWTH ON (001) $Cd_{0.96}Zn_{0.04}Te$

Growing II-VI semiconductor layers such as CdTe, HgTe or $Cd_{1-x}Hg_xTe$ on top of II-VI substrates such as CdTe or $Cd_{0.96}Zn_{0.04}Te$ implies low misfits, i.e. below $2.3 \ 10^{-3}$.

For these systems, there appears to be a critical thickness of the order of 400 nm over which part of the elastic energy stored in the layer is relaxed via formation of misfit dislocations (Fontaine et Al, 1987, Chami et Al, 1988 (2)).

Fig. 4 a is a weak-beam micrograph of the (001) CdTe/(001) $Cd_{0.96}Zn_{0.04}Te$ system. There appears to be very few dislocations in the layer even close to the interface, which had also been inferred from the small width of Double Crystal X-Ray Diffraction peaks. At the interface lie 60° misfit dislocations which are dissociated over part of their length. This correlates R.B.S. measurements of the same epitaxial system (Chami et Al, 1987).

From $\vec{g}.\vec{b}$ analysis, we could show that, where the dislocation is dissociated, the 30° partial lies at the interface while the 90° lies within the layer, at a distance of approximately 15 nm. This is consistent with the dissociation sense expected from relaxation of a layer under a compressive stress (a layer > a substrate).

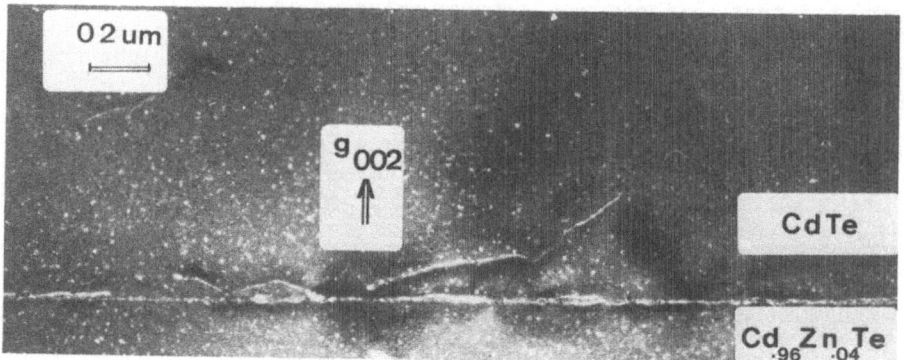

Fig. 4a. Misfit dislocations at the CdTe/$Cd_{0.96}Zn_{0.04}$Te interface.

Fig. 4 b is a high-resolution <110> lattice image of the same interface. It is clear that finding the exact position of the interface is not feasible, but at least one can assure that the interface is coherent over large distances. However note the existence of residual impurities that delineate the interface and which were also detected by S.I.M.S. analysis.

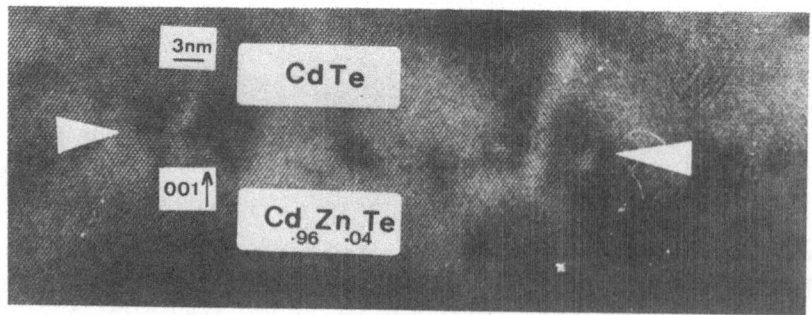

Fig. 4b. lattice image of the CdTe/$Cd_{0.96}Zn_{0.04}$Te interface showing interface decoration by impurities.

(111) CdTe growth can also be achieved on (111) $Cd_{0.96}Zn_{0.04}$Te but the density of twins running parallel to the interface and therefore of twin boundary dislocations make it difficult to have a comprehensive view of how elastic strain is relaxed.

Common II-VI semi-conductors span a very wide range of energy-gaps and many types of heterostructures can be envisaged that would be of interest both for their potential applications and for their fundamental transport and electrooptic properties (Panish, 1987).

CdTe layers confined between ZnTe barriers

Fig. 5a is a <110> lattice image of a 25 Å thick (001) CdTe layer (Eg = 1.4 eV) buried in between two (001) ZnTe barriers. In the case where CdTe grows coherently onto the first ZnTe barrier, CdTe and ZnTe lattice parameters match in the interface plane and thus CdTe is tetragonally distorted in the growth direction : this is clearly evidenced by observation that {111} CdTe lattice fringes are somehow more bent towards the [001] growth direction than are the corresponding {111} lattice fringes in ZnTe. This is schematized in Fig. 5b and the corresponding angle is drawn on Fig. 5a. This was used to determine the layer thickness (2.5 mm) and we found it to be in good agreement with R.B.S. measurements (Chami A.C; and Ligeon E., private communication). 400 KeV <100> HREM images would also allow to assess this thickness and furthermore to image interface roughness on an atomic scale. However <110> HREM images have this advantage that, if relaxation has occurred, misfit dislocations would appear end-on.

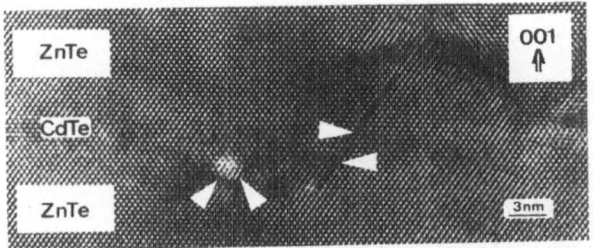

Fig. 5a. CdTe quantum well between ZnTe barriers.

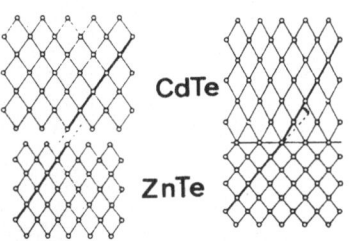

Fig. 5b. lattice plane bending due to tetragonal deformation.

As indicated in Fig. 5a, partial relaxation has actually happened, and 60° or Lomer dislocations are present at the ZnTe/CdTe interface, at a distance of approximately 40 nm from each other. This would not be expected from a simple elasticity theory (Fontaine et Al, 1987) where one would predict a 20 nm critical thickness for this 6% misfit system. Note, however that this model was devised for low misfit epitaxy. At least, our observations suggest that no instant relaxation has occurred for this high misfit system, and that strained layer superlattices are feasible as long as the thickness of the individual layers remains very small. Observation of very thin quantum well (below 2 nm) are under way and should prove very efficient to understand how lattice strain is relaxed in this sort of high misfit systems.

CdTe/ZnTe superlattices

(001) CdTe/ZnTe strained layer superlattices (S.L.S.) were grown on top of $Cd_{0.96}Zn_{0.04}Te$ substrates with equal nominal individual layer thicknesses of the order of 1.5-2 nm.

In order to make sure that free standing superlattices were grown, the number of periods was chosen large enough for the S.L.S. to take its own equilibrium lattice parameter.

Two types of buffers were tried before deposition of the S.L.S. : either a single CdTe buffer or a multi-layer buffer with stepped Zn composition as detailed above in § II.2. In this latter case, the last buffer was chosen to tentatively match the S.L.S. lattice parameter.

Fig. 6 represents the <110> lattice image of a typical ZnTe/CdTe S.L.S. As in the case of the quantum well above, it is clear that {111} lattice fringes are distorted on passing from one layer to the other, upon tetragonal deformation. No dislocations were ever found at interfaces within the superlattice.

But misfit dislocations, mainly of 60° type, were detected at the S.L.S./CdTe buffer interface. In this case these dislocations could arise from partial relaxation of the first ZnTe layer (cf previous §) or from relaxation of the S.L.S. as a whole. As in the case of the high misfit systems such as (001) ZnTe/GaAs and (001) CdTe/GaAs described above, many stacking-faults are present that extend from the interface into the S.L.S.

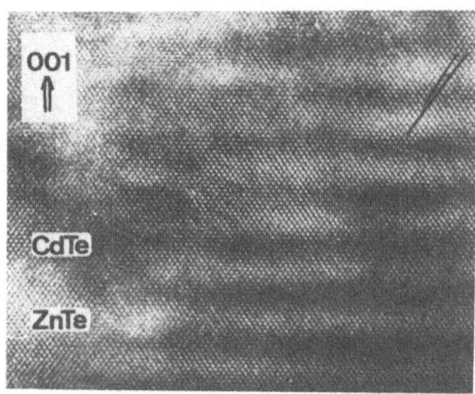

Fig. 6.   (001)CdTe/ZnTe superlattice.

When the S.L.S. is deposited onto a $Cd_{0.5}Zn_{0.5}Te$ buffer, the successive layers are alternately under tension and under compression. No misfit dislocations can be seen at the S.L.S./buffer interface. In this case, we found, by measurement on lattice images and on the electron diffractogram, that the S.L.S. mean lattice parameter was fairly well matched to that of the $Cd_{0.5}Zn_{0.5}Te$ buffer. Such a system does not exhibit stacking-faults at the S.L.S./buffer interface.

The superlattice period (p=4 nm) in Fig. 6 was determined by the distance between satellite spots on the electron diffractogram rather than by direct observation of the lattice image because of the apparent roughness and of the poor contrast available in the <110> observation orientation. It was found to be in good agreement with Double Crystal Diffraction and R.B.S. estimations.

CdTe-HgTe superlattices

In this sort of superlattice, successive layers experience a very small lattice mismatch ($3 \cdot 10^{-3}$). One can grow thicker layers than in the CdTe/ZnTe case while retaining perfectly coherent interfaces.

Fig. 7a is a <110> lattice image of a 3.4 nm/6.7 nm CdTe/HgTe superlattice (Di Cioccio et Al, 1987) grown on top of (111) CdTe. Dislocation could be seen at interfaces within the superlattice. Occasional 60° dislocations with their (111) extra half-plane parallel to the interface were found at the superlattice/CdTe substrate interface and were found to be associated with impurity segregation on the CdTe surface.

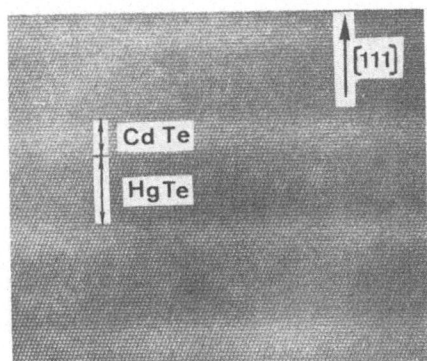

Fig. 7a. (111) HgTe/CdTe superlattice

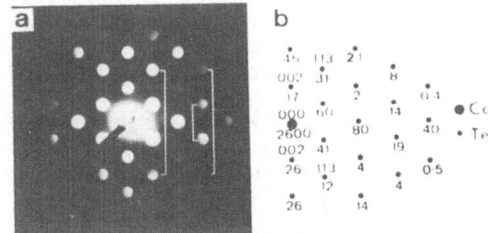

Fig. 7b electron diffractogram of CdTe showing assymmetry in spot intensities.

In the same study, the polarity of (111) CdTe was directly assessed by accurate determination of the diffraction spot intensity (Hewat et Al, 1988). This is of much importance if one wants to know which of the (111) A face (triply bonded Cd face) or the ($\overline{1}\overline{1}\overline{1}$)B face (triply bonded Te face) is the best for further epitaxy. As outlined above, it is also highly relevant when one is concerned with understanding how heteroepitaxy proceeds and might be necessary in order to determine the atomic structure of defects (Di Cioccio et Al, 1987).

The experiment lies on the fact that, when multiple scattering is involved for non centrosymmetric crystals (zinc-blende type) of finite thickness, the intensities of diffraction spots g and $\overline{g}$ are different. The intensities of diffraction spots recorded on a wedge shape selected area are compared to those calculated using a multi-slice theory (Fig. 7b). The diffraction patterns were consistent with a ($\overline{1}\overline{1}\overline{1}$) B face (Te dangling bonds) as the best face for epitaxy which agreed with R.B.S. polarity measurements (Chami et Al, 1988 (1)).

CONCLUSIONS

II-VI layers in the (001) orientation grown on top of (001) GaAs are typical of high misfit systems : most interfacial dislocations have their Burgers vector in the interface plane, stacking-faults and/or microtwins are present in the vicinity of the interface, their partials often being pinned by dislocation reactions, and finally a large density of grown-in dislocations lie within the layers. We have shown that the defect concentration in (001) CdTe layers could be greatly reduced by appropriate use of ZnTe thin buffer layers and of $Cd_xZn_{1-x}Te$ multilayer buffers with stepped Zn composition.

CdTe has this advantage that it provides the possibility of growing (111) layers on top of (001) substrates yielding unique heteroepitaxial relationships that we have analysed. Twinning is present parallel to the interface but studies presently carried-out tend to show that it is possible for the twins to be eliminated.

CdTe epitaxial growth on $Cd_{0.96}Zn_{0.04}Te$ leads to low misfits which are accomodated by dissociated $60°$ dislocations at the interface. The sense of the partials was shown to correspond to that expected from relaxation of the built-in compressive stress. The good crystalline quality of these layers has motivated further growth of heterostructures among which single quantum wells and superlattices.

In particular, we have demonstrated that partial lattice relaxation might occur even for layer thicknesses much less than the expected critical thickness and has to be born in mind if one wants to avoid any non-radiative trap in II-VI based electrooptic systems.

The structure of Strained-Layer-Superlattices of the type ZnTe/CdTe was detailed and we found that it bears a resemblance to that of either low-misfit or high-misfit single layer systems according as the S.L.S. is grown respectively on $Cd_{0.5}Zn_{0.5}Te$ or on CdTe buffers. (111) HgTe/CdTe superlattices were shown to have rather flat interfaces with no interface dislocations despite $60°$ ones associated with impurities.

Finally, it is demonstrated how an accurate determination of crystal polarity in non centrosymmetric materials with the zinc-blende structure is made possible by thorough exploitation of electron diffractograms.

Through one example, we have also pointed out that extensive use of <100> cross-sections is very powerful when one is concerned with interface roughness, stacking sequences at heteroepitaxial interfaces and crystal polarity; we intend to extend this approach to all (001) oriented confined layers and superlattices.

ACKNOWLEDGEMENTS

The author wishes to thank A. Bourret, J. Thibault-Desseaux, L. Di Cioccio, E. Hewat and M. Dupuy for very fruitful discussions on the electron microscopy results ; he is also very grateful to the whole II-VI epitaxy team headed by J.L. Pautrat and Y. Merle d'Aubigné and he is indebted to C. Martin and C. Bouvier for their everyday technical assistance.

REFERENCES

Panish, M.B., 1987, "Materials for Infrared Detectors and Sources", 3. Ed. Farrow R.F.C., J.F. Schetzina, J.T. Cheung, M.R.S. Symposia proceedings

Ponce, F.A., Anderson, G.B., Ballingall, J.M., 1987, "Materials for Infrared Detectors and Sources", 199 Ed. Farrow R.F.C., J.F. Schetzina, J.F., J.T. Cheung, M.R.S. Symposia proceedings

Lu, G., Cockayne, D.J.H., 1986, Phil. Mag. A53, (3) 307

Marée, P.M.J., Barbour, J.C., Van Der Veen, J.F., Kavanagh, K.L., Bulle-Lieuwma, C.W.T., Viegers, M.P.A., 1987, J.A.P., 62, (11) 4413

Ourmazd, A., Tsang, W.T., Remtschler, J.A., Taylor, D.W., 1987, A.P.L., 50, (20), 1417

Bourret, A., Rouvière, J.L., Spendeler, J., 1988, Phys. Stat. Sol. (a) 107, 481

Million, A., Di Cioccio, L., Gailliard, J.P., Piaguet, J., 1988

Cohen-Solal, G, Bailly, F., Barbé, M., 1986, A.P.L. 49, 1519

Chami, A.C., Ligeon, E., Danielou, R., Fontenille, J. (1) 1988, A.P.L. 52 (18), 1502

Fontaine, C., Gailliard, J.P., Magli, S., Million, A., Piaguet, J., 1987, A.P.L., 50, (14) 903

Chami, A.C., Ligeon, E., Danielou, R., Fontenille, J., Magnea, N., Mariette, H. (2), 1988, A.P.L. 52 (22), 1974

Chami, A.C., Ligeon, E., Fontenille, J., Danielou, R., 1987, J.A.P., 62 (9), 3718

Di Cioccio L., Hewat, E.A., Million, A., Gailliard, J.P., Dupuy, M., 1987, in "Microscopy of Semiconducting Materials", Inst. of Phys. Conf. Ser. n°87, 243

Hewat, E.A., Di Cioccio, L., Million, A., Dupuy, M., Gailliard, J.P., 1988, J.A.P., 63 (10) 4929

HIGH RESOLUTION ELECTRON MICROSCOPY STUDY OF INDIUM DISTRIBUTION IN InAs/GaAs MULTILAYERS

C. D'Anterroches
Centre National d'Etude des télécommunications, CNS
Chemins du Vieux Chêne, BP 98, 38243 Meyan, Cedex

J.M. Gerard, and J.Y. Marzin
Centre National d'Etude des télécommunications, Paris B
196 av. H. Ravera, 92220 Bagneux

ABSTRACT

Two InAs/GaAs multilayers have been studied using X-Ray diffraction (XR), photoluminescence (PL) and high Resolution Transmission Electron Microscopy (HRTEM) in order to determine the Indium location. X-Ray diffraction has provided the thickness and periodicity of the multilayers. The ones chosen were respectively A : 0.9 monolayer (mL) and B : 1.7 mL thick according to XR measurements. From comparison of their structure we conclude that Indium intermixes with Gallium and gives rise to a thicker film, InGaAs, the Indium proportion being at least 50 %. The interface InAs/GaAs is atomically flat, whereas the interface GaAs/InAs is extremely rough. This may be a way of decreasing the elastic energy.

INTRODUCTION

The optoelectronic properties of InAs/GaAs multilayers are such as to induce much interest in the growth of this material. The problem is the large lattice misfit (7.2 %). Thus, after having obtained good ternary compound multilayers, many groups have achieved InAs/GaAs multilayers. The growth techiques were either Metalorganic chemical vapor deposition (MOCVD) (1-3) or molecular beam epitaxy (MBE) (4-9). Such a lattice mismatch can be partly accomodated by a misfit dislocations network, or the InAs film can be entirely strained. In this paper this last kind of film is studied. During MBE (the technique used) the growth is controlled by RHEED. A thick GaAs sublayer is grown between two InAs films, to smooth a possible surface roughness. The authors had previously shown that the GaAs layers of this kind of multilayer are locally strained (10) due to the GaAs/InAs interface roughness. The purpose of this paper is to determine the Indium distribution in the InAs layer from X-Ray diffraction, photoluminescence and HRTEM analysis.

GROWTH

The growth of pseudomorphic InAs layers on GaAs is particularly difficult due to the large lattice mismatch between InAs and GaAs (7 %). When InAs films thicker than a critical limit h_c are deposited on GaAs, a shift from bidimensional (2D) deposition to a three dimensional (3D) growth mode is observed by RHEED. This critical thickness h_c, close to 2 or 3mL (6 to 9 A InAs), depends on growth conditions.

In this work strained-layer Superlattices (SLS) A and B are both grown by a modified MBE technique, at 350°C, which alternate deposition of column III species, and As_4. We adapted recently this so called Migration Enhanced Epitaxy technique (MEE), first introduced by Horokoski and coworkers (12) in the GaAs/AlAs system, to the growth of highly strained heterostructures such as InAs wells in GaAs (13) or InAs/GaAs SLS on InP substrates (14).

This growth technique allows to enhance noticeably the critical thickness h_c, and thus extends the range of pseudomorphic deposition of InAs on GaAs.

RHEED is used throughout the growth, to monitor first the thermal oxide desorption of GaAs (001) substrates at 620°C, and then control the deposition of a 0.5 μm thick GaAs buffer layer under standard MBE conditions (T = 600°C). The sample is then cooled down to 350°C, during a growth interruption before the MEE growth of the SLS takes place. Particular attention is paid during the deposition of the InAs sublayers, to observe by RHEED an eventual shift to 3D growth.

Relatively thick GaAs layers (350 A to 500 A) are grown between each quantum well, to smooth the surface and optimize the overall crystalline quality. SLS A and B consist of 6 periods, which is sufficient to allow characterization experiments (X-ray diffraction) and optical studies.

EXPERIMENTAL RESULTS

The growth was controlled by RHEED. The RHEED pattern abruptly changes when small amounts of In ($\simeq$0.1 mL) are deposited on a GaAs surface. The reconstruction streaks of the c 4x4 pattern observed for GaAs at 350°C disappear, and only integer order streaks are observed during the deposition of the InAs film. Diffuse reconstruction streaks appear when GaAs is deposited on top, and fully recover their intensity over only 5 ml GaAs growth. No spots were observed during the deposition of InAs, which confirms the bidimensional character of the growth.

X-ray double diffraction investigations allowed to check the designed sample parameters. The profiles obtained for SLS A and B indicate that the large GaAs confining layers are essentially unstrained. When 3D growth of InAs films occurs, GaAs sublayers are strained, and the existence of large strain inhomogeneities are revealed by the assymmetry of the profile (8). We can deduce the period of the SLS from the angular spacing between satellites. The SLS mean lattice parameter Lw along the [001] direction is also extracted from the position of one particular diffraction order of the SLS. This measure allows to determine the total In quantity deposited per SLS period, within 0.1 ml. It can be shown (8) that this estimate is essentially independent of the actual In composition profile within a period and thus on an eventual degree of intermixing between GaAs and InAs. This estimate leads to Lw = 0.9 ml (SLS A) and Lw = 1.7 ml (SLS B).

PL confirms the qualitative conclusion deduced from RHEED and XR analysis. Both PL spectra obtained at 8°K for SLS A and B are shown figure 1. A single peak is related to SLS emission, which displays a small spectral width (12 meV full width at half maximum (FWHM) for both SLS). The important broadening ($\simeq$ 50 meV) and shift to lower energy ($\simeq$ 100 meV)

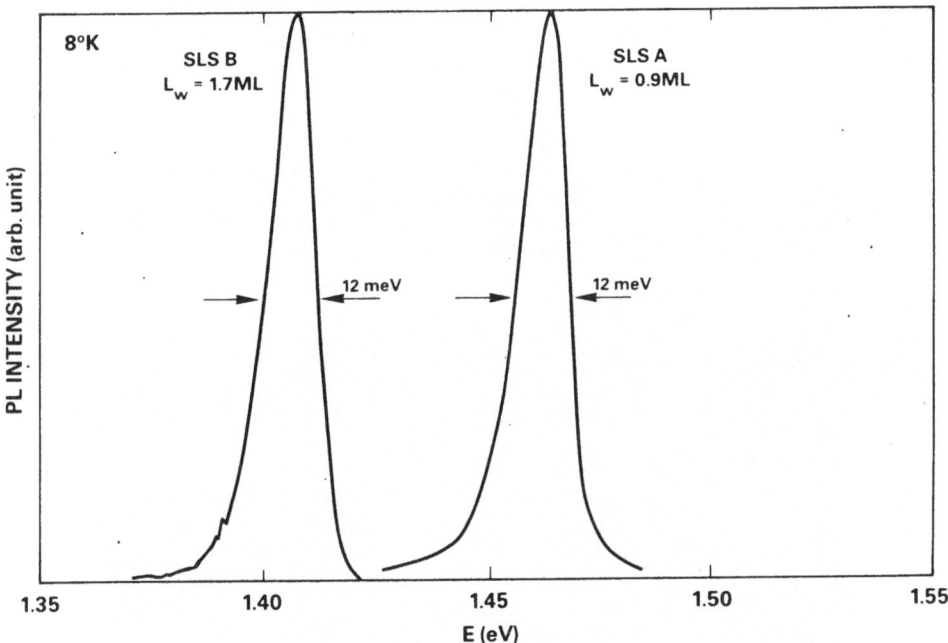

Fig. 1 Low temperature (8°k) PL spectra for SLS A and B.

characteristic of 3D grown structures (15) are not seen for SLS A and B. The bidimensional growth of these SLS is thus confirmed.

We therefore conclude from RHEED observations, and from X-ray diffraction and PL characterization that a 2D growth of these InAs/GaAs SLS has been obtained. As a result, X-ray diffraction profiles and PL spectra are qualitatively close to what would be expected for a perfect SLS. This means mainly however that these techniques are essentially insensitive to residual inhomogeneities and imperfections which are still observed in these layers, as shown in the following.

ELECTRON MICROSCOPY RESULTS

These multilayers are too strained to obtain appropriate samples for planar view analysis. Cross-sectional views show that they are free of dislocations within the detection limit i.e. 10^7 cm^{-2}. No dislocation network, to compensate for the lattice mismatch, was detected showing that the two multilayers are elastically strained.

The 1.7 ml thick film (fig 2a) appears thicker than the 0.9 ml (fig 2b), but the resolution is low and the accuracy does not allow the thickness of the film to be measured. Thus high resolution images have been studied.

From our measurements we can deduce that the accuracy in the periodicity deduced from X-Ray diffraction is about 2 monolayers.

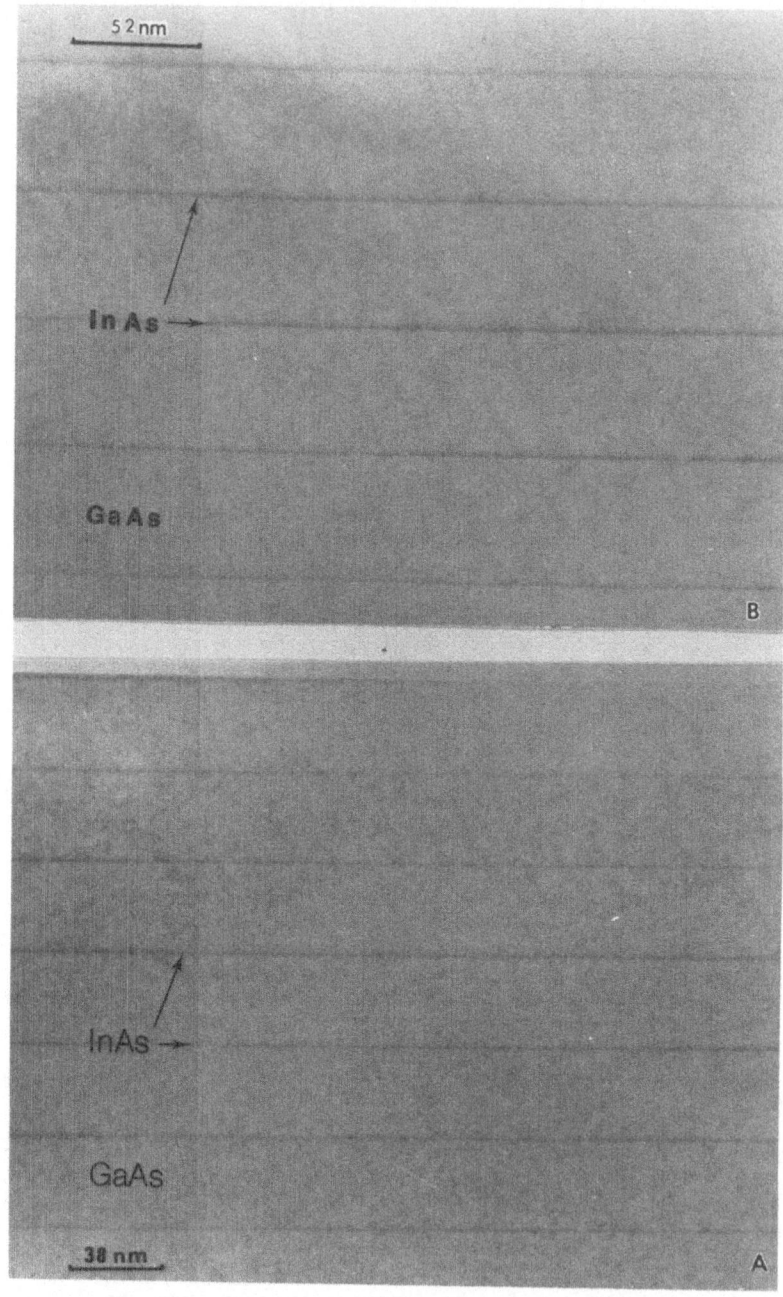

Fig. 2   Cross-sectional view of SLS A and B.

Figure 3 shows that we can distinguish the two interfaces :

- the first : InAs/GaAs, the Surface of In deposition, is atomically flat. The steps which are detected at this interface are due to the misorientation of the GaAs surface. The step distance corresponds to a 0.2° to 0.7° misorientation from the (100) plane.

- the second : GaAs/InAs, is on the contrary very rough and less well defined. The boundary between the light and dark areas cannot be clearly seen.

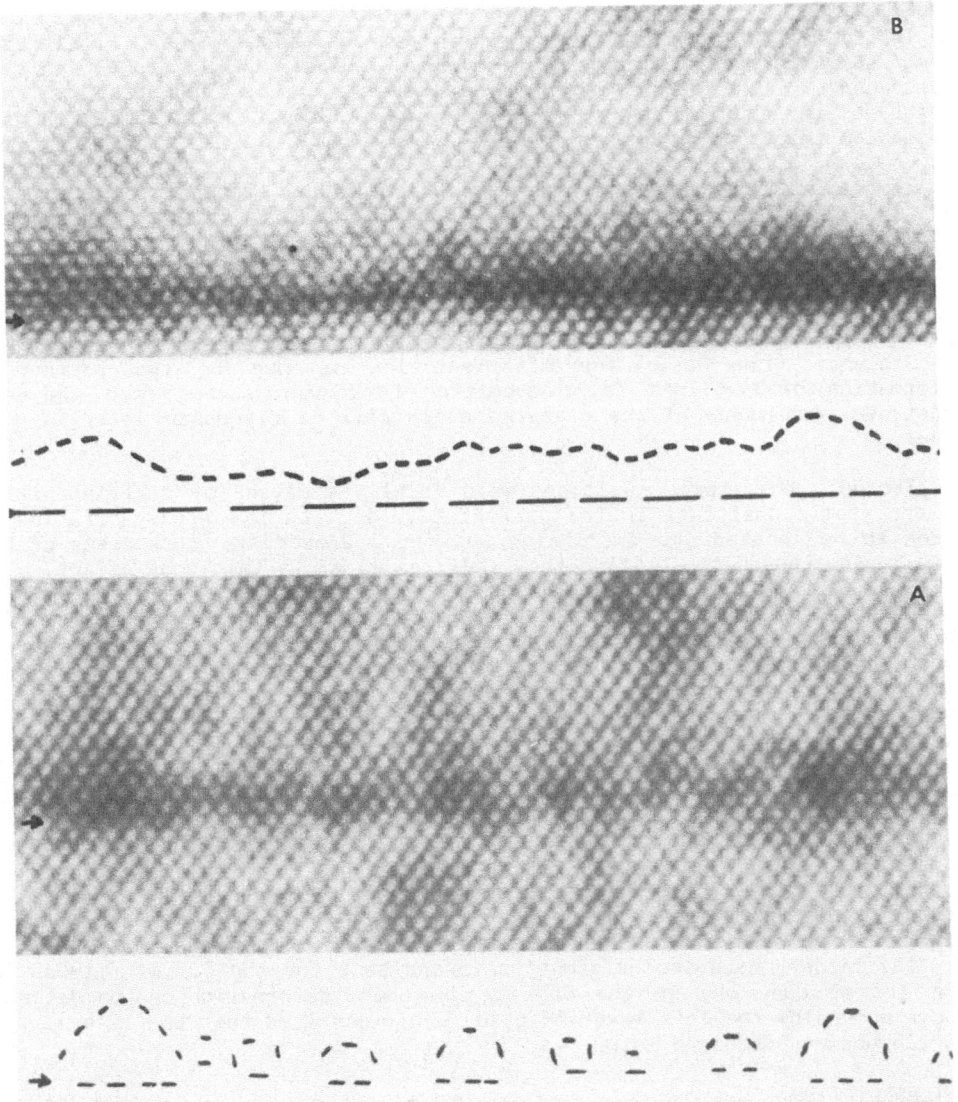

Fig. 3   GaAs/InAs interface roughness for both SLS A and B and the deduced Shape of the InAs film.

From high magnification images (fig 3a), taking into account the darker area, it can be deduced that the roughness is such that the film thickness of the so-called 1.7 ml film varies from 1 mL to 5 mL (insert schemas).

Figure 3b is a detail of the 0.9 ml film. This appears less continuous than the previous one, but its roughness is similar. Indeed its thickness can reach 4 ml.

How can we be sure that the dark areas correspond exactly to deposited Indium ? Indeed, during the thinning process, GaAs is often irregularly ejected and the local thickness variations imply a local contrast variation. For example in this Figure 3 there are areas in the GaAs layer which appear to be as dark as the InAs film.

To identify the In location, two methods can be used : either a comparison with simulated images which could indicate the In proportion ; or measurement of the deformation. Since the InAs lattice constant is very different from that of GaAs, the deformation is directly measurable on high resolution images as described below.

To measure the strain on high resolution images a comparison has to be made in terms of plane orientation and atomic position between the perfect GaAs lattice and the supposed InAs layer.

First the (111) plane orientation was analysed. When the film thickness is lower than 3 ml it cannot be measured to the required accuracy. With at least 3 ml we measured a 2.5° misorientation between (111) GaAs and (111) InAs planes (fig. 4a). The misorientation is due to the tetragonal deformation of the InAs layer submitted to planar stress from the GaAs substrate. The value of the measured angle will be discussed later is this paper.

Secondly the atomic positions were locally analysed by superimposition of the atomic positions in the perfect crystal with the areas where Indium seems to be located. No distortion was found around the dark areas of the GaAs layer, thus demonstrating that they really are a thickness effect.

On the other hand large distortions were measured in the InAs layer. The perfect lattice deduced from the area below the InAs layer is superimposed, in the bottom left, on the InAs layer and top GaAs layer. The deformation is then directly measurable. It is not parallel to the [100] direction, showing that there is not only a tetragonal distortion. The two components of the strain were measured : 4.3 % ± 0.3 % along [100] and varying from - 0.9 % to + 0.9 % along [011] (fig. 4a).

The roughness of the GaAs/InAs interface was analysed in the following manner. For example the rough area is shown in Figure 4b. In the left there is a good fit between the atomic positions in the GaAs top layer and the superimposed lattice of the GaAs substrate from plane P, whereas in the bottom right area there is no fit.

The largest measured deformation is the same for the 0.9 ml film as for the 1.7 ml one, but in the Case of 0.9 ml a deformation can be detected above and below the InAs layer (Fig 4b). This confirms that the layer is not continuous as discussed later.

INTERPRETATION

The main subject of discussion will be the Indium identification and the strain measurements concerning the film thickness and substrate orientation :

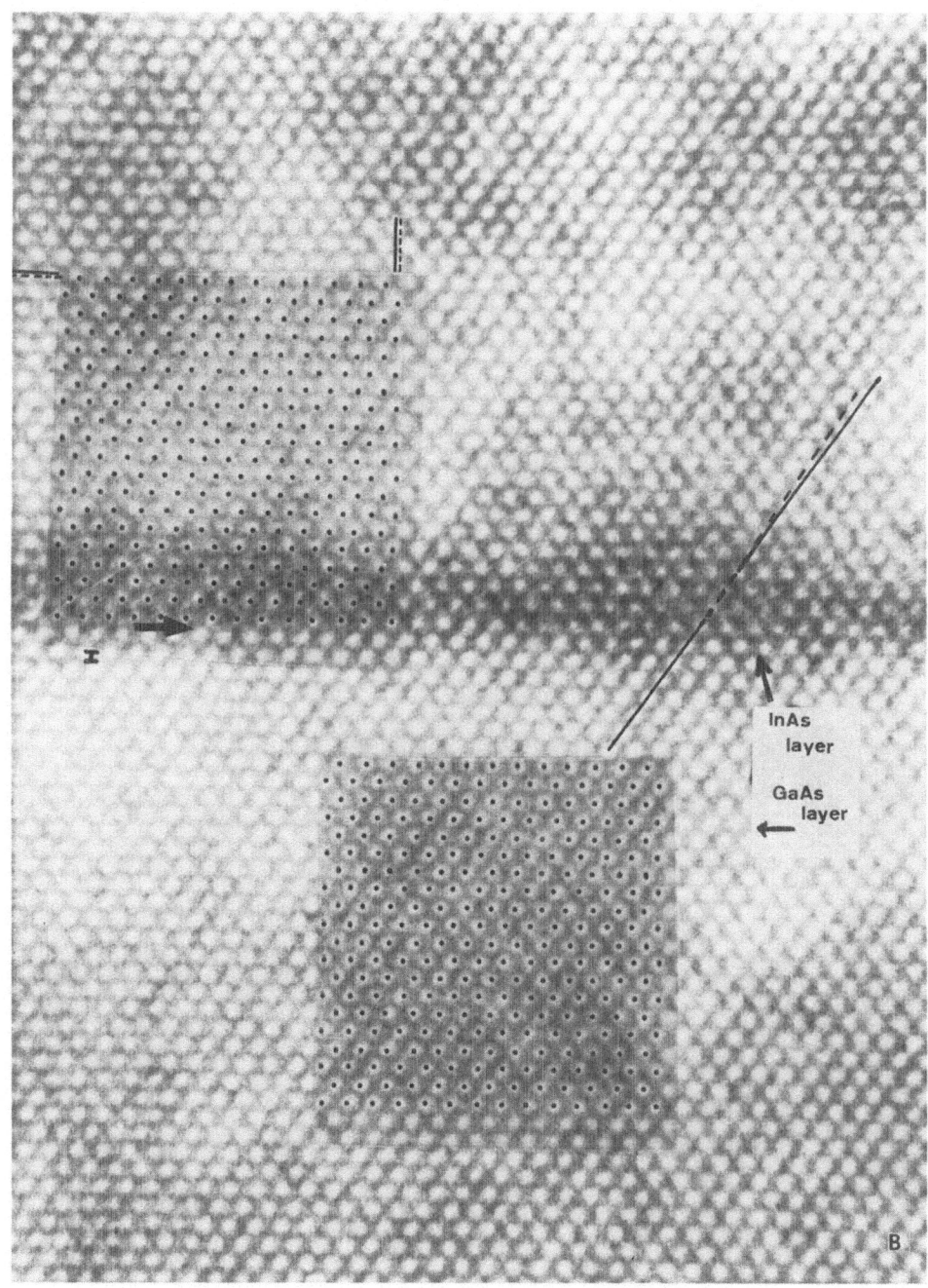

Fig. 4a   Superimposition of GaAs buffer layer atomic positions, above and below InAs layer (4a) : SLS B, (4b) : SLS A. (cont.)

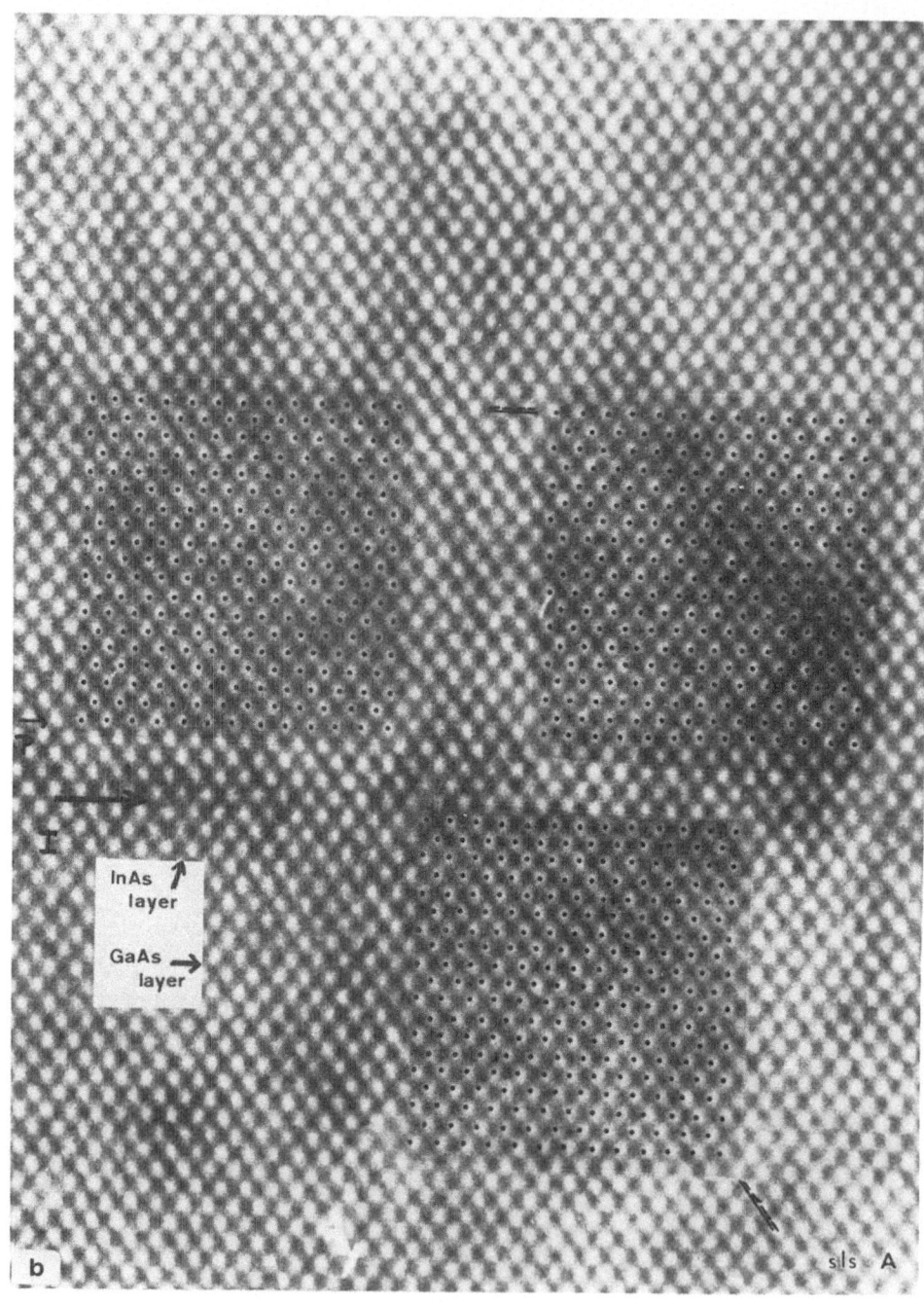

InAs
layer

GaAs
layer

b

s|s   A

Fig. 4b

Film roughness

In the case of the expected 1.7 mL film the thickness reaches 6 ml and consequently instead of 1.7 mL the mean value of the thickness is 3 mL. The accuracy of the measurement is dependent on the integration over the thickness of the specimen, it might be about 0.5 mL. Such an extension would imply that there is no InAs film but either a $In_{0.57} Ga_{0.43}$ As film (0.57 ± 0.05) or a 1mL InAs and $In_{0.35} Ga_{0.65}$As on top. This question can only be answered by analysis of the distortions.

Misorientation measurements

InAs submitted to the tetragonal deformation from the GaAs substrate is in compression in the (100) plane and in tension in the [100] direction. Its lattice constant a_{ZI} in the growth direction becomes according to the elastic theory : a_{ZI} = 6.499 A

Thus the (111) InAs/(100) GaAs angle is : 58°46, i. e 3°61 more than for the unstressed crystal.

The measured 2.5° misorientation leads to : a_{ZI} = 6.211 A. There are no misfit dislocations thus the stress is entirely elastic and the change of lattice constant may be attributed to a change in Indium composition.

If a_{ZI} = 6.211 A , then a_I = 5.92 A

If we apply the linear law for lattice constants in case of ternary compounds :

$$n = \frac{a_I - a_{0G}}{a_{0I} - a_{0G}}$$

thus : n = 63 % and the ternary compound would be : $In_{0.63} Ga_{0.37}$ As

The measurement accuracy is ± 0.25°, leading to an error in n which is about ± 0.05

Distortion measurements

Two components of the strain were measured their maxima are : + 4.3 % along [100] and ± 0.9 % ± 0.3 % along [011].

A 4.3 % distortion along [100] corresponds to the ternary compound $In_{0.61} Ga_{0.39}$ As, if we take into account only the tetragonal strain.

It is more difficult to analyse the component parallel to [011]. It is very small and is present over 20 monolayers. It is thus very difficult to detect whether it is homogeneous over these planes or if it decreases as it should. For the 0.9 mL film we obtained opposite values of Δa below and above the expected Indium plane. Thus the model of a Spherical inclusion explains these results, and there is no continuous Indium plane but some clusters. Then the distortion must be the result of superpositions of positive and negative strains.

From roughness, misorientation, and distortion measurements we have deduced that the InAs film does not appear to be exactly InAs but a ternary compound the mean value of the composition being around $In_{0.6} Ga_{0.4}$ As with an accuracy of n = 0.6 ± 0.05 if it is homogeneous in composition. But this value has to be discussed in terms of elastic field. It has been assumed that the stress is tetragonal ; in fact, given the shape of the Indium deposited film, it is submitted to a tridimensional stress. Thus, the corresponding error in In proportion estimation can only by evaluated in knowing the strain field. This calculation is in progress.

DISCUSSION

The dependence of the PL peak energy on the thickness L_w of the quantum well has been recently described (13). The PL peak energy decreases from 1.48 eV to 1.395 eV when L_w varies from 0.9 ml to 3 ml (fig 5a). It should be noted that, after some rapid decrease, the PL peak energy variation is much smaller between 1.7 and 3 ml. Simple calculations (effective mass or tight binding models) are not likely to predict these PL peak energies within a few meV accuracy for such thin wells. They indicate however that such a saturation is fully unexpected.

Curve C1 (see fig 5a) is obtained in an effective mass approach, assuming no intermixing between In and Ga. The conduction band discontinuity ΔEc between GaAs and strained InAs was used as single fitting parameter. When ΔEc varies, calculated transitions always stay below curve C2. Some satisfying fit is thus obtained for the thinnest wells, whereas it is impossible to account for the results obtained when L_w > 2 ml. When some exchange is introduced, curves such as C3 can be obtained ; here 1.2 mL In have been swept over 30 A GaAs. It remains however clearly impossible to account for all experimental data simultaneously.

Our results attest therefore that some spreading of the deposited In actually occurs. This phenomenon may concern more than the last deposited In ml. The number of displaced In ml and the thickness over which In is incorporated in GaAs should moreover increase with increasing Lw.

Figure 5b displays the FWHM obtained for a series of SLS, including sample A and B. Since PL is excitonic for these SLS (13), FWHM gives some insight on the inplane homogeneity of these films. An increase of the FWHM is observed for the last samples when Lw is increased, which should indicate an increase of the interface roughness, or compositional inhomogeneity of the wells.

C. Guille and al. (11) have recently demonstrated In/Ga intermixing by Auger and X-Ray photoemission spectroscopies. They found that no significant intermixing occurs at the InAs/GaAs interface, whereas nearly one monolayer of InAs is driven to the surface during deposition of the first GaAs layer, and gradually dissolves in the next 7 layers of GaAs. The calculated atomic exchange was E = 0.8 ± 0.15.

HRTEM images have shown that the InAs/GaAs interface is atomically flat, and the steps at the interface are due to substrate misorientation. The other interface is very rough, not so well defined, thus confirming the exchange.

According to the Auger experiments during deposition, the last Indium plane would exchange with the Ga plane. This would lead to a complete exchange of the 0.9 mL SLS. That is, the ad-layers would have a maximum of 20 % Indium. In fact, for this multilayer we found distortions corresponding to a 50 % In layer. Thus, as the error in the strain measurement leads to an under estimation of its value, the exchange cannot be 0.8.

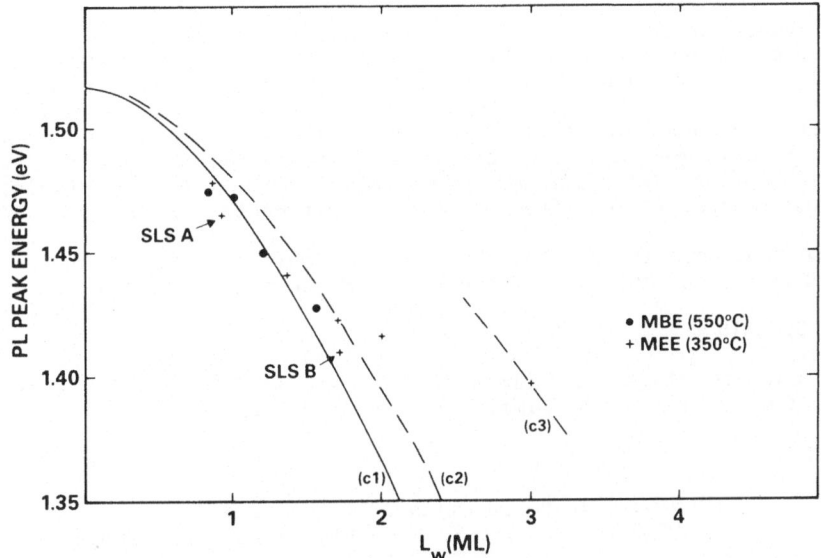

Fig. 5a PL peak energy is plotted as a function the InAs well thickness Lw
for MBE (.) and MEE (+) grown samples. Theoretical calculations
leading to curves C_1, C_2, C_3 are detailed in the text.

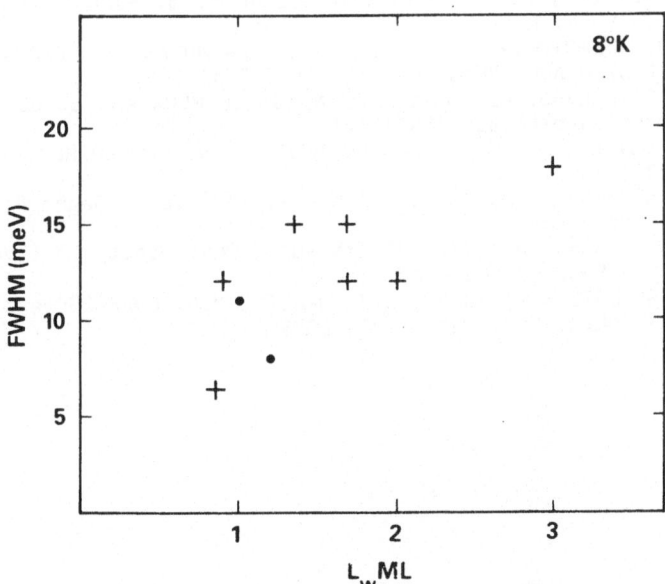

Fig. 5b PL FWMM obtained at 8° K for various InAs/GaAs SLS is plotted as a
function of the well thickness Lw.

CONCLUSION

Our experiment thus confirms the previous result concerning the exchange, but leads to the following model : the deposited Indium exchanges with Gallium during deposition ; during the exchange there are areas which grow rich in Indium : during deposition of the following layer, there is competition between In segregation and In/Ga exchange. Thus instead of having one InAs monolayer, we obtain a distribution of about $In_{0.5} Ga_{0.5}$ As., the GaAs/InAs interface being very rough. This model also explains the Auger experiments. Indeed, from the Auger experiments the measured value for the Indium distribution is the mean value throughout the InAs film. The interface roughness is such that half of the layer is InAs. If there is only 50 % Indium in this half layer, the measured exchange is then 0.75.

ACKNOWLEDGMENTS

The authors thank J. Primot for X-ray analysis, J.C. Pfister for fruitful discussions and M. Timmins for reading the manuscript.

REFERENCES

1 _ N.K WAGNER, Thin Solid Films 38 (1976) 353.

2 - H.A WASHBURN, J.R. SITES, H.H. WIEDER, J. Appl. Phys. 50 (1979) 4872.

3 - T. FUKUI, H. SAITO, Jap. J. of Appl. Phys. 24 (1985) L774.

4 - J.D. GRANGE, E.H.C. PARKER and R. M. KING J. Phys. D12 (1979) 1601.

5 - A.C. GOSSARD, Thin solid Films 57 (1979) 3.

6 - C.A. CHANG, C.M. SERRANO, L.L. CHANG, and L. ESAKI, Appl. Phys. Letters 37 (1980) 538.

7 - R.S. WILLIAMS, B.M. PAINE, W.J. SCHAFFER and S.P. KOWALCZYCK, J. Vacuum Sci. Technol. 21 (1982) 386.

8 - M. QUILLEC, L. GOLDSTEIN, G. LE ROUX, J. BURGEAT and J. PRIMOT, Appl. Phys. Letters 55 (1984) 2904.

9 - F.J. GRUNTHANER, H.Y. YEN, M.A. MADHUKAR, R. FERNANDEZ and J. MASERJIAN Appl PHYS. Letters 46 (1985) 983.

10 - C. D'ANTERROCHES, J.Y. MARZIN, G. LE ROUX and L. GOLDSTEIN J. of Crystal Growth 81 (1987) 121.

11 - C. GUILLE, F. HOUZAY, J.M. MOISON and F. BARTHE surf. Sci. 189 (1987) 1041.

12 - Y. HOROKOSHI, M. KAWASHIMA and M. YAMAGUCHI, Japan J. Appl. Phys. 25 (1986) L868.

13 - J.M. GERARD, and J.Y. MARZIN Appl. Phys. Lett. 53 (1988) 568.

14 - J.M. GERARD unpublished.

15 - L. GOLDSTEIN, F. GLAS, J.Y. MARZIN, M.N. CHARASSE and G. LE ROUX. Appl. Phys. Lett. 47 (1985) 1099.

CONVERGENT BEAM ELECTRON DIFFRACTION STUDIES OF DEFECTS, STRAINS AND

COMPOSITION PROFILES IN SEMICONDUCTORS

D. Cherns

H.H. Wills Physics Laboratory
University of Bristol
Tyndall Avenue
Bristol, BS8 1TL, UK

SUMMARY

This paper shows how convergent beam electron diffraction has been used at Bristol to study strains, defects and composition profiles in plan-view semiconductor multilayers. It is shown that epitaxial strains in bicrystals and multilayers can be measured down to $\sim$ 0.1% and that varying strain fields near dislocations and interfaces can be investigated with high sensitivity. It is also shown that convergent beam diffraction gives a powerful new method of examining superlattice reflections from both periodic and irregular multilayer structures and studies of single quantum well samples of AlGaAs/GaAs and InP/InGaAs, which give well thicknesses to near monolayer precision, are also described.

INTRODUCTION

The materials problems associated with semiconductor multilayers include the characterisation of composition profiles, layer strains and the presence of inhomogeneities and defects. The characterisation of composition and strain profiles may be accomplished by glancing x-ray diffraction, through analysis of the rocking curves obtained as the crystal is rotated about the incident beam. However as relatively large areas are sampled i.e. by glancing beams $\sim$ 1mm across, information is necessarily averaged over any inhomogeneities present.

In this paper the ability to use convergent beam electron diffraction to generate rocking curves is stressed. It will be shown that electron diffraction rocking curves also contain detailed information on composition and strain profiles and that, as in x-ray diffraction, a relatively simple kinematical treatment can often be used to analyse the results. Moreover, since convergent beam patterns can be obtained from very small probes, down to, say, 50A° across, the influence of micro-structure on strain and composition profiles can be examined.

TECHNIQUES

In order to explain how rocking curves are generated and how spatial information can be obtained by convergent beam diffraction it is useful first to discuss the diffraction techniques used in our work. In the conventional convergent beam diffraction method, henceforth referred to as CBED, the incident electron beam is focussed on the specimen. The resulting electron diffraction pattern then consists of a series of diffraction discs. Disc overlap occurs when the convergence half-angle of the incident beam exceeds the Bragg angle, effectively limiting the convergence to avoid confusion in the patterns. Since, in electron diffraction, the diffraction angles are relatively small and the Ewald sphere is approximately flat, the diffraction discs show the rocking curve behaviour approximately along the beam direction. For example, for a film of thickness t where the film normal is along the beam direction, and where multiple diffraction routes may be ignored, the rocking curve seen for reflection g varies as

$$I_g = I_o \frac{\sin^2 \pi t s_{eff}}{(\pi s_{eff})^2} \tag{1}$$

where $s_{eff} = \sqrt{s^2 + \frac{1}{\xi_g^2}}$ (eg see ref(1)), s is the deviation parameter

and s_g is the extinction distance. This gives rise to subsidiary fringes

on each side of the main diffraction contour as illustrated in fig 1(a). In the case of a bicrystal or multilayer, information on the composition profile and on layer strains is present as structure in the reciprocal lattice along the growth direction. Thus it will be seen that convergent beam diffraction can examine multilayer composition and strain in plan-view specimens rather than in cross-section as required, for example, for high resolution studies.

In the large angle convergent beam diffraction technique[2] referred to henceforth as LACBED, the incident probe is brought to a focus either above or below the specimen as shown in fig 1(b) when the objective focus is set at the incident probe focus, such that diffracted beams for different reflections are spatially separated. A selected area aperture can be used to select a single reflection. The diffraction pattern then consists of one diffracted disc with other, possibly overlapping, discs removed. This method has a number of advantages over CBED:

(1)   Since overlapping discs are removed from the convergent beam pattern, the convergence half angle is no longer limited by the Bragg angle and is only limited by microscope optics. For example, for the Bristol Philips 300kV EM430 microscope operating at 200-300kV in "nanoprobe" mode with a condenser 2 lens current ~0.8 Amps a convergence half-angle of about 3° is achieved.

(2)   The selected area aperture limits the acceptance angle for inelastically scattered electrons about the chosen reflection. In our work, the acceptance half-angle through a 5 micron or 2 micron selected area aperture may be reduced to about 5×10^{-4} rad i.e. less than a tenth of a typical Bragg angle. The reduction in inelastic scattering enables weak structure in the rocking curves from multilayer samples, essential for our analysis, to be detected. The selected area aperture thus plays a similar role to the objective aperture in dark field imaging where the reduction in inelastic scattering enhances image contrast and allows weak beam imaging to be carried out[3].

(3)   Since the illuminated area of the specimen is much larger than the incident probe, an image of the specimen is recorded in the convergent beam disc. The area illuminated depends on the extent of defocus but for

a normal defocus of 10-20 microns (fig 1(b)), is about 1-2 microns across. This enables spatial variations in the rocking curves to be examined.
Some of the above points will be illustrated in the next section.

DIFFRACTION FROM STRAINED BICRYSTALS AND MULTILAYERS

Fig 2 shows a CBED pattern from a plan-view sample of $Si/(Si/Si_{0.6}Ge_{0.4})_s$ where the s refers to a periodic superlattice with alternating 30A° layers. The misfit in this sample was predominantly accommodated by elastic strain with occasional misfit dislocations, possibly accommodated between the Si substrate and the superlattice. The diffraction pattern in fig 2 is recorded with the angle between the beam direction and [001] sample normal (i.e. growth direction) about 10°. The sample is relatively thick such that individual discs due to elastic scattering are indistinct owing to substantial inelastic scattering. This, however, enables us to see a series of diffracting lines from various sets of crystal planes, such as $33\bar{1}$ (labelled). Rocking curves, obtained by taking sections perpendicular to each diffraction line, are seen to consist usually of 2 main peaks, the peak separation increasing with the angle between the relevant diffracting planes and [001] (arrowed).

Fig 3 shows LACBED patterns from a $NiSi_2/(001)Si$ sample. The sample consisted of islands of epitaxial $NiSi_2$ about 500-1000A° thick and typically 1-2 microns across on a continuous Si substrate. Most or all of the 0.4% misfit between $NiSi_2$ and Si was accommodated elastically.

Figs 3(a) shows a LACBED pattern taken from a region where the specimen normal was close to the beam direction. The pattern shows an image of a $NiSi_2$ island about 1 micron across. The Bragg angle, at which the central disc and 200 discs in the CBED pattern begin to overlap is also indicated. Fig 3(b) shows part of the bright field disc from a region where the sample has been tilted such that the angle between the [001] sample normal and the electron beam direction was 45°. An image of a $NiSi_2$ island is seen superimposed on a 331 diffraction contour running approximately left to right. The 331 contour is seen to split into 2 peaks on crossing the island. The same behaviour is seen in the 331 dark field LACBED pattern taken at the same foil orientation and shown in fig 3(c). In the dark field disc, the subsidiary fringes around the main peak or peaks are also more clearly visible than in bright field. The patterns in figs 3(a)-(c) appear closely similar to images obtained from buckled (domed) samples, but it is worth pointing out that the samples, in this case, were approximately flat.

The peak splitting in figs 3(b) and (c) can be understood qualitatively using a simple kinematical argument. The misfit stress in $NiSi_2/(001)Si$ leads to an opposite crystal distortion in the $NiSi_2$ and Si layers such that inclined lattice planes which are parallel in the unstrained cubic crystals rotate in opposite senses. The relative angle of rotation is given by

$$\delta\theta = \frac{\eta}{2} \frac{(1 + \nu) \sin 2\theta}{(1 - \nu)} \tag{2}$$

where η is the natural mismatch and θ is the angle of inclination of the planes involved to the sample normal (fig 4). The maximum relative rotation is thus for planes at $\theta = 45°$. Kinematically we thus expect 2 main peaks at angles where the incident beam coincide with the Bragg

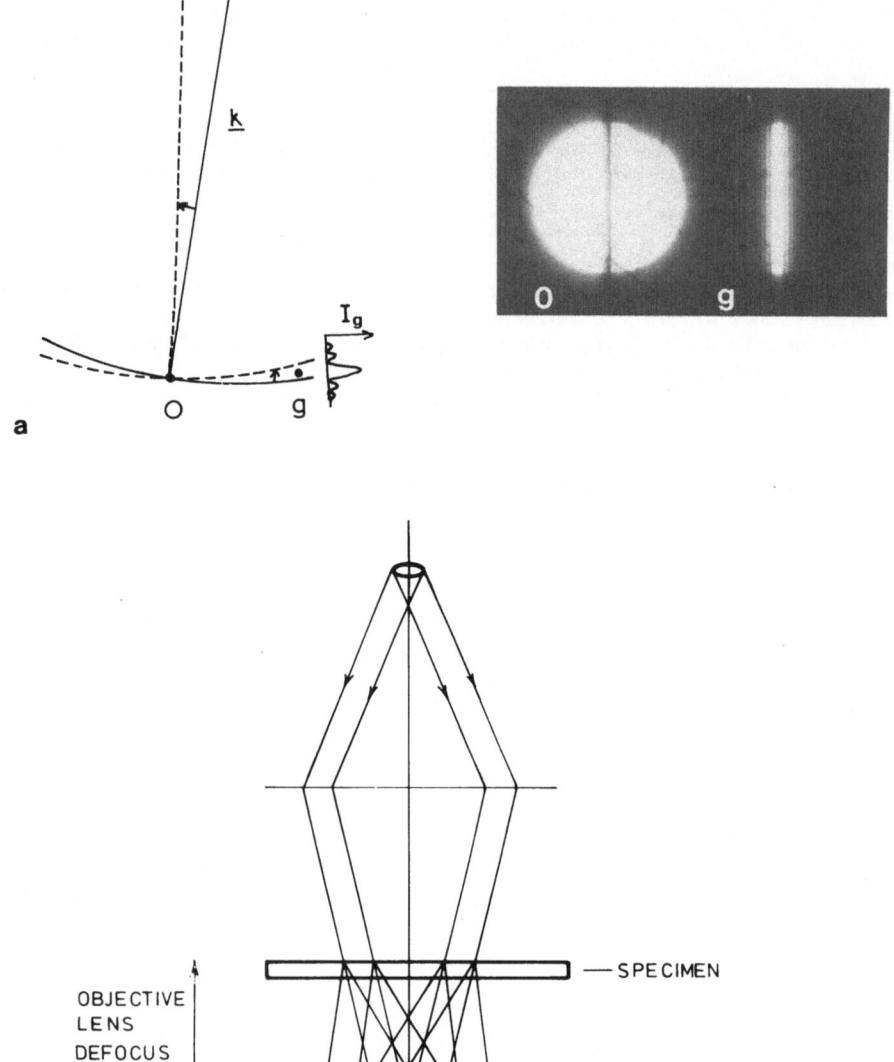

Fig.1 (a) As the direction of the incoming wave $\underline{k}$ varies in a convergent incident beam, the Ewald sphere is swept through a reflection $\underline{g}$. An intensity profile of the type illustrated schematically is seen in the experimental pattern for Si, $g=220$ [courtesy A.R. Preston]. (b) The LACBED technique (see text).

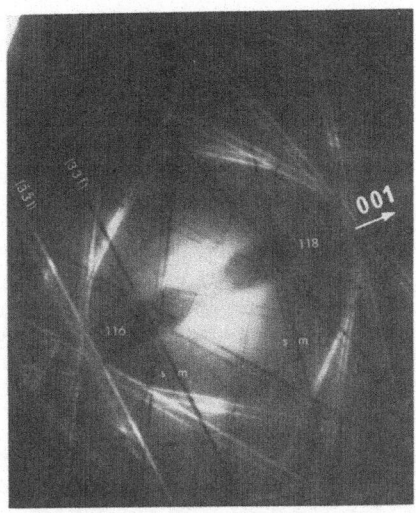

Fig 2. CBED pattern from a Si/(Si$_{0.6}$Ge$_{0.4}$)$_s$ (s=superlattice) sample showing diffraction contours which are split due to misfit strains (Cherns and Legoues: unpublished).

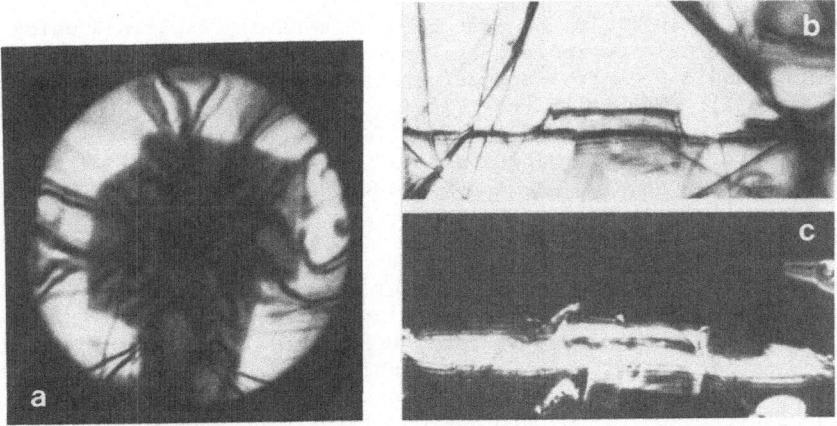

Fig 3. LACBED patterns from NiSi$_2$/(001)Si,(a) bright field disc with [001] approximately along the optic axis,(b) detail of bright field disc with the foil tilted by 45° wrt (a) and showing a 331 contour crossing a NiSi$_2$ island,(c) detail of 331 dark field disc corresponding to (b).

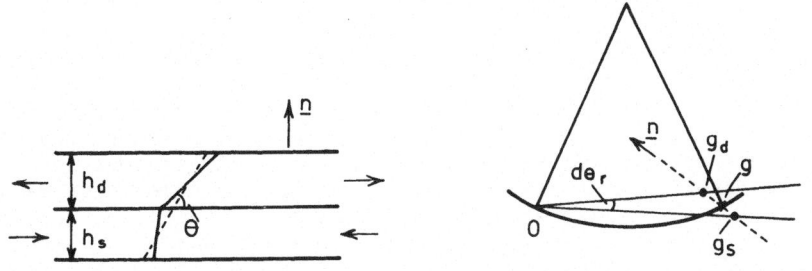

Fig 4. Tetragonal distortion in NiSi$_2$/(001)Si due to misfit strains.

angle for planes in the deposit and substrate. Alternatively, as shown
in fig 4, we may view the Ewald sphere as passing through slightly
separated spots for the $NiSi_2$ and Si. This argument is not correct, even
kinematically, when the diffracted amplitudes for the two spots begin to
overlap. The full kinematic sum is

$$A_{hkl} = \int F_{hkl}(z) e^{-2\pi i(\underline{g}.\underline{R}(z)+sz)} dz \qquad (3)$$

where F(z) is the structure factor for the hkl reflection, z is the depth
in the foil, s is the deviation parameter and R(z) represents any crystal
displacement, for example a rigid shift of diffracting planes at the
$NiSi_2$/(001)Si interface or the varying strain field due to a defect.

Equation (1) would predict a single diffraction peak as the rotation angle
is reduced (see ref [4] fig 8). Moreover, as the diffraction amplitudes
overlap, dynamical interactions need to be considered, clearly so when
the extinction distance for the relevant reflection becomes comparable
to the foil thickness. However, despite these problems the simple
assumption that the observed peak separation is equal to the relative
rotation angle for inclined planes appears reasonable for $NiSi_2$ in figs

3(b), (c). In fact, it appears that this assumption can be used to
determine strains in bicrystals down to ∿ 0.1%[4].

The results in fig 2 can also be qualitatively explained using
equation (3). For a periodic multilayer the maximum in the rocking curve
goes from a split peak to a single peak as the multilayer period is
reduced (fig 5). The split peaks in fig 2 probably arise, therefore, from
the Si substrate (1 peak) and the Si/SiGe multilayer (1 peak). The
angular separations of the main peaks (∿ 0.15° for 331) appear in
reasonable agreement with experiment (see ref [4] for further details).

STRAIN AT INTERFACES AND DEFECTS

The rocking curves from bicrystals should also contain information on
rigid body displacements which are included in the R(z) term in equation
(3). The LACBED method has, in fact, been used in this way to examine
displacements at stacking faults in single crystal material i.e. the
case where $F_{hkl}(z)$ is a constant. The method can be used simply to
give the fault type[5],[6]. Determination of the magnitude of the fault
vector requires a proper dynamical calculation and the method by which
this may be achieved has been outlined recently by Eaglesham et al[7],[8].

The LACBED method can also be used to analyse non uniform strain
fields due to defects such as dislocations. The ability in convergent
beam diffraction to identify relatively high order reflections (large gs)
means that we may expect great sensitivity to small strains since
contrast depends on $\underline{g}.\underline{R}$ (see equation (3)). Cherns and Preston[9],[10] have
examined the behaviour of higher order lane zone (HOLZ) deficiency lines
in bright field LACBED patterns on approaching dislocations, an example
of which is shown in fig 6(a). The kinematical treatment in equation (3)
may indeed be used to simulate the line splittings for these high index
contours and an example of such a calculation is also shown (fig 6(b)).
The number of subsidiary fringes into which the main contour splits can
be used to determine the dislocation Burgers vector. The high value of
$\underline{g}$ means that dislocations with rather small Burgers vectors, for example,
stair rod dislocations can be examined[4]. Fig 6(c) shows the behaviour
of a relatively low index reflection on crossing misfit dislocations in
$NiSi_2$/(111)Si. The behaviour is qualitatively similar although a

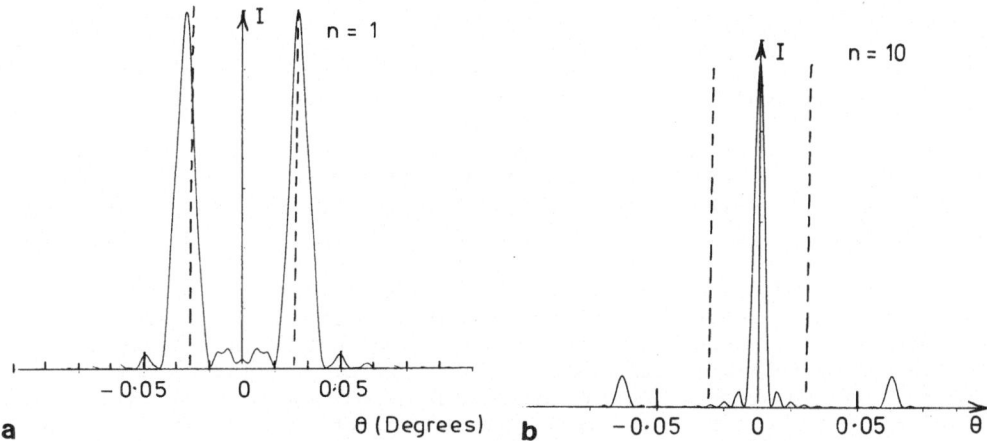

a

θ (Degrees)

b

Fig 5. Kinematical calculation of scattered intensity from (a) a bicrystal and (b) a 10-period multilayer, both of total thickness=5000A°. In both cases there is a relative plane rotation of 0.05° between adjacent layers. Equal layer thicknesses and scattering factors are assumed. [courtesy A.R. Preston].

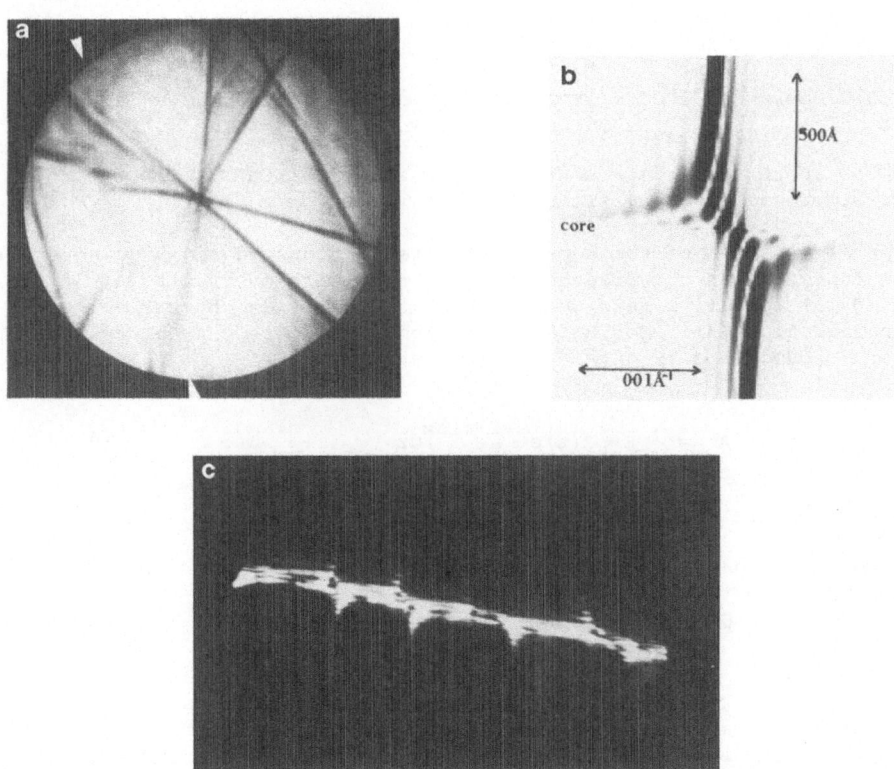

Fig 6. LACBED patterns, (a) a dislocation (arrowed) crossing HOLZ deficiency lines in the bright field disc from a FeNiCr alloy (<114> zone axis), (b) simulated dark field pattern for a dislocation with |$\underline{g}.\underline{b}$| =6, (c) misfit dislocations in $NiSi_2$/(111)Si crossing a low index diffraction contour.

dynamical treatment would be required to achieve a quantitative explanation in this case. Clearly the method could be used to investigate the reduction in strain in a bicrystal or multilayer due to misfit dislocations although this has not, in fact, been done.

Fig 7 shows a bright field LACBED pattern from a cross-section of $NiSi_2$/(001)Si. In producing a thin cross-sectional sample of a crystal containing misfit stresses, surface relaxation leads to non-uniform bending of crystal planes perpendicular to the surface. This, of course, is a major factor in imaging composition fluctuations or spinodal decomposition in III-V semiconductors, as described elsewhere in this volume, and is also a problem in interpreting high resolution images from cross-sectional samples. The high index contours in fig 6(c) detect the effect of this stress relaxation through the splitting of contours as the interface is approached. Again, since high gs are used, the rocking curves are very sensitive to strain and the effects are seen in fig 7 up to about 2000A° from the interface.

DIFFRACTION FROM MULTI-QUANTUM WELLS

Over the past year in Bristol, the LACBED method has been used to examine composition profiles on a range of multi-quantam well (MQW) structures. Studies have been carried out on AlGaAs/GaAs [11,12] InP/InGaAs [12] and Si/SiGe [13]. In all cases TEM samples were prepared by backthinning from the substrate side such that all multilayers were seen in plan-view. For a periodic multilayer, we expect superlattice satellites nq to be grouped around the main reflections such that q is parallel to the growth direction, as shown schematically in fig 8. For a multilayer of period λ, $|q| = \lambda^{-1}$.

Fig 9 shows a 200 dark field LACBED pattern taken from a lattice-matched InP/$In_{0.53}Ga_{0.47}$As multilayer grown by MOCVD. The multilayer period was about 445Å comprising 350Å InP and 95Å InGaAs. The superlattice sidebands nq are visible out to $n \sim 17$.

The intensities of the superlattice reflections in fig 9 do not fall off monotonically as n increases but fluctuate with every 5th satellite (n = 5,10,15) appearing very weak. This may be easily understood by applying equation (3). For a lattice-matched and defect-free crystal equation 3 reduces to

$$A_s = \int F_{hkl}(z) e^{-2\pi i s z} dz \tag{4}$$

The structure factor F_{hkl} for a unit cell in the sphalerite structure is given by

$$F_{hkl} = 4 (f_{cation} \pm f_{anion}) \tag{5}$$

where f is the scattering factor per atom. For reflections hkl with h+k+l = 4m+2 such as 200 (m=0) the cation and anion scattering factors subtract giving a large difference ΔF between the structure factors for InP and $In_{0.53}Ga_{0.47}$As; for g = 200, $\Delta F \cong 9.2$A°. The amplitudes of the superlattice reflections depend on ΔF. Assuming an infinite periodic multilayer (i.e. to avoid thickness oscillations and no composition gradient between layers, equation (4) gives the relative amplitudes A_n of the superlattice reflections as

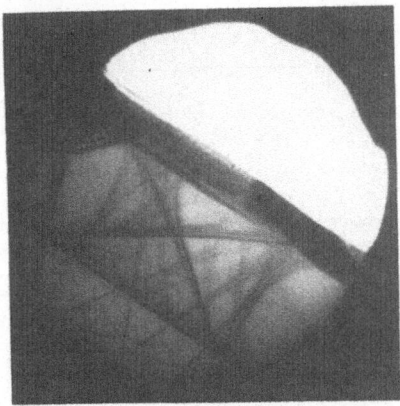

Fig 7. LACBED bright field disc showing $NiSi_2$/(001)Si cross-section. Splitting of diffraction contours near the interface implies bending of planes due to relaxation of misfit stresses.[courtesy of A.R. Preston].

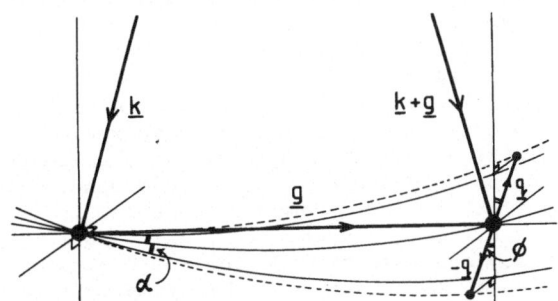

Fig 8. Schematic diagram showing the disposition of superlattice reflections around a reflection g for a plan-view multilayer (after Vincent et al.[11]).

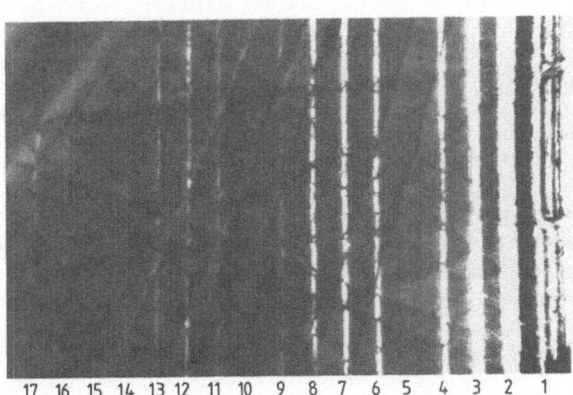

17 16 15 14 13 12 11 10 9 8 7 6 5 4 3 2 1

Fig 9. 200 dark field LACBED pattern from an InP/$In_{0.53}Ga_{0.47}As$ multilayer of period 445Å. Superlattice sidebands $n\underline{q}$ up to n=17 are visible.[courtesy of Miss J. Wang].

$$A_n \; \alpha \; \left(\frac{\sin n \pi \frac{\lambda_1}{\lambda}}{n \pi} \right) \Delta F \qquad \qquad (6)$$

where λ_1 is the thickness of one of the component layers. Since the multilayer in fig 9 has $\lambda_1/\lambda \sim 0.2$ we expect every 5th satellite to be very weak as indeed observed.

$InP/In_{0.53}Ga_{0.47}As$ examined in $g = 200$ represents a favourable case for detecting superlattice reflections. In contrast, reflections such as 220 where the scattering factors f_{cation} and f_{anion} add in equation (5), $\Delta F \sim 0.4 \; \overset{\circ}{A}$ for $InP/In_{0.53}Ga_{0.47}As$ such that superlattice reflections in $g = 220$ are very weakly excited.

Since all the superlattice reflections $n\underline{q}$ in fig 9 are clearly well separated from the intense and possibly dynamical region around $s = 0$, $17\underline{q}$ being equivalent to $s = 4 \times 10^{-2}\overset{\circ}{A}^{-1}$, we might expect the kinematical formula (equation (3)) to be reasonably good for calculating superlattice reflection intensities. Some care, however, needs to be taken as multiple diffraction leads also to dynamical sidebands whether or not the sample is a multilayer. This effect is seen more easily in fig 10 which shows examples of 200 dark field patterns from an AlGaAs/GaAs multilayer of $200\overset{\circ}{A}$ period. Since the structure factor difference $\Delta F \sim 1.4\overset{\circ}{A}$ is much less than that for the InP/InGaAs specimen illustrated in fig 9, the dynamical sidebands due to multiple scattering involving systematic row reflections, 400, 600, $\overline{2}00$ etc are relatively more prominent. The first dynamical sideband occur at $s=\pm g^2/k$ and are comparable to the intensity in the first superlattice reflection $\underline{q}$. However, since the positions of the dynamical sidebands only depend on the Ewald sphere radius, distinguishing superlattice and dynamical sidebands is relatively easy. Thus, as the foil is tilted about the [200] axis, as illustrated in fig 10 the superlattice sidebands move towards the $s = 0$ band as the projection of $\underline{q}$ along z is reduced. Alternatively the dynamical sidebands may be shifted by varying the voltage which changes the Ewald sphere radius. The situation where the dynamical and superlattice sidebands coincide, and where dynamical effects on the superlattice sidebands are therefore at a maximum, is of interest and some experiments have been carried out in Bristol to investigate this case (Qin and Steeds, private communication).

The LACBED patterns in figs 9 and 10 should show any spatial variations in sideband intensities since different parts of the patterns arise from spatially separated regions as explained earlier. One problem is that for any particular satellite, the variation is one-dimensional, i.e. along the line of the sideband, and different sidebands come from different regions of the sample. However, having characterised the diffracted intensity for a given reflection by LACBED, it has proved possible to identify low order superlattice reflections directly in dark field imaging. An example of a 200 dark field image from the AlGaAs/GaAs multilayer illustrated in fig 10 and with q strongly excited is shown in fig 11. In this superlattice image an interesting structure is seen which is not apparent in either the 400, s=0 image or the dynamical sideband image (see ref (11)). The structure is seen to have a scale which is elongated along one of the surface <110> directions.

Direct superlattice images showing similar structure to that in fig 11 have now been obtained from samples grown both by molecular beam epitaxy as in fig 11 and by organo-metallic chemical vapour deposition[12] Hence it is tempting to associate this structure with the fact that

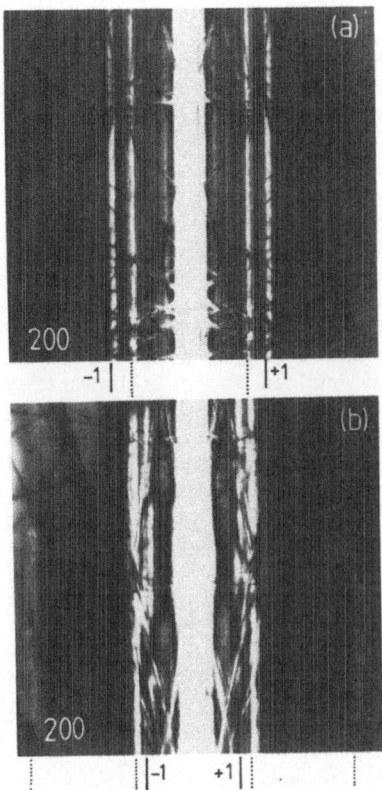

Fig 10. 200 dark field LACBED patterns from an $Al_{0.3}Ga_{0.7}As/GaAs$ multilayer of period 210A°. In (a) the sample was approximately flat, whereas in (b) the sample was tilted by about 45° towards [011] such that the projection of $\underline{q}$ along z is reduced (courtesy of Dr. R. Vincent).

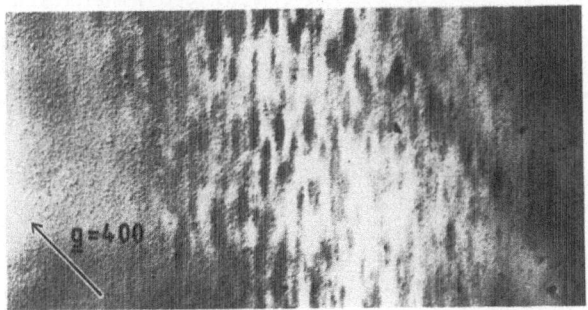

Fig 11. The AlGaAs/GaAs multilayer illustrated in fig 10 now imaged in the first superlattice sideband reflection about the 400 reflection i.e. $\underline{g}_{400}+\underline{q}$ (courtesy of Dr. R. Vincent).

step densities on the (100) surface during growth are probably different in the 2 <110> directions. However it is not yet clear whether the contrast arises from changes in the average value of q, changing the value of s at which q is excited, or fluctuations in q through the foil which would reduce the peak intensity. Variations in total film thickness and possible local strains may be ruled out on the grounds that the contrast only appears in superlattice reflections. By observing image changes which occur as the sample is progressively tilted it appears that the average value of q varies (e.g. see Vincent et al[12], fig 4). Images such as that in fig 11 should in fact be very sensitive to changes in q with variations down to $\sim$ 1% or about 2A° expected to produce visible changes in contrast.

The fact that many orders of superlattice sideband have been observed in LACBED patterns from AlGaAs/GaAs and InP/InGaAs multilayers suggests that the method should give useful information on composition profiles in cases where either the multilayer is not periodic or where composition gradients exist. Recent studies suggest that irregular structures may indeed be analysed. Fig 12 shows an example of an AlGaAs/GaAs sample composed of a s-period multilayer surrounded by cladding layers (of AlGaAs). The sample was prepared initially by backthinning the GaAs substrate with a selective etch to AlGaAs. In the region illuminated in the LACBED pattern in fig 12, a Gatan precision ion miller (PIMS) was used to etch a hole through the backthinned sample. Away from the hole the LACBED pattern shows a structure in reasonable agreement with that computed kinematically (see simulation). The superlattice sidebands show 3q to be weak in agreement with equation (6), the splitting of individual sidebands being attritutable to the presence of the cladding layers. The fact that there are five regular periods of superlattice leads to three subsidiary maxima between neighbouring reflections nq, the number of subsidiary fringes being given by x-2 where x is the number of periods. As the hole in the sample is approached, the progressive removal of these subsidiary fringes occurs as layers are removed. Eventually a single crystal AlGaAs sample remains with side-bands falling off monotonically as given by equation (1).

DIFFRACTION FROM SINGLE QUANTUM WELLS

The LACBED method has recently been applied to studies of 3-layer single quantum well (SQW) structures in AlGaAs/GaAs[14] and InP/In$_{0.53}$Ga$_{0.47}$As[15]. Rocking curves calculated kinematically

(equation (3)) for a SQW structure are illustrated in fig 13. These show oscillations similar to those for a single crystal as in equation (1), and spaced at $\Delta s = t^{-1}$ where t is the sample thickness. However the oscillations are modulated in amplitude at a frequency which depends on the depth of the quantum well in the sample. In fact modulation frequencies $\Delta s = t_1^{-1}$ are present where t_1 is the thickness of any of the layers. The most obvious period in fig 13 is given by $\Delta s = t_1^{-1}$ where t_1 is the thickness of the thinner cladding layer ($t_1 = 1.5$ microns). Less obvious periods are given by $\Delta s = t_3^{-1}$ and $\Delta s = t_2^{-1}$ the latter being only visible at much larger values of s not shown here.

The behaviour illustrated in fig 13 has already been verified experimentally for an Al$_{0.4}$Ga$_{0.6}$As/GaAs sample[14]. The same behaviour

has been observed in InP/In$_{0.53}$Ga$_{0.47}$As and a recent example is shown in fig 14. Despite the fact that the In$_{0.53}$Ga$_{0.47}$As layer is only 30A°

thick in 2000A° InP the fringe modulation is quite dramatic, being much larger than that for AlGaAs/GaAs owing to the greater difference in structure factors between the layers (see earlier).

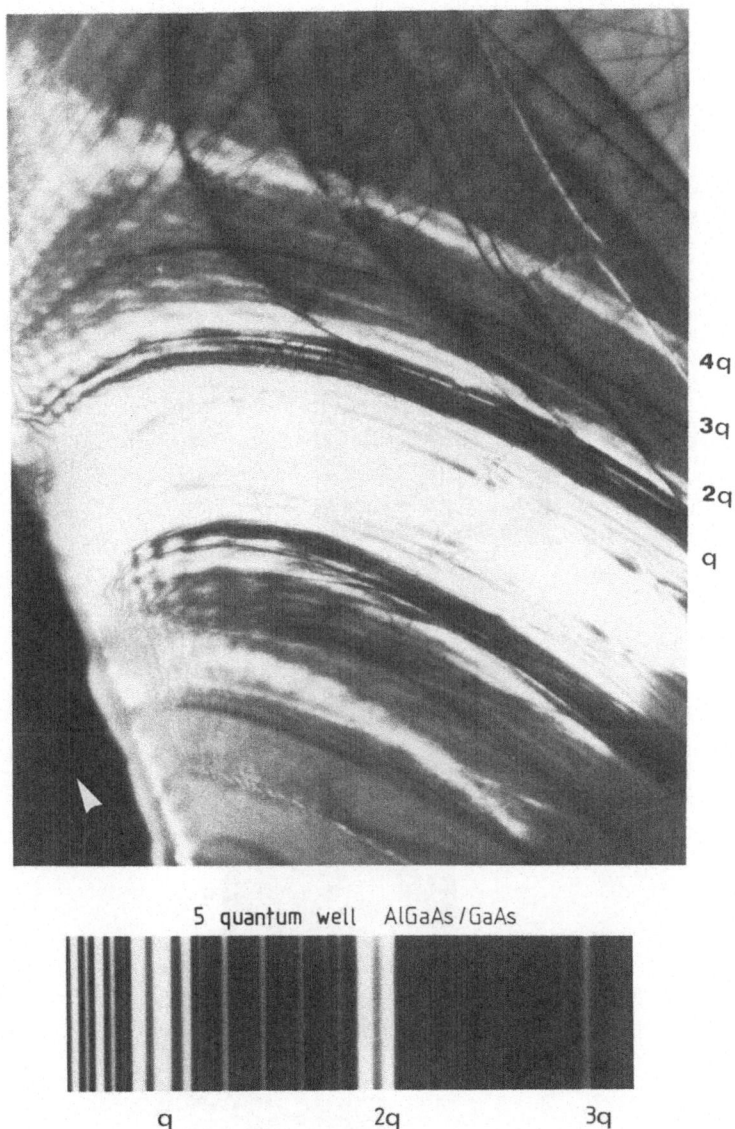

Fig 12. 200 dark field LACBED pattern from a 5-quantum well sample containing 5 GaAs layers of width 55A° separated by 175A° $Al_{0.35}Ga_{0.65}As$, the whole enclosed by 1500A° cladding layers of $Al_{0.35}Ga_{0.65}As$. The pattern shows an area (arrowed) which has been locally thinned to perforation in a Gatan precision ion miller. A kinematical simulation of the expected rocking curve is also shown.

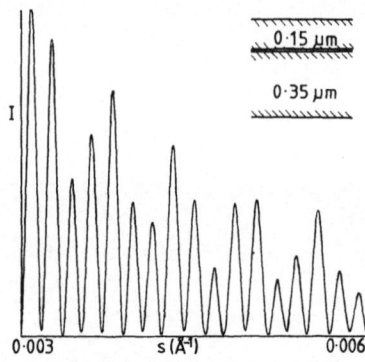

Fig 13. Simulated rocking curve for a 30A° layer of GaAs in 5000A° $Al_{0.3}Ga_{0.7}As$ as illustrated (courtesy of Dr R. Vincent).

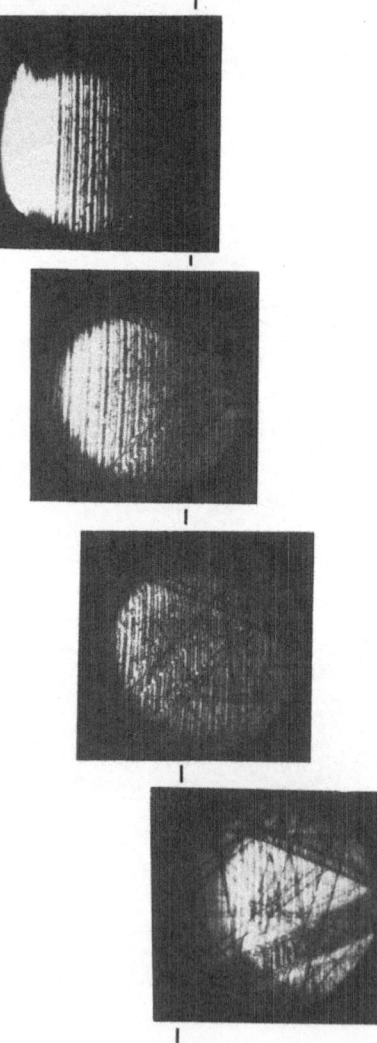

Fig 14. 200 dark field LACBED patterns from a nominal 1000A°InP/40A° $In_{0.53}Ga_{0.47}As$/800A°InP sample showing the behavior out to large s. The dashed line indicates where the fringe modulation passes through a minimum at $s=0.027A°^{-1}$, equivalent to a 37A° InGaAs layer (courtesy of I. Jordan).

The sensitivity of LACBED patterns like those in fig 14 to changes in quantum well thickness is currently being investigated both experimentally and theoretically. Kinematical calculations show that the most direct method of determining t_2 is to examine modulations of the pattern at the frequency $\Delta s = t_2^{-1}$. At values of $s = t_2^{-1}$, $2t_2^{-1}$, $3t_2^{-1}$ etc we expect the modulation to be absent ie zero amplitude. This can be seen in the experimental pattern at the arrowed position corresponding to $s = t_2^{-1}$, the modulation becoming apparent on moving to either smaller or larger s. The point at which the modulation disappears can be located to perhaps 10% accuracy in s, implying that we can measure this nominal 30Å or near-monolayer accuracy.

This method for determining quantum well thicknesses has been applied successfully to 2000A° thick $InP/In_{0.53}Ga_{0.47}As$ samples with InGaAs layers down to ~ 15A° thickness. As this requires rocking curve detail out to very large values of s, i.e. $s \geq 0.07Å^{-1}$ for a 15Å well, certain experimental precautions were required to record pattern detail.

(1)   In order to reduce inelastic background a small (2 micron) selected area aperture was used to reduce the acceptance angle to

$\leq 5 \times 10^{-4}$ rad (see section (2)).

(2)   Samples $\leq$ 2000Å total thickness were also used. The option of cooling samples to reduce inelastic background has been investigated but the need for very long exposure photographs (see below) and the need for good sample stability meant that cooling experiments have been unsuccessful to date.

(3)   In order to achieve realistic film exposures, $\leq$ 15mins maximum, it was necessary to use a large probe 500-1000Å to achieve sufficient pattern intensity at large s. Microscope operation under these conditions was with a tungsten hairpin filament. Since the spatial information in LACBED depends on the focussed probe size, information on film structure variations has been lost.

An alternative method of determining quantum well thickness which is less stringent on imaging requirements appears to be by fitting the amplitude of the modulation observed at smaller values of s ($s \ll t_2^{-1}$).

This is also found to be quite sensitive to variations in t_2 under some conditions and recent calculations suggest that monolayer variations in well thickness should also be visible by this route.

DISCUSSION

It has thus been shown how both uniform and non-uniform strains in bicrystals and composition profiles in a variety of multilayer samples can be examined by convergent beam electron diffraction and particularly by the large angle (LACBED) technique. An important point is that samples can be examined in plan-view rather than in the cross-sectional geometry. This has a number of advantages.

(1)   In samples with misfit strains, the plan-view geometry avoids surface relaxation which leads to non-uniform plane bending in cross-sectional samples.

(2) Plan-view samples enable information to be gained in 2 dimensions rather than in one dimension for cross-sections. Thus images such as that in fig 11 promise information on growth phenomena which would be hard to extract from studies of cross-sections.

(3) The plan-view geometry is appropriate to studies of luminescence (cathodoluminescence, see Steeds this volume) or electrical properties (EBIC, see Sieber this volume). The ability to characterise the composition profile in the same studies raises the interesting possibility of correlating structural and electronic properties.

In comparison with x-ray rocking studies the LACBED technique gives potentially more information on higher order satellites from MQW structures if spatial averaging which should act to attenuate the higher order satellites can be avoided. It is, of course, the higher order satellites which are most sensitive to the composition profile. A problem here, as noted in the previous section, is that the focussed probe size, over which averaging must occur, must be increased to achieve the weaker high order intensity features. Thus beam intensity imposes a limitation on the resolution of the LACBED method for composition profile determination.

ACKNOWLEDGEMENTS

This paper describes work carried out by various members of the Microstructural Group of the Bristol Physics Department in the last few years. The author wishes to thank Dr. R. Vincent, Dr. C.J. Kiely, Miss J. Wang, A.R. Preston and I.K. Jordan for provision of figures.

REFERENCES

1. P.B. Hirsch, A. Howie, R.B. Nicholson, D.W. Pashley and M.J. Whelan, "Electron Microscopy of Thin Crystals", Krieger, New York (1977).
2. M. Tanaka, R. Saito, K. Ueno and Y. Harada, J. Electron Microsc. 29 (1980) 408.
3. D.J.H. Cockayne, I.L.F. Ray and M.J. Whelan, Phil. Mag. 20 (1969) 1265.
4. D. Cherns, C.J. Kiely and A.R. Preston, Ultramicroscopy 24 (1988) 355.
5. D. Cherns and A.R. Preston, J. Electron Microscope Technique: in press.
6. M. Tanaka and T. Kaneyama, Proc. 11th Int. Cong. in Electron Microscopy, Kyoto 1986 ed. T. Imura et al. Vol. 1, p 203.
7. D.J. Eaglesham, C.J. Kiely, D. Cherns and M. Missous, Phil. Mag.: submitted.
8. D. Cherns, D.J. Eaglesham and C.J. Kiely, Proc. 11th Int. Congress on Electron Microscopy, Kyoto 1986, ed. T. Imura et al. Vol. 1 p 207.
9. D. Cherns and A.R. Preston, Proc. 11th Int. Congress on Electron Microscopy, Kyoto 1986, ed. T. Imura et al Vol. 1, p 721.
10. A.R. Preston and D. Cherns, Inst. Phys. Conf. Ser. No. 78 (1986) 41.
11. R. Vincent, D. Cherns, S.J. Bailey and H. Morkoc, Phil. Mag. Letters 56 (1987) 1.
12. R. Vincent, J. Wang, D. Cherns, S.J. Bailey, A.R. Preston and J.W. Steeds, Inst. Phys. Conf. Ser. No. 90 (1987) 233.
13. D. Cherns and F. Legoues: unpublished.
14. D. Cherns, I.K. Jordan and R. Vincent, Phil. Mag. Letters 58 (1988) 45.
15. I.K. Jordan: unpublished.

HOLZ DIFFRACTION FROM SEMICONDUCTOR SUPERLATTICES

H. Gong, C.D. de Haan and F.W. Schapink

Delft University of Technology, Laboratory of Metallurgy
Rotterdamseweg 137, 2628 AL Delft, The Netherlands

ABSTRACT

Superlattice higher-order Laue zone (HOLZ) rings of diffraction are observed to occur in CBED patterns taken in plan view from GaAs/AlAs superlattices. The fine structure of these superlattice reflections is characteristically different from the corresponding structure of fundamental reflections originating from the average lattice. These diffraction effects, induced by composition modulation, are discussed and compared with strain modulation effects occurring in CBED patterns from other systems such as GaAs/InGaAs or Si/GeSi.

1. INTRODUCTION

In recent years semiconductor superlattices have become very important devices in semiconductor science and technology, and consequently much attention is being devoted to the elucidation of such structures. In semiconductor materials research employing TEM and electron diffraction, extensive use has been made both of cross-sectional specimens and plan-view thin specimens. In TEM and electron diffraction studies the former type of specimens were thought to give more detailed results and have frequently been preferred, although their preparation is much more difficult. In the field of electron diffraction several studies employing convergent-beam electron diffraction (CBED) have been performed in recent years on both types of specimens. Detection of local strains has been attempted in cross-sections of strained-layer superlattices; the interpretation of such experiments is however complicated by elastic surface relaxation effects introduced in the samples [1]. More recently, CBED patterns were investigated using plan-view specimens. Here, in principle, two effects contribute to diffraction from higher-order Laue zones (HOLZ). Firstly, the composition modulation along the superlattice axis is expected to introduce extra HOLZ rings (referred to as superlattice HOLZ). Secondly, the matching of the lattices at the interfaces causes a (periodic) strain modulation, and this modulation gives rise to certain diffraction effects in CBED (e.g. shifts in HOLZ lines [2]). We will discuss the HOLZ effects in this paper, with emphasis on the compositional modulation in GaAs/AlAs-type superlattices, since strain effects are expected to be small in this system.

2. SINGLE AlGaAs LAYERS

Let us first consider briefly the description of electron diffraction from a [001] oriented GaAs (or a related III-V compound) thin specimen, because this orientation will be employed throughout the paper. Since high-energy electrons propagate in crystals as Bloch waves [3] the question is which states describe the electron behaviour. It has been shown that for GaAs the

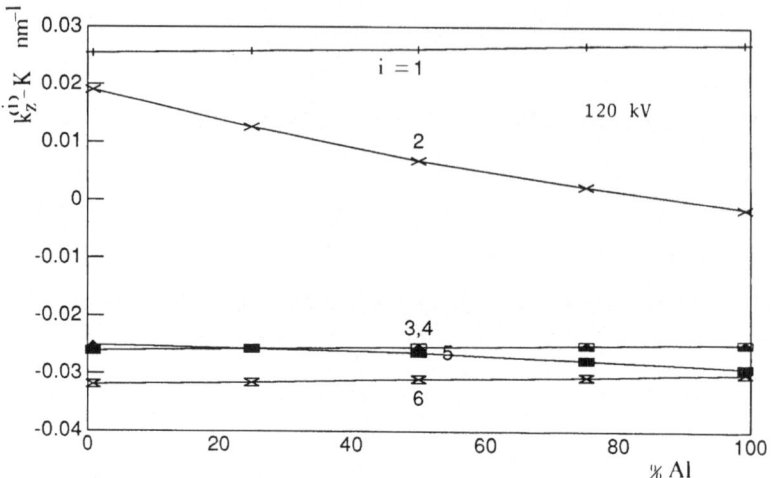

Fig. 1. Variations of the wave vector component Δk_z for different Bloch states in [001] $Al_xGa_{1-x}As$ diffraction, with Al content.

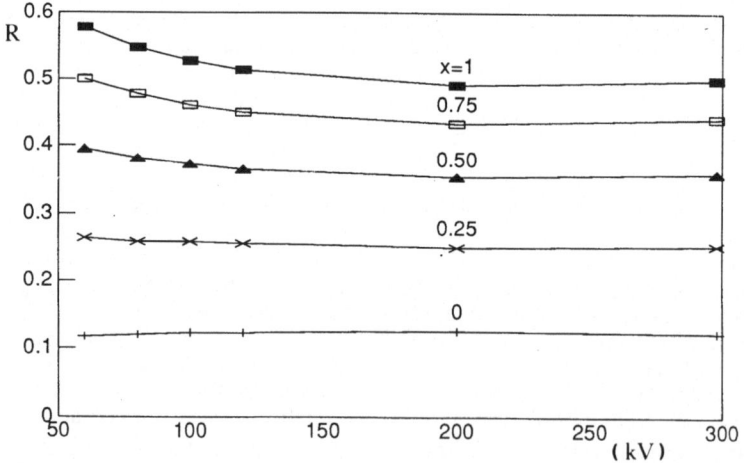

Fig. 2. Variation of the parameter $R = \left(k_z^{(1)} - k_z^{(2)}\right) / \left(k_z^{(1)} - k_z^{(5)}\right)$ with accelerating voltage (kV) in $Al_xGa_{1-x}As$, for different x.

most important Bloch states can be classified according to atomic state symmetries associated with different strings; for [001] diffraction there are three important states labelled as 1s (As), 1s (Ga) and a hybridized 2s (Ga + As). These Bloch states will be indicated as (1), (2) and (5), respectively. Now the different states are localized on different strings along [001] and each Bloch state has a different potential energy in the well associated with a particular string. Since the total energy is a constant for elastic scattering, different potential energies of Bloch states imply different kinetic energies and, consequently, different values for $k_z^{(i)}$, where $k_z^{(i)}$ is the wave-vector component of state (i) along [001]. These different states $k_z^{(i)}$ appear as separate lines in HOLZ diffraction discs and are directly related to the strength of the projected crystal potential. For [001] GaAs it has been shown [4] that only two lines appear in first-order Laue zone (FOLZ) discs, corresponding to the 1s (Ga) and 1s (As) states (which are too close together to be observed separately) and a hybridized 2s (Ga + As) state, respectively.

When Al is dissolved in GaAs, part of the Ga sites will be occupied by Al atoms. It has been found that the above states associated with atomic strings in AlGaAs are modified as follows [4,5]. Bloch state (2), which should now be indicated as a 1s (Ga/Al) state, has a lower value for k_z and the lowering is a function of the Al content. Fig. 1 depicts the change in wave-vector component $k_z^{(i)}$ for states (1), (2) and (5) as a function of Al content. In fig. 1 the various branches of the zero-layer dispersion surface shown were computed by dynamical calculations involving 69 beams from the zero-order Laue zone. For AlGaAs only branches (1), (2) and (5) are excited to a considerable extent in FOLZ discs, as was first pointed out by Eaglesham and Humphreys [4]. It is seen that the location of state (2), relative to (1) or (5), can be employed as a measure of the Al content in an AlGaAs specimen. We have also investigated the effect of accelerating voltage of the incident beam on the location of these branches in AlGaAs. Fig. 2 shows the parameter $(k_z^{(1)} - k_z^{(2)}) / (k_z^{(1)} - k_z^{5})$ computed as a function of accelerating voltage (V) for different Al concentrations in AlGaAs. It is seen that for small Al content (up till about 25 %) there is little dependence on V, whereas for large Al content this parameter increases with decreasing voltage. This computed behaviour is compared with experimental values in the next section, where it will be shown that experimental values show a downward tendency with decrease in V (cf. table I).

3. GaAs/AlAs MULTILAYERS [6,7]

In this section some results obtained on CBED patterns taken in plan view from multilayer specimens of the AlAs/GaAs type will be described and discussed. In particular attention will be focussed on the superlattice effects in HOLZ diffraction. Since these effects depend on the superlattice spacing, results for two specimens with 6.7 nm and 12.1 nm superlattice period, respectively, will be analyzed. Also, effects of a change in accelerating voltage will be reported.

Before discussing the CBED patterns in more detail, let us briefly consider the diffraction effects to be expected from a 1-D superlattice, consisting of AlAs and GaAs layers, with the incident electron beam oriented parallel to the [001] superlattice axis. In this case two types of HOLZ reflections are expected to occur. First of all, the very small difference in lattice constant for GaAs (a=0.56532 nm) and AlAs (a=0.5660 nm) gives rise effectively to a single average lattice for the multilayer, if the strains caused by the small difference in lattice parameter are neglected. This average lattice generates rings of HOLZ reflections in CBED zone-axis patterns. Secondly, the periodic modulation in Al/Ga concentration along the superlattice [001] axis introduces a periodic modulation in the structure factor along [001], and this leads to the formation of extra Laue zone reflections (cf. fig. 3), which may conveniently be referred to as superlattice HOLZ rings of reflections (abbreviated as sHOLZ).

3.1 The 6.7 nm AlAs/GaAs Multilayer Specimen

As has been remarked already, the modulation in Al/Ga concentration along the [001] superlattice axis causes superlattice HOLZ (sHOLZ) rings of reflections to occur. Their approximate location is given by the intersection of Ewald's sphere with the higher-order zones derived from the superlattice period, as indicated in fig. 3. Apart from these reflections, we have the HOLZ reflections associated with the average lattice of the multilayer specimen, i.e. derived from an AlGaAs single layer with the same chemical composition as the superlattice. The 6.7 nm multilayer specimen consists of layers of 1.7 nm GaAs and 5.0 nm AlAs; thus the overall composition is given approx. by $Al_{.75}Ga_{.25}As$. Fig. 4 shows a [001] zone-axis pattern, where two rings of sHOLZ reflections and the FOLZ ring associated with the average lattice may be clearly observed. The location of these rings is in agreement with the equation [8]:

$$R = (2KH)^{1/2} \tag{1}$$

where R is the projected distance of the HOLZ ring from the origin (see fig. 3), K is the electron wave vector and H is a multiple (m) of the reciprocal of the superlattice period, i.e. $H = mq$, where $q = (6.7)^{-1}nm^{-1}$. For the sHOLZ rings in fig. 4 we have m = 1 or 2. Apart from these rings (which may be considered to be associated with the fundamental reflections of the ZOLZ) we have sFOLZ reflections associated with fundamental FOLZ reflections from the average lattice, i.e. at locations given by

$$H_{sF} = a^* + mq = nq \tag{2}$$

where a^* is the reciprocal of the average lattice parameter a and it is assumed that the superlattice is commensurate with the average lattice, that is: $a^* = a^{-1} = kq$ (k and n are integers). In fig. 4 we may observe faint superlattice rings associated with the FOLZ, for which $m = \pm 1$.

The location of FOLZ and sHOLZ reflections can directly be deduced from the Bravais lattice of the average structure, which is F-centred, the same as for GaAs. As a consequence fundamental HOLZ reflections projected onto the zero layer should either coincide with zero-order reflections, or be located on centred positions of the zero layer. This has been verified, and e.g. fundamental FOLZ reflections in fig. 4 are in centred positions. On the other hand, reflections of the sHOLZ type project onto zero-layer reflections, for the first and second rings in fig. 4.

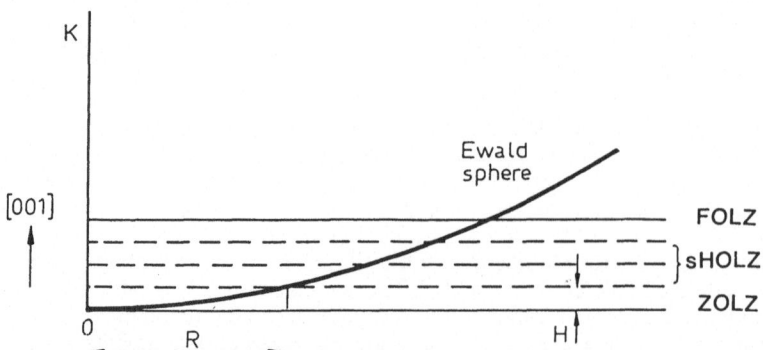

Fig. 3. Schematic diagram of a reciprocal lattice cross-section containing the incident wave vector K. The higher-order Laue zones (HOLZ) include superlattice zones (sHOLZ); for clarity only a few sHOLZ are shown.

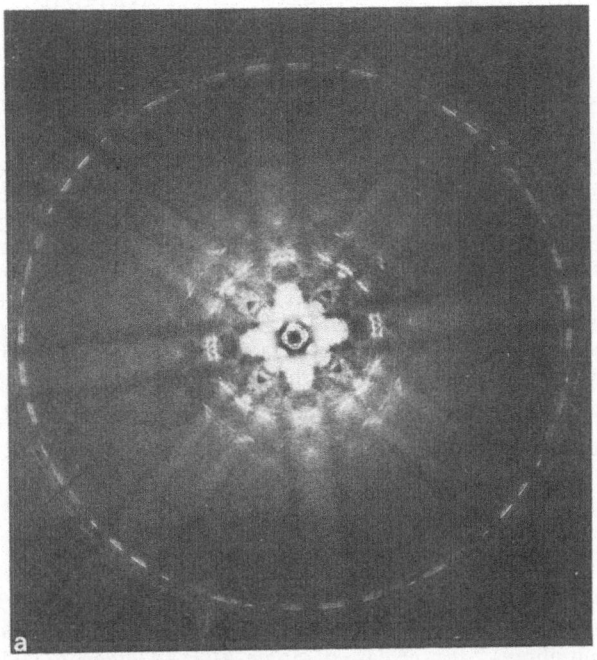

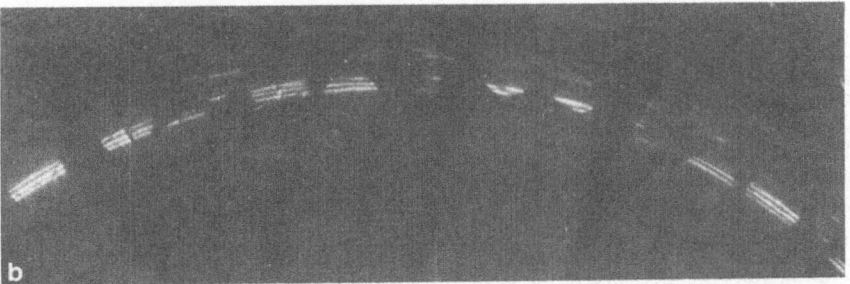

Fig. 4a. CBED [001] zone-axis pattern from a 6.7 nm superlattice GaAs/AlAs specimen, taken at 120 kV. Details of the FOLZ (near the periphery of the pattern) are shown enlarged in b.

Table I. Comparison between calculated and experimental values of Δk_z for the 6.7 nm specimen containing 75% Al

Accelerating voltage (kV)	$k_z^{(1)}-k_z^{(5)}$ (nm^{-1})		$(k_z^{(1)}-k_z^{(2)})/(k_z^{(1)}-k_z^{(5)})$	
	experiment	calculation	experiment	calculation
60	$(6.9\pm0.1)\times10^{-2}$	9.6×10^{-2}	0.38 ± 0.03	0.50
80	$(6.3\pm0.1)\times10^{-2}$	7.4×10^{-2}	0.41 ± 0.03	0.48
100	$(5.5\pm0.2)\times10^{-2}$	6.2×10^{-2}	0.44 ± 0.04	0.46
120	$(5.5\pm0.2)\times10^{-2}$	5.4×10^{-2}	0.45 ± 0.04	0.45

It may be observed from fig. 4 that there is a characteristic difference between the fine structure of fundamental FOLZ reflections and superlattice reflections. Whereas the former consist of 3 closely spaced bright lines, the latter contain only 2 bright lines having a considerable larger separation. In order to understand these differences in fine structure we first consider the fundamental FOLZ reflections. Since these originate from the average structure, it is expected that the fine structure is the same as for a single AlGaAs layer having identical chemical composition, i.e. 75 % Al in the case of the 6.7 nm superlattice specimen. This explains the occurrence of three lines, representing the intersection of the free-electron sphere, associated with a particular FOLZ reflection, with Bloch states (1), (2) and (5) of the zero-layer dispersion surface in AlGaAs (cf. fig. 1). The separation Δs of two lines in a HOLZ reflection H is simply related to Δk_z from fig. 1 via the relation

$$\Delta s = \left(\frac{K}{2H}\right)^{1/2} \Delta k_z \tag{3}$$

which is easily derived from eqn. (1). The separation Δs between states (1) (or (5)) and (2) is a function of the overall Al-composition in the superlattice; this was first pointed out by Eaglesham and Humphreys [4] for the case of single AlGaAs layers. In table I a comparison between computed and experimental values of Δk_z for branches (1), (2) and (5) is presented for the 6.7 nm superlattice. The computed values of Δk_z have been obtained from dynamical

computations of the zero-layer dispersion surface (cf. fig. 1) of a single AlGaAs layer, assuming the Al-content to be equal to the overall Al composition of the multilayer. On the other hand, experimental values of Δk_z were derived from the separation Δs of the branches in relevant FOLZ discs and employing eqn. (3) for converting Δs values into Δk_z values. Comparison of computed and experimental Δk_z for different accelerating voltages shows good agreement at 120 kV, whereas differences increase with decreasing voltage. The origin of the latter effect is not known at present, and should be further investigated.

Let us next discuss briefly the fine structure of sHOLZ reflections, consisting of two lines at much larger separation compared with the FOLZ reflections (cf. fig. 4). First consider the existence of two lines in superlattice reflections. This phenomenon can be explained from the amplitude of the sHOLZ reflections as determined by the appropriate Fourier components of a set of modified potentials [9]. Each modified potential consists of the product of a conditional projected potential $U^{(n)}(\underline{R})$ (where $\underline{R}$ is a position vector in the projected unit cell) and the amplitude distribution $\tau^{(j)}$ of Bloch state j. Now, for the fundamental FOLZ reflections the (1s) Bloch state in AlGaAs is localized both on (Al/Ga) and As strings in the unit cell, and the modified potential will be similar to $U^{(n)}$. Together with the hybridized 2s Bloch state this gives rise to 3 lines in FOLZ reflections. However, different conditions exist for sHOLZ reflections. In this case the Fourier components of $U^{(n)}$ are determined only by the compositional modulation on (Al/Ga) strings along [001], and thus represent a potential for which the As string is effectively absent. Multiplication of this

Table II. Comparison between calculated and experimental values of Δk_z for the 12.1 nm specimen containing 25% Al

Accelerating voltage (kV)	$k_z^{(1)}-k_z^{(5)}$ (nm^{-1})		$(k_z^{(1)}-k_z^{(2)})/(k_z^{(1)}-k_z^{(5)})$	
	experiment	calculation	experiment	calculation
90	$(5.8\pm0.3)\times10^{-2}$	6.6×10^{-2}	0.21 ± 0.04	0.26
100	$(4.9\pm0.3)\times10^{-2}$	5.9×10^{-2}	0.21 ± 0.05	0.26
110	$(4.7\pm0.2)\times10^{-2}$	5.5×10^{-2}	0.21 ± 0.03	0.26
120	$(5.7\pm0.3)\times10^{-2}$	5.1×10^{-2}	0.22 ± 0.03	0.25
300	$(4.2\pm0.2)\times10^{-2}$	2.9×10^{-2}	0.26 ± 0.03	0.25

potential by $\tau^{(j)}(\underline{R})$, the Bloch wave amplitude at the As string, yields a modified potential that produces zero diffracted amplitude. Consequently branch (1) will be absent in sHOLZ reflections, and only two lines will be observed. Their separation Δs will be considerably larger according to eqn. (3), because H in the factor $(K/2H)^{1/2}$ is much smaller for sHOLZ reflections. For the 6.7 nm superlattice this factor, comparing the line separation for the first sHOLZ ring (m = 1) with the corresponding line separation in the FOLZ ring, is equal to 3.44.

Finally, it seems worth while to point out that all superlattice reflections close to the transmitted beam (for which m = 1) have similar intensities, as can be seen from fig. 4. It might have been expected that different sHOLZ reflections would show different intensities; in particular a weak sHOLZ reflection may be expected to be associated with a (600) fundamental reflection (for which h+k = 4n+2), because then the (Al/Ga) and As strings scatter in anti-phase. However, according to the explanation suggested above the As contribution to a sHOLZ reflection is absent and hence this effect should not arise.

3.2 The 12.1 nm AlAs/GaAs Multilayer Specimen

It is of interest to extend the results of the previous section to specimens with considerably larger superlattice spacings. Bird [10] has analyzed the situation theoretically. He showed that the effective extinction distance ξ for [001] diffraction determines the behaviour of electrons in a [001] superlattice with spacing L. When $\xi \gg L$, the usual approximation [3] of first projecting the full crystal potential and then treating the HOLZ interactions separately is valid. This is the case discussed in the previous section. However, when ξ becomes of the same magnitude as L, the above approximation will no longer hold and a full 3-D treatment of the diffraction problem appears necessary, which allows for interference between different layers of the reciprocal lattice. According to Bird, ξ = 17.7 nm for 120 kV electrons in GaAs, and this value for ξ would imply considerable 3-D diffraction effects in a specimen with 12.1 nm superlattice spacing. Our computations, based on fig. 1, give the following somewhat different results for ξ, similar to some earlier results [5]:

Voltage (kV)	80	120	300
Extinction distance (nm)	13.9	19.5	34.5

Irrespective of the precise value for the extinction distance, it is clear from these computed values for ξ that interesting 3-D diffraction effects may be expected to occur for a 12.1 nm superlattice, especially when the voltage is not too high.

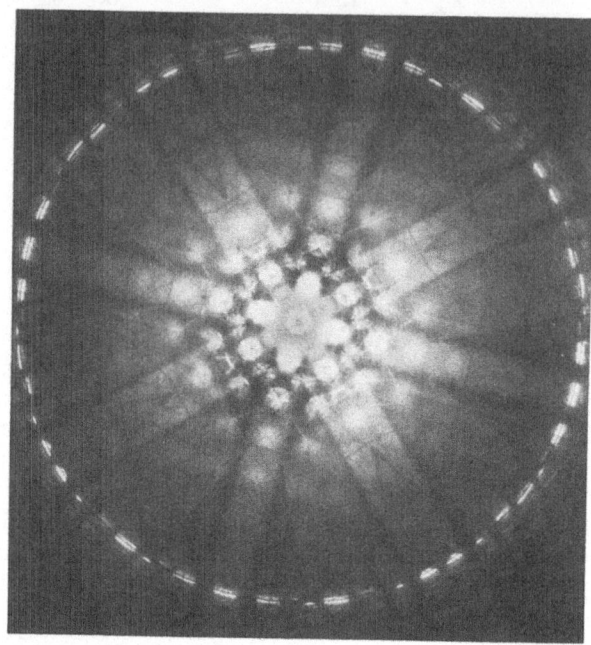

Fig. 5. CBED [001] zone-axis pattern of the 12.1 nm superlattice GaAs/AlAs specimen, taken at 120 kV.

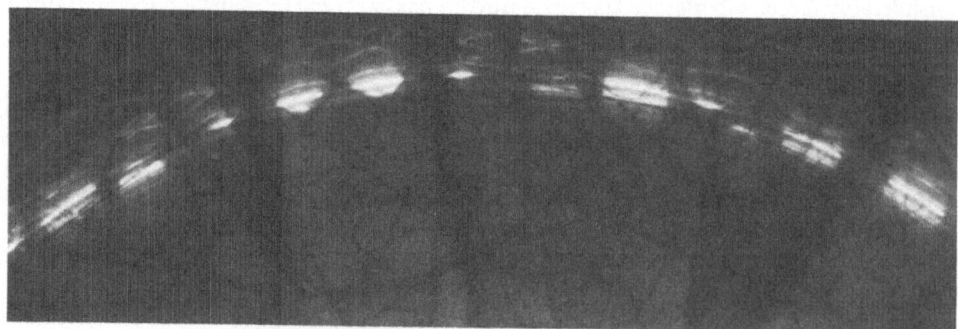

Fig. 6. Enlargement of part of the FOLZ ring from fig. 5.

Fig. 5 shows a [001] zone-axis pattern of the 12.1 nm multilayer specimen, taken at 120 kV. In comparison with corresponding micrographs of the previous specimen (with smaller superlattice spacing) the following differences may be noted.

(i) the specimen consists of a sequence of 8.8 nm GaAs and 3.3 nm AlAs layers; thus the overall Al content is about 25 % Al, much lower than the Al content in the specimen discussed in the previous section. This implies that branches (1) and (2) of the zero-layer dispersion surface (cf. fig. 1) are much closer, as can be observed from a comparison of relevant FOLZ discs from both specimens.

(ii) the larger spacing of the superlattice decreases the values of H for the reciprocal lattice in eqn. (1) and consequently the diameter of the sHOLZ rings becomes smaller, as can be deduced from fig. 5. Also, the smaller Al content would imply a larger separation of the two lines corresponding to branches (2) and (5) in sHOLZ rings close to the transmitted beam. The latter effect is difficult to observe in fig. 5, since the diameter of the different discs in the CBED pattern is such that part of the rings fall outside the discs. Also, the intensity of one of the components of the double sHOLZ rings appears to be weaker than for the superlattice discussed in section 3.1, so that at first sight the sHOLZ rings may appear to consist of single lines.

(iii) as a consequence of the larger superlattice spacing the sHOLZ reflections associated with the fundamental FOLZ (given by eqn. (2)) are closer to the FOLZ lines. In fact the separation of branches (1) and (5) (about 0.5 nm^{-1}) becomes of the same order of magnitude as the spacing between fundamental and superlattice lines in FOLZ, given as .76 nm^{-1} by eqn. (3) (see fig. 6). Hence the enumeration of different lines may become difficult in FOLZ reflections; however, the most prominent lines are still caused by branches (1), (2) and (5) of the dispersion surface.

In table II a comparison between calculated and experimental values of Δk_z is made for the voltage range 90-300 kV. The behaviour of the experimental values of $\Delta k_z = k_z^{(1)} - k_z^{(5)}$ is somewhat peculiar. From general arguments an increase in extinction distance is expected with increasing accelerating voltage. This implies a decrease in Δk_z with voltage. However, from table II there appears to exist a maximum in the experimental value of Δk_z at about 120 kV for the 12.1 nm specimen.

4. STRAIN MODULATION EFFECTS

Thus far we have described HOLZ diffraction effects caused by compositional modulation in a superlattice. Generally there are also strains involved in the coherent matching of two lattices at the interface(s), which we have neglected for the GaAs/AlAs system. The nature of these strains in epitaxial layers of III-V compounds has been discussed by Hornstra and Bartels [11], taking into account the anisotropic elasticity. They showed that for (001) GaAs there are two effects: (i) a difference in lattice plane spacing between layer and substrate; this effect is a maximum for lattice planes parallel to the interface, and (ii) a different tilt of lattice planes ($\Delta\theta$) inclined to the interface. The latter effect is a maximum for $\theta = 45°$ and zero for θ equal to 0 and 90°. Quite recently strain effects in the GaAs/InGaAs system (in which compositional effects could be neglected) have been investigated using CBED in plan view [12]. It has been found that so-called sidebands occur in HOLZ reflections in a 6 % In alloy when the incident electron beam is along [102] (26° from the symmetrical [001]). These sidebands are visible as line segments in HOLZ reflections, and up to 5 line segments have been observed in particular fundamental FOLZ reflections, with the sidebands (first and second-order) sometimes stronger than the fundamental reflection (no sidebands are associated with reflections belonging to the [001] zone). It was verified that the sideband separation is in agreement with the expected value from the superlattice spacing. However, the explanation of these sidebands in terms of the strain modulation seems somewhat in doubt, since it has been calculated that the kinematic intensity of the sidebands goes rapidly to zero for superlattice spacings of 50 nm or smaller [13].

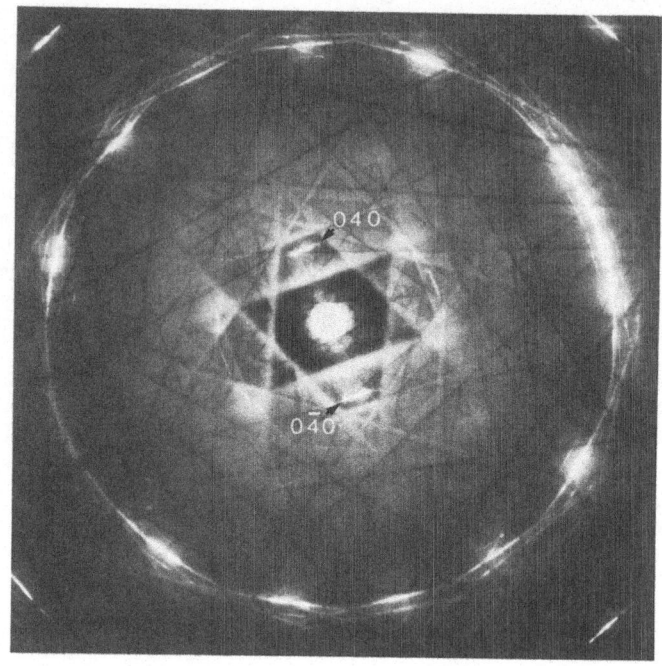

Fig. 7. CBED [102] pattern from the 12.1 nm specimen, taken at 120 kV.

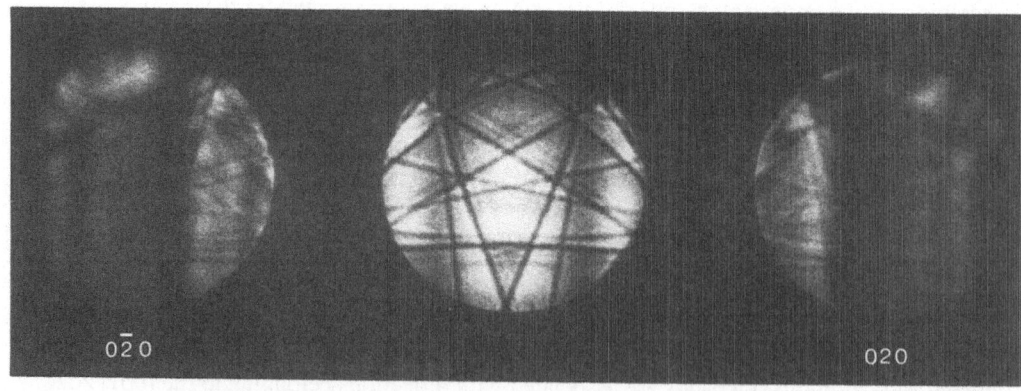

Fig. 8. HOLZ lines in bright-field disc of [103] pattern from the 6.7 nm specimen, taken at 100 kV.

In view of these recent results on strain modulation effects we have investigated similar patterns from our GaAs/AlAs multilayer specimens. Fig. 7 shows a [102] pattern from the 12.1 nm spacing specimen discussed in section 3.2. It may be seen that this pattern contains superlattice reflections associated with the ZOLZ reflections, as well as weak superlattice reflections close to the fundamental FOLZ. The fine structure of the FOLZ reflections in fig. 7 is much simpler compared with the [001] zone-axis pattern, because there is no splitting of the dispersion surface for the [102] incident beam orientation. These results are entirely as expected from a compositional modulation along [001] in the specimen; in particular the superlattice reflections associated with the 040 and $0\overline{4}0$ reflections in fig. 7 should be noted. No evidence for strain effects, as reported in ref. 12, could be seen.

Some off-axis CBED patterns have also been taken for the 6.7 nm spacing specimen discussed in section 3.1. Apart from similar sHOLZ reflections as found for the 12.1 nm specimen, fig. 8 shows the (000) disc from a [103] pattern. The bright-field HOLZ lines in this disc clearly show a splitting which does appear similar to the phenomenon observed in ref. 12.

5. DISCUSSION AND CONCLUSIONS

In this paper specific HOLZ diffraction effects from semiconductor superlattices have been shown to exist. In particular it has been shown that superlattice HOLZ rings of reflections occur in [001] CBED patterns, taken from plan-view specimens with the superlattice axis parallel to the electron beam. The fine structure of these superlattice reflections, consisting of two bright lines as opposed to three bright lines in fundamental reflections, has been qualitatively explained. However, it should be noted that the detailed behaviour of the superlattice reflections is not yet well understood, for instance differences in intensity occur for different specimen thicknesses. At present computer generation of CBED patterns is being employed in order to compare the detailed experimental and simulated patterns under different conditions.

With regard to the origin of the diffraction effects from a superlattice, in general strains and composition fluctuations act as two contributing factors. Let us briefly consider these two factors separately.

In the GaAs/AlAs superlattice system as discussed in this paper, the main superlattice effects result from Al/Ga composition fluctuations along [001] in the specimens, arising on the Ga sublattice of the GaAs structure. These fluctuations can qualitatively explain the difference in fine structure of superlattice and fundamental reflections in [001] zone-axis patterns, as indicated above. We also investigated the effect of overall Al composition in the specimen on the location of branches (1), (2) and (5) of the zero-layer dispersion surface of [001] AlGaAs. From a comparison of computed and experimental values of Al-content (cf. tables I and II) it is concluded that the Al composition can be reliably determined from a (multilayer) specimen provided the voltage is sufficiently high, i.e. at about 100 kV.

However, the detailed behaviour of the Δk_z values for different voltages obtained for the 12.1 nm specimen remains unexplained, and this generates some uncertainty in the determination of Al content.

The influence of strains has, to a first approximation, been neglected in the AlAs/GaAs specimens studied in this paper. Fung et al.[12] have recently investigated strain modulation effects in GaAs/InGaAs multilayer specimens, in which the composition modulation could be neglected. It was shown that sidebands, due to strain modulation, could be associated with reflections in off-axis patterns not belonging to the [001] zone-axis of the specimen. Thus the main difference between composition and strain modulation appears to be the absence of superlattice reflections (or sidebands) associated with reflections belonging to the [001] zone-axis in the case of strain modulation. Also, the explanation of the effects originating from strains is not clear at present, since recent calculations[13] indicate that the strain effects rapidly decrease with decreasing superlattice spacing, say below 50 nm spacing.

Some preliminary [102] and [103] patterns, similar to those from Fung et al.[12], taken from the GaAs/AlAs 6.7 nm specimen (fig. 8) have shown some indication of a strain effect in the split HOLZ lines observed in bright-field. However, more work is needed before any firm conclusions can be reached.

Acknowledgements

The authors would like to thank Mr. H. van 't Blik (Philips Research Laboratories, Eindhoven) for providing the high-quality GaAs/AlAs multilayer specimens used in this investigation.

References

1. H.L. Fraser, D.M. Maher, C.J. Humphreys, C.J.D. Hetherington, R.V. Knoell, and J.C. Bean, The detection of local strains in strained layer superlattices, Inst.Phys.Conf.Ser.No.76:307 (1985).
2. E.P. Kvam, D.J. Eaglesham, C.J. Humphreys, D.M. Maher, J.C. Bean, and H.L. Fraser, Heteroepitaxial strains and interface structure of Ge-Si alloy layers on Si(100), Inst.Phys.Conf.Ser.No.87:165 (1987).
3. C.J. Humphreys, The scattering of fast electrons by crystals, Rep.Prog.Phys.42:1825 (1979).
4. D.J. Eaglesham and C.J. Humphreys, A new technique for microanalysis using CBED: model study of (Al/Ga)As, in: 'Proc. XIth Int. Cong. on Electron Microscopy, Vol. 1', Japanese Society of Electron Microscopy, Kyoto, p. 209 (1986).
5. C.J.D. Hetherington, D.J. Eaglesham, C.J. Humphreys, and G.J. Tatlock, TEM compositional microanalysis in III-V alloys, Inst.Phys.Conf.Ser.No.87:655 (1987).
6. R. Gat and F.W. Schapink, Convergent-beam electron diffraction from GaAs/AlAs superlattices, Ultramicroscopy 21:389 (1987).
7. G.M. Pennock and F.W. Schapink, Convergent-beam electron diffraction from GaAs/AlAs multilayers, Inst.Phys.Conf.Ser.No. 87:219 (1987).
8. J.W. Steeds, Convergent beam electron diffraction, in: "Introduction to Analytical Electron Microscopy", J.J. Hren, J.I. Goldstein, and D.C. Joy, ed., Plenum Press, New York (1979).
9. R. Vincent, D.M. Bird, and J.W. Steeds, Structure of AuGeAs determined by convergent-beam electron diffraction II. Refinement of structural parameters, Phil.Mag. A50:765 (1984).
10. D.M. Bird, Characterization of superlattices by convergent beam diffraction, Inst.Phys.Conf.Ser.No.87:225 (1987).
11. J. Hornstra and W.J. Bartels, Determination of the lattice constant of epitaxial layers of III-V compounds, J.Cryst.Growth 44:513 (1978).
12. K.K. Fung, P.K. York, G.E. Fernandez, J.A. Eades, and J.J. Coleman, Convergent-beam electron diffraction study of strain modulation in GaAs/InGaAs superlattices grown by metal-organic chemical vapour deposition, Phil.Mag.Lett.. 57:221 (1988).
13. D. Cherns, C.J. Kiely, and A.R. Preston, Electron diffraction studies of strain in epitaxial bicrystals and multilayers, Ultramicroscopy 24:355 (1988).

DETERMINATION OF COMPOSITION AND IONICITY BY CRITICAL VOLTAGE AND OTHER

ELECTRON DIFFRACTION METHODS

J. Gjønnes, H. Matsuhata* and K. Gjønnes

Department of Physics
University of Oslo
Blindern, Oslo, Norway

Abstract   Several methods for determination of structure factors/
structure parameters by convergent beam electron diffraction (CBED) can
be described in terms of the gap, $(\gamma^j-\gamma^l)_{min}$, at the dispersion surface.
Most accurate may be those based upon measurement of the condition for
zero gap, revaled by zero contrast of a Kikuchi or Kossel line. By
measurement in non-systematic cases, measured either as a critical
voltage or as a diffraction condition, the scope of the method is
increased. Application of non-systematical critical voltage measurement
to various types of semiconductor structures: ZnS, diamond, rutile type
is shown.

Introduction and theory

In structure characterization of semiconductors the emphasis is on
details, at the local or defect level or in the average structure: hence
sensitivity is essential. The unique facility of electron microscopy for
observation of defects and interfaces is well recognised; the
advantages of electron scattering in the detailed study of the average
structure may not be appreciated to the same extent. For determination
of valence electron distribution, site occupancies, thermal parameters
etc, one has usually turned to x-ray or neutron diffraction methods.

However, electrons have useful properties also for such studies: High
sensitivity to valence electron distribution through the scattering
factor $(Z-F^X)/s^2$, ($s=\sin\theta/\lambda$, F^X the atomic scattering factor for X-rays
for atom Z); high sensitivity also to coordinates and thermal parameters
through the large $\sin\theta/\lambda$-range available; absolute measurement of low-
order structure factors can be applied to crystals of dimensions
appreciably less than one μm.

These properties have been demonstrated in a variety of effects and
methods for determination of structure factors (see e.g. Goodman &
Lehmpfuhl 1967; Watanabe, Uyeda & Fukuhara, 1968; Gjønnes & Høier, 1971;
Voss, Lehmpfuhl & Smith, 1980; Sellar, Imeson & Humphries (1980);
Vincent, Bird & Steeds, 1984; Taftø & Gjønnes, 1985) – often applied to
semiconductors. Such applications may still appear limited – but are now

---

*Present address: Toyota Technological Institute, Tempaku, Nagoya, Japan

increasing, due to the growing use of the technique of convergent beam electron diffraction, CBED. There the two dimensional rocking curve, $I_g(k_x,k_y)$, is measured within disks for each reflection g. This is a much more precise measurement than can be obtained form the rather poorly defined spot intensities in the traditional SAD spot pattern. The intensity distributions $I_g(k_x,k_y)$ can be expressed also as function of angles or of excitation errors for the reflections, but the most convenient variables may be the wave vector components k_x,k_y in the plane normal to the most prominent zone axis in the pattern. Measurements of $I_g(k_x,k_y)$ can be used in various ways, e.g:

- direct comparison of the distribution or part of it with model calculations, which has been tried mainly for the one-dimensional distribution for reflections in a systematic row.

- measurement of the intensity level at corresponding points in the CBED disks (Olsen, Goodman & Whitfield, 1985)

- focus on special, mainly "two-wave" features, which we shall discuss here. They include Kossel line fringes, IKL (intersecting Kikuchi line) split, critical effects - which is our main theme; they may be used also for obtaining precisely defined intensities, I_g, which can be compared with dynamical scattering calculations.

We shall here discuss these features in a Bloch wave description, emphasising the dispersion surface, which we represent by the variation of an eigenvalue $\gamma(k_x,k_y)$, through a two-dimensional section in wave-vector space. We shall focus the attention on the two-wave like regions appearing around Brillouin zone boundaries and stress the concept of the "gap", $(\gamma^i-\gamma^j)_{min}$, which plays a role comparable to the band gap in the electron theory of transport properties. The gap at the the dispersion surface can be interpreted as an "effective Fourier potential", U^{eff}, its inverse is an extinction length, . The analogy with band theory may be apparent in the usual form of the eigenvalue equation in the forward scattering approximation. On taking the z-axis normal to the entrance surface of the crystal, we may write the fundamental equations for the Bloch waves in matrix form (see e.g. Reimer, 1984)

$$A\ \underline{C} = 2k\gamma\ \underline{C} \qquad\qquad (1)$$

where the eigenvalues $\gamma^j = \underline{K}_{oz}{}^j - \underline{k}_z$ are the differences between the z-components of the vacuum wave vector, $\underline{k}$, and the wave vector $\underline{K}_o{}^j$ for Bloch wave j, with components $C_g{}^j$. The elements of the matrix A are

$$A_{gh} = U_{gh} = U_{g-h}; \quad A_{gg} = 2ks_g = k_o{}^2 - (\underline{k}_o+g)^2 = -2\underline{k}_og - g^2 \ ,$$

where g are reciprocal lattice vectors. U_g are the Fourier component of the periodic potential in the crystal. The excitation error s_g which measures the deviation of reflection g from Bragg condition is seen to be a linear function of a horizontal component of the incident wave. Hence the "empty lattice" solution of (1), which obtains for $U_{gh} = 0$ will appear as a set of straight lines.

It has been pointed out by several authors (Buxton, 1976; Høier, 1972; Gjønnes, Gjønnes, Zhu & Spence, 1988) that many intensity features can be represented to a good approximation by a pair (i,j) of Bloch waves and two-beam like expressions for e.g. the separation between the two branches

$$k(\gamma^i-\gamma^j) \sim \sqrt{(ks)^2+U_g{}^2} \qquad\qquad (2a)$$

and the intensity profile

$$I_g \sim \frac{U_g^2}{(ks_g)^2 + U_g^2} \sin^2[\pi z \sqrt{s_g^2 + (U_g/k)^2}\,] \qquad (2b)$$

with an effective Fourier potential

$$U_g^{eff} = k/\xi_g = (k/2)(\gamma^i - \gamma^j)_{min} \qquad (2c)$$

where ξ_g is the corresponding extinction length.

Another useful formula is the integrated intensity (Blackman, 1939)

$$\int I_g\, ds_g = \int J_o(x)dx \qquad (2d)$$

which has the low thickness or kinematical limit $z^2 U_g^2$, and the high thickness or dynamical limit $|U_g|$.

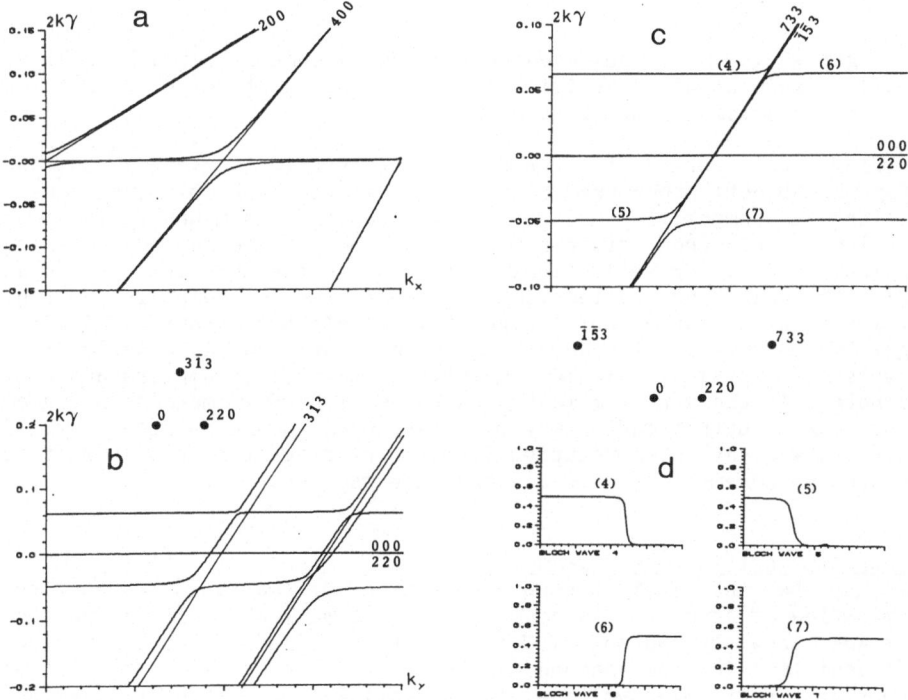

Fig. 1. Examples of calculated dispersion surface sections: $2k\gamma$ for selected branches as function of the wave vector component k_x (a) and k_y (b and c) and excitation errors $2ks_g$ (the straight lines) a: around 400; systematics only; b: g = 220, h = $\bar{3}13$; c: g = 220, h = 733, f = 153. d: excitation $|C_o|^2$ for main branches in (c). Multiple beam calculations with 10-15 beams for GaAs at 200kV.

Such expressions may apply for the main intensity features near the gaps $(\gamma^j - \gamma^l)_{min}$ at the dispersion surface even when many reflected beams are excited, cf the calculated dispersion surface sections shown in Fig. 1. Further analysis shows that the profile across the different Kossel line segments in patterns like the one reproduced as Fig. 2 can indeed be described to a good approximation by the two-wave like intensity expression above.

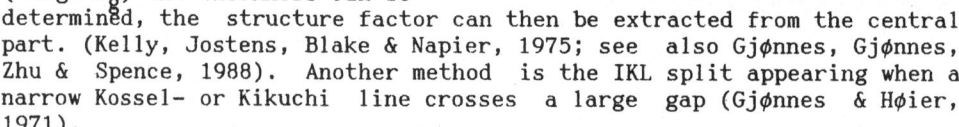

Fig. 2. CBED Kossel pattern taken with large aperture. Rutile, 113.

We may distinguish between three cases:

. Small gap - where an integrated intensity according to Eqn (2d) can be extracted, e.g. from a scan across the Kossel line segment.

. Large gap - with an extensive Kossel fringe pattern. From the outer part (large s_g) the thickness can be determined, the structure factor can then be extracted from the central part. (Kelly, Jostens, Blake & Napier, 1975; see also Gjønnes, Gjønnes, Zhu & Spence, 1988). Another method is the IKL split appearing when a narrow Kossel- or Kikuchi line crosses a large gap (Gjønnes & Høier, 1971).

. Zero gap - which is observed as vanishing contrast of a Kikuchi or Kossel line segment at a "critical voltage" or particular diffraction condition, is a main theme of this article.

But before we proceed to these and other effects, let us consider briefly the object: structure details in relatively simple structures: Variations in composition or occupancy, ionicity and other features in the valence electron distribution can be revealed by accurate determination of inner reflections. Referring to the ZnS-structure as an example, the weak inner reflections are sensitive to composition, e.g. substitution of Al for Ga and to ionicity, or electron transfer. Bonding charges may be revealed in the strong reflections, 400, 111. Reflections at high $\sin \theta/\lambda$ values will be sensitive to thermal parameters and atom coordinates. In the very simplest structures, like FCC metals, measurement of one structure factor may be interpreted in a meaningful way. In all other cases any interpretation in terms of structure details must be based upon measurement of several structure factors.

Zero gap: The critical voltage methods.
These may be the most accurate electron diffraction methods for determination of structure factors. The systematical critical voltage effect was shown by Watanabe, Uyeda & Fukuhara (1968). The contrast of the Kikuchi line for the second order of a strong inner reflection vanishes at a particular voltage, due essentially to a three beam effect which leads to a vanishing gap, $\gamma^j - \gamma^l = 0$ at the dispersion surface. Sellar, Imeson & Humphreys (1980) showed that an accuracy of a few tenths of a per cent in determination of a strong structure factor in a metal could be obtained by using CBED instead of Kikuchi patterns. Other structure factors and temperature factor must be known. Only a few low order structure factors can be obtained in this way - and even this depends on a million volt microscope.

Therefore one is looking for other "critical effects", which can yield comparable accuracy. Buxton, Loveluck & Steeds (1978) studied critical voltages appearing at zone axis position. Gjønnes & Høier (1971) showed that any three beams 0,g,h in a noncentrosymmetric case will produce a vanishing gap at the dispersion surface and hence a vanishing Kikuchi (or Kossel) line contrast at position defined by the excitations errors for the two reflections g and h:

$$2ks_g = U_g(U_{g-h}/U_h - U_h/U_{g-h})$$

$$2ks_h = U_h(U_{g-h}/U_g - U_g/U_{g-h}) \qquad (3)$$

This follows from the dispersion equation, $|A| = 0$, which in the three beam case can be written:

$$(2ks_g - 2k\gamma + U_g^2/2k\gamma)(2ks_h - 2k\gamma + U_h^2/2k\gamma)$$
$$= (U_{g-h} + U_g U_h/2k\gamma)^2 \qquad (3a)$$

which represents an hyperbola in the s_g, s_h plane. The condition (3) corresponds to the degenerate case which obtains when the right hand side of (3a) is zero. In the systematic, second order critical voltage $g = 2h$, $U_{g-h} = U_h$. Then $2ks_g = 0$ from the first of Eqn (3), whereas the second equation is satisfied only at the critical voltage, through the factor m/m_0 in the Fourier potentials U_g.

Recently we have extended this analytical treatment to a general four beam case. Take a_{ij} as off-diagonal elements and 0, x, y, z as diagonal elements of A and define new variables:

$$X = x + a_{12}^2/\gamma - \gamma \; ; \; Y = y + a_{31}^2/\gamma - \gamma \; ; \; Z = z + a_{41}^2/\gamma - \gamma$$

The dispersion equation then takes the form

$$XYZ + pX + qY + tZ + C = 0, \qquad (4)$$

where

$$p = - a_{13}^2 a_{14}^2 (1/\gamma + a_{34}/a_{13} a_{14})^2$$

$$q = - a_{12}^2 a_{14}^2 (1/\gamma + a_{24}/a_{12} a_{14})^2$$

$$t = - a_{12}^2 a_{13}^2 (1/\gamma + a_{23}/a_{12} a_{13})^2$$

$$C = \sqrt{-2pqt}$$

When $Z = 0$ the degeneracy is found for

$$X = \sqrt{-qt/p} \; ; \; Y = \sqrt{-pt/q} \; ; \; Z = \sqrt{-pq/t} \qquad (5)$$

- which can be regarded as a parametric representation of a curve in x,y,z-space (x,y and z define the three excitation errors). For a given voltage there will be a relation between these excitation errors (viz: the Ewald sphere), which may cut this curve at certain points which mark the degeneracies. If one of the excitation errors, e.g. z becomes very large, the three beam case above is retrieved; the four beam case may include up to four degeneracies, but not all of these may be attainable. The case $Z = 0$ which can be treated separately may include degeneracies in symmetrical cases, as in the four-beam case discussed below.

In order to be useful in structure characterization, the degeneracies must be susceptible to precise measurement. Gjønnes & Høier (1971) found that rather few cases satisfied this requirement, with the diamond configuration of spots as a prime example. Below we shall discuss this and other symmetrical cases in some detail, based on the three- and four beam equations above and consideration of Bloch wave symmetry at special points. We shall use the symmetry notation by Cochran (1952), see Gjønnes & Taftø (1978)

Three examples

In the four beam case of Fig. 3, around a 2mm point, it is readily found that the projected Laue points for the degeneracies must lie on a mirror line. We shall treat this case by inspecting the fundamental equations (1) for the four beams o, g,f,h with $s_h = 0$, (the centre of the Laue circle at the horizontal mirror line):

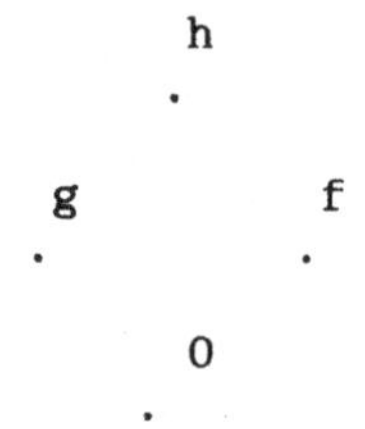

Let us write the matrix equation

$$
\begin{vmatrix}
-2k\gamma & U_h & U_g & U_g \\
U_h & -2k\gamma & U_g & U_g \\
U_g & U_g & 2k(s_g-\gamma) & U_m \\
U_g & U_g & U_m & 2k(s_f-\gamma)
\end{vmatrix}
\begin{vmatrix}
C_o \\
C_h \\
C_g \\
C_f
\end{vmatrix}
= 0 \qquad (6)
$$

h
.

g   f
.   .

0
.

Fig.3. Beams for (6)

There will be one antisymmetrical Bloch wave (m') with coefficients:

$$c_o = -c_h, \quad c_g = c_f = 0; \quad \text{and eigenvalue } \gamma_3 = -U_h \qquad (6a)$$

and three symmetrical Bloch (m) with:

$$c_o = c_h, \quad \text{from the equations:}$$

$$
\begin{vmatrix}
U_h - 2k\gamma & \sqrt{2}U_g & \sqrt{2}U_g \\
\sqrt{2}U_g & 2ks_g-2k\gamma & U_m \\
\sqrt{2}U_g & U_m & 2ks_f-2k\gamma
\end{vmatrix}
\begin{vmatrix}
C_o \\
C_g \\
C_f
\end{vmatrix}
= 0 \qquad (6b)
$$

The dispersion equation corresponding to (6b) is

$$(U_h - 2k\gamma)(2ks_g - 2k\gamma)(2ks_f - 2k\gamma) + 4U_g^2 U_m - (U_h - 2k\gamma)U_m^2$$

$$- 2(2ks_g - 2k\gamma)U_g^2 - 2(2ks_f - 2k\gamma)U_g^2 = 0 \qquad (6c)$$

A condition for a degenerate eigenvalue is then found by inserting $\gamma_3 = -U_g$ in this equation:

$$(2ks_g + U_g - U_g^2/U_h)(2ks_f + U_h - U_g^2/U_h) = (U_m - U_g^2/U_h)^2 \qquad (7)$$

which can be used to determine the position of the degeneracy along the Kikuchi line h. We may express the two excitation errors as

$$s_{g,f} = s(1 +/- x)$$

where s is the excitation error at the symmetrical position in the centre of the four-beam configuration in Fig. 3 and x the distance from this position along the mirror line s_g=0. The two positions of the degenerate points on that line is found by inserting these expressions for the excitation errors in (7):

$$(2ks)^2 x^2 = 4k^2(s + U_h - U_m)(s + U_h + U_m - 2U_g^2/U_h) \qquad (7a)$$

The two points will merge into one degeneracy, at the symmetrical point, for a "non-systematical critical voltage" given by

$$2ks = 2U_g^2/U_h - U_h - U_m. \qquad (7b)$$

If $U_g > U_h$, as in the FCC-case above, e.g. (h = 422, g = 220, f = 202, m = 022), 2ks must be positive, for (7a,b) to be satisfied. This means that the reflections g and f should be inside the Laue circle, i.e. that $|\underline{h}| > |\underline{m}|$. It follows that in the case above no degenerate points are found at the other mirror line: this four beam case includes two degeneracies below the critical voltage given by (7b), one at this voltage and no degeneracy at higher accelerating voltages. A dispersion surface section corresponding to equation (6) $(s_h=0)$ is sketched in Fig. 4a.

Similar cases may be obtained in other centered projections. A related case obtains in projections of symmetry pmg. There the degeneracies for the second order of the forbidden reflection (i.e. 02), will appear in a configuration similar to Fig. 3, but with the two reflections g and f outside the Laue circle.

Several observations have been made of the extinctions on the 422-line in FCC, for Si, GaAs, ZnS. For determination of relation between structure factors of the type (7a or b) one may either measure the position of the degeneracies, as in the original measurement by Gjønnes & Høier (1971) in Kikuchi patterns taken at 100kV, or the voltage at which the degeneracies coincide at the symmetrical position (Matsuhata & Gjønnes, 1987). Fig. 4b shows convergent beam patterns from ZnS taken of 242 at voltages below, near and above the critical voltage defined by (7b). Dispersion surface sections from multiple beam calculations for ZnS at the same voltages are shown in Fig. 5. Although the shape of the branches appears quite different from the four-beam result (Fig. 4a), the position of the degeneracies are very similar, cf. table 1.

a

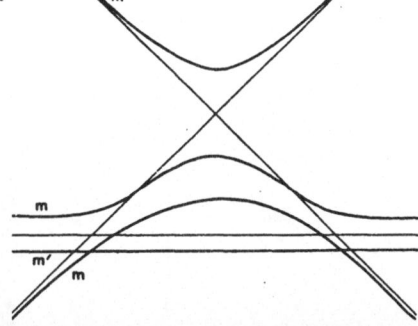

Fig. 4a) Section of four beam dispersion surface corresponding to Eq (6) $(s_h=0)$

b

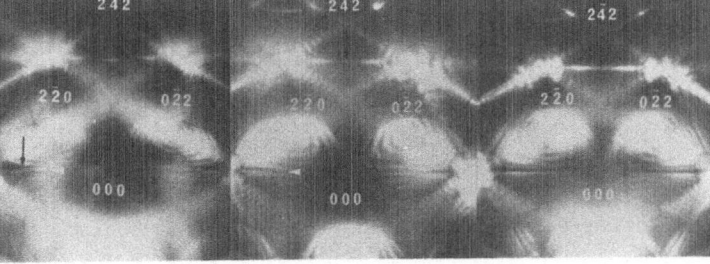

b) CBED patterns from ZnS at 102, 142 and 203 kV primary voltage

93

Fig. 5. Calculated dispersion surface sections for ZnS at three voltages, along the two mirror lines $(s_{422}=0; s_{220}=s_{202})$.

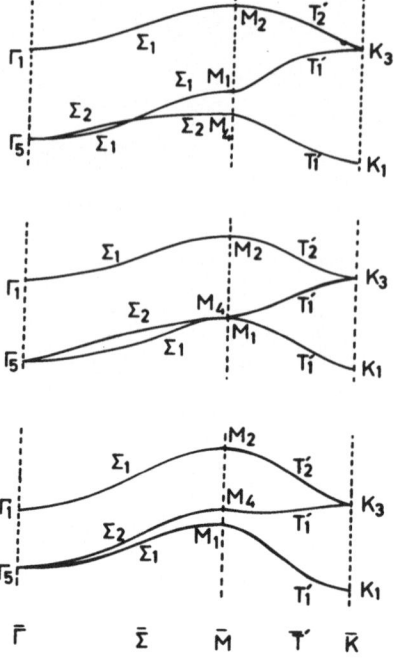

Table 1

Calculated critical voltages in the non-systematic cases, Figs. 4 and 6(below); ca 100 beams. Doyle-Turner (1968) scattering factors and available Debye-Waller factors.

a)			b)		
ZnS	165	kV	Cu	151	kV
" obs	152± 5		" obs ca	120	
GaAs	139		Al	514	
Ge	149		Ge	391	
Si	293		Si	807	
Cu	532		ZnS	395	
Al	1345		GaAs	370	

Another symmetrical case is represented by Fig. 6. Analytical calculations may be performed with the five beams 000, 200, 020, 420, 240, in a square projection. Along the symmetry line, where $s_{200} = s_{020}$ the solution can again be separated in two antisymmetrical Bloch waves, (with $C_O = 0$) and three symmetrical Bloch waves, $C_{200} = C_{020}$, $C_{420} = C_{240}$. A degeneracy leading to vanishing contrast feature may appear between the latter, at a particular voltage. An expression for this can be obtained from a reduced three-beam matrix, following the three-beam treatment by Gjønnes & Høier. The vanishing contrast shown in Fig. 6 appears at a particular voltage, as seen in the CBED pattern.

a   b

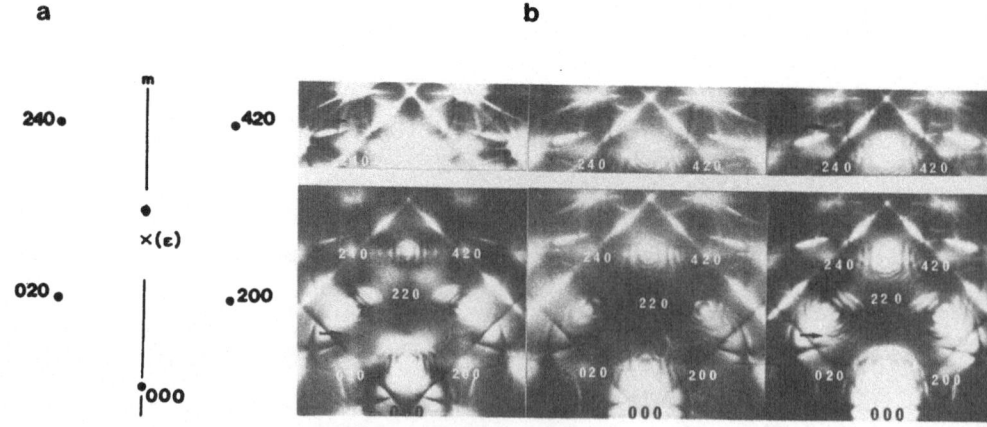

Fig. 6a) schematic five beam case. b) CBED patterns from Cu taken at voltages 82, 122 and 203kV.

Application to the rutile type structure of SnO_2

Only in very simple structures, where accurate temperature factors are available will one or two such critical voltages be sufficient for determination of structure factors or structure parameters. As a slightly more complicated example we have studied the rutile type SnO_2, where the ions may exist in several valence states. A set of degeneracies leading to critical voltage were investigated; see Figure 7, including a systematic case, a zone axis critical voltage, Fig. 9, and a two fold rotation case. The latter may be a very useful configuration, since it can easily be found in any non-rectangular projection with a centre of symmetry.

From calculated values for the critical voltages, Table 2 it is seen that these are indeed sensitive to the valence states of the ions, see also Fig. 8. These calculations are based on free, spherical ions and isotropic temperature factors. An interpretation in terms of a particular ionic state is therefore at best tentative; a full treatment should include deformation of the electron clouds as well as anistropic temperature factors. Instead we have attempted to evaluate structure factors from the measured critical voltages, using different ionicities for other structure factors entering the calculations. Examples of results are shown in Table 3, based on the diamond case critical voltage used to determine the 110 structure factor. Similar calculations were performed for the other configurations in Fig. 7. As might be expected the different structure factors lead to different ionicities when compared with calculations based on free ions.

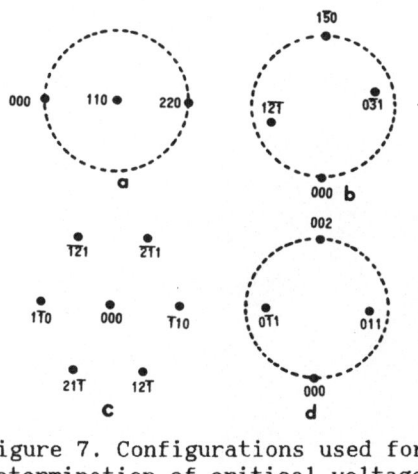

Figure 7. Configurations used for determination of critical voltages in SnO_2.

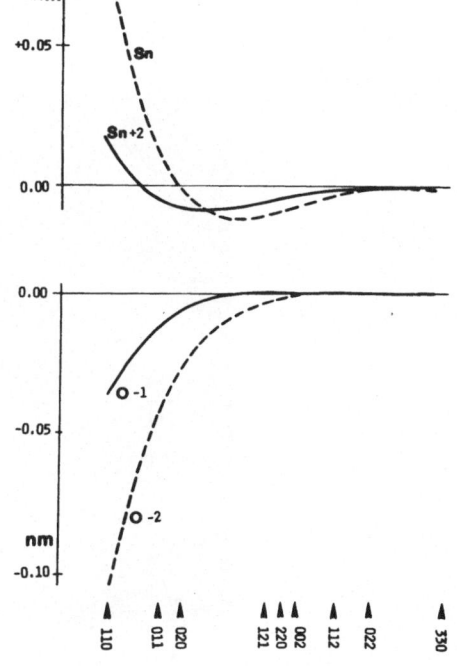

Figure 8. Scattering factors for ions and neutral atoms in SnO_2, with position of reflections shown.

Table 2. Calculated and experimental critical voltages for different cases in SnO_2, in kV.

	SnO_2	$Sn^{+2}O_2^-$	$Sn^{+4}O_2^{-2}$	exp
110 systematic, 13 beam	209	197	74	146+/-3
150 at [513], 84 "	173	183	207	179+/-4
113 zone axis 99 "	182	181	150	164+/-6
200 at [100] 198 "	261	250	114	153+/-7

Table 3. Estimated structure factor for 011

Experimental values:
SnO$_2$ assumed for higher order reflections · 4.905 x 10^{-4}nm

$Sn^{+2}O^{-2}$ "   "   "   "   4.888

$Sn^{+4}O^{-2}_2$ "   "   "   "   4.701

Calculated values:
SnO_2 4.504

$Sn^{+2}O^-_2$ 4.525

$Sn^{+4}O^{-2}_2$ 4.851

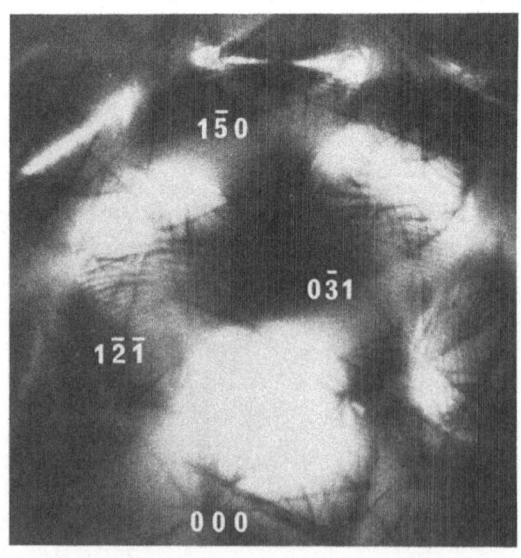

Fig. 9. CBED pattern from SnO_2 in 531 zone, near critical voltage for 150.

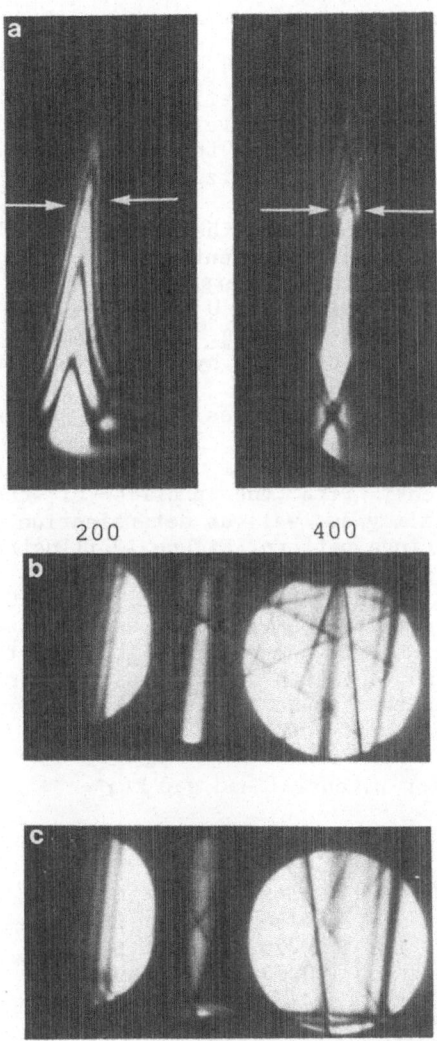

Fig. 10a) Large angle CBED patterns at an GaAs/Ga$_{1-x}$Al$_x$As interface: b,c CBED patterns of 200 and 400 in the Ga$_{1-x}$Al$_x$As and GaAs respectively.

Small gap: Measurement of integrated intensity

The critical voltage and related methods, where either accelerating voltage or a diffraction condition corresponding to a Bloch wave degeneracy is measured has been found best suited for determination of the larger structure factors. This applies even more to the methods based on large gaps at the dispersion surface, viz: Kossel fringes and the meaurement of intersecting Kikuchi line split. There is thus an apparent need to extend these two groups of methods of measurements based on small gaps, in practice of an integrated intensity. A number of configurations can be used, relating to inner, superstructure reflections as well as to outer reflections, e.g. the HOLZ line intensity measurements used extensively by the Bristol group, see Vincent, Bird & Steeds (1984) or the measurement of intensities of higher order systematics by Taftø & Metzger (1985).

These measurements may be based on the assumption that the intensity profile across a Kossel line segment is given by the gap at the dispersion surface and hence that the expression of the form (2b) applies with a suitable effective potential, U_g^{eff}. This can be approximated by some perturbation expressions, e.g. the Bethe potential, interband scattering (Howie, 1963) or Bloch wave hybridization (Buxton, 1976).

Application to the ionicity in GaAs was shown by Gjønnes, Gjønnes, Zhu & Spence (1988), where the measurement in a systematic row is discussed in detail. The structure factor of 200 could be determined with an accuracy of a few per cent, with the profile of the 400 reflection providing intensity scaling as well as determination of thickness from the outer part of the fringe pattern. Figure 10 illustrates how this may be applied also to e.g. GaAs/Ga$_{1-x}$Al$_x$As. The LACBED patterns from 200 and 400 are taken so as to show the interface. Normal CBED patterns from either side of the interface, Fig. 10b and c, can be used for quantitative determination of composition through the 200 structure factor. Table 4 shows tha variation of U_{200} and the corresponding gap at the dispersion surface with x in Ga$_{1-x}$Al$_x$As.

Table 4. The Fourier potential and gap $k(\gamma^1-\gamma^2)$ for Ga$_{1-x}$Al$_x$As.

x	$U_{200}(\text{A}^-2)$	$k(\gamma^1 - \gamma^2)$
0.0	.00143	.00158
0.1	.00184	.00204
0.2	.00226	.00251
0.3	.00268	.00298

Discussion

A variety of well defined measurements relating to structure factors/ structure parameters can be obtained from CBED patterns. Many of the magnitudes can be interpreted in terms of the gap at the dispersion surface, or an effective potential, or an extinction length. The methods ar conveniently divided in large gap, zero gap and small gap methods; the most accurate ones may be those based on zero gap or Bloch wave degeneracies. The use of selected non-systematic cases provides a considerable extension of the method and does not depend upon high voltage instruments. The condition for the degeneracy can be determined either by measuring the voltage for extinction appearing at a particular, symmetrical position or by measuring the position at a known voltage. The measurements can be performed to an accuracy of a few kV, which may correspond to half a per cent or better in the structure factor for electrons. On translating from electrons. $(Z-F^x)/s^2$ to X-ray scattering factors, accuracies in the 10^{-3} range are then achieved for the inner reflections.

In order to translate this level of accuracy into structure information, other structure factors must be known to sufficient accuracy, in particular thermal parameters. These may be obtained by other diffraction techniques, but integrated intensities across Kossel line segments in CBED patterns are also seen as a possibility for collecting a sufficient amount of data for a complete refinement of e.g. the valence electron distribution in simple structures. Combination of small gap and large gap method offers the possibility of scaling the former.

In semiconductors such CBED methods can be used to determine ionicities and other features of the electronic structure in the material as well as composition, within areas of a few tens of nm.

REFERENCES

Blackman, M. (1939) Proc. Roy. Soc. A29, 68 - 82.
Buxton, G.F. (1976) Proc. Roy. Soc. A 300, 335-361.
Buxton, G.F., Loveluck, J.E. and Steeds, J.W. (1978) Phil. Mag. A 38, 259
Cochran, W. (1952) Actra Cryst. 5 630-633.
Doyle, P.A. and Turner, P. (1968) Acta Cryst. A24, 390-397.
Gjønnes, J. & Høier, R. (1971) Acta Cryst. A27, 313-316.
Gjønnes, K., Gjønnes, J.,Zhu, J. and Spence, J.C.H. (1988) Acta Cryst.
Gjønnes, J. & Taftø, J. (1978) Int. Conf. Electron Diffraction, London 1978, Bristol: Inst.Phys.p150-155.
Goodman, P. and Lehmpfuhl, G. (1967) Acta Cryst. 22, 14-24.
Howie, A. (1963) Proc. Roy. Soc. A271, 268-287.
Høier, R. (1972) Phys. Stat. Sol. A11, 597-610.
Kelly, P.M., Jostens, A., Blake, R.G. and Napier, J.G. (1975). Phys.Stat. Sol. (a) 31, 771-780.
Matsuhata, H. & Gjønnes, J. (1988) EUREM 88, Inst. Phys. Conf. Ser. No 93, Vol 2 19-20.
Moodie,A.F. (1979) Chemica Scripta 14, 21-22.
Olsen, A., Goodman, P. and Whitfield, H. (1985) J. Sol. State Chem. 60, 305-15.
Reimer, L. "Transmission Electron Microscopy" Springer: Berlin 1984.
Sellar, J.R., Imeson. D. and Humphreys, C.J.(1980) Acta Cryst. A36 686-696.
Taftø, J. & Gjønnes, J. (1985) Ultramicroscopy 17, 329-334.
Taftø, J. and Metzger, T.H. (1985) J. Appl. Cryst. 6, 110-113.
Vincent,R., Bird, D.M. and Steeds, J.W. (1984) Phil. Mag. A50, 765-86.
Voss, R., Lehmpfuhl, G. and Smith D.J. (1980) Z. Naturforsch. 59, 973-984.
Watanabe, D., Uyeda, R. and Fukuhara, A. (1968) Acta Cryst. A25 138-140.

MEASUREMENT OF STRUCTURE-FACTOR PHASES BY ELECTRON DIFFRACTION

FOR THE STUDY OF BONDING IN NON-CENTROSYMMETRIC SEMICONDUCTORS

J.C.H. Spence, J.M. Zuo and R. Hoier*

Department of Physics, Arizona State University, Tempe, Az.
85287 U.S.A.
*Dept. of Physics University of Trondheim-NTH, 7034
Trondheim, Norway

INTRODUCTION

A quantity of fundamental interest for the study of semiconductors is the ground-state charge-density distribution. This is surprisingly difficult to measure with sufficient accuracy to reveal bonding effects in crystals, since the bond charge typically represents less than 0.01% of the total charge-density. For semiconductors containing a center of symmetry for which large single crystals can be grown (such as silicon) , X-ray diffraction techniques can produce rather accurate results[1]. An urgent need exists, however, for a method which can be applied to non-centrosymmetric semiconductors and other materials which are crystalline only on a sub-micron scale.

Spectroscopic techniques which are sensitive to charge-transfer effects suffer from the difficulty that it is neccessary to disentangle excitonic effects from those of ionicity. To the extent that "elastically" scattered Bragg beam intensities are measured, one is able to probe the true ground state of the crystal. In some of our experiments we have approached this ideal by detecting energy filtered elastically scattered electrons.

In this paper we address one aspect of this problem - the accurate measurement of the phases of the structure factors. In centro-symmetric crystals these have values 0 or π (for an origin on the center of symmetry). In non-centrosymmetric crystals these phases may have any value, and these must be measured accurately in order to obtain a charge-density map. In this paper we therefore give an example of phase determination in the non-centrosymmetric CdS structure, using the three-beam convergent-beam electron diffraction (CBED) method, together with many-beam Bloch-wave calculations. Limitations on the accuracy of the method are also discussed.

Many researchers[2,3,4,5,6,7,8] have contributed to the development of electron crystallography and convergent-beam electron diffraction (CBED). We cite here a very few of the many papers in the history of this subject. Very briefly, the use of the two-beam expression (which does not preserve phase information) for structure analysis was first analysed by MacGillavry[3], the enhaced sensitivity of low-order reflections to bonding (by comparison with X-ray reflections) was emphasised by Cowley[2], and the critical voltage method has also been developed and applied with considerable success[4,9] . The use of the rocking-curve information in the systematics orientation has also been developed[10,6,8], the use of weak higher order reflections has been advocated and applied successfully [7], and the Intersecting Kikuchi Line (I.K.L) method has also been developed and applied[11]. On the theoretical side, a review of the Bethe Bloch wave theory of transmission electron diffraction has recently been given[12], while the extension of this to the three-dimensional case (including HOLZ effects) is described elsewhere[13]. The analyses reported in this work required a further extension of this theory to include the case of three-dimensional dynamical transmission electron diffraction in a parallel-sided slab of non-centrosymmetric crystal inclined to the incident beam, with absorption[14].

The problem of phase-determination using dynamical three-beam effects in X-ray diffraction is the subject of a recent book[15]. For electrons, the classic work of Kambe[16] established that three-beam CBED intensities are sensitive to the sum of the phases of the three relevant structure factors. We call this sum the three-phase structure invariant. It is independant of the choice of origin. Fourteen years later, it was shown[17] that, for this non-systematics three-beam case, a degeneracy point exists at which the intensity is zero for centro-symmetric crystals. (This point is labelled "minimum" in figure 2). The position of this point (either as shown or at q) indicates immediately whether the three-phase structure invariant sums to 0 or π. A method of determining both amplitudes and phases in centrosymmetric crystals has been described[18], which depends on finding lines in a three-beam pattern along which the intensity expression reduces to two-beam form. For non-centrosymmetric crystals, the intensity "zero" becomes a minimum of intensity, and indicates the region in a CBED pattern most sensitive to phase[19]. Approximate expressions have also been given for the three-phase invariant[19] based on the second Bethe approximation, and based on a single scattering approximation[20]. The non-centrosymmetric case recieved less attention until recently, however methods for the determination of the three-phase invariant in these crystals have recently been described[21,22].

Our aims have been : (1) to develop quantitative methods for recording one and two-dimensional transmission electron diffraction data directly into a computer for analysis, and (2) To develop the necessary computational strategy for the analysis of these intensities. We have concentrated on the systematics orientation (for energy-filtered one-dimensional data) and on the three-beam geometry (not filtered). The non-systematics three-beam geometry provides a general method of phase determination, but requires two-dimensional data handling and makes energy filtering difficult. The systematics orientation may also sometimes be used to determine phases[23].

In recent work[24], we have used comparisons of (systematics) CBED rocking curves from crystalline GaAs with many-beam calculations to refine the low-order structure factor amplitudes. If Debye-Waller factors are taken from accurate neutron diffraction work , and the phases of two odd reflections taken from pseudo-potential calculations for a GaAs crystal, it is possible to synthesise the charge density along the Ga-As bond, as shown in figure 1. This shows the partially ionic and partially covalent nature of the GaAs bond. The amount of charge found to be in the bond (0.071 $\pm$ 0.045 electrons) is found to be in good agreement with theory.

PHASE DETERMINATION IN CBED THEORY

Our approach has been to use the approximate solutions to the three-beam dynamical diffraction problem obtained by Kambe[16] to indicate the regions in a three-beam CBED pattern which are most sensitive to structure-factor phase. Then a many-beam Bloch-wave calculation is matched to the intensity along this region. Figure 2 shows the general form of a three-beam CBED pattern. Choosing a point in any CBED disc allows the conjugate point in the central disc to be defined, since these are connected by a reciprocal lattice vector. This point in the central disc then defines the incident beam direction and thus the entire family of excitation errors. For CdS we take g = (41-2) , h = (41-4) and h-g = (00-2), all in the [-140]   ZOLZ. Lines of high intensity are expected where the Bragg condition is satisfied along the Kikuchi lines KL. Here the excitation errors S_g and S_h are zero. Dynamical effects produce a splitting of

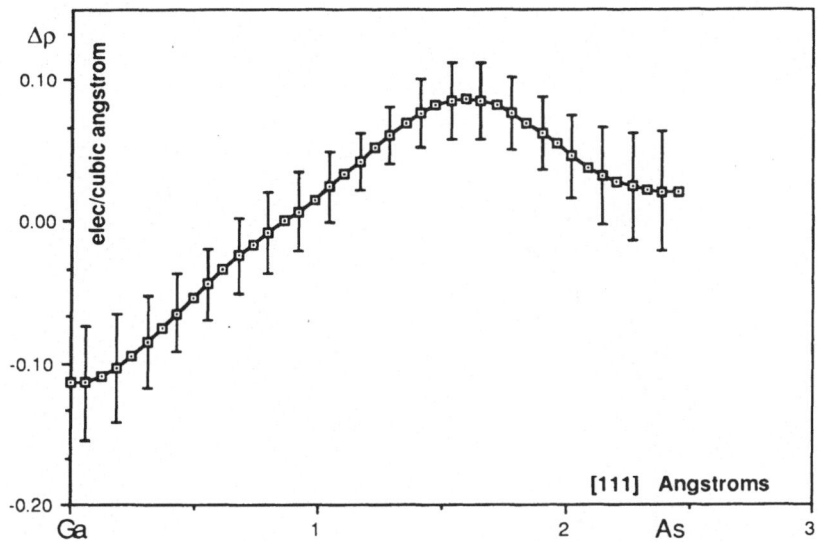

Figure 1.   Experimental measurement (by CBED structure factor refinement) of the charge difference $\Delta\rho$ along the Ga - As bond in GaAs. This is the difference between the measured charge and that given by the neutral-atom scattering factors in the International Tables. Charge-transfer (ionic) effects can be seen from the electron deficit at the Ga nucleus and surplus at As, and covalent effects from the pile-up near mid-bond[24].

the intensity onto the two hyperbolae AB and A'B', defined[25,16] by a co-ordinate $S_{\pm} = 0$. Along these hyperbolae the incident beam direction is constrained to move in such away that

$$S_h = |U_{h-g}|^2 /(4K^2 S_g)$$

1

The distance between these two hyperbolae measured along the line $S_g = S_h$ shown is $|U_{h-g}|/K$, and this forms the basis of the Intersecting Kikuchi line method for measuring $|U_{h-g}|$. In figure 2, S_g =0 near B and B', and goes to a large negative value near A, and a large positive value near A'.

It is the intensity along these hyperbolae which shows the greatest sensitivity to changes in the three-phase invariant ψ. In X-ray work, this is the sum of the phases of the three structure factors which, for CdS, are given by

$$F_{hkl} = (f_{Cd} + f_S exp2\pi ilu)[exp2\pi i(2h/3 + k/3) + exp2\pi i(h/3 + 2k/3 + l/2)]$$

2

Here k - h = 3n (n an integer) in the [-140] ZOLZ.

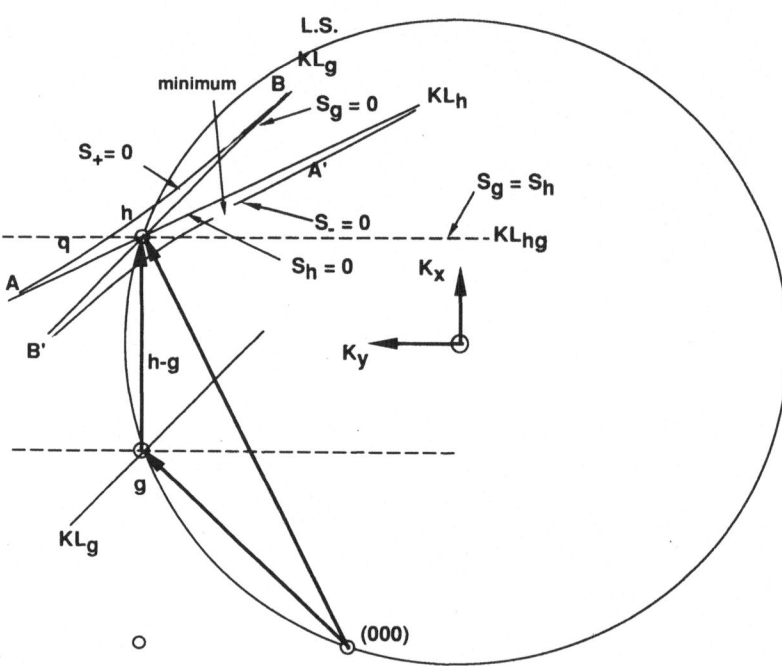

<u>Figure 2.</u>　　　Three-beam interactions. The Laue circle L.S. is shown passing through points g and h at the exact Bragg condition, defining a set of points, one in each CBED disk. For other incident beam directions (corresponding to different points in the central CBED disk) the center of the L.S. moves and its radius changes. Kikuchi lines KL_h and KL_g (along which the excitation errors S_h and S_g are zero) are shown. Superimposed on this diagram is the general form of the three-beam CBED intensity distribution for disc h, which has extrema on the hyperbolae where $S_+ = 0$ and $S_- = 0$ shown. The intensity approaches the two-beam value at A and A' and fades toward B and B'. For the CdS example, g = (41-2), h = (41-4) and h-g = (00-2).

In the "strong-coupling" approximation where $|U_{h-g}| >> |U_g|$ or $|U_h|$ the intensity along the hyperbolae (where $S_\pm = 0$) in a crystal which is not centrosymmetric may be expressed as[25]

$$I_h = \frac{(2KS_g)^2}{|U_{h-g}|^2 + (2KS_g)^2} \sin^2\left\{\frac{\pi t|U_h^{eff}|}{K}\right\}$$

3

With

$$|U_h^{eff}|^2 = |U_h|^2 \frac{(2KS_g)^2}{|U_{h-g}|^2 + (2KS_g)^2} \left\{ (1 - \frac{|U_g||U_{h-g}|}{2KS_g|U_h|} \cos \Psi)^2 + (\frac{|U_g||U_{h-g}|}{2KS_g|U_h|} \sin \Psi)^2 \right\}$$

4

Here the electron wave-vector is K, the structure-factors $U_g = K/\xi_g = 2m|e|V_g/h^2$ (with V_g a Fourier coefficient of crystal potential), and the three-phase invariant is Ψ. For electron diffraction this must be taken as the sum of the phases of the three relevant electron "structure factors" U_g (not the X-ray structure factors F_{hkl}, which have different phases). Using equation 1, equations 3 and 4 can also be expressed entirely in terms of S_h.

In equation 3, S_g is negative on the upper hyperbola AB and positive on the lower, but falls to zero on the line KL_g.. The prefactor in equation 3 is independent of phase, and accounts for a slow reduction in the intensity of I_h near B and B' where $S_g = 0$. The intensity approaches the two-beam value near A and A'. From equation 3 we see that for thicknesses $t = (n + 1/4) \xi_h$ the intensity is most sensitive to changes in U_h^{eff}, and hence to Ψ. Here the slope of the "Pendellosung" curve is also steepest. The intensity along the hyperbolae has either a maximum on the upper hyperbola ($S_g < 0$) and a minimum on the lower ($S_g > 0$), or the converse, depending on whether $\cos \Psi$ is greater or less than zero. The variation of the effective potential U_h^{eff} with excitation error for several values of the three-phase invariant is shown in figure 3. Values of U_g have been taken from tables[26]. Experimentally it is difficult to measure the electron intensity along the hyperbolae, rather, we have taken line scans parallel to KL_{hg} in figure 2 at several places cutting both hyperbolae, and compared the results with many-beam calculations. In this way a value of Ψ may be refined. It is clear that the most sensitive region for such a scan is at the minimum shown in figure 3.

EXPERIMENTAL RESULTS

Crushed samples of single-crystal hexagonal CdS were examined in a Philips EM400T electron microscope at room temperature. CBED patterns were obtained using a probe size of about 100nm, and recorded on film. The processed negatives were read into a VAX 750 computer using a CCD camera to minimize field distortion. This method is quick and convenient and takes advantage of the large storage capacity of film. However the resulting patterns include an inelastic background. For the systematics orientation, where one-dimensional data is used we have found an energy loss spectrometer useful for recording the elastic intensity[24]. The pattern is scanned, under computer control, over the spectrometer entrance slit. We have also developed a liquid nitrogen cooled YAG-CCD detection system with large dynamic range for parallel detection on the electron microscope[27]. Using this system, which reads two-dimensional data directly into a computer, we expect increased accuracy in phase determination because of its larger dynamic range (14 bits).

The subtraction of the background due to inelastic scattering presents special problems in two-dimensional patterns. For this work the background was treated as follows. A point diffraction pattern taken from the same region used for anaylsis was recorded under identical conditions, and read into the computer. The resulting peaks were then fitted to the Lorentzian function which describes small angle scattering by electronic excitations, plasmons and some phonons[28].This was convoluted with a top-hat

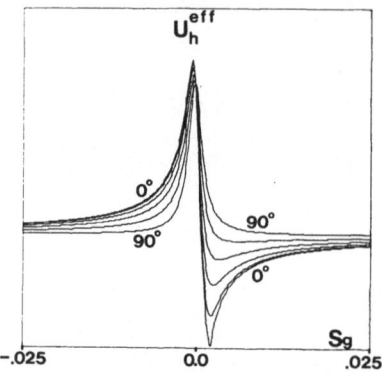

<u>Figure 3.</u>   Variation of the effective potential U_h^{eff} with excitation error for equal increments in the phase invariant between 0 and 90°. This quantity is related to the intensity in three-beam CBED patterns along AB $(S_g < 0)$ and B' A' $(S_g > 0)$ (see figure 2).

function representing the incident beam-divergence (for the point pattern), and the result convoluted with the results of the many-beam calculations. This procedure avoids the noise amplification problems which are well known to be associated with deconvolution.

Figure 4(a) shows the pattern used for analysis, while figure 4(b) shows an enlarged view of the (41-4) CBED disc, and the positions of two line scans taken across it. These lines run parallel to KL_{hg} in figure 2. The central intensity minimum in the upper hyperbola is due to an additional interaction (the (00-6)), which is fully included in the many-beam calculations.

DISCUSSION AND CONCLUSIONS

The many-beam Bloch-wave calculations for the intensity along X-X' and Y-Y' in figure 4(b) depend on the following parameters, which were found as follows : 1. The accelerating voltage was determined from an analysis of HOLZ line positions. 2. Absorption coefficients for reflection g were obtained by matching the asymmetry in the (000) disc against calculations with reflection g at the Bragg angle. We find $U'(0,0,-2)/U(0,0,2) = 0.08 \pm 0.005$ and $U'(0,0,6)/U(0,0,6) = 0.1$. This allows a parametric fit to be made to the absorption potential[6] of the form

$$U'_g/U_g = -0.13g + 0.03g^2 \qquad\qquad 5$$

This expression was used to obtain values for the other U'_g required in the many-beam calculation. Note that since CdS is non-centrosymmetric, both U'_g and U_g are complex. By taking their ratio to be a real constant, we assume that the phases of the

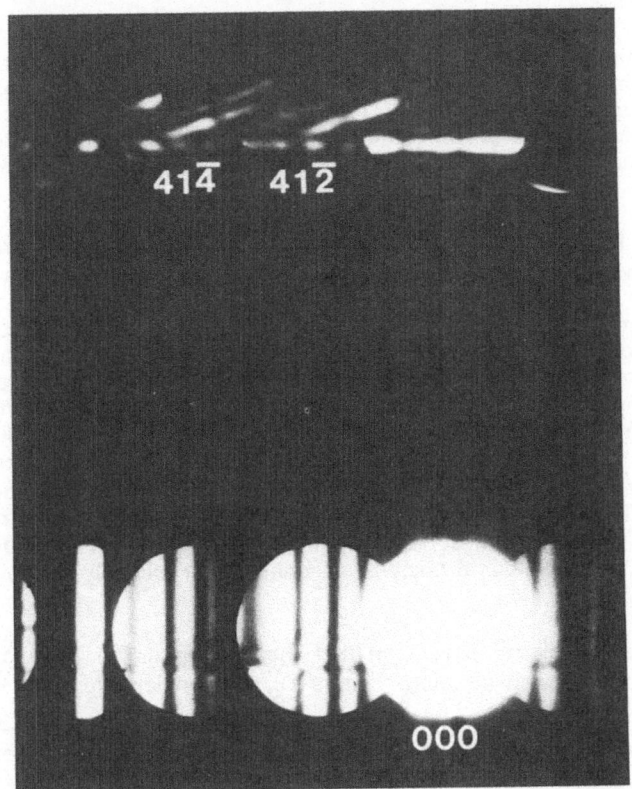

Figure 4(a). Small camera-length view of the CBED pattern used to determine a three-phase invariant in CdS. The three strong beams are indexed. All others carrying appreciable intensity are also included in the calculations shown in figure 5.

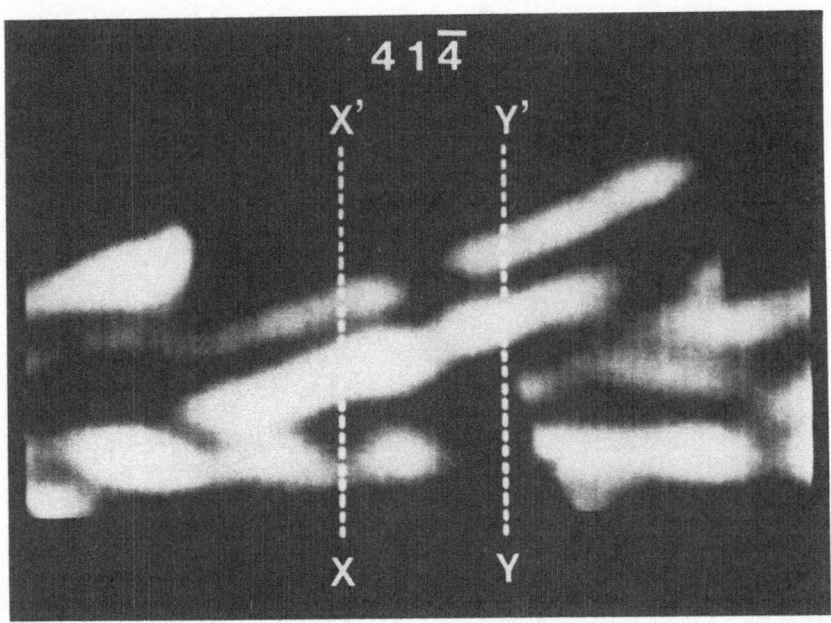

Figure 4(b). Enlarged view of the (41-4) CBED disc used for analysis. The lines indicate the positions of the intensity profiles shown in figure 5.

absorption potential's coefficients are equal to those of the real (elastic scattering) potential. 3. The specimen thickness was found to be 86.5 ± 0.5 nm from a comparison of 32-beam calculations with the (00h) systematics - in particular the outer thickness-sensitive fringes of the (00-4) disc were used. Data was read from film into the computer, again using a CCD camera. 4. Debye-Waller factors were taken from recent accurate X-ray work[29].

Figures 5 (a) and (b) shows a comparison of the experimental intensity (crosses) and the results of fifteen-beam calculations for two cuts across the hyperbolae. Calculations are shown for several values of the three-phase invariant, differing by 5°. Unfortunately the most sensitive region could not be used, since it is disturbed by the (4,1,0) interaction, which causes the gap in figure 4(b). The calculations solve the time-independant Schroedinger equation by the eigenvalue (Bloch wave) method for a 120kV electron traversing a thin slab of parallel-sided non-centrosymmetric crystal which may be inclined to the beam. Absorption is included. The renormalised eigenvector method is used[13], and all HOLZ reflections included. The FORTRAN source code has been published[14]. In fact, only the phase of the (002) structure factor has been changed in figure 5. Since three-beam theory depends only on the sum of the three relevant phases, this procedure is strictly correct only to the extent that the many-beam pattern is three-beam like. (For a general many-beam pattern, the intensity depends on individual phases).

From figure 5 we find that the sum ψ of the phases of the (41-4), (41-2) and (00-2) electron structure factors U_g (dimensions length $^{-2}$) in hexagonal CdS is 49.6 ± 5°. The value of the position parameter assumed was 0.37717[29], which also gives a theoretical value of $\Psi = 49.6°$ if neutral atom scattering factors are used.

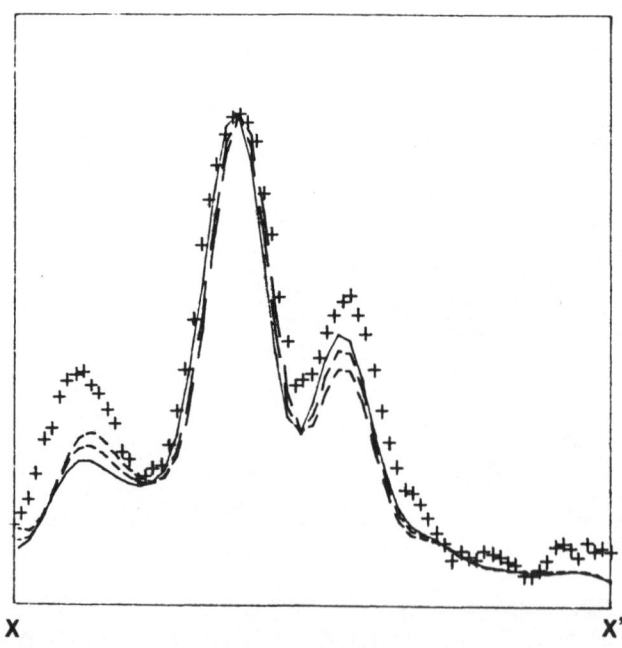

X   X'

<u>Figure 5(a)</u> Comparison of experimental intensity (crosses) and the results of fifteen-beam dynamical calculations for the intensity along the lines X-X' indicated in figure 4(b) for several values of the three-phase invariant (49.6°, 54.6°, 59.6°). The best fit is obtained for $\Psi = 49.6°$.

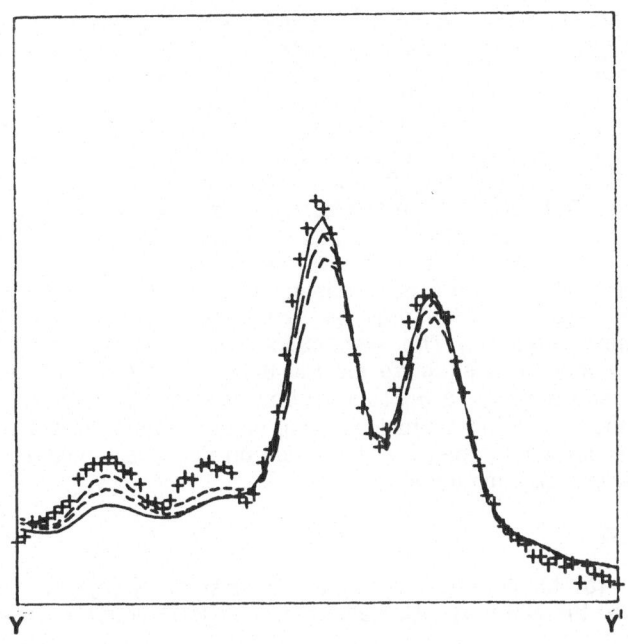

Y   Y'

Figure 5(b). Similar to figure 5(a) but for the line Y-Y' in figure 4(b).

We may conclude that: (1) the three-beam non-systematics CBED geometry provides a useful general method for obtaining approximate values of the three-phase structure invariants. Because we were not able to use the most sensitive region of the CBED pattern in this work, we are unable to assess its accuracy fully. (2) Assuming that accurate Debye-Waller factors are available, the most important limitation to the accuracy of this method is the uncertainty in the estimate of background due to inelastic scattering, which has a two-dimensional variation, and the possibility of accidental reflections obscuring the sensitive region of the pattern.

Similar information may be obtained from electron channelling patterns. (For an analysis of the three-beam case in non-centrosymmetric crystals and its application to channelling, see [30]). These structure invariants may be used as starting values for structure refinement by other methods, for which they provide useful constraints.

Our most recent research[23] also suggests that, in particular cases, the systematics geometry may also be used for accurate phase measurements. This in turn would allow the refinement of atom positions and measurements of bonding charge distributions. For CdS (which is a one-parameter structure) it appears possible to determine the phase of U(00-2) by this method with an accuracy of about 0.5° if the position parameter is assumed known. Alternatively, if an ionicity is assumed, it would be possible to determine the dimensionless atomic position parameter to within about ± 0.0005. These ionicity and atomic co-ordinate effects might be disentangled from a series of patterns emphasising different orders. For example, we find that the (004) structure factor phase is very sensitive to u, whereas the phase of the (002) depends more strongly on bonding.

In comparing some of the various methods which have been proposed for electron crystallography, our experience suggests that the three-beam non-systematics method is the most generally useful for non-centrosymmetric crystals requiring phase determination. However, it requires the handling of large two-dimensional data sets, and is limited in accuracy by the two-dimensional nature of the background which must be subtracted. Energy filtering is not usually possible. The systematics geometry facilitates energy filtering, and any remaining (phonon) background may be estimated from scans taken outside the CBED discs, since this background is also one-dimensional. However only in some cases[23] is sensitivity to phase obtained in the systematics geometry. (To the extent that the rocking-curve in a satisfied reflection is two-beam like, it is not sensitive to phase. However the perturbation acting on a first-order reflection from a satisfied second order reflection may be extremely sensitive at certain voltages in non-centrosymmetric crystals.) The systematics geometry also has the advantage of providing many independent structure factors, unlike the more accurate critical voltage method[9], which provides only a relationship between structure factors. The intersecting Kikuchi line method[11] can also provide useful approximate values of structure factors, and is by far the easiest to apply since it relies on distance measurements taken from film, rather than intensity measurements.

Acknowledgements

We are thank Prof M.O'Keeffe for useful discussions. Supported by N.S.F. grant DMR8741208, and the N.S.F.-A.S.U. National Center for Electron Microscopy.

REFERENCES

1. P.J.E.Aldred and M.Hart, Proc Roy. Soc. Lond. A332, 223 (1973)
2. J.M.Cowley, Acta Cryst. 6, 516 (1953).
3. C.H.MacGillavary, Physica 7, 329 (1940).
4. D.J.Smart and C.J.Humphreys, Inst.Phys. Conf. Ser. 41, 14 (1978).
5. P.Goodman. Acta Cryst. A32 7932 (1976).
6. R.Voss, G.Lehmpfuhl and D.J.Smith Z.Naturforsch 59, 973 (1980).
7. R.Vincent, D.M.Bird and J.W.Steeds, Phil. Mag. A50, 765 (1984).
8. T.Shishido and N.Tanaka , Phys Stat. Sol. (a)383, 453 (1976).
9. J.R.Sellar, D.Imeson and C.J.Humphreys, Acta Cryst. A36, 686 (1980).
10. K.Gjonnes,J.Gjonnes,J.Zuo and J.C.H.Spence,Acta Cryst(1988) in press.
11. J.Tafto and J.Gjonnes Ultramicros. 17, 329 (1985). See also H. Matsuhata, Y.Tomokiyo, H. Watanabe and T. Eguchi. Acta. Cryst. B40, 544 (1984).
12. For a review ,see C.J.Humphreys. Rep. Prog. Phys. 42 ,1825 (1979).
13. A.L.Lewis, R.E.Villagrana and A.J.F.Metherell, Acta Cryst. A34,13 (1978)
14. J.M.Zuo K. Gjonnes and J.C.H.Spence. J. Micros. Technique. (1988) in press.
15. S.Chang, Cryst.Reviews, 1, 87 (1987).
16. K. Kambe, J.Phys.Soc.Jap.12, 1 (1957)
17. J.Gjonnes and R.Hoier,Acta Cryst. A27, 313, (1971)
18. Hurley, A.C. and Moodie, A.F. (1980) Acta Cryst. A36, 737
19. Hoier, R. and Marthinsen. Acta Cryst. (1983) A39, 854.
20. D.Bird, R.James and A.R. Preston,Phys.Rev.Letts. 59, 1216 (1987).
21. Marthinsen, K., Matsuhata, H., Hoier, R. and Gjonnes, J. (1987) Austr. J. Phys. In Press.
22. R. Hoier, J.M.Zuo, K.Marthinsen and J.C.H.Spence , Ultramicros. (1988) In Press.
23 J.M. Zuo, J.C.H.Spence and R. Hoier. Ultramicros. (1988) in press.
24. J.M.Zuo, J.C.H.Spence and M. O'Keeffe (1988). Phys. Rev. Letts 61, 353.
25. J.M.Zuo, R. Hoier and J.C.H.Spence (1988) Acta Cryst. In press.
26. International Tables for X-ray Crystallography. Vol 4. (Eds. J.A.Ibers and W.C.Hamilton, Kynoch Press, Birmingham) 1974.Tables 2.2A and 2.4.6A.
27. J.C.H.Spence and J.M.Zuo. J.Sci. Instr. (1988). In press.
28. R.F.Egerton. Electron Energy Loss Spectroscopy in the Electron Microscope. Plenum, (1986).
29. A.W.Stevenson, M. Milanko and Z. Barnea (1984). Acta Cryst. B40, 521.
30. K.Marthinsen and R. Hoier (1988). Acta Cryst. A44, 588

EDX AND EELS STUDIES OF SEGREGATION IN STEM

J.M. Titchmarsh and I.A. Vatter

Fracture Studies Group
Harwell Laboratory
Didcot, Oxon, OX11 0RA, UK

INTRODUCTION

Segregation in materials can be broadly divided into two types; equilibrium (ES) and non-equilibrium (NES). In the former[1] the segregating species is assumed to have reached a steady-state equilibrium at a particular temperature such that the rate of capture at a sink exactly balances the rate of evaporation from the sink by thermal excitation. Subsequent rapid cooling to room temperature does not significantly alter the segregation profile. A simple concentration step change can be assumed to occur at the matrix-sink interface, with no significant concentration gradients present in the adjacent matrix. With NES, the concentration profile at the boundary is determined by the capture of solute atoms during quenching from an elevated temperature[2] and so solute concentration gradients occur in the matrix adjacent to the boundary. The extent of the profiles is determined by the diffusion rates of the migrating species, and these can also be on the scale of inter-planar spacings. Much wider depletion and segregation profiles can also be produced by precipitation reactions at grain boundaries during high temperature anneals. Although point defects and linear defects can trap solute atoms, in this paper we shall consider sinks to be two-dimensional, i.e. grain boundaries, precipitate/matrix interfaces.

In the field of metallurgy, segregation can be both beneficial and deleterious. For example, the toughness of many low-alloy ferritic steels can be reduced by the phenomenon of reversible temper embrittlement, caused by the ES at grain boundaries of minor impurity elements such as phosphorus, tin and antimony[3]. The sensitisation of grain boundaries to corrosive attack in stainless steels is due to chromium depletion in the matrix adjacent to grain boundaries[4], caused by the growth of chromium-rich precipitates on the boundaries. Boron segregation can improve creep ductility in steels[5], and rare earth segregation to grain boundaries can reduce oxidation and spallation rates from stainless steels[6].

The relevance of segregation studies in the field of semiconductor materials characterisation is not as obvious. In silicon device technology the development of very high purity single-crystal wafers and homoepitaxial growth has completely avoided grain boundary problems in many instances. However, the use of polysilicon, the recrystallisation of silicon rendered amorphous during processing by ion-implantation, and metallisation/contact processes can all produce interfaces where segregation might conceivably affect device integrity. ES is often assumed to occur within one or two atomic distances of a boundary. Present MBE and MOCVD methods are capable of making III-V devices with layer thicknesses on this scale. Consequently, the measurement of grain boundary segregation in metal alloy systems by analytical electron microscopy (AEM) is then a similar problem to the measurement of composition changes in such epitaxial structures. Indeed, in some respects the semiconductor problem should be easier to analyse because the structure is simple and the chemical species known, whereas a grain boundary in a steel is generally curved, decorated by precipitates, contains unexpected chemical species and image interpretation is generally more difficult.

In this paper we shall describe the general features relating to the measurement of interfacial segregation by Energy-Dispersive X-ray Analysis (EDX) and Electron Energy-Loss spectroscopy (EELS) by AEM. Whether the specimen is metallic, ceramic or semiconducting is usually of little importance when considering the relevent parameters. Features specific to semiconductors will be emphasised where appropriate. It is assumed that the reader has a basic understanding of the principles of EDX and EELS, detailed descriptions of which can be found in many publications[7,8].

SPECIMEN CONSIDERATIONS

In order to derive meaningful quantitative information about segregation it is important to optimise and control the experimental conditions. Concentration gradients will be a maximum in a direction normal to an interface. If a specimen contains small particles which are completely embedded then the electron probe samples regions of varying concentration and detailed quantitative information is very difficult to deconvolute. Experiments are usually performed with selected interfaces which extend right through the foil and which are flat. Double-tilting stages are preferable so that the specimen can be tilted until the interface plane is parallel to the incident beam direction (Fig.1). In practice there is always likely to be a small misorientation the size of which will be related to the local thickness of the foil and the imaging conditions. It has been suggested[9] that a realistic orientation error in a conventional TEM/STEM AEM can be +/- 4°, but this seems very pessimistic. In a dedicated STEM we can routinely minimise boundary contrast widths to less than 2nm in foils of 100nm thickness (Fig.2), and orientation asymmetries can be noted from bright-field phase-contrast image detail when going through focus. Under such conditions a tilting accuracy of +/- 1° or better is probably achievable. For EDX analysis additional constraints are imposed by the tilting ranges over which a direct line of sight occurs between the point of analysis and the x-ray detector, whereas the full tilting range is usually available for EELS.

Surface films are almost always present on electron microscope specimens (Fig.1) as a consequence of preparation methods and exposure to the atmosphere. The ideal microscope would have an in-situ ion-milling facility to remove these layers immediately prior to analysis. Silicon, germanium and some compound semiconductors are probably covered by an oxide coating of minimal thickness, but compounds containing aluminium, for example, could attract thick films. Many semiconductor device samples, ion-milled as transverse sections, could be covered by a thin film of sputtered products, and great care must be taken with final preparation to minimise this. Many illustrations can be found in the high-resolution EM

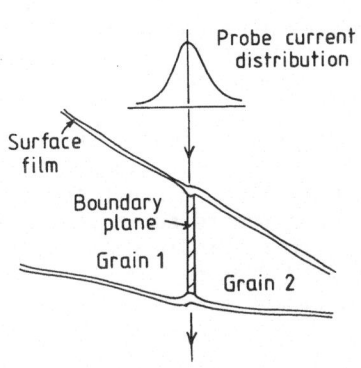
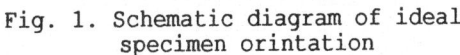

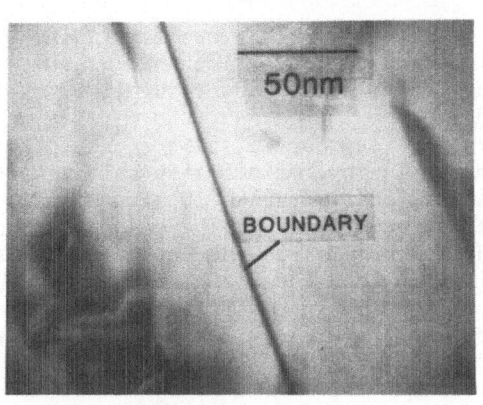

Fig. 1. Schematic diagram of ideal specimen orintation

Fig. 2. Boundary in austenitic steel oriented for analysis

literature which clearly show the presence of amorphous material beyond the crystal structure contrast in thin films at the edge of the hole in the specimen. Provided that the foil thickness is much greater than the surface film thickness, or the thickness and composition of surface layers can be determined by additional measurements, such layers should not prevent measurements of interfacial segregation, although accuracy will obviously be limited. An exception to this can occur when the interface is grooved along the surface during foil preparation and subsequently becomes a site for deposition of spurious material which cannot be quantified.

For both EDX and EELS it is advisable to avoid strongly diffracting conditions for several reasons. First, in polycrystalline materials the boundary contrast is clearer when strong diffraction contrast from matrix bend contours, thickness fringes or defects is absent. Second, channelling effects[10] can cause large variations in relative characteristic edge ionisation rates which greatly complicate data analysis. Third, the presence of coherent bremsstrahlung peaks could obscure the detection of small characteristic peaks from segregated species. Unfortunately, when analysing semiconductor epitaxial growth defects and quantum well structures it is often necessary to excite strongly the 200 reflections in order to see clearly the features of interest, and to ensure that the interface planes are closely parallel to the beam[11]. However, many-beam dynamical calculations suggest that the channelling effects in ordered alloys which could occur under such conditions become negligible provided that the electron probe convergence angle is greater than a few milleradians, which is usually the case for practical analysis[12].

The choice of foil thickness is often limited by various factors beyond the control of the analyst, eg. precipitation or interface curvature. When possible a compromise must be reached between increasing the foil thickness, both to improve the counting statistics and to reduce the relative contribution from surface artefacts, and decreasing the thickness to minimise "beam broadening" (for EDX) or multiple inelastic scattering (for EELS). A more detailed discussion of sensitivity and statistics will be given below.

A further problem is the reduction of drift during analysis. Ideally, adequate time should always be given for complete stabilisation of the stage and power supplies, but significant drift is still possible during prolonged analysis periods when working with high spatial resolution. For EDX this can be checked and partly corrected either manually, by periodically halting acquisition to reposition the probe, or automatically using either a one-dimensional[13] or a two-dimensional[14] image correlation system. The one-dimensional system will not correct for any drift parallel to the boundary. For serial signal recording in EELS, drift is a more serious problem than for EDX because it is highly possible that characteristic edges are recorded from slightly different locations on the specimen. Parallel data recording[15,16] will significantly reduce drift-related errors in EELS.

Although semiconductor specimens are usually stable during electron microscope investigation, under an intense, static electron probe it is possible to cause damage; holes can be drilled through InP[12], for example. Significant sputtering from the specimen surface can also occur at incident electron energies well below those required for bulk Frenkel pair production[17]. Moreover, sputtering rates are different for the component species of an alloy, and this is likely to affect high spatial resolution analysis in many compound semiconductor systems as smaller, brighter electron probes are used with increasing energy.

ELECTRON PROBE CURRENT DISTRIBUTION

In Fig.1 the electron probe is represented schematically by a normal current distribution centred at some distance, x, from the boundary plane. This is clearly an idealised representation, but one which is easy to use for modelling and calculating segregation. ES can be detected and measured with probes formed using thermal electron emission[18,19], but the current is very small unless the probe diameter is tens of nanometers; although the errors due to drift are then negligibly small, the size of the segregant signal relative to that from the matrix decreases as the probe diameter increases, and characteristic peaks become lost in the background. In addition, NES and diffusion profiles which can be very narrow, require the use of probe diameters significantly smaller than the profile width for meaningful measurements to be acquired. For these reasons the sensitivity will improve as the probe size falls, and it is therefore important to consider the shape of the electron current in very small probes when estimates of sensitivity limits are required for EDX and EELS.

Wave optics calculations[20-23] can be used to determine the theoretical distribution of probe current as a function of the electron beam energy, the energy-spread of the beam, the distance from the Gaussian focal plane in the axial direction, and the aberration coefficients of the electron optical system. A point object source in usually assumed, which implies that the Gaussian image of the source has no radial extension. While this might be close to reality for some optical configurations of a STEM with a field emission source, increased signal yields are often obtained by using

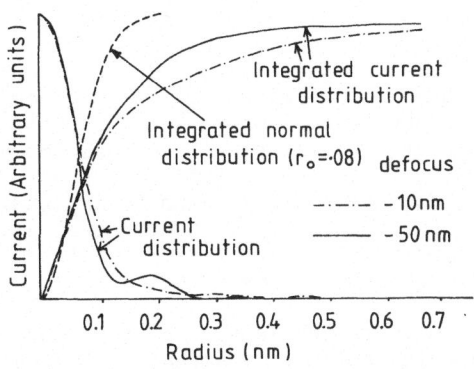

Fig. 3. Examples of point-spread functions and integrated
current distributions for 300keV electrons.

probes with a finite Gaussian image. The wave-optical, point-source
distribution must then be convoluted with the Gaussian image of the source
to derive a more realistic radial current distribution[23]. Examples of
point-source spread functions are shown in Fig.3 for a 300keV beam with
different amounts of defocus, using an objective lens with a spherical
aberration coefficient of 1mm. Such a system should be available in the
near future. The principal features of these distributions are a large
axial peak only weakly dependent on defocus, and an oscillating tail, the
fluctuations of which depend critically on the defocus. A normal
distribution can be fitted to the axial peak with an r_0 of ~0.08 nm. (r_0^2
is the variance of the normal curve). However, the distributions of
current integrated as a function of radial distance are different, the
normal curve being much narrower than the point-spread functions. If the
probe "diameter" is defined as that distance within which a given
percentage of the current lies (usually taken as 80 or 90%) then a small
change in focus can greatly affect the probe size. The integrated current
curves for the point-spread functions still retain shapes which are
similar to that for the normal curve close to the axis, but deviate with
increasing r. It is not possible to fit another integrated normal curve
which accurately models the integrated current distributions over the full
range of r. Even so, these curves suggest that analysis on the scale of
the inter-planar spacing in many materials will soon be feasible,and
recent images obtained using the large-angle, annular dark-field detector
in a FEG-STEM with an objective lens spherical aberration coefficient of
1.2mm, at an accelerating voltage of 100keV, support this prediction[24].

The effect of chromatic aberration and the spread of electron energy
in the beam can also be predicted using wave optics. For the conditions
used to calculate the curves in Fig.3, an energy spread of 0.5eV and a
chromatic aberration coefficient of 3mm would not change significantly the
current distributions. The stability of the microscope power supplies
would probably be of greater importance.

When an extended Gaussian image of the source is used and the point-
spread function is convoluted with this image, the general result is that
any fluctuations in the tail of the point-spread function are smoothed. If

the size of the Gaussian image is greater than the central peak of the point-spread function then the resultant probe current distribution tends to assume the shape of the Gaussian image. Thus, if the common assumption is made that the extended source image has a normal current distribution, it is reasonable to assume that a normal distribution of current can be used to model, to a first approximation, the measurement of interfacial segregation. However, the elastic scattering of the fast electrons as they pass through the foil can change the intensity and radial distribution of the probe, and affect the accuracy of measurements. Allowance must be made for this "beam-broadening" effect using Monte Carlo or similar calculations, and this will be discussed below.

A final point to note is that when the probe current is high it is possible to use very thin foils for examination and still maintain adequate counting statistics. Not only is this advantageous for reducing beam-broadening, but the range of variation in the radial extent of the probe current distribution between entrance and exit surfaces arising as a consequence of focussing a very narrow probe is limited. A further advantage is that any diffraction-broadening of the probe[25] will also be minimised. These factors will be important when trying to achieve the ultimate sensitivity and spatial resolution.

The accurate measurement of probe current distribution is very demanding and relatively inaccurate, particularly when the diameter is <5nm and the current ~1nA. Very few AEM reports can be found in the literature which show the results of probe size measurements, and in many cases the nominal probe size, as stated by the equipment manufacturer is assumed without any attempt to confirm such numbers. It is most important that measurements of probe size are made if reasonably accurate estimates of segregation concentrations and sensitivity limits are required, particularly when working with very small probe diameters.

MODELLING

For both EDX and EELS, spectrum analysis yields an atomic or weight concentration estimate, corrected for various factors such as absorption and fluorescence (EDX), or multiple scattering (EELS). The problem is then to relate such compositional data to the real segregation profile by a suitable model which incorporates the relevant parameters, e.g. segregation distribution, probe current distribution, foil thickness, sample geometry, matrix composition, electron scattering within the foil[26,27]. The uncertainties in some of these parameters are always large enough to ensure that any calculation is, at best, only a good estimate of the real situation. Foil thickness is measured most conveniently in the microscope using EELS, with an accuracy better than 10% in many cases[28], and the matrix composition determined during the course of the experiment with better accuracy still. Uncertainties in geometry mainly affect the accuracy of EDX absorption corrections, and are likely to have only a small effect. The distribution of segregation, the probe current distribution and the detailed scattering behaviour of fast electrons in crystals at arbitrary orientation are the most important variable factors. The probe size probably exceeds the thickness of any ES, and the latter can be assumed to occupy some fraction of one or two planes of atoms. (Such an assumption is supported in the case of ferritic steels by surface analysis experiments.) A normal probe current distribution, the limited justification for which has already been discussed, is usually assumed for mathematical convenience, and the scattering is modelled according to one of several possible expressions for differential angular cross-sections. By assuming, a priori, the shape of the segregation distribution, the model can predict the fractional boundary layer coverage. More complex models for segregation profiles, e.g. a normal distribution, lead to a continuous range of possible solutions. Diffusion profiles on a scale much larger than the probe diameter are hardly worth modelling as the experimental results provide a fairly accurate distribution. When the scale of NES or a diffusion profile is similar to the probe size, however, the greatest difficulties arise because the statistical accuracy of the experimental data is unlikely to be good enough to distinguish between small changes in the assumed shapes of current and chemical profiles.

For ES we have chosen to use a Monte Carlo method to determine the distribution of scattered electron trajectories in the segregated layer and the matrix. The Monte Carlo programme is similar to that developed by others for thin foil AEM applications[29], employs a screened Rutherford scattering cross-section, and can incorporate a wide range of specimen geometries. This has been used to predict profiles of measured composition as the probe is moved across boundaries with different widths, amounts of segregation and orientation in a range of foil thicknesses[23]. A linear least-squares method is then used to obtain the optimised fit to a given set of experimental data, together with the best estimate of the fraction of a monolayer of segregated species at the boundary. The accuracy of this approach has recently been confirmed by direct comparison with surface analysis[30].

A principal result of such calculations is that the effect of high-angle elastic scattering is negligible in degrading the apparent spatial resolution of profiles of ES, even in a foil of thickness equal to several mean free paths of the elastic scattering. This is illustrated for the case of a 25% monolayer of phosphorus segregation in iron in Fig.4. The principal effect of elastic scattering is to reduce the maximum of the profile, and to extend the tailing of the profile. These and other calculations suggest that the total integrated area of the profile is approximately constant for a given amount of segregation, no matter what probe size, orientation or foil thickness is used[23]. Hence, if the statistical accuracy of the data points in an experimental profile was sufficient, it would not be necessary to determine these parameters experimentally, but simply to scale the measured integrated profile area to a single calculated profile area in order to determine the fractional monolayer coverage of the interface. However, the statistical accuracy is rarely good enough except for large amounts of segregation; in practice, it is usually more accurate to align the boundary, use a known probe size and measure the local foil thickness, and then compare the experiment with a calculation made for the specific, measured parameters.

In very thin foils the effects of high-angle elastic scattering are negligibly small to the point where a simple analytic calculation can be used to estimate the amount of ES[31]. The measured profile is a simple convolution of the incident probe current distribution and the (assumed) atomically-sharp segregation profile; this simply gives the probe current profile projected into a diametral plane. For a radially symmetric probe with a normal distribution, this projection is also a normal distribution which can be represented as:

$$i = (i_o / x_o (2 \pi)^{1/2}) . \exp (-x^2 / x_0^2) \qquad (1)$$

This has an integrated area equal to unity and a second moment (variance) of x_0^2. The fractional ratio, R, of electron trajectory path lengths in the segregation and in the matrix can be written as:

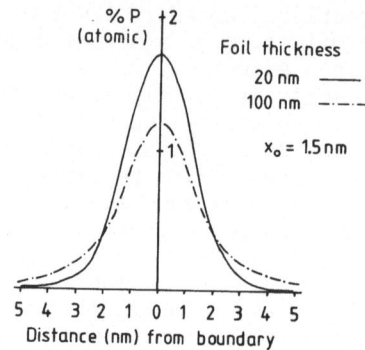

Fig. 4. Monte Carlo calculations of
concentration profiles of
P segregated in Fe

$$R = (f \delta / x_0 (2 \pi)^{1/2}) / (1 - f \delta / x_0 (2\pi)^{1/2})$$
$$\sim f \delta / x_0 (2 \pi)^{1/2} \qquad\qquad (2)$$

when $f < 1$, and $x_0 \gg \delta$. f is the fractional concentration of the
segregant atoms in the boundary layer of thickness δ. R can be related
directly to the atomic concentrations derived from the analysis of the
experimental spectrum to estimate f. Alternatively, the ES can be equated
to a uniform distribution of solute under the probe, such that $R = n_s / n_m$
where n_s and n_m are the solute and matrix atomic densities, respectively:
this equivalence will be used later to derive an estimate for the
detection limit.

STATISTICAL CONSIDERATIONS

When measuring ES in particular, it is important to estimate the
confidence limits and statistical errors associated with the detection of
a small peak, S, on a large background, B. A detailed treatment of this
problem has been given elsewhere[32], but we shall employ a simpler, less
rigorous analysis to estimate detection limits. In Fig.5 are shown,
schematically, an EDX peak and an EELS ionisation edge. In both cases, S
is found by subtracting the best estimate of B from the total counts, T,
in the appropriate energy window of the spectrum. The statistical variance
of S, var(S), is then the sum of the variances of T and B.

Then: $$\mathrm{var} (T) = T = S + B \sim B \qquad\qquad (3)$$

when S is very small, so that:

$$\mathrm{var} (S) \sim B + \mathrm{var} (B) \qquad\qquad (4)$$

The signal-to-noise ratio, SNR, is defined as:

$$SNR = S / (B + \mathrm{var} (B))^{1/2} \qquad\qquad (5)$$

and the limit for signal detection at a confidence level of >99% is usually given by SNR = 3. Thus, an estimate of the variance of B allows an estimate of the detection limit to be made from any spectrum containing statistically significant peaks from segregated species.

Alternatively, theoretical estimates of detection limits for ES can be made based on the methods used previously to derive detection limits for uniformly distributed chemical species[33,34], but incorporating additional features specific to the situation of ES. To achieve this an estimate of var(B) is first required. We shall assume that the backgrounds in Fig. 5 are both linear; this is probably a realistic assumption for many EDX peaks, but less so for EELS. The estimation of var (B) for a more accurate mathematical form for the background shape for EELS, as well as the linear approximation, have been considered by Egerton[8]. The linear background assumption has the advantage of algebraic simplicity while giving estimates of variance similar to those for the more rigorous analysis.

In Fig.5 the zeroes of the energy scales are chosen to simplify the algebra by eliminating covariance terms from the statistical analysis. B and S are determined by optimising the interpolation of the background under the peak for EDX, and extrapolation for EELS. The form of the background in both cases is written as:

$$B = a_0 + a_1 E \qquad\qquad (6)$$

so that: $\mathrm{var}\ (\ B\ )\ =\ (dB/da_0)^2\ \mathrm{var}(a_0)\ +\ (dB/da_1)^2\ \mathrm{var}\ (a_1) \qquad (7)$

For EDX (Fig.5a) the background interpolation is over n channels under the peak, using m adjacent background channels on each side of the peak. For EELS (Fig.5b) the background is fitted over m channels preceding the ionisation edge, and extrapolated for n channels under the edge. Standard

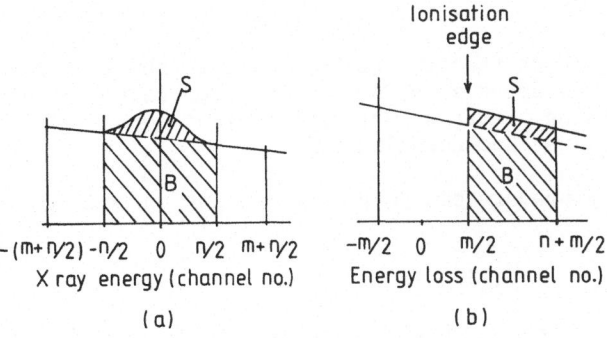

Fig. 5. Windows limits for var(B) calculations: (a) EDX and (b) EELS.

statistical analysis[36] then predicts:

$$\text{var (B)} = n^2 \sigma^2/2m \qquad \text{(EDX)} \qquad (8)$$

and:

$$\text{var (B)} = n^2 \sigma^2(1 + 3(1 + n/m)^2) / m \qquad \text{(EELS)} \qquad (9)$$

σ^2 is the typical variance of a single channel (i.e. $\sigma^2 = B/n$), so that when n = m,

and:
$$\text{var (B)} = B/2 \qquad \text{(EDX)},$$
$$\text{var (B)} = 13B \qquad \text{(EELS)} \qquad (10)$$

Combining Eq. 5 and Eq. 10 gives:

$$\text{SNR} = S/ (1.5 B)^{1/2} \qquad \text{(EDX)}$$
and:
$$\text{SNR} = S/ (14 B)^{1/2} \qquad \text{(EELS)} \qquad (11)$$

Thus, the SNR estimate is smaller for EDX than for EELS by a factor of about three, for similar numbers of counts, which simply reflects the greater accuracy of interpolation compared with extrapolation. For EDX the value of S can be calculated using standard expressions for x-ray production and detection. Similarly, B can be calculated using a suitable expression for the bremsstrahlung cross-section for the matrix composition[36]; alternatively, the bremsstrahlung cross-section can be measured experimentally relative to the matrix cross-section for characteristic x-ray production, and scaled expressions for matrix x-ray intensities used in Eq.11. Thus:

$$S = n_s I \tau t \sigma_s w_s a_s e_s \Omega \qquad \text{and} \qquad B = n_m I \tau t \sigma_m{}^s e_s \Omega \qquad (12)$$

where: I is the incident electron flux, τ is the analysis time, t is the foil thickness, Ω is the fractional solid angle subtended at the specimen by the detector, e_s is the detector efficiency at the energy of the signal characteristic energy, w_s is the x-ray fluorescent yield of the ionisation event for chacteristic signal x-rays, a_s is the partition function of the signal characteristic line, σ_s is the ionisation cross-section for a signal atom ionisation, and $\sigma_m{}^s$ is the cross-section for bemsstrahlung produced by the matrix and integrated under the signal peak. Combining Eq.2, Eq.11 and Eq.12, with the assumptions that SNR = 3, and R = n_s / n_m yields an expression for the minimum detectable fraction of a monolayer, f_{min}, which can be detected using EDX.

$$f_{min} = 3x_0 (2\pi h \sigma_m{}^s)^{1/2} / \delta\sigma_s w_s a_s (I\tau t \ n_m \ e_s \ \Omega)^{1/2} \qquad (13)$$

It can then be shown that the probe diameter from a thermal electron source needs to be about an order of magnitude larger than that from a cold field emission electron source to achieve equal sensitivity for a given foil thickness and counting time.

The same procedure can be used to derive an equivalent equation for EELS.

$$f_{min} = (3x_0/\sigma_s\delta) (2h\pi\sigma_B{}^s /n_B I\tau t)^{1/2} .\exp(t/2\lambda_e) \qquad (14)$$

σ_s and $\sigma_B{}^s$ are now, respectively, the partial differential cross-section for the ionisation edge of the segregated species, and the partial

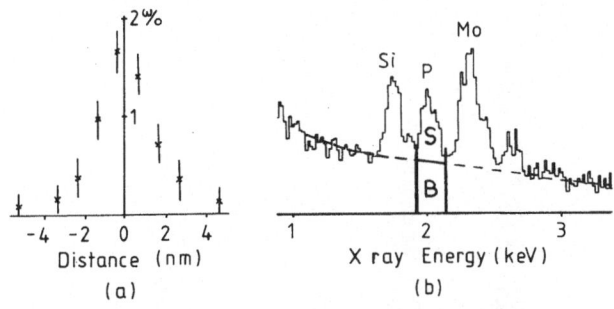

Fig. 6. Phosphorus segregation in a ferritic steel: (a) measured profile, and (b) part of spectrum with probe on boundary.

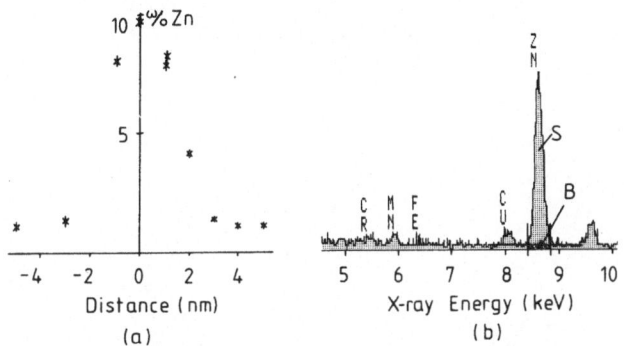

Fig. 7. Zinc segregation in an aluminium alloy: (a) measured zinc profile (b) part of spectrum with probe positioned at grain boundary.

differential cross-section of the background from the matrix, both integrated over the appropriate collection half-angle and the same energy window at the characteristic edge of the segregated species. The factor $\exp(t/2\lambda_e)$ allows for the proportion of the total electron beam elastically scattered outside the collection aperture[8]. (λ_e is the mean free path for elastic scattering). τ is typically a fraction of a second for serial data collection, or many seconds for parallel data collection, the latter giving a much lower value of f_{min}.

COMPARISON OF EXPERIMENT AND THEORY

The experimental results shown in this section were all recorded

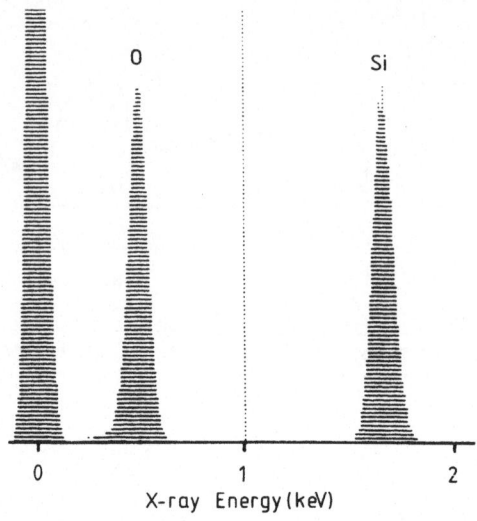

Fig. 8. Low-energy EDX spectrum from amorphous
silica showing relative sizes of O-K
and Si-K characteristic peaks.

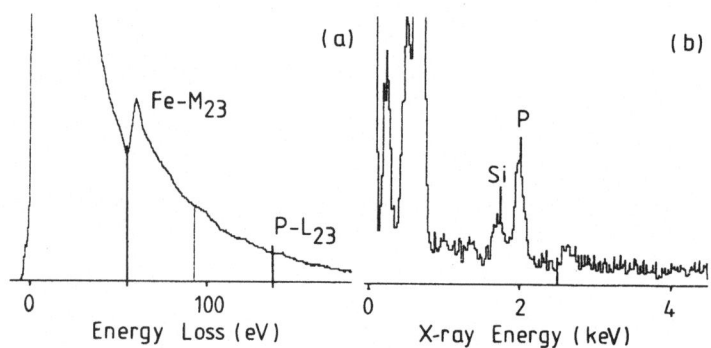

Fig. 9. Comparison of signals from P segregated at a grain boundary
in a ferritic steel: (a) P-L_{23} in EELS and (b) P-K in EDX.

using a VG Microscope HB501 dedicated STEM with a cold field emmission
source. An EDX composition profile showing ES of phosphorus at a grain
boundary in a ferritic steel is shown in Fig.6a. In Fig.6b is shown part
of the spectrum obtained with the probe right at the boundary; the
phosphorus peak has a measured SNR of 15.4, or about five times greater
than the detection limit. Monte Carlo modelling for this experiment, using
the measured foil thickness of 18nm, gave a best estimate of 0.42 atom
layers of phosphorus in the boundary plane. The estimate of f_{min} in this
case is, therefore, about 0.08 atom layers. The profile in Fig. 6a can be

used to obtain an estimate of the probe size of $x_o = 1.5$nm. Using Eq.13 and the relevent experimental parameters, the best estimates of which are listed in Table 1, a theoretical value of $f_{min} = 0.057$ atom layers can be calculated. A second example of ES, namely Zn in Al (Fig.7), gave a measured SNR of about 40, with a Monte Carlo estimate of 0.50 atom layers of zinc at the boundary. This suggests a detection limit of about 0.04 atom layers, while the the corresponding theoretical estimate for f_{min} is about 0.023 atom layers (using the parameters listed in Table 1.). The experimental detection limits, therefore, correspond to ~100 atoms of phosphorus and ~50 atoms of zinc, respectively. For both examples the values of f_{min} could have been lowered by a factor of two or three by counting for longer and by increasing the thickness of the foils, and the future availability of a probe similar to that depicted in Fig.3 would reduce the values by an order of magnitude, making the detection of less than 1% of an atomic layer of segregation routine for many materials.

Table 1.   Parameters used to calculate f_{min}.

Symbol (Units)		P in Fe (EDX)	Zn in Al (EDX)	O in Si (EDX)	P in Fe (EELS)
σ_s	m²	2 x 10^{-25}	2.5 x 10^{-26}		
w_s		0.07	0.40	7.5 x 10^{-27}	
a_s		1	0.88		
δ	nm	0.2	0.2	0.2	0.2
h		1.5	1.5	1.5	14
n_m	m⁻³	8 x 10^{28}	8 x 10^{28}	5 x 10^{28}	8 x 10^{28}
t	nm	18	50	50	40
Ω		0.08	0.08	0.08	
e_s		0.9	1.0	0.3	
τ	sec.	100	60	100	0.2
I	el/sec	5 x 10^9	5 x 10^9	5 x 10^9	5 x 10^9
σ_m^s	m²	7 x 10^{-27}	8 x 10^{-28}	5 x 10^{-27}	6.8 x 10^{-24}
σ_B^s	m²				8.8 x 10^{-24}
λ_e	nm				17

In view of the development of "windowless" EDX detectors capable of detecting k-shell x-rays from elements of low atomic number (>=5), it is interesting to consider what might be the possible f_{min} for segregation of an element such as oxygen in polycrystalline silicon. Fig.8 shows a spectrum from amorphous silica acquired with such a detector, from which it is possible to deduce an effective k-ratio[37] of 1.14 and, hence, an approximate value for the product $\sigma_o w_o a_o$, which is listed in Table 1. The resulting value of f_{min} is 0.12.

The use of Eq.14 to calculate f_{min} for EELS is complicated by relatively large uncertainties in the integrated partial cross-sections σ_s and σ_B^s, and also λ_e. For example, in the case of phosphorus segregated in a ferritic steel, the P-L_{23} edge lies on the tail of the Fe-M_{23} edge, which cannot be calculated using the commercial software packages presently available, and any multiple scattering perturbations. The value of σ_B^s can be estimated by indirect methods; it can be scaled experimentally to the Fe-L_{23} partial cross-section which can be calculated using the SIGMAL2 code[8]; this method has been used to derive the value in Table 1. The value of λ_e has been calculated from an empirical formula[8].

The estimate for f_{min} for the parameters listed in Table 1 is ~0.17. Experimental results comparing EELS and EDX for ES of phosphorus in a 9%Cr ferritic steel are shown in Fig.9. The energy-loss spectrum was acquired using serial detection, a 0.2 second dwell/channel to compromise the conflicting requirements of maximising counts and minimising drift, an energy window of 100eV, and a collection semi-angle of 9mrad. The spectrum in Fig.9a shows a possible $P-L_{23}$ edge, but the SNR=0.9, and so detection is not certain. Using the same probe configuration and current the EDX spectrum, acquired in 100 seconds, showed a P-K peak with a SNR of ~40. Monte-Carlo calculations suggested a boundary segregation of ~0.9 atom layers, which gives an EDX f_{min} similar to that of the previous example (Fig.6b) in a different alloy. There is a clear inconsistency here between the EDX and EELS estimates because the calculation using Eq.14 suggests that EELS should be able to detect the phosphorus with the conditions employed. Some of the discrepancy could be explained by uncertainties in several of the listed parameters, as already indicated, and clearly, for this particular case, EDX is superior to EELS. However, the use of parallel data recording, with an acquisition time of 100 seconds to equal that of the EDX analysis, had it been available, would have given an experimental SNR of of ~20, comparable with the EDX result.

CONCLUSIONS

The estimation of detection limits for interfacial ES for both EDX and EELS analysis requires knowledge of physical and experimental parameters which often can only be estimated with limited accuracy. The the shape and the magnitude of the probe current, and the distribution of the segregation probably introduce the largest errors.

Specific theoretical and experimental estimates of detection limits for EDX agree to within a factor of two.

For the case of phosphorus in iron, EDX is superior to EELS using serial data recording, but parallel EELS data recording will greatly influence this observation.

Significant improvements in detection limits are possible by using a higher accelerating voltage and objective lenses with lower coefficients of spherical aberration. It is likely that 1% of an atom layer of ES will routinely be detected for many element combinations in the near future.

ACKNOWLEDGEMENTS

This work was undertaken as part of the Underlying Research Programme of the UKAEA.

REFERENCES

1.   D.McLean, "Grain Boundaries in Metals",O.U.P., London,(1957).
2.   T.M.Williams,A.M.Stoneham and D.R.Harries,The segregation of boron
        to grain boundaries in solution treated type 316 austenitic
            stainless steel, Met. Sci. 10:14 (1976).
3.   H.L.Marcus and P.W.Palmberg,Auger fracture surface analysis of a
        temper embrittled 3340 steel, Trans. Met. Soc. AIME 245:1664 (1969).
4.   E.C.Bain, R.H.Aborn and J.J.B.Rutherford, The nature and prevention
        of intergranular corrosion in austenitic stainless steel, Trans. ASM
        21:481 (1933).
5.   J.K.Lai, A set of master curves for the creep ductility of type 316
        stainless steel, J. Nucl. Materials 82:123 (1979).
6.   M.J.Bennett, J.A.Desport, M.R.Houlton, P.A.Labun and J.M.Titchmarsh,
        Inhibition of scale growth on 20Cr-25Ni-Nb stabilised stainless
        steel by yttrium ion implantation revealed by analytical electron
        microscopy, Mater. Sci.Tech. 4:1107 (1988).

7. D.B.Williams,"Practical Analytical Electron Microscopy in Materials Science",Philips Electronic Instruments Inc.,Electron Optics Publishing Group, Mahwah,New Jersey, (1984).

8. R.F.Egerton," Electron Energy-Loss Spectroscopy in the Electron Microscope", Plenum Press, New York, (1986).

9. P.Doig and P.E.J.Flewitt, Measurement of solute profiles across inclined grain boundaries using STEM-EDS microanalysis, in: "EMAG '87 - Analytical Electron Microscopy", G.W.Lorimer, ed., Institute of Metals, London, (1988).

10. J.C.H.Spence and J Tafto, Alchemi: a new technique for locating atoms in small crystals, J.Microscopy 130(II):147 (1983).

11. P.Petroff, Transmission electron microscopy of interfaces in III-V compound semiconductors, J. Vac. Sci. Technol. 14:973 (1977).

12. J.F.Bullock, STEM analysis of nanometre-scale inhomogeneities in semiconductors,D.Phil. Thesis, University of Oxford, (1988)

13. C.R.M.Grosvenor, P.E.Batson, D.A.Smith and C.Wong, As segregation to grain boundaries in Si, Phil. Mag. A 50:409 (1984).

14. S.H.Vale and P.J.Statham, STEM image stabilisation for high resolution microanalysis, in: "Electron Microscopy 1986", proc. XI Int. Congress on Electron Microscopy, T.Imura, S.Maruse and T.Susuki, eds., Japanese Society of Electron Microscopy, 573 (1986).

15. O.L.Krivanek, C.C.Ahn and R.B.Keeney, Parallel detection electron spectrometer using quadrupole lenses, Ultramicroscopy 22:103 (1987).

16. H.Shuman, Parallel recording of electron energy loss spectra, Ultramicroscopy 6:163 (1981)

17. D.Cherns, The surface structure of (111) gold films sputtered in the high voltage electron microscope: A theoretical model, Phil. Mag. 36:1429 (1977).

18. J.R.Michael and D.B.Williams, An analytical electron microscope study of the equilibrium segregation of bismuth in copper, Met. Trans. A 15:99 (1984).

19. P.Doig and P.E.J.Flewitt,The detection of monolayer grain boundary segregation in steels using STEM-EDS x-ray microanalysis, Met. Trans. A 13:1397 (1982).

20. C.Colliex and C.Mory, Quantitative aspects of scanning transmission electron microscopy, in: "Proc. of 25th SUSSP",J.N.Chapman and A.J.Craven, eds., Edinburgh University Press 25:149 (1983).

21. C.Mory,Etude theorique et experimentale de la formation de l'image en microscopie electronique a balayage par transmission, Ph.D. Thesis, Universite de Paris-Sud, Centre D'Orsay, (1985).

22. E.Munro,Calculation of the combined effects of diffraction, spherical aberration, chromatic aberration and finite source size in the SEM, Proc. VIIIth ICXOM, Boston, R Ogilvie and D.Wittry, eds., NBS Washington D.C., paper no. 19 (1977).

23. J.M.Titchmarsh, Materials analysis by STEM-EDX at high spatial resolution, in: "Microbeam Analysis 1988",D.E.Newbury,ed., San Francisco Press Inc., San Francisco, 65 (1988).

24. S.J.Pennycook and L.A.Boatner, Structural and chemical imaging of high T_c superconductors by high resolution STEM, Proc. of Symp. on High Resolution Microscopy of Materials at 1988 Fall Meeting of RMS, Boston, W.Krakow, F.A.Ponce and D.J.Smith, eds., MRS Publications, (1989), in press.

25. L.Marks, Direct observations of diffractive probe spreading, Ultramicroscopy 16:261 (1985).

26. P.Doig and P.E.J.Flewitt, The role of specimen and instrumental parameters in STEM-EDS x-ray microanalysis of thin foils, J. Microscopy 130:377 (1983).

27. A.J.Garrett-Reed, Some considerations of the ultimate spatial resolution acheivable in scanning transmission electron microscopy, in: "SEM/1985/I",O.Johari, ed., SEM Inc., AMF O'Hare,Chicago, 21 (1985).

28. T.F.Malis, S.C.Cheng and R.F.Egerton, The EELS log-ratio technique for thickness measurements in the TEM, J. Elecron Microscopy Techniques 8:193 (1988).

29. D.E.Newbury and R.L.Myklebust, A Monte Carto electron trajectory simulation for analytical electron microscopy, in: "AEM 1981", R.H.Geiss, ed., San Francisco Press Inc.,91 (1981).

30. I.A.Vatter and J.M.Titchmarsh, Measurement of grain boundary segregation by STEM-EDX, Ultramicroscopy (1989), in press.

31. J.M.Titchmarsh, Metallurgical applications of analytical electron microscopy with high spatial resolution, in: "Proc. XIth ICXOM", J.D.Brown and R.H.Packwood, eds., ICXOM-11, London, Ontario 337 (1987).

32. P.Trebbia, Unbiassed method for signal estimation in electron energy loss spectroscopy, concentration measurements and detection limits in quantitative microanalysis: methods and programs, Ultramicroscopy 24:399 (1988).

33. D.C.Joy and D.M.Maher, Sensitivity limits for thin specimen x-ray analysis, in: "SEM/1977/I", O. Johari, ed, SEM Inc., AMF O'Hare, Chicago,325 (1977).

34. D.C.Joy and D.M.Maher, EELS: detectable limits for elemental analysis, Ultramicroscopy 5:333 (1980).

35. N.R.Draper and H.Smith, "Applied Regression Analysis", 2nd Edition, Wiley, New York (1981).

36. J.N.Chapman, C.C.Gray, B.W.Robertson and W.A.P.Nicholson, X-ray production in thin foils by electrons with energies between 40 and 100 keV, X-ray Spectrom. 12:153 (1983).

37. G.Cliff and G.W.Lorimer, The quantitative analysis of thin specimens, J. Microscopy 103:203 (1975).

TEM-CATHODOLUMINESCENCE STUDY OF SINGLE AND MULTIPLE QUANTUM WELLS

OF MBE GROWN GaAs/AlGaAs

J.W. Steeds, S.J. Bailey*, J.N. Wang and C.W. Tu**

Physics Department
University of Bristol
Bristol BS8 1TL
United Kingdom

*Materials Research Laboratories
University of Illinois at Urbana-Champaign
Urbana, Illinois 61801, USA

**Bell Laboratories
Room MH 7B-410
Murray Hill, NJ 07974, USA

INTRODUCTION

Luminescence spectroscopy is a singularly powerful technique for characterising semiconductor materials. For high quality materials great sensitivity exists to trace impurities and in the case of quantum wells luminescence spectra give a very clear indication of the quality of the structures which have been grown.

In spite of this undoubted versatility and utility, spectroscopy is inevitably an exercise in interpretation of peak shapes, positions, widths and fine structure. In the context of quantum wells problems of interpretation can unfortunately arise. Even for ideal quantum well structures the energies of peaks in the emission spectra have to be calculated on the basis of information about the well and barrier widths and composition. There is a measure of uncertainty about each of these factors. The energies of impurity-related peaks are dependent on calculations based on assumptions about the impurity location within the quantum wells. In addition new defects exist, the interface steps, which are not present in bulk material. When one adds in the uncertainties associated with some of the methods of calculation it becomes apparent that microstructural information such as that provided by transmission electron microscopy (TEM) can only aid the process of assessment of quantum well structures. The combination of TEM with microscopic cathodoluminescence (CL) in the same instrument offers an interesting prospect for obtaining new insight into the interpretation of spectral details.

It was with this thought in mind that, many years ago, Dr P.M. Petroff established a facility at Bell Labs[1] for STEM CL experiments. Not long after his initiative we undertook a similar exercise in Bristol[2] and more recently we have used this facility to study quantum well structures[3]. This contribution is a review of the results we have obtained.

Experiments performed by use of STEM CL are naturally interpreted with reference to the vast literature which exist on characterisation of quantum wells by photoluminescence (PL). PL is in many ways the obvious technique for this exercise. It is relatively cheap to set up, non- destructive in nature and has several important advantages over CL[4]. One of the most important of these is the ability to perform excitation spectroscopy by tuning the exciting wavelength in the region of the spectral features to be investigated. In particular, this technique permits the measurement of the Stokes shift between related absorption and emission peaks, and this shift gives an important indication of the interface quality of the quantum well structure[5]. Another important advantage is the freedom from radiation damage or contamination which can affect CL experiments. Finally, since the samples may be immersed in liquid helium below its lambda point, lower temperatures can be achieved in PL experiments which can be advantageous.

It will help the purposes of this review if we start by identifying the various sources of spectral detail in quantum well emission spectra, largely deduced by PL spectroscopy. The first obvious step is to distinguish intrinsic and extrinsic emission processes. The increase in exciton binding energy and the relative lack of importance of impurities make the luminescence spectra from quantum wells relatively simple in form, especially at room temperature: spectra are dominated by the heavy-hole exciton peak. There are nevertheless a number of distinct processes of an intrinsic nature associated with the excitonic emission. The first and most frequently encountered is a small peak of higher energy associated with light-hole excitons. Its presence is well-width and temperature-dependent. The well width is important because this determines the magnitude of the light-hole/heavy-hole splitting; the temperature is important because this determines the statistics of occupation of the light-hole band[6]. In practice, the effect was readily distinguished as the only process giving rise to a peak of higher energy than the main heavy-hole exciton peak. Other intrinsic effects which have been reported, such as the excitonic 2s state, bi-excitons and phonon replication have not been observed in the samples which we have studied. In any case, phonon replication has only been reported for InP/InGaAs quantum wells and we shall restrict our comments to the GaAs/GaAlAs system in this review.

There are many possible sources of extrinsic luminescence. Structure may be observed in PL spectra from certain samples because of monolayer variations of the layer width on a scale large compared with exciton size[7] : we return to this point later in the review. The ledges at the interfaces can act as traps for the excitons, limiting their freedom to diffuse in the quantum wells. The density and purity of these ledges affects the exciton peak position in the emission spectrum. Point defect impurities have a further degree of complexity in quantum wells on account of the defect location within the well. The ionization energy of donors and acceptors at first rises as the well width decreases and the ionization energy is higher for impurities at the well centre rather than the well edge[8]. As a result, free to bound transitions are well width and impurity position-dependent. Neither donor nor acceptor-bound excitons are reported in quantum well systems because the ledge spacing is much smaller than the impurity spacing and the excitons are therefore trapped at the ledges instead. Further extrinsic luminescence effects are associated with dislocations, stacking faults and oval defects: these have been studied in this laboratory and the results will be summarised in this review.

EXPERIMENTAL DETAILS

The STEM CL system used for the results presented here is capable of high spatial (0.1 μm) and good spectral resolution over a wide range (300nm –1.8μm). The normal operating temperature using liquid helium cooling was about 30K. The system is capable of both spectral acquisition and monochromatic imaging. Further details of the system are given elsewhere [9]. Time resolved operation was not available although it has been demonstrated that very good time resolution can be achieved by performing CL in a scanning electron microscope [10]. For acquisition of CL spectra a microscope operating voltage of 120kV was normally chosen. At this voltage a reasonable beam current was achieved in a 100nm probe with the minimum amount of beam spreading in the sample. It was found that this operating voltage gave the highest spatial resolution in monochromatic images as well as high quality spectra: the beam current was kept at the lowest possible level consistent with reasonable acquisition times (normally not greater than one hour).

The specimens studied were generally plan view, prepared using a selective etching technique to remove the GaAs substrate from the overlying AlGaAs layer. Thin areas were typically 1mm in diameter of uniformly thin epitaxial layer. If these were not sufficiently transparent for good defect resolution at 120kV the specimen was transferred after CL characterisation to a TEM operating at 300kV. Lattice displacement damage at the higher operating voltage precluded further subsequent investigation of the specimen by CL.

This method of specimen preparation has many advantages. The quantum wells, lying parallel to the surface, prevent the escape of excitation to the surfaces. As a result of this anisotropic diffusion the spectra obtained from bulk and selectively-etched samples were identical and also very similar to results obtained from bulk samples by PL. The large thin areas make it possible to evaluate the specimens on a macroscopic scale comparable with device dimensions. In practice it was found that all samples contained extended defects but these were not uniformly distributed. Instead they were clustered in small areas representing a tiny fraction of the whole region examined. In a sense, then, most of the results reviewed here are unrepresentative as they were obtained from a few specially selected regions. The samples had to be mounted by careful glueing at one corner and this is one reason for the relatively high temperatures achieved with the helium stage. Even so, repeated thermal cycling of the specimens invariably led to catastrophic failure through fracture. In this respect oval defects were a particular problem as their shape and the local stress concentrations caused them to act as natural sources for cracks.

Although several different samples were studied in this work we found that it was necessary to limit our attention to only the highest quality samples available. For poorer samples the defect density was sometimes so high that one could not study a particular defect in isolation without the influence of a neighbouring defect. In addition, the spectral effects associated with extended defects were so variable and complex as to defy generalisations. Details of the specimens studied are given in Fig 1. They were grown by molecular beam epitaxy. Most of the results discussed here were from samples A, B and C; some reference is made to results from sample D; sample E gave results which were too variable to permit generalisation.

It is fortunate that the local details of the quantum well structures in the plan view samples can be deduced by new techniques of

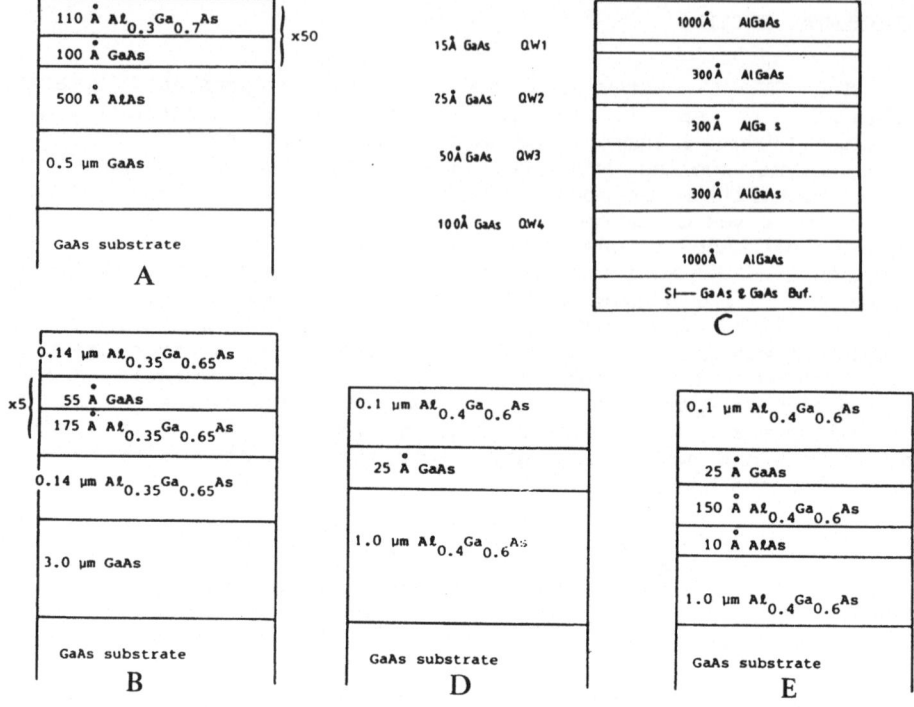

Fig 1.   Schematic diagrams of the five QW structures investigated.

convergent beam electron diffraction developed in this laboratory. This work, closely associated with the work reviewed here, is discussed in the companion paper in these proceedings by Dr Cherns.

RESULTS AND DISCUSSION

All results were obtained at low temperature ($\sim 30K$) unless stated otherwise.

(a)   Luminescence from regions free of extended defects

Sample B, with 100A quantum wells, invariably showed a weak peak on the high energy side of the heavy hole exciton peak with about 10% of its intensity (Fig 2). The peak had an energy of 11meV greater than that of the heavy hole peak, as is predicted for the light-hole exciton in wells of this size[11]. Sample A, with 55A well widths, lacked a light-hole satellite at low temperature (Fig 3) but on warming to room temperature one appeared about 20meV on the high energy side of the main peak. This is the calculated energy difference for 55A wells, and the increase of separation explains the absence of the peak at low temperature. Both samples A and B had very weak tails on the long wavelength side of the heavy-hole peak. By increasing the gain the tails were sometimes found to be structured, with broad weak peaks at about 1% of the heavy-hole intensity. In both A and B two broad peaks were sometimes discernible; for A at approximately 18 and 38meV below the heavy-hole peaks and for B at approximately 21 and 40meV below the

heavy-hole peak. The peak at 40meV from the heavy-hole emission of B
was broad and of variable intensity; it is not present in Fig 2. The
interpretation of such ill-defined information must necessarily be
speculative. The large energy differences imply emission from the
conduction band to neutral acceptors . Since carbon is a well-known
acceptor impurity in MBE grown material and it generates an emission
peak about 20meV below the excitonic peak in bulk GaAs, it is the
natural candidate to consider. The value of 20meV would be increased
for carbon atoms at the centre of quantum wells to a value of about
35meV for 55A wells and about 23meV for 100A wells according
to theoretical calculations[12]. Carbon at the edge of the wells in
the two cases would give emission lines at about 20meV and 13meV
respectively[13]. It may be that carbon is responsible therefore for
three of the background peaks of the two samples, leaving only the
40meV peak of the B well without a plausible explanation. Bulk GaAs
containing silicon acceptors has a band-acceptor peak about 32meV below
the exciton peak. If allowance is made for some increase in this value
of 100A wells for silicon impurities at the well centres this might
account for the observed broad emission from sample B. Work of Miller
et al[5] indicated that for broader wells impurities were predominantly
at the well centres, while for narrower wells they were more often at
the well edges.

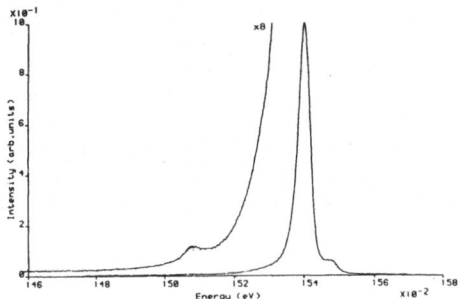

Fig 2. CL spectra from unfaulted
crystal of sample B.

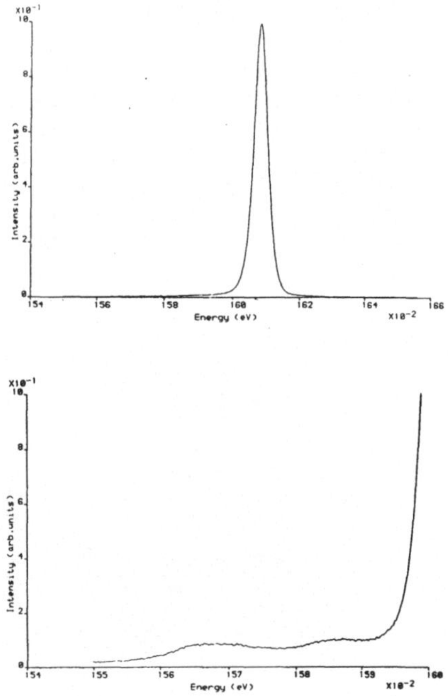

Fig 3. CL spectra from unfaulted
crystal of sample A
showing the n=1 (e-hh)
peak (top left) and weak
structure on the low
energy side (left).

(b)   Growth interrupted samples

Sample D contained four single quantum wells and was prepared with
growth interruption at both the GaAs and AlGaAs interfaces. As a
result the four different single quantum wells each revealed fine
structure (Fig 4) which may be interpreted as coming from individual
regions within the wells varying by monolayer steps in thickness[7]. One
consequence of the flat interfaces is to make easier the lateral
diffusion of excitons in the quantum wells so that excitation flows
from the narrower to the broader regions of the wells, biassing the low
excitation spectra in favour of the lower energy peaks[14]. A check
therefore of the interpretation of the spectra is to increase the

excitation level when increasingly more emission is expected from the narrow portions of the wells. Experiments were performed to confirm this explanation for the fine structure.

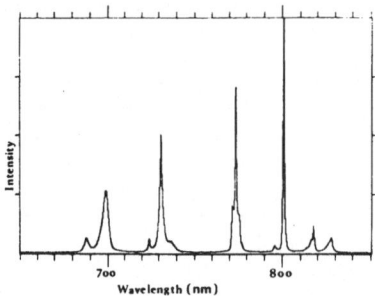 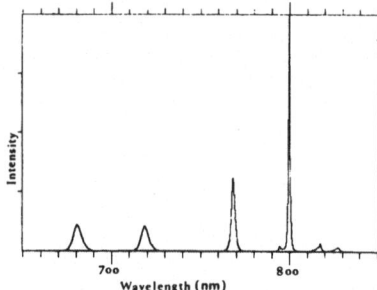

Fig 4. CL spectra from unfaulted crystal of sample C with interruption growth (left) and without interruption growth (right).

There then existed the interesting possibility of generating monochromatic CL images in each of the separate peaks associated with a particular single quantum well. We repeated the earlier experiment of Petroff and co-workers[15]. Images were obtained with marked spatial variation of intensity (Fig 5) and it may be seen that there is a high degree of anticorrelation between the images as would be expected. Any given region has thickness of a given number of monolayers. More elaborate experiments of this type have been performed by Christen and Bimburg et al[16]. They found that samples produced at slightly different growth temperatures had markedly different plateau sizes. They also performed time resolved experiments in which the excitation was observed to spread across particular plateaux as the time delay increased.

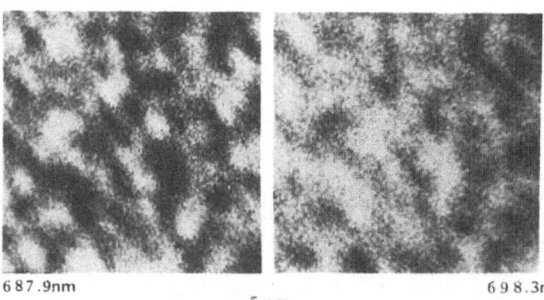

Fig 5. Monochromatic CL images of sample D with interruption growth at indicated wavelength.

687.9nm   698.3nm

5 μm

There remain some areas of clarification to pursue before these interesting new results can be regarded as completely satisfactory. Anti-correlation between the images is not perfect and the plateaux sizes are rather larger than might have been expected. These points might be explained by the exciton diffusion and the time resolved results do indeed show a finer scale of structure at shorter times[16]. One also has to take account of the possible overlap of impurity peaks from narrow regions with emission peaks from wider regions. Impurities might well play a more important role when the interfaces are so flat. Such effects could account for some of the anticorrelation failures. One final puzzling result comes from our own work. We found that the structured images were not reproduced in successive cold runs on the same specimens although the spectra were apparently unchanged. A possible explanation of this result might be the gradual disordering of the planar interfaces by electron irradiation. If the plateaux widths were reduced below the resolution of our experiment ($\sim 0.3\,\mu$m) but remained larger than the exciton size ($\sim$20nm) then the result could be explained.

(c)   Stacking faults

Of the various forms of stacking fault observed in our samples we concentrated on two classical forms[17]. One of these, the pyramidal stacking fault, has alternating {111} faces of intrinsic and extrinsic character with stair rod dislocation between. The other, a folded back stacking fault, consisted of two close parallel stacking faults, one of each type. Detailed analysis by diffraction contrast experiments revealed that the extrinsic faults lay on arsenic faces, and the intrinsic faults on gallium faces. The diametrically opposite intrinsic parts of the pyramidal stacking faults were found to be associated with growth anomalies in the epitaxial layers of specimen B. Similar observations have been reported previously[18]. These anomalies are regions of reduced epilayer thickness where the intrinsic stacking faults emerge at the surface. Both pyramidal and folded back stacking faults were found to originate at points on the substrate surface or very close to it.

There were very few stacking faults in sample A but a reasonable number in sample B. In consequence most of the results we obtained were from sample B. CL spectra obtained from regions with pyramidal stacking faults showed three reasonably strong broad subsidiary peaks on the long wavelength side of the heavy-hole exciton peak (Fig 6). Two of these peaks, at 9 and 14 meV from the heavy-hole exciton, were of variable strength between 10% and 30% of the heavy-hole exciton emission intensity: they were specifically related to the stacking fault. The third peak amounted to an enhancement of the background intensity at around 21meV from the heavy-hole exciton peak. Monochromatic images formed in the various peaks yielded interesting results (Fig 7). Both light-hole and heavy-hole images showed exciton quenching in the vicinity of the pyramidal fault. This quenching was strongest near the places where the quantum wells intersected the intrinsic parts of the pyramid. The 9meV emission was strongly variable in intensity but gave monochromatic images with strong emission from the quenched regions of the heavy and light-hole electron maps. The 14meV emission was less variable in intensity and when weak gave rather a complex monochromatic image elongated in the sense of the extrinsic faults. When the 14meV emission was much stronger than the 9meV emission the two monochromatic maps were rather similar in intensity distribution to the monochromatic map previously described for the 9meV emission: intensity was concentrated near the positions where the quantum wells intersected the intrinsic faults. Images formed in the 21meV emission band showed general enhancement of intensity in the region of the pyramidal fault.

By contrast, the folded back fault showed strongly enhanced emission in the broad peak at 21meV away from the heavy-hole exciton peak (Fig 8), and the monochromatic images simply showed exciton quenching at the fault and enhanced 21meV emission.

There are many pieces of evidence to indicate that these interesting effects were the results of impurity contamination of the stacking fault.

133

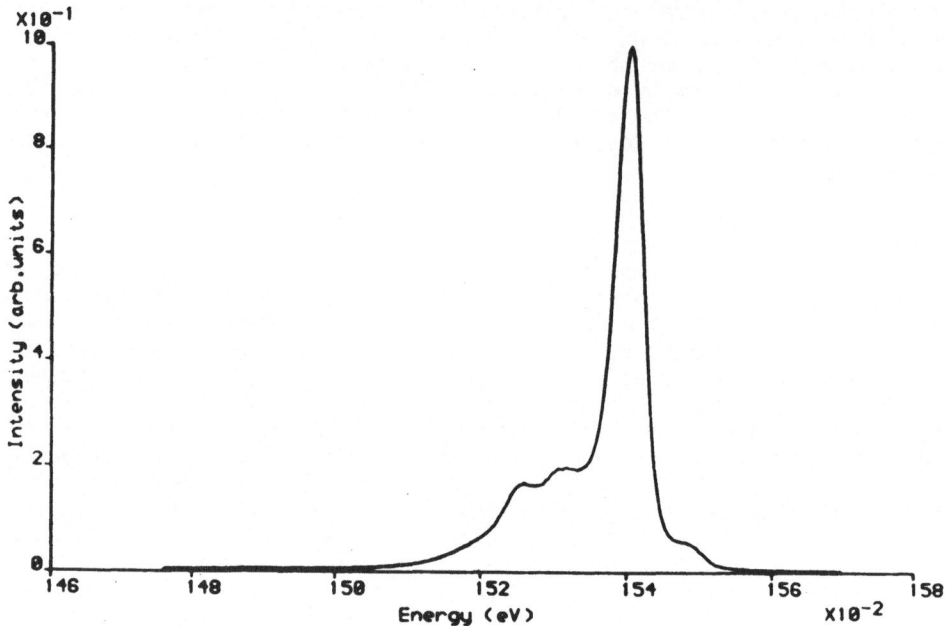

Fig 6. CL spectrum from a pyramidal
stacking fault in sample B.

(i)   Similar experiments performed on stacking faults in
       GaAs/AlGaAs quantum wells of poorer optical quality showed
       greatly enhanced and very variable emission on the
       long-wavelength side of the heavy hole-exciton peak.

(ii)   A sample with an AlAs layer grown to accumulate impurities
       prior to the quantum well growth had reduced long wavelength
       emission in the vicinity of stacking faults (sample D).

(iii) The growth impairment associated with the intrinsic parts of
       the stacking fault pyramids is indicative of impurity
       involvement.

(iv)   Certain areas of Sample D revealed an extended cellular
       structure when imaged in the long wavelength tail to the main
       exciton emission (Fig 9). This cellular structure was not
       apparent at a casual glance by transmission electron
       microscopy but could be discerned faintly by careful
       examination of some of the negatives. The stacking faults
       were invariably located in the cell walls of this structure.

     There is evidence from other quarters that stacking faults are
decorated with impurity. X-ray topography of stacking faults in
diamond and diffraction contrast experiments on intrinsic stacking
faults in silicon both indicate that small supplementary displacements
exist. Moreover, a few experiments by time of flight field ion
microscopy have revealed directly the presence of impurity atoms
contaminating stacking faults. It appears from our experiments that
excitons bind to the impurities and/or quantum well steps with
different energies at places where the intrinsic and extrinsic stacking
faults cross the quantum wells. As a result a different sense of
elongation was observed in either case. In addition the background
impurity level was enhanced in the vicinity of the stacking faults,

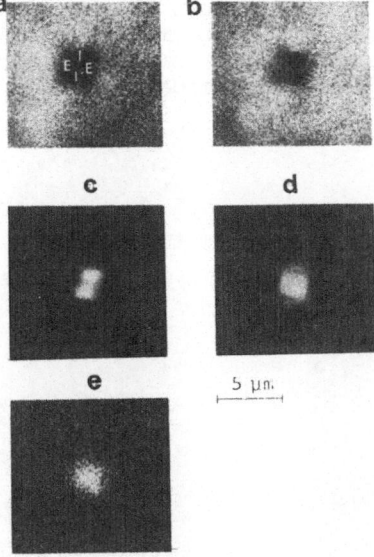

Fig 7. Monochromatic CL images of a pyramidal stacking fault in sample B. a) n=1 (e-lh) emission. b) n=1 (e-hh) emission. c),d),e) 9,14 and 21meV below the n=1 (e-hh) emission.

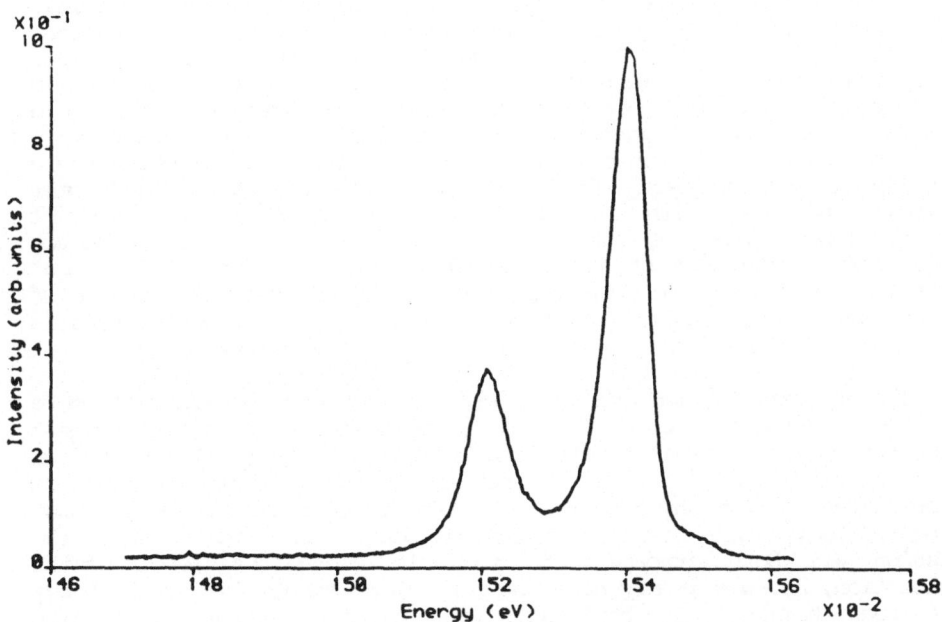

Fig 8. CL spectrum from a folded back stacking fault in sample B.

giving enhanced emission in the band displaced by 21meV. The folded back faults, having a much smaller volume to contain the extra impurity (approximately one hundred times smaller) showed much greater background enhancement than the pyramidal faults.

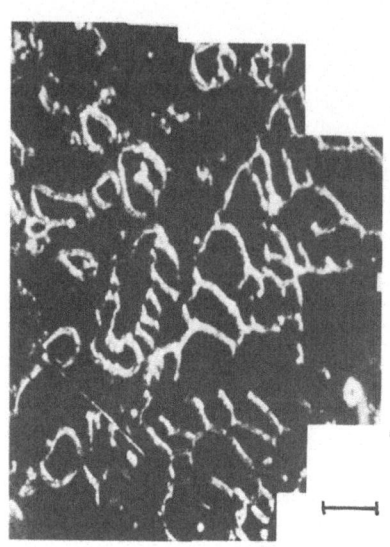

Fig 9. Monochromatic CL image of sample D showing cellular structure. The line is 20μm long.

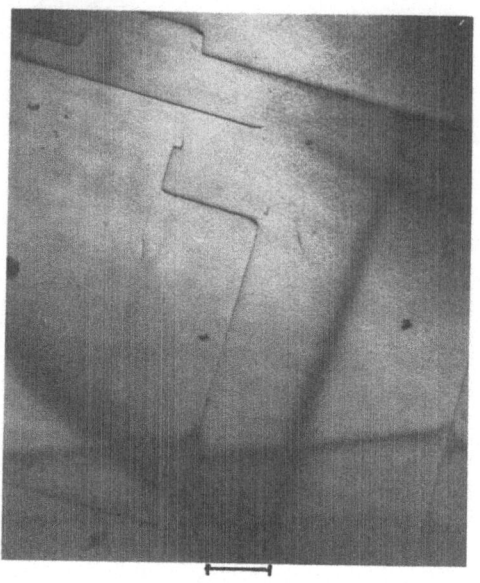

Fig 10. BF TEM micrograph showing 60° misfit dislocation in sample A. The line is 2μm long.

(d)   Misfit dislocations

Sample A contained a low density of misfit dislocations (Fig 10). These were predominantly of 60° character at the substrate/AlGaAs interface (see Fig 1). The selective etch, in removing the substrate eliminated these misfit dislocations and they could only be observed in the annular ring at the periphery of the circular specimens where some substrate remained. Occasional segments of misfit dislocation were also observed at the interfaces of the quantum wells, of which there were five in the specimen. These segments were of both 60° and Lomer Cottrell character with the latter in the majority. They were of variable length from 1-50 μm and were sometimes observed to reduce their length drastically under examination. We concentrated our attention on these dislocations for which no previous reports of cathodoluminescence exist, although Petroff et al [19] reported results on misfit dislocations at $Ga_{1-x}Al_xAs_{1-y}P_y$ interfaces.

The experimental results which we obtained were considerably more variable than those reported for the stacking faults. In the simplest cases the spectral detail on the long wavelength tail of the exciton emission was simply a small enhancement of the general background at large distances from any defects: the associated peaks were only about 1% of the heavy hole exciton emission peak. In other cases the emission was both stronger and variable along the length of the dislocation, but was in any case not more than about 10% of the heavy hole peak height. By contrast, lower quality specimens containing dislocations, also part of this study, gave widely varying results and local emission which exceeded the strength of the heavy hole exciton emission.

136

The dislocations which gave the simple background enhancement of CL emission were generally short, a few microns in length. The monochromatic images formed in the heavy hole exciton peak showed a single narrow line (half-width ∿ 0.5 μm) of reduced contrast at the dislocation with a wide band of slightly enhanced emission at distances of a few microns (Fig 11a). Images formed in the two background peaks 20meV and 40meV from the heavy hole peak showed two parallel lines of strongly enhanced emission (half width ∿ 0.5 μm) with a narrow minimum of intensity (half width ∿ 0.3 μm) along the dislocation line (Fig 11b).

a   **b**

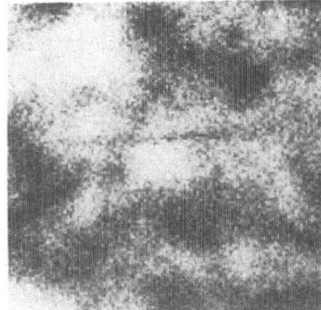 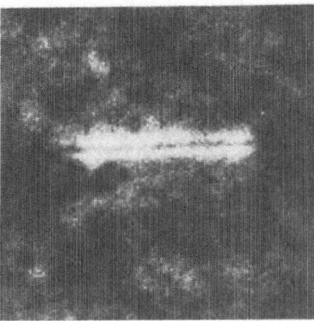

Fig 11. Monochromatic CL images of dislocation in sample A. a) n=1 (e-hh) emission, b) 20meV below the n=1 (e-hh) emission. The line is 2μm long.

An example of more complicated behaviour is shown in Fig 12. In this case the image varies strongly along the dislocation length, as do the spectra acquired at different positions along the dislocation (Fig 13). The dislocation, which is somewhat longer than in Fig 11, has stronger emissions and reveals a doubled minimum of intensity at the heavy-hole emission wavelength. The enhanced tail emission gives a strong single patch of intensity at either end of the dislocation. At 20meV from the heavy-hole emission two fine bright lines of emission about 1 μm apart occur either side of the central part of the dislocation. Related examples involving longer dislocations of 50 μm in length show irregular contrast jumps along the dislocations, and in one case five such jumps were observed[6]. One other feature typical of these results on longer dislocations with more complex emission was that the region of bright emission in monochromatic images, formed by the long wavelength tail of the emission spectrum, was the tendency for the width of the bright region to reduce as the energy difference from the heavy hole exciton peak increased. At the same time the resolution of the microstructure evident in the material near to the dislocation became progressively sharper.

The interpretation of these results is necessarily speculative at this stage. However it appears that some progress can be made by proposing the formation of a Cottrell atmosphere of impurities around the dislocations. This atmosphere would enhance near the dislocation the background emission in the long wavelength tail and clean up more distant regions leading to enhanced excitonic emission. At the dislocation itself a narrow depletion zone would result from the high impurity content there and would be non-radiative. To explain the more complex results there are a number of additional factors to take into account. We know that the dislocations being studied lie close to the quantum wells in the samples, but we do not know the precise location of the dislocation cores. Previous work by cross-sectional TEM has revealed that such dislocations run along parallel to the GaAs/AlGaAs interface for a while and then step through to the next interface in staircase fashion. Clearly the emission pattern will depend strongly on whether the dislocation core lies locally in the quantum well itself

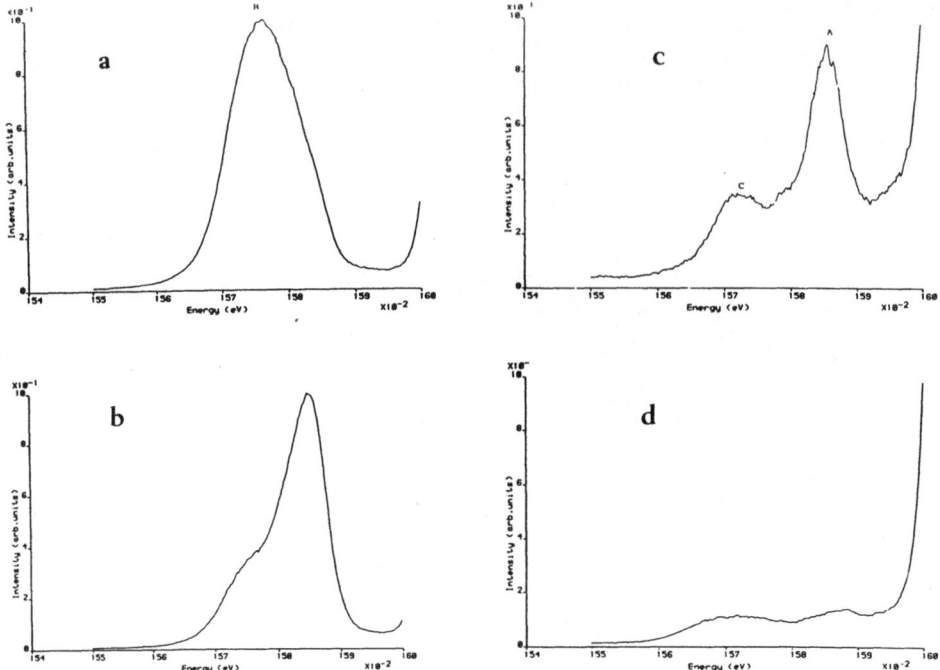

Fig 12. CL spectra from different position of a misfit dislocation in sample A. a) one end b) middle c) another end d) unfaulted crystal.

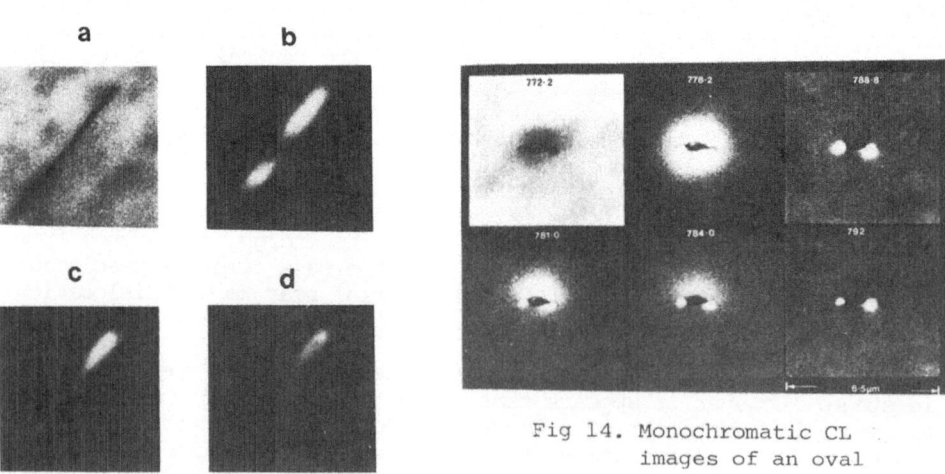

Fig 14. Monochromatic CL images of an oval defect.

5 μm

Fig 13. Monochromatic CL image of the misfit dislocation in sample A (spectra see Fig 12). a) n=1 (e-hh) emission, b),c) and d) at the energies marked A:B:C on Fig 12.

or in the barrier layer. Equally it is suspected that in the case of a multiple quantum well structure not all the quantum wells are equally active in contributing luminescence. Hence a high concentration of impurity at a dislocation remote from the most active quantum well could result in strong tail emission without quenching at the projected position of the dislocation core. Also the dislocation steps through the quantum wells themselves provide new and unique sites for impurity trapping and exciton binding. Some of the changes of intensity along the longer dislocation lines are likely to be the consequence of these steps. In this respect it is interesting to note that the largest number of contrast anomalies recorded (5) was just that of the number of quantum wells in the sample. In further support of the idea that Cottrell atmospheres play an important part in the interpretation of our results is the observed shrinkage of contrast onto the dislocation core as the wavelength selected for the monochromatic map shifts to larger values. It is well known for bulk semiconductors that there is a red shift of photo emission from highly doped semiconductors[20](the so called red shift resulting from band-gap renormalisation). If we assume that a similar effect occurs in highly doped quantum wells, and there is some evidence for it, then by moving to wavelengths far into the long wavelength tail of the exciton emission we are automatically selecting the highly doped regions necessarily close to the dislocation core. It might be possible in the future to map out concentration profiles associated with dislocations by exploitation of this effect.

Quite apart from the effort to understand the luminescence processes associated with dislocations there is an important practical application of the work we have done. It is clearly helpful to be able to determine whether a particular growth run has produced misfit dislocations. From the work reported here it is apparent that macroscopic non-destructive evaluation of wafers can be performed with a cold SEM CL system. In this case, by tuning to the exciton peak of the bulk AlGaAs emission, one can reveal the misfit dislocations lying at the substrate interface as a rectangular array of dark lines[6] and by tuning to the long wavelength tail of the quantum well exciton peak one can reveal misfit dislocations associated with the quantum wells as bright lines.

(e) Oval Defects

A wide variety of oval defects has been studied. These include regions which contain particles such as dust particles, Ga_2O_3 , or multiply-twinned polycrystalline GaAs particles. In addition some oval defects were simply local regions where growth had not occurred: any associated particles which might once have existed had dropped out. Other such defects were the sites of dense dislocation tangles of uncertain origin, but lacked any identifiable particle or inclusion.

On the whole the variety of results obtained defy generalisations. One exception was our work on the oval defects associated with dense dislocation tangles: this has recently been the subject of an independent publication[21] . The other is the tendency for enhanced background peaks to occur near oval defects in the long wavelength tails of the quantum well emission. The idea that a higher concentration of impurities exists near oval defects is only what one would suspect. However, it was also noted that as monochromatic images were formed further into the long wavelength tail, so the emission was concentrated closer to the margins of the oval defects (Fig 14). This observation, which closely resembles our results on dislocations, is taken to indicate a higher concentration of impurity with an associated large red shift close to the oval defects.

CONCLUSIONS

TEM CL experiments are able to provide a great deal of detailed information about intrinsic and extrinsic luminescence processes in quantum well structures. The results obtained are not well understood at present and a good deal of further effort is required to elucidate the basic processes involved. At a more practical level, the information obtainable by this technique offers considerable promise for effective non-destructive evaluation of epitaxial layers and devices in the future. The extension of the work described here to quantum wells in quantum dots has already been started and quantum wires can also be investigated by this technique [22].

REFERENCES

1. P.M. Petroff, D.V. Lang, J.L. Strudel & R.A. Logan, "Scanning Transmission Electron Microscopy Techniques for Simultaneous Electronic Analysis and Observation of Defects in Semiconductors". Article in Scanning Electron Microscopy Vol. 1, O. Johari, ed. SEM Inc. Chicago (1978) p.325.

2. S.H. Roberts, "Cathodoluminescence Spectrometer Design for the TEM". Article in Institute of Physics Conf. Ser. No. 61 (EMAG 81), London & Bristol (1982) p.51.

3. J.W. Steeds & S.J. Bailey, "High Resolution Cathodoluminescence Studies in a Transmission Electron Microscope", Atti del XVI Congresso di Mic. Elect. Bologna (1987) p.107.

4. J.W. Steeds, "Performance and Applications of a STEM-Cathodoluminescence System", to be published in the Proceedings of the Workshop on Beam Injection Assessment of Defects in Semiconductors by Journal de Physique.

5. G. Bastard, C. Delalande, M.H. Meynadier, P.M. Frijlink & M. Voos, "Low-temperature Exciton Trapping on Interface Defects in Semiconductor Quantum Wells", Phys. Rev. B29 : 7042 (1984).
   R.C. Miller, A.C. Gossard, W.T. Tsang & O. Munteanu, "Extrinsic Photoluminescence from GaAs Quantum Wells", Physica 117 and 118B : 714 (1983).

6. C. Weisbuch, R.C. Miller, R. Dingle, A.C. Gossard & W. Wiegmann, "Intrinsic Radiative Recombination from Quantum States in GaAs-Al$_x$Ga$_{1-x}$As Multi-Quantum Well Structures", Solid State Commun. 37 : 219 (1981).
   P. Dawson, G. Duggan, H.I. Ralph & K. Woodbridge, "Free Excitons in Room-Temperature Photoluminescence of GaAs-Al$_x$Ga$_{1-x}$As Multiple Quantum Wells", Phys. Rev. B28 : 7381 (1983).

7. T. Fukunaga, K.L.I. Kobayashi & H. Nakashima, "Photoluminescence from AlGaAs-GaAs Single Quantum Wells with Growth Interrupted Hetero-interfaces Grown by Molecular Beam Epitaxy", Jap. Journ. Appl. Phys. 24 : LS10 (1985).

8. G. Bastard, "Hydrogenic Impurity States in a Quantum Well. A Simple Model", Phys. Rev. B24 : 4714 (1981).

9. S. Myhajlenko, "Near Infra-red Cathodoluminescence Assessment of Semiconductors in a TEM". Article in Institute of Physics Conf. Ser. No. 68 (EMAG 83), London & Bristol (1983) p.51.

10. D. Bimberg, H. Munzel, A. Steckenborn & J. Christen, "Kinetics of Relaxation and Recombination of Non-equilibrium Carriers in GaAs: Carrier Capture by Impurities", Phys. Rev. B31 : 7788 (1985).

11. R.C. Miller, D.A. Kleinmann, W.T. Tsang & A.C. Gossard, "Observation of the Excited Level of Excitons in GaAs Quantum Wells", Phys. Rev. B24 : 1134 (1981).

12. R.L. Greene & K.K. Bajaj, "Shallow Impurities in Semiconductor Quantum Well Structures", Solid State Commun. 53 : 1103 (1985).

13. C. Delalande, "Optical Studies of Shallow Impurities in Semiconductor Quantum Well Structures", Physica 146B : 112 (1987).

14. C.W. Tu, R.C. Miller, P.M. Petroff, R.F. Kopf, B. Deveaud, T.C. Damen & J. Shah, "Intrawell Exciton Transport in Monolayer-flat GaAs/AlGaAs Single Quantum Wells Grown by Molecular Beam Epitaxy", J. Vac. Sci. Technol. B6 : 610 (1988).

15. P.M. Petroff, J. Gibert, A.C. Gossard, G.J. Dolan & C.W. Tu, "Interface Structure and Optical Properties of Quantum Wells and Quantum Boxes", J. Vac. Sci. Tech. B5 : 1204 (1987).

16. D. Bimberg, J. Christen, T. Fukunaga, H. Nakashima, D.E. Mars & J.N. Miller, "Direct Imaging of the Columnar Structure of GaAs Quantum Wells", Superlattices & Microstructures 4 : 257 (1988).

17. G.R. Booker, "Crystallographic Imperfections in Silicon", Disc. Faraday Soc. 38 : 298 (1964).

18. Y.G. Chai, Y-C Pao & T. Hierl, "Elimination of Pair Defects from GaAs Layers Grown by Molecular Beam Epitaxy", Appl. Phys. Lett. 47 : 1327 (1985).

19. P.M. Petroff, R.A. Logan & A. Savage, "Non-radiative Recombination at Dislocations in III-V Compound Semiconductors", Phys. Rev. Lett. 44 : 287 (1980).

20. A. Haufe, R. Schwabe, H. Fieseler & M. Ilegems, "The Luminescence Lineshape of Highly Doped Direct-gap III-V Compounds", J. Phys. C : Solid State Phys. 21 : 2951 (1988).

21. J. Wang, J.W. Steeds & C.W. Tu, "The Investigation of Impurity Distributions Around an Oval Defect in Molecular Beam Epitaxy AlGaAs/GaAs Single Quantum Wells by Transmission Electron Microscopy and Cathodoluminescence" to be published in the Proceedings of the Third International Conference on Shallow Impurities in Semiconductors, Linkoping, Sweden 1988 by the Institute of Physics.

22. P.M. Petroff, A.C. Gossard, R.A. Logan & W. Wiegmann, "Towards Quantum Well Wires : Fabrication and Optical Properties", Appl. Phys. Lett. 41 : 635 (1982).

EBIC STUDIES OF INDIVIDUAL DEFECTS IN LIGHTLY DOPED SEMICONDUCTORS:

CdTe AS AN EXAMPLE

B. Sieber

Laboratoire de Structure et Propriétés de l'Etat Solide, UA 234
Bâtiment C6, Université des Sciences et Techniques de Lille
59655 Villeneuve d'Ascq, Cédex, France

INTRODUCTION

Electron beam induced current (EBIC) experiments performed in the scanning electron microscope (SEM) are well-known to provide unique information, at a local scale, on bulk inhomogeneities and on electrically active extended defects in semiconductors[1]. The EBIC current arises from the collection of minority carriers created by the incident electron beam which are drifted by the electric field of a Schottky diode or of a p-n junction; they have been created in the space charge region (SCR) of the junction or they have reached the SCR by diffusion in the bulk of the semiconductor. The EBIC current is therefore material dependent through the minority carrier diffusion length L and through the SCR width W (W decreases when the doping level increases). Only the Schottky diode configuration where the junction is parallel to the surface and perpendicular to the electron beam, will be discussed in this paper, as it allows both imaging and quantitative characterization of bulk parameters of the semiconductor, as well as of extended defects. The accelerating beam voltage E_o used in EBIC experiments is also an important parameter, as it controls the electron penetration depth R of incident electrons in the material, and thus the depth from which the electrical information comes. The minority carriers created at a depth from the surface greater than W+L do not contribute to the collected current. Thus, the EBIC image is, for a semiconductor such as GaAs or CdTe (where L is of the same order of magnitude as R), a rapid and straightforward tool of characterization of its local inhomogeneities: for instance, at high accelerating voltages ($E_o \approx 30$ kV), the areas which exhibit the highest EBIC current can be directly identified to those with the highest diffusion length. A local quantitative determination of L and W can futhermore be made at a scale of the order of the generation and diffusion volumes of electron-hole pairs: the EBIC current is collected as a function of E_o; the variation of the collection efficiency e_{cc} with E_o (e_{cc} is the experimental gain to the theoretical gain ratio) is representative of the SCR width for small E_o values, and of the diffusion length for high E_o values[2].

The bulk diffusion length is limited by impurities and point-defects present in the semiconductor, and the recombination of carriers can be either radiative or non-radiative. Such a process is locally enhanced by dislocations, grain-boundaries, clusters, precipitates present in the specimen. As a matter of fact, it has been demonstrated quite a long time ago that such extended defects can act as recombination centres for electron-hole pairs. This can occur via the core of the defect, if it introduces for instance levels in the band gap of the semiconductor, or via impurities which have segregated around it. The EBIC mode of the SEM provides an unique way to image these defects which usually give rise to dark contrasts when they are scanned by an electron beam. They appear as dark spots if they are dislocations perpendicular to the surface or precipitates and clusters located under the surface; dislocations parallel to the surface and GBs are displayed on the EBIC image as dark lines. The resolution, of the order of one micron, decreases when E_o increases. This could be considered as a disadvantage in comparison with other electron microscopy techniques; but it is the only one, with cathodoluminescence[3,4] which can bring local information on the electrical activity of defects.

In contrast to the bulk parameters which can be determined by routine experiments from now about 10 years, the identification of dark spots is quite recent. The first EBIC contrast theory of defects has been described by Donolato[5] in 1978/79. Based on a phenomenological model, it allows the characterization of dark spots in semiconductors in which the SCR width W can be neglected in comparison with the electron penetration depth R. But this assumption does not remain valid for all the doping levels of semiconductors; therefore, this model has been extended by Sieber[6] to 'lightly' doped semiconductors where the SCR width is of the same order of magnitude as R; CdTe was taken as a example. This extension is quite necessary, since it has been shown experimentally in silicon and CdTe that recombination at extended defects can take place even in the presence of an external electric field[7-12].

In the following we will describe these EBIC models, emphasizing, in each case, how routine experiments can be conducted in the SEM in order to assess the nature of the dark spots. It will be shown that, if such an identification can be performed in the case of 'doped' semiconductors by varying only one parameter, namely E_o, another one is necessary in the case of 'lightly' doped semiconductors; it will be demonstrated that the reverse bias applied to the junction is an appropriate parameter, as it acts on the SCR width. This will be illustrated by experiments made on a n-type CdTe specimen.

EBIC CONTRAST OF DEFECTS

Continuity Equation

The generation of electron-hole pairs, their diffusion and their recombination are described by the well-known continuity equation which, in the absence of any external electric field and under steady-state and low injection conditions is written, for a n-type semiconductor:

$$D \text{ div grad } \Delta p(\underline{r}) - \frac{\Delta p(\underline{r})}{\tau(\underline{r})} = - g(\underline{r}) \tag{1}$$

D is the minority carrier diffusivity, $\Delta p(\underline{r})$ the excess minority carrier density and $\tau(\underline{r})$ the minority carrier lifetime such that $L=(D\tau)^{1/2}$.

$\Delta p(\underline{r})/\tau(\underline{r})$ is the recombination term and $g(\underline{r})$ is the generation rate of electron-hole pairs.

Equation (1) can be reduced to a one-dimensional equation in an homogeneous medium:

$$D \text{ div grad } \Delta p(z) - \frac{\Delta p(z)}{\tau} = - g_2(z) \qquad (2)$$

$g_2(z)$ is the depth-dose function. $\tau(\underline{r})$ is usually taken as a constant τ.

The expression of $\Delta p(z)$ which satifies eqn(2) as well as boundary conditions taking into account the geometry of the system, can be quite easily derived, even if calculations are lengthy; therefore, the EBIC current can be theoretically expressed as a function of the diffusion length L. For example, in the geometry described in fig.1, where the SCR is not negligible, the boundary conditions are:

$$\Delta p(z) \Big|_{z=W} = 0$$

$$\Delta p(z) \Big|_{z\infty} = 0 \qquad (3)$$

The bulk EBIC current density is given by:

$$J_{BO} = - eD \frac{d\Delta p(z)}{dz} \Big|_{z=W} \qquad (4)$$

The EBIC current density in the SCR is:

$$J_{DO} = - e \int_0^W g_2(z)dz \qquad (5)$$

if it is assumed that all the minority carriers created by the electron beam are collected by the electric field of the SCR.

An electrically active defect present in the generation volume locally decreases the EBIC current, giving rise to a contrast which can be expressed as:

$$c = \frac{I_{DD} + I^*}{I_{DO} + I_{BO}} \qquad (6)$$

I_{DO} and I_{BO} are the background currents taken far from the defect. I_{DD} and I^{BO} are the recombination currents at the defect in the SCR and the bulk region respectively.

The defect is described[5] as a volume V_D of reduced minority carrier lifetime τ_D; equation (1) thus becomes:

$$D \text{ div grad } \Delta p'(\underline{r}) - \frac{\Delta p'(\underline{r})}{\tau} = - g(\underline{r}) + (\frac{1}{\tau_D} - \frac{1}{\tau}) e(\underline{r}) \Delta p'(\underline{r})$$

$$(7)$$

$$e(\underline{r}) = \begin{cases} 0 \text{ if } \underline{r} \notin \text{ defect} \\ 1 \text{ if } \underline{r} \in \text{ defect} \end{cases}$$

145

$\Delta p'(\underline{r})$ is the new carrier density. Any problem encountered in the establishment of an EBIC contrast theory of defects comes from the fact that continuity equation like eqn(7) cannot be generally reduced to a one-dimensional equation like previously. If, furthermore, a three-dimensional generation function is taken (fig.1), which is far much more realistic than a constant generation, I_{BO} and I_{DO} will be expressed as:

$$I_{BO} = - eD \iint_{\Sigma} \frac{\partial \Delta p(\underline{r})}{\partial r} \bigg|_{z=W} d\Sigma \tag{8}$$

$$I_{DO} = - e \iiint_{SCR} g(\underline{r}) \, d^3 r \tag{9}$$

I^* can be calculated once $\Delta p'(\underline{r})$ is known. Assuming that all the carriers created inside the volume V_D of the defect recombine, I_{DD} can be expressed as a function of $g(\underline{r})$:

$$I_{DD} = - e \iiint_{V_D} g(\underline{r}) \, d^3 r \tag{10}$$

$I^* = I_{BO} - I_{BD}$ where I_{BD} is the current from which the defect is imaged. It can be written as[6] :

$$I^* = - eD \iiint_{V_D} \text{grad } \Delta p'(\underline{r}) \, d^3 r \tag{11}$$

Doped semiconductors

In such semiconductors, the SCR width can be neglected, and the collecting barrier Σ is the metal-semiconductor interface. The EBIC contrast of defects is:

$$c = \frac{I^*}{I_{BO}} \tag{12}$$

Donolato[5] has treated the case of a 'point-like' defect (precipitate, cluster) with a spherical symmetry, and that of a dislocation perpendicular to the surface which can be described as a row of 'point-like' defects. The generation was assumed to be a constant, and the excess minority carrier density $\Delta p'(\underline{r})$ in presence of the defect to be equal to $\Delta p(r)$. Resolution of eqns(1) and (7), with boundary conditions for $\Delta p(r)$ similar to those of eqns(3) led to the following conclusions:
    - the EBIC contrast curve of a 'point-like' defect as a function of incident beam voltage E_O ($c=f(E_O)$) goes through a maximum (fig. 2a).
    - the EBIC contrast of a dislocation perpendicular to the surface decreases when increasing E_O (fig. 2b).
Dark spots in bulk doped semiconductors can therefore be easily identified by taking EBIC images for a limited number of accelerating beam voltages.

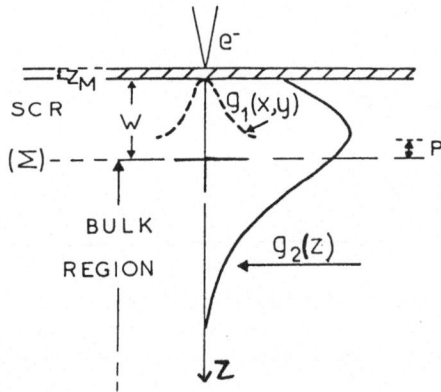

Fig.1 Specimen geometry. The hatched top layer represents the metal thickness z_M of the Schottky diode. The origin is at the metal SCR interface and below the incident electron beam. The bulk region is semi-infinite. $g_1(x,y)$ describes the lateral generation of electron-hole pairs (eqn.16), while $g_2(z)$ is the depth dose function (eqn.17).

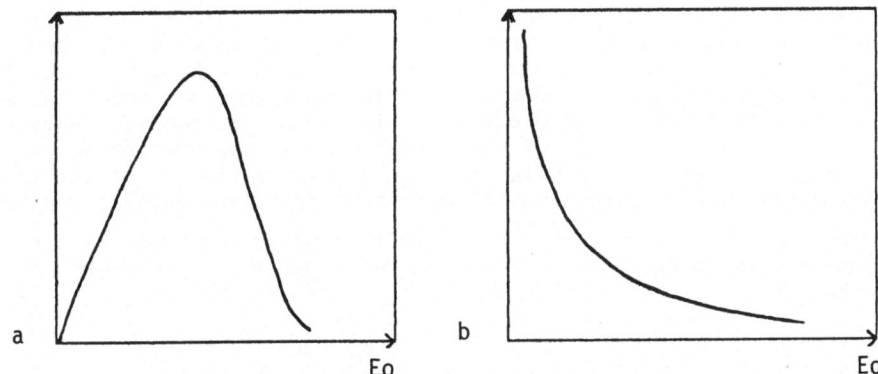

Fig.2 'Doped' semiconductor. EBIC contrast curves as a function of the accelerating voltage E_0 when the SCR is negligible in comparison with the electron penetration R^5.

   a- 'point-like' defect located in the bulk. The position of the maximum depends on the defect depth.

   b- dislocation perpendicular to the surface.

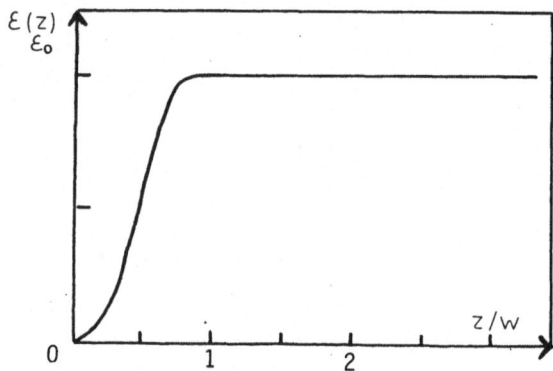

Fig.3 'Lightly' doped semiconductor. Schematical depth dependence of
the radius ε of the cylinder which describes the dislocation
perpendicular to the surface, when the SCR width is no more
negligible.

'Lightly' doped semiconductors

Now the SCR width can no more be neglected, and eqn(6) which gives
EBIC contrast has to be fully calculated[6]. In the bulk material, the
dislocation perpendicular to the surface is described by a recombination
cylinder of constant radius ε_0 around the dislocation line[13] inside which
the minority carrier lifetime is reduced to τ_D. This allows an 'easy'
resolution of the continuity equation. The same description can be made
when the dislocation is in the SCR, as it can act as an efficient
recombination centre. Nevertheless, due to the presence of the Schottky
field, the radius of the cylinder is z-dependent. This is due to the fact
that the electric field of the dislocation can compete more and more
efficiently with that of the diode when the latter decreases. Therefore,
the recombination probability of the dislocation in the SCR increases with
depth from about zero to its bulk value. The exact variation of the radius
with depth can only be solved numerically by taking into account the band
structure of the dislocation[14]; a quite rough, but good analytical
approximation has been found to be given by a gaussian variation of $\varepsilon(z)$
(fig. 3):

$$z < z_G \qquad \varepsilon(z) = \varepsilon_0 \exp \left(- \left(\frac{z_G - z}{\sigma_2(E_0)} \right)^2 \right) \qquad (13)$$

$$z > z_G \qquad \varepsilon(z) = \varepsilon_0 \qquad (14)$$

The three-dimensional generation function can be approximated by

$$g(\underline{r}) = g_1(x,y) \cdot g_2(z) \qquad (15)$$

148

$$g_1(x,y) = \exp\left(- \frac{x^2 + y^2}{\sigma_1^2(E_O)}\right)$$ (16)

is the lateral spread of the beam. It is a Gaussian function centred on the beam axis. Its width σ_1 increases with E_O. $g_2(z)$ is the depth-dose function as derived by Kyser[15] for GaAs:

$$g_2(z) = A \exp\left(- \left(\frac{z-z_O}{\Delta z(E_O)}\right)^2\right) - B \exp\left(- \frac{bz}{z_O(E_O)}\right)$$ (17)

z_O and Δz increase with E_O. A,B and b are constants; the A/B ratio is given.

Under such assumptions it has been theoretically found that the recombination currents in the SCR and in the bulk behave like the background currents with respect to the generation and to the material parameters (they increase with E_O, and the bulk currents increase with the diffusion length L)[6]. Furthermore, they depend on the SCR width, as well as on dislocation parameters:

$$I_{DD} = - e \pi \varepsilon_O^2 \, f(\sigma_1, \Delta z, z_O, W, \sigma_2)$$ (18)

$$I^* = - e \gamma \frac{\sigma_1^2}{2D} \, f(\Delta z, z_O, W, L)$$ (19)

where $\gamma = \pi \varepsilon_O^2 (1/\tau_D - 1/\tau)$ is the dislocation strength $(cm^2 s^{-1})$[5].

A typical variation of the EBIC contrast of a dislocation perpendicular to the surface with E_O is shown in fig.4; on the x axis is reported R/W ratio (R the electron penetration depth) instead of E_O, as it

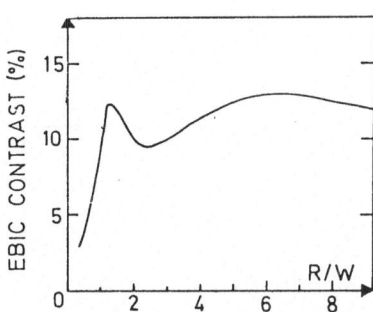

Fig.4 'Lightly' doped semiconductor. Typical shape of EBIC contrast curve as a function of R/W ratio for a dislocation perpendicular to the surface. The simulation has been made for the following values of the parameters:
generation σ_1=0.2R, Δz=0.35R, z_O=0.125R; material L=0.5 μm;
dislocation ε_O=56.5 nm, σ_2=0.2 nm, z_G=0.1 μm (z_G/W=0.2), τ_D/τ=0.1.

is more meaningful, though it is equivalent. The value of ε_0 which gives an EBIC contrast of few percents has been estimated to $\simeq 50$ nm; it is of the same order of magnitude as the Debye-Hückel length λ_D which depends on the doping level of the material through the relation:

$$\lambda_D = (2 \varepsilon_0 \varepsilon_L \ kT \ / \ n_0 \ e^2)^{1/2} \tag{20}$$

$\varepsilon_0 \varepsilon_L$ is the static permittivity, k the Boltzmann's constant and T the absolute temperature. At 300K λ_D ranges from 35 nm to 11 nm in CdTe for n_0 equal to 10^{15} and 10^{16} cm^{-3} respectively.

It can be immediately noticed that the EBIC contrast variation with E_0 is very different when contribution of the SCR is negligible (fig.2b) or not (fig. 4). The first increase of contrast is due to the increased recombination probability at the dislocation in the SCR with depth. The first maximum in fig.4 occurs when the dislocation current I_{DD} in the SCR is close to its maximum value. When the background current I_{DO} in the SCR reaches its maximum value, the contrast is a minimum. Then, the contrast depends only on the currents in the bulk region, and when the contribution of the SCR becomes less and less important, its behaviour with R/W is similar to that shown in fig.2b.

For a fixed value of z_G, the shape of the curves c=f(R/W) depends on the bulk diffusion length of the material (fig.5) as well as on one parameter which describes the dislocation : τ_D/τ ratio (fig.6). This does not happen in the case of doped semiconductor.

EBIC contrast experiments have been performed on dislocations introduced at room temperature by microhardness in a n-type CdTe specimen (n=1.6x10^{16} cm^{-3}; W=0.3 µm); roughly two types of contrast behaviours have been evidenced as shown in fig.7, which agree quite well with theoretical curves. The bulk material around defect n°2 in fig.7 could have a diffusion length between 1 and 0.5 µm ('active' defect,fig.6); or, if L=1µm, the τ_D/τ ratio is between 0.01 and 0.1 ('less-active' defect, fig.6).

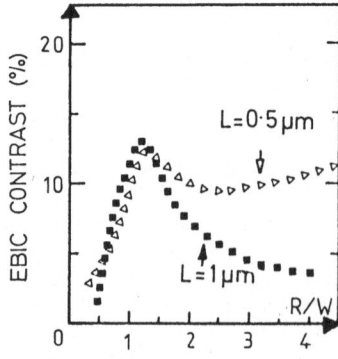

Fig.5   Lightly' doped semiconductor. Influence of the diffusion length on the EBIC contrast curves of a dislocation perpendicular to the surface. Values of L=0.5 and 1 µm are typically observed in CdTe. Other parameters are as in fig.4.

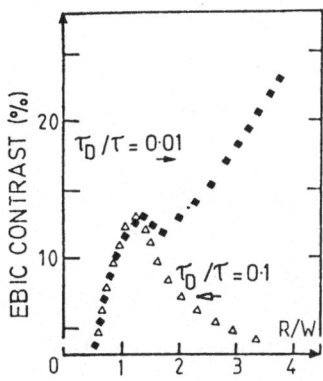

Fig.6 'Lightly' doped semiconductor. Influence of the τ_D/τ ratio. Dislocation perpendicular to the surface. $\tau_D/\tau=0.1$: the dislocation can be named as 'less-active' dislocation.

$\tau_D/\tau=0.01$: 'active' dislocation. L=1µm. The other parameters are as in fig.4.

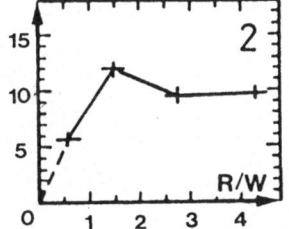
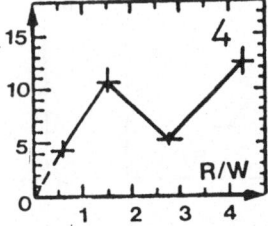

Fig.7 Lightly' doped semiconductor. Experimental EBIC contrast curves c=f(R/W) of deformation-introduced dislocations in a n-type CdTe specimen (n=1.6x10^{16} cm^{-3}; W=0.3 µm). The y axes show contrast (%). Two kinds of behaviours are evidenced. The accelerating voltages E_o are 10, 15, 20 and 25 kV; they correspond to a R/W ratio of 0.58, 1.53, 2.78 and 4.3 respectively.

A 'point-like' defect is described by a cylinder centred at the defect; when it lies in the SCR, at a distance P from its bottom (fig.1), its radius is $\epsilon(W-P)$ and its height $2\epsilon(W-P)$. Therefore, its recombination probability increases with depth. The theoretical EBIC contrast passes through a maximum and then decreases when the ratio R/W increases (fig.8). The position of the maximum of contrast depends on the depth of the defect; when it is close to the bottom of the SCR, the c=f(R/W) curve, as simulated in fig.8 can be identical to that of a dislocation perpendicular to the surface (fig.5: L=1µm or fig.6: $\tau_D/\tau=0.1$).

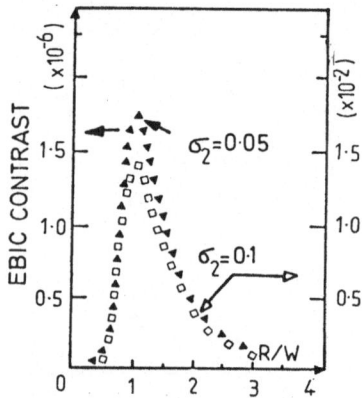

Fig.8 'Lightly' doped semiconductor. EBIC contrast curve as a function of R/W. 'Point-like' defect located in the SCR at a depth W-P. The parameters of the generation function are as in fig.4. L=1μm. ε_0=56 nm, z_G=0.1 μm (z_G/W=0.2), P/W=0.2.

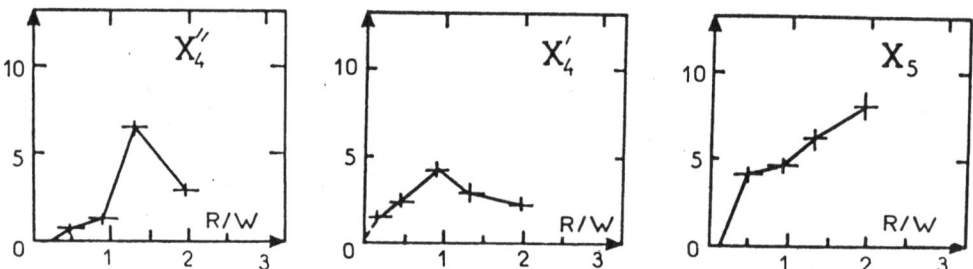

Fig.9 Lightly' doped semiconductor. Typical experimental c=f(R/W) curves of grown-in defects in a n-type CdTe specimen (n=1.5x10^{15} cm^{-3}; W=0.9 μm) imaged as dark spots in the EBIC mode. The y axes show EBIC contrast (%).

Experimental contrast curves c=f(R/W) have been recorded on grown-in defects in a n-type CdTe specimen (n=1.5x10^{15} cm^{-3}; W=0.9 μm); three kinds of behaviours have been evidenced (fig.9). Defect X_5 can be identified as

a 'point-like' defect located in the bulk, by analogy with fig.2a, as the maximum of contrast has not been reached yet. By contrast, it is quite impossible to decide unambiguously whether defect X'_4 and X''_4 are

'less-active' dislocations perpendicular to the surface (fig.6) or 'point-like' defects located at the bottom of the SCR. Therefore, this kind of identification cannot be made, as in the case of 'doped' semiconductors, by recording the EBIC contrast as a function of E_0 which only changes R in the R/W ratio; it needs the use of another parameter, namely the bias V_r applied to the diode, which can change W in the R/W ratio. V_r can, on the opposite to E_0, act on the recombination efficiency of the defect; therefore, the influence of E_0 and of V_r on the contrast should be very different.

IDENTIFICATION OF DARK SPOTS IN 'LIGHTLY' DOPED SEMICONDUCTORS.
AN EXAMPLE:CdTe.

Experimental

Experiments have been performed on grown-in defects in an indium-doped CdTe specimen ($n=2.8 \times 10^{15}$ cm^{-3}; W=0.6 μm) on which have been made an ohmic contact on the back side and a gold (thickness $\simeq$ 50 nm) Schottky diode on the front surface. The diffusion length, equal to $1 \mu m^{16}$, was of the order of magnitude of the SCR width W. The possibility to apply a reverse bias to the diode has been first used to determine a more realistic electron range R than that derived by Kanaya and Okayama[17].It has been found that the measured R value is $\simeq$ 0.7 times smaller than the R_{KO} range, and that it is very close to the depth at which the modified gaussian depth-dose function[15] is equal to 10% of its maximum value. This new range will be used on the following.

In order to define EBIC imaging experiments which can, in routine, allow the identification of dark spots in 'lightly' doped semiconductors ($< 5 \ 10^{16}$ cm^{-3}), let us first come back to fig.3 which displays the variation of the cylinder radius of the dislocation with depth. It can be shown that the global shape of the $\varepsilon(z)$ remains unchanged when increasing the SCR width by applying a reverse bias[18] (fig.10). The radius has been determined as following: the radial electric field of the dislocation E_D

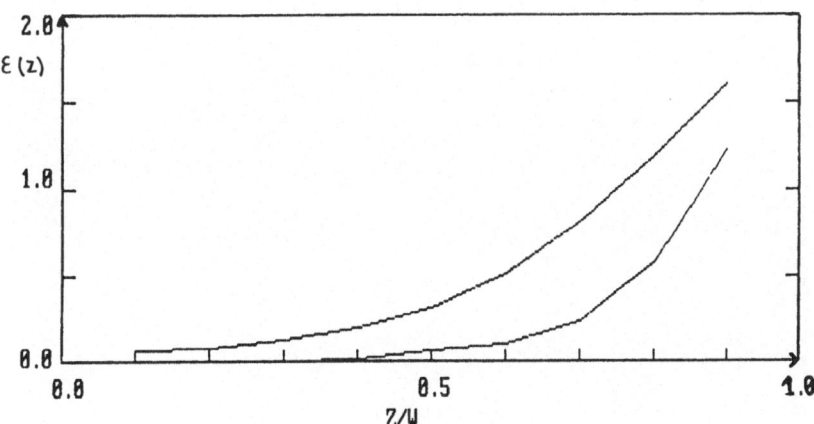

Fig.10 'Lightly' doped semiconductor. Variation of the radius $\varepsilon(z)$ (in λ_D units) with increasing reverse bias V_r of the diode[18]. T=300K, $n=2.8 \times 10^{15}$ cm^{-3}; dislocation level located at 0.2 ev from the top of the valence band. a- V_r=0V b- V_r=2V. See text for details.

has been calculated at different depths in the SCR in the Debye-Hückel approximation. E_D is a maximum at the dislocation line and tends towards zero at a distance of about $3\lambda_D$ from the dislocation line (λ_D= Debye-Hückel length). $\varepsilon(z)$ has been taken as the distance from the dislocation line at which E_D was equal to the field of the Schottky diode. As this field decreases in the SCR with increasing depth, the radius increases with depth. It can be assumed that a 'point-like' defect located in the upper-half of the SCR is not any longer a recombination centre, since the Schottky field is too high in that region.

Theoretical EBIC curves of dislocations perpendicular to the surface and of 'point-like' defects located at the bottom of the SCR have been previously shown on fig.5, 6 and 8. Let us now define (E_o, V_r) conditions for which it will be possible to distinguish between a 'less-active' dislocation and a 'point-like' defect (fig.8 and fig.5 or 6).
It can be first noticed, on theoretical curves, that all types of defects must be visible for R/W=1. At higher R/W values set by changing only R, and whatever they are, 'active' dislocations alone will be visible as their EBIC contrast curve is M-shaped. The negative effect of the bulk on the contrast of 'less-active' dislocations could be suppressed by increasing the SCR width and by keeping a constant accelerating beam voltage. R/W decreasing, it can be expected that the contrast of these dislocations is enhanced, while that of a 'point-like' defect is not, due to the greater strength of the SCR field.

Results

In fig.11a, taken for R/W=1.2 (13 kV, 0 V), all the defects are in contrast. Only S defects remain visible when a high reverse bias is applied to the diode (fig.11b; (13 kV, 2.5 V); R/W=0.6). The SCR width is so large (W=1.2 μm) that electron-hole pairs are created in its upper-half. Therefore, S defects cannot be recombination centres located in the specimen. They must be located on the CdTe surface (being tellurium

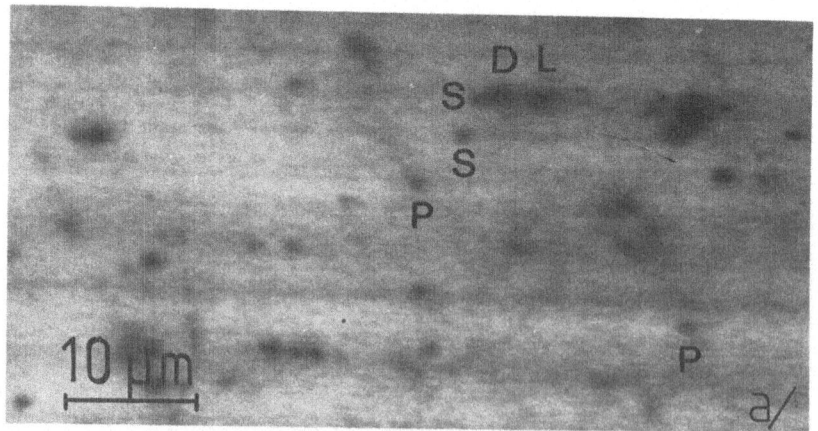

Fig.11 EBIC micrographs of dark spots in an indium doped CdTe bulk specimen (n= 2.8×10^{15} cm^{-3}; W=0.6 μm).
a- E_o=13 kV, V_r=0 V, R/W=1.2. All the defects, S, D, L and P are visible.

precipitates for instance), which locally modify the backscattering coefficient. Their disappearance in fig.11c, taken at (17 kV, 0 V) confirms this assumption.

At (21 kV, 0 V), L defect is out of contrast (fig.11d; R/W=2.6); it could be either a 'point-like' defect or a 'less-active' dislocation. Its nature is determined by applying a 2.6 V reverse bias to the diode (fig.11e; R/W=1.6): L is again in contrast, and, as previously assumed, it is identified as a 'less-active' dislocation. P defects, which become invisible when increasing the SCR width, are 'point-like' defects located in the lower-half of the SCR at V_r=0 V. D defects, which are visible whatever is E_O, are 'active' dislocations.

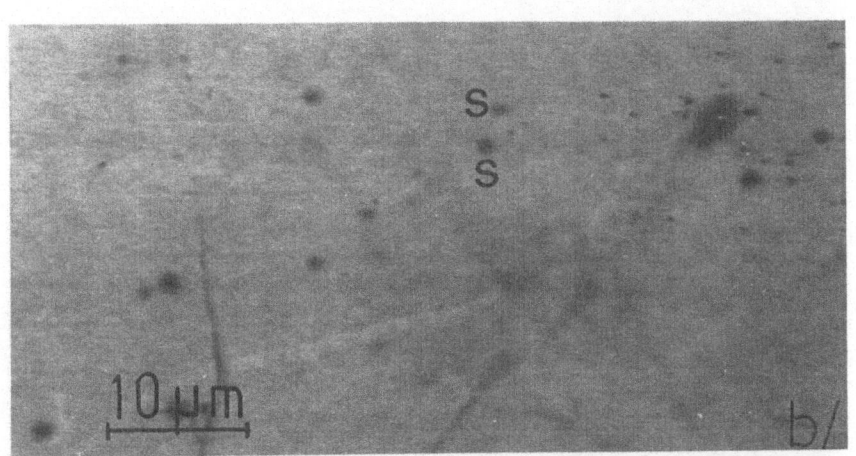

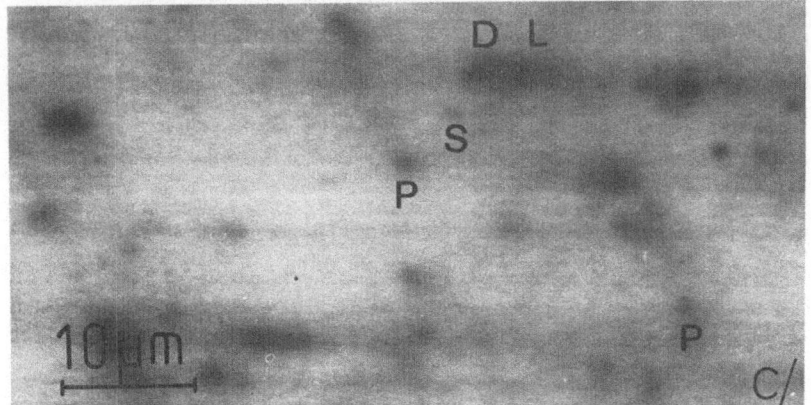

Fig.11   b- E_O=13 kV, V_r=2.5 V, R/W=0.6. Only S defects remain
        visible. They must be precipitates located on the specimen
        surface.
                c- E_O=17 kV, V_r=0 V, R/W=1.9. S defects are invisible.

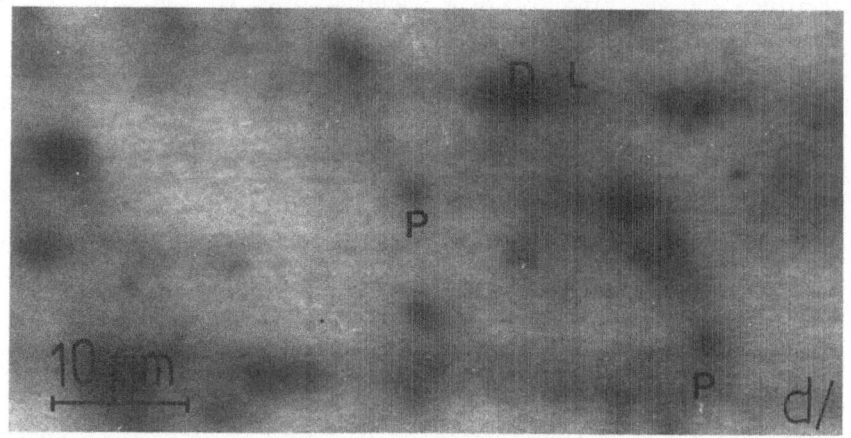

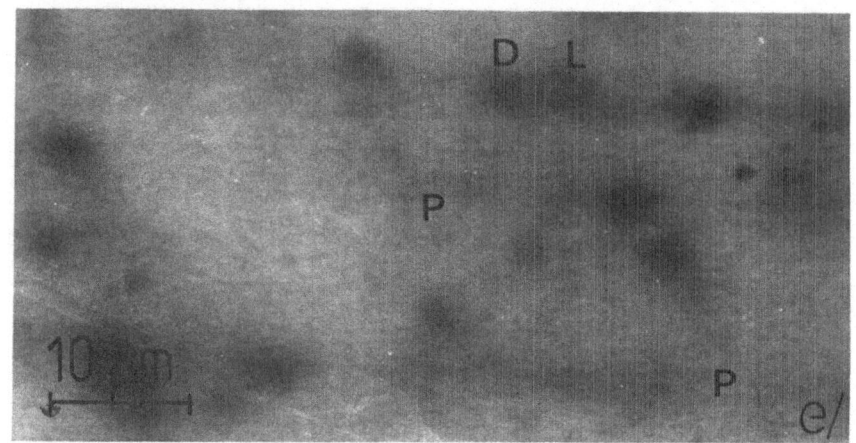

Fig.11   d- E_O=21 kV, V_r=0 V, R/W=2.6. Only D and P defects
        remain visible.
              e- E_O=23 kV, V_r=2.6 V, R/W=1.6. L defect ('less-active'
        dislocation) is again in contrast; P defects are invisible
        ('point-like' defects). D is an 'active' dislocation.

CONCLUSIONS

Theoretical calculations of the EBIC contrast of defects have been necessary to provide routine experiments from which the nature of the dark spots can be assessed.

This assessment can be experimentally made in 'doped' semiconductors by varying only one parameter, such as the beam accelerating voltage E_0. In 'lightly' doped semiconductors, both the SCR and the bulk contribute to the EBIC contrast. So, EBIC images taken as a function of E_0 only do not allow a complete characterization of the dark spots. A reverse bias, which increases the SCR width, has to be applied to the diode, if one wants to make the distinction between 'less-active' dislocations perpendicular to the surface and 'point-like' defects located at the bottom of the SCR.

It has been found experimentally that grown-in defects in n-type CdTe are mainly 'active' dislocations and surface defects which could be tellurium precipitates.

REFERENCES

1. International workshop on Beam Injection Assessment of Defects in Semiconductors (BIADS 1988). 18-20 july 1988, Meudon Bellevue, France. To be published in Rev. Phys. Appl.
2. C.J. Wu and D.B. Wittry, J. Appl. Phys. 49:2827 (1978).
3. J.W. Steeds, this issue.
4. P.M. Petroff, this issue.
5. C. Donolato, Optik, 52:19 (1978/79); Appl. Phys. Lett. 34:80 (1979).
6. B. Sieber, Philos. Mag. B 55:585 (1987).
7. M. Kittler, Krist. Teknik. 15:575 (1980).
8. M. Kittler and W. Seifert, Phys. Stat. Sol. (a) 66:573 (1981).
9. H. Leamy, L.C. Kimerling and S.D. Ferris, Proc. 8th Int. Conf. on X-ray Optics and Microanalysis, Boston, p 625 (1977).
10. S. Mil'shtein, D.C. Joy, S.D. Ferris and L.C. Kimerling, Phys. Stat. Sol. (a) 84:363 (1984).
11. D.C. Joy and C.A. Pimentel, Inst. Phys. Conf. Series n° 76, 355 (1985).
12. B. Sieber and J. Philibert, Philos. Mag. B 55:575 (1987).
13. C. Donolato, J. Phys. Paris, 9:C4-269 (1983).
14. J.L. Farvacque and B. Sieber, BIADS 1988, to be published in Rev. Phys. Appl.
15. D.F. Kyser, Proc. 6th Int. Conf. on X-Ray Optics and Microanalysis, Osaka, Ed G. Shinoda et al (University Tokyo Press) p 147 (1971).
16. B. Sieber and J.L. Farvacque, Inst. Phys. Conf. Series n° 87, 739 (1987).
17. K. Kanaya and S. Okayama, J. Phys. D 5:43 (1972).
18. J.L. Farvacque and B. Sieber, unpublished results.

ELECTRONIC STRUCTURE AND FERMI LEVEL PINNING

OBTAINED WITH SPATIALLY RESOLVED ELECTRON ENERGY LOSS SCATTERING

P.E. Batson

IBM Thomas J. Watson Research Center
Yorktown Heights, New York 10598

INTRODUCTION

The electron microscope has made great strides towards obtaining direct structural images of buried defects and interfaces in metals and semi-conductors. In principle, electronic structure may also be obtained directly from the same areas by observing the electron energy loss scattering. Currently at IBM, the high resolution electron spectrometer on the HB501 scanning transmission electron microscope (STEM) is producing core loss spectra which show directly changes in electronic structure at defects and interfaces. This report describes briefly the basis for the technique, and an application to the Al/Si(111) interface. At this interface, new electronic states appear within the Si gap and the Si conduction bandstructure a few eV above the conduction band minimum is modified. These modifications are intimately related to the establishment of the Schottky Barrier, allowing a direct measurement of the local pinning of the Fermi level.

The instrument has been described in detail elsewhere.[1,2] In brief, it consists of a VG Microscopes HB501 STEM with a Wien filter electron spectrometer and a Princeton Applied Research diode array detector. The spectrometer system replaces the original VG chamber top plate and sector magnet spectrometer. The Wien filter is located within an electrode which is held within a few volts of the STEM gun potential. Scattered electrons from the sample region are transferred to the spectrometer electrode by a doublet quadrupole lens and then decelerated to about 100eV energy on entering the high voltage electrode. Energy analysis is accomplished at this low energy to obtain high resolution. The electrons are then reaccelerated on exiting the spectrometer electrode. Finally they come to a focus inside a small chamber at the extreme top of the instrument. Spectra may be obtained either in serial mode, using a single slit and photomultiplier combination, or in parallel, using the diode array. Spectrometer alignment, bright field imaging, and low energy loss spectrometry utilize the single slit. Core loss spectra are obtained with the parallel array. Use of the double detection arrangement allowed a smooth transition to parallel detection. At present, as well, the serial detection produces a higher resolution and a lower background than the parallel system. In situations that do not require the very high efficiency, therefore, the serial scanning system is preferable.

For these studies, the spectrometer was configured to give an energy resolution of 0.35eV with an acceptance half angle of about 8mR. This resolution included about 0.28eV from the field emission source, about 0.15eV from the spectrometer angular aberrations, and about 0.1eV from parallel detector distortions. The STEM was operated to obtain 1Namp into a 0.8nm probe size using a beam convergence of 8mR. Thus, the spectrometer was fairly well matched to the beam convergence to maximize efficiency for forward scattered electrons.

BULK Si 2p RESULTS

The Si 2p edge consists of a threshold at 99.86eV followed by a delayed maximum near 120eV and ultimately decreasing in intensity towards 200eV. Since the threshold is small and at a fairly low energy loss where the background due to valence scattering is large, prior work has tended to emphasize the intensity variations on a 10-20eV scale. In this work, we are concerned with conduction band changes, so we must obtain variations on an energy scale of 0.1 to 2eV. Therefore, we typically obtain the inelastic scattering over a much smaller energy range than in the past. Figure 1 shows a 2p edge for the energy range 90 to 140eV to show the overall behavior. The expanded inset shows the range of interest in the electronic measurements. Within this energy range, we obtain the scattered intensity with an accuracy of about 0.5% in intensity and ±20meV in energy position. These results are obtainable now with the parallel array in a minute or two, allowing systematic investigation of the edge shape as a function of position. The spectra are automatically normalized for beam current fluctuations and recording time, so that a comparison of scattering intensity between two scans gives a measure of the relative number and strength of scattering centers.

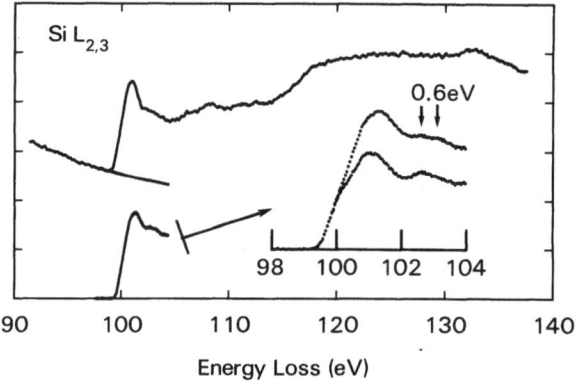

Figure 1. Si 2p scattering showing the onset at 99.86eV, various structure between 100 to 110eV (including a probable SiO_2 contribution at 106eV), and the delayed maximum between 120 and 130eV. After background subtraction between 98 to 104, the data are replotted in the inset. Next, the $2p^{1/2}$ part is removed by deconvolution of the 0.6eV spin orbit splitting to extract the $2p^{3/2}$ part of the data.

Variations in the final density of states will be reflected in variations of the shape of the edge. However, the core level density of states also contributes to the shape. In particular, the spin orbit splitting of the Si 2p core electrons gives an absorption edge which is made up of two identically shaped contributions which are shifted by 0.6eV. I follow the work of Brown, et. al.,[3] and remove the $2p^{1/2}$ contribution by deconvolution of two Kronecker delta functions which are displaced by 0.6eV and which have a relative weighting of 2:1. The result of this correction is shown in Figure 1 to allow a comparison with the raw data. In the expanded inset, the spin orbit splitting in the raw data may be seen as a doubling of the peak at 103eV. In the simple $2p^{3/2}$ result, this splitting has been eliminated to show the conduction band density peak at 102.7eV. All of the following figures will have the $2p^{1/2}$ part stripped away to better show the variations due to the final density of states.

The $2p^{3/2}$ results are replotted in Figure 2 and compared with the total density of states for the Si conduction bands.[4] On the basis of this comparison, the various peaks and inflection points in the data may be associated with various critical points in the Si bandstructure. Interestingly, the measured data do not reproduce very well the intensity of the total density of states. It has been suggested that this is due to core-hole interaction, or a core-hole exciton.[5] Recently, ground state calculations for Si suggest that the disagreement between the theoretical and experimental results may actually be a projection effect, in that selection rules do not allow transitions to final states having p-symmetry. Therefore the relevant final density of states should be the s- and d- projected density of states. When this is examined, better comparisons with the data result.[6] In either case, it is agreed that for Si, the observed structure is loosely identifiable with the conduction band density of states. Thus we can identify peaks in the data with transitions to Δ_1, to L_1 and to L_3 in the Brillouin Zone. Transitions to $\Gamma_{1,5}$ are optically forbidden. Between 98.78eV and 99.86eV there often is scattering which may be identified with final states lying within the 1.08eV Si gap. Some of this intensity in Figure 2 is likely a result of surface states. As the specimen thickness changes, the prominence of this intensity changes relative to the bulk absorption at 99.86eV. Similar results are obtained in GaAs and diamond. It can also be verified by constant dose experiments that this in-gap intensity remains constant as the thickness changes, while the bulk contribution varies predictably with the thickness. Finally, there is an orientation effect wherein (111) type surfaces show more scattering within the gap than (110) surfaces.

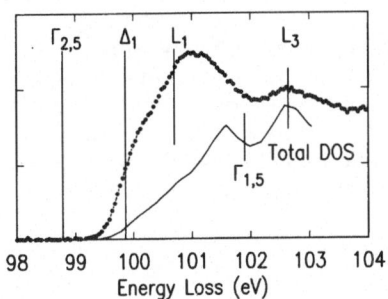

Figure 2. Comparison of $2p^{1/2}$ intensity with the total density density of states. Experimental features occur at Δ_1 (the band minimum in the (100) direction), L_1 (the minimum in the (111) direction), and at L_3 (a higher minimum in the (111) direction). Transitions to $\Gamma_{1,5}$ are dipole forbidden.

SUM RULE CONSIDERATIONS

The bulk intensity at the onset is rather small, reflecting the fact that most of the Si density of states occurs well away from the band edges. A sum rule analysis performed for Si has indicated that only about 0.005 electrons per atom contribute to the intensity within 0.3eV of the $2p^{3/2}$ absorption edge.[3] In a typical experiment, a 0.8nm diameter probe is focussed onto a sample having a thickness of about 25nm. Therefore, about $4 \times 10^{-21} cm^3$ of material is probed, corresponding to only 200 atoms for Si. Thus, a dangling bond defect level which has a strength of 1 electronic state, should give a differential scattering intensity equal to that produced by the bulk at 0.3eV energy resolution. At first glance, this estimate seems to be unrealistically large. However, estimates for the GaAs direct interband scattering give very similar results.[7] In that case, a calculation for the differential scattering cross section for a single defect state gave a result which was 100 times bigger than the cross section for direct inter-band transitions (on a per-atom basis).

If a defect state is present within the gap of a semi-conductor, then the spectral density of the bulk must be modified in some way. In a simple picture, we may think of a defect state as arising from a local distortion of a bulk lattice. Thus the shape of the bulk loss will be modified. If the defect has a simple symmetry, then only those bulk transitions having similar symmetry will be modified. The extent of the modifications will be governed by the electronic sum rules. As we will see below, the energy loss results generally show that scattering intensity within the gap is accompanied by modifications to the shape of the bulk edge.

ORIENTATION AND CHANNELING

Recently, calculations have been performed to estimate the amount of probe spreading in crystalline samples using the STEM imaging geometry.[8] It was found that, when the beam was aligned with a high symmetry zone axis, the beam current very rapidly formed fine filaments of high density running down the atom columns. This is a more general case of the classic two beam scattering condition using a small positive deviation parameter.[9] Thus, a 0.8nm diameter probe becomes a set of several very narrow filaments whose intensities follow an envelope which is roughly 0.8nm in diameter. In this situation, the envelope does not spread as the fast electrons traverse the sample. In contrast, if the incident beam direction does not correspond to a direction of high symmetry, then any filaments of high intensity do not propagate parallel to the incident beam, and the amount of probe spreading will be very large. In the past, it has been felt that strong diffraction conditions should be avoided in analytical conditions, in the hope that coherent, nonlinear effects might be avoided. On the basis of the recent calculations, it appears that the coherent effects may be useful to avoid probe spreading. In the case of core loss scattering, the zone axis channeling may increase the amount of scattering because the peak intensity at the atom columns will be several times higher than the probe envelope intensity.

Al/Si(111) INTERFACE

The above arguments suggest that it must be possible to obtain direct electronic structure information from individual defect states in standard high resolution electron microscope samples. In practice, of course, other mechanisms (surface states, amorphous surface layers, finite volume effects, and probably more) will likely conspire to make interpretation difficult. Some of these effects have been described elsewhere.[10] In Figure 3, I show several spectra from an Al/Si(111) interface. They are taken at various distances from the interface in a sample that has been thinned in a (110) plane to produce a cross-section sample with the (111) interface plane perpendicular to the sample surface. The sample was oriented so that the interface was parallel to the incident beam direction. Then it was tilted about an axis perpendicular to the interface to eliminate strong diffraction. As was discussed above this probably produced probe spreading in the direction parallel to the interface. This will be checked in future experiments.

For the present, the spectra show quite readily several variations which have not been observed before. First it should be noted that these spectra were obtained under several constraints that were not present for the data in Figure 2 above. Those results were obtained from a large, uniform bulk region with little restriction on the total integration time. In Figure 3, each spectrum was acquired for a uniform electron dose in a time which was limited to control specimen mechanical drift. Also the probe size was carefully controlled, limiting the total beam current. Therefore, the statistical quality of the results in Figure 3 is necessarily poorer than that of Figure 2. Even so, the total electron dose during the 20sec acquisition time for each spectrum was about $10^{10}e^-/\text{Å}^2$.

Referring to the Figure, the bulk $2p^{3/2}$ shape is reproduced at distances greater than about 5nm from the interface. Closer to the interface, extra intensity appears within the Si gap. This intensity appears to be of two types. First, at distances between 1 and 5nm from the interface, fairly large features are present. These are not accompanied by large changes in the shape of the Si $2p^{3/2}$ edge. Next, at distances within 1nm of the interface, the onset of the bulk edge shifts downwards in energy. This is a fairly subtle effect, requiring very good statistics to observe it. More data, using longer integration times, are discussed below. The downwards shift of the onset is accompanied by changes in the shape of the bulk features associated with the L points in the Brillouin Zone. Specifically, the peak at 102.8eV shifts down to 102.2eV, while a 104eV peak appears to move down to 103.4eV. The position of the Δ_1 shoulder, and the L_1 peak at 101eV are not modified. In addition to these systematic changes, randomly occuring gross modifications occur, as exemplified by the last curve in the Figure.

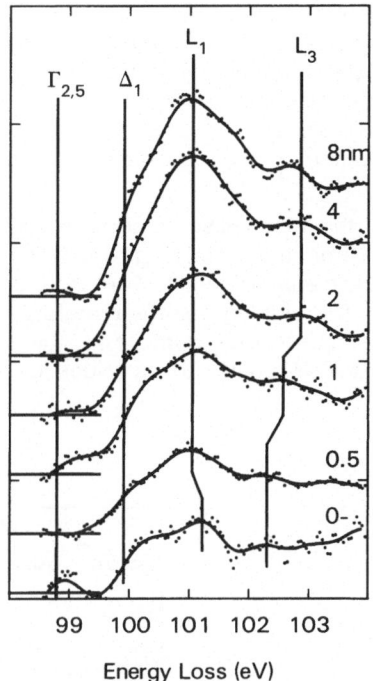

Figure 3. Sequence of spectra as a function of position near the Al/Si(111) interface. Within 2nm of the interface, changes occur which are probably related to the formation of a Schottky barrier.

Thus there appear to be at least three kinds of electronic structure changes observed -- 1) rather gross effects within the gap without changes in the bulk absorption shape, 2) subtle shifts in the bulk absorption onset accompanied by shifts in bulk peaks associated with L points, and 3) very gross in-gap peaks accompanied by large changes in the bulk absorption. At this point, a firm identification of these effects is difficult.

However, a highly speculative explanation might be the following. It is well known that electronic states within the gap can result from the presence of impurity atoms within the bulk. These impurity related states may or may not affect the local valence and conduction bands depending on their identity and location within the lattice. They likely will be quite strong, since they will involve a one electron state isolated on a single impurity atom. Therefore, considering the arguments above regarding the strength of defect scattering, the features 1) and 3) may be impurity atom related scattering. On the other hand, the spectra showing type 2) features are rather more subtle. In addition, they show a well defined progression from the bulk to the interface. Recently, S. Louie and M. Cohen[11] showed that the bulk Si conduction band is expected to be substantially modified close to an ideal Al/Si(111) interface, even in the absence of gross structural or compositional variations. They found that within about 0.5nm of the interface, Metal Induced Gap States (MIGS) were introduced within the Si gap. In addition, changes in the DOS at higher energies were observed as a consequence of the shift of state density of mainly p-character into the gap. Since the band edge at Δ_1 is composed of mainly s-like states, the initial onset of the conduction band was not much modified. The present observation appears to match this prediction quite closely.

If this mechanism is correct, then the Fermi level pinning point may be obtained directly from the initial, small onset of intensity within the gap. In Figure 4, I compare better quality statistical results from the bulk and the interface. A clear onset at 99.2eV is present. The pinning point is therefore measured to be 99.20-99.78=0.42eV above the valence band maximum, and the resulting Schottky Barrier for this interface is 1.08-0.42=0.66eV. These values are in good agreement with accepted values.[12]

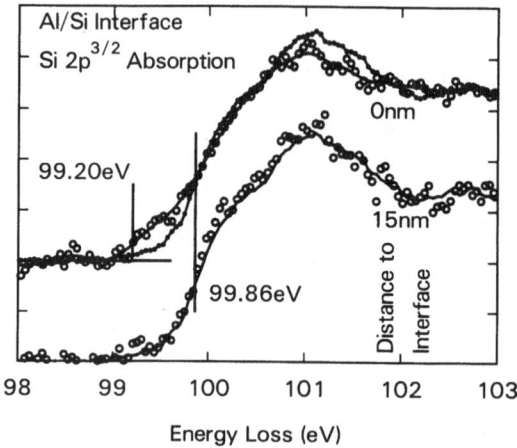

Figure 4. Better quality results showing a comparison between the bulk and interface results. The lower curves show a comparison between two bulk results having different statistical quality to show reproducibility. The upper curves are a comparison between the interface and the better quality bulk result. The Schottky barrier pinning position is probably indicated by the small onset of intensity at 99.2eV.

Thus we are led to the following picture -- that the interface pinning for this system is well described within the metal induced gap states model. But there exist, as well, isolated defect states, possibly due to impurities, which may pin the Fermi level locally at grossly different positions. In this case these impurities may be Al atoms in the Si matrix, oxygen atoms introduced from an initial native oxide, or possibly the boron atoms used to dope the Si p-type. It seems possible that in uncontrolled growth conditions, the density of these impurity states may be large enough to dominate the interface behavior. From the data in Figure 3, the Fermi level should be pinned near the valence band edge in that case, leading to a very high Schottky Barrier. This behavior has, been observed,[13] but not exclusively. Apparently the barrier can be increased or decreased depending on the identity of the impurity.

CONCLUSIONS

These studies are the first with this instrument that have shown such rich detail which is related directly to the electronic structure of the interface. In the future, collaborative work will relate the electronic structure obtained by energy loss to the atomic structure obtained by high resolution transmission electron microscopy. It should then be possible to calculate electronic properties for the atomic structure, and thus to compare predicted electronic properties with the measured properties in known structures.

ACKNOWLEDGEMENTS

I wish to acknowledge conversations with J. Tersoff and M. Wittmer. The Al/Si(111) cross section sample was kindly loaned by F. LeGoues.

REFERENCES

1. P.E. Batson, Rev. Sci. Instrum. 57 (1986) 43.
2. P.E. Batson, Rev. Sci. Instrum. 59 (1988) 1132.
3. F.C. Brown and O. Rustgi, Phys. Rev. Lett. 28 (1972) 497.
4. J.R. Chelikowski and M.L. Cohen, Phys. Rev. B10 (1974) 5095.
5. M. Altarelli and D.L. Dexter, Phys. Rev. Lett. 29 (1972) 1100.
6. X. Weng, O.L. Sankey and P.Rez, Proc. 46th E.M.S.A., (ed. Bailey, San Fransisco Press, 1988), p. 506.
7. P.E. Batson, K.L. Kavanagh, J.M. Woodall, and J.W. Mayer, Phys. Rev. Lett. 57 (1986) 2729.
8. R.F. Loane, Proc. 46th E.M.S.A., (ed. Bailey, San Fransisco Press, 1988), p. 820.
9. P.B. Hirsch, A. Howie, R.B. Nicholson, D.W. Pashley, and M.J. Whelan, "Electron Microscopy of Crystals," (London, Butterworths, 1965), p. 215.
10. P.E. Batson, Ultramicroscopy, in press.
11. S.G. Louie and M.L. Cohen, Phys. Rev. B13 (1976) 2461.
12. J. Tersoff, J. Vac. Sci. Tech. B3 (1985) 1157.
13. M. Wittmer, private communication.

EPITAXIAL NiSi$_2$ AND CoSi$_2$ INTERFACES

R. T. Tung, A. F. J. Levi, F. Schrey, and M. Anzlowar

AT&T Bell Laboratories
Murray Hill, New Jersey, 07974, U. S. A.

I. INTRODUCTION

Epitaxial NiSi$_2$ and CoSi$_2$ have attracted much scientific and technological attention in recent years. Scientifically, epitaxial silicide interfaces are the only single crystal metal-semiconductor interfaces that are available. They are ideal material systems for the study of Schottky barrier height (SBH). Technologically, epitaxial metal-semiconductor structures may be an important part of the next generation vertical integration of microelectronic devices. Also, the long electron mean free path of CoSi$_2$ has rekindled people's interest in ballistic transistors. Work in epitaxial silicide began more than a decade ago. Early works involved growth of epitaxial silicides with conventional Si processing techniques such as e-beam evaporation and furnace annealing.[1] [2] [3] Much improved results were obtained more recently in studies involving growth under ultrahigh vacuum (UHV) conditions.[4] [5] [6] [7] [8] [9] [10] [11] [12] The epitaxial NiSi$_2$/Si and CoSi$_2$/Si interfaces have very high structural perfection. These two cubic disilicides have the fluorite lattice structure and good lattice matching with silicon, with mismatches of -0.4% and -1.2% respectively. On Si(111), two epitaxial orientations are possible. Type A silicide has the same orientation as the silicon substrate; type B silicide shares the surface normal <111> axis with Si, but is rotated 180° about this axis with respect to the Si.[13]

II. GROWTH OF EPITAXIAL SILICIDES

UHV procedures for the growth of epitaxial silicide structures can be categorized into three main growth techniques. The first technique is the "reaction technique" which is also referred to as the solid phase epitaxy (SPE) technique. This involves the deposition of a layer of metal at room temperature followed by annealing in UHV to allow the silicide reaction to take place.[5][6][8] The second UHV growth technique is molecular beam epitaxy (MBE). In this technique, metal and silicon of the correct stoichiometric ratio are co-evaporated onto the clean Si substrate which is held at an elevated temperature (usually ~ 450-650°C).[4][8] The third technique is the "template technique". This name was coined during the study of $NiSi_2$ growth on Si(111) and Si(100).[14] [15] This technique is essentially a two step process. It involves firstly the growth of an ultrathin (usually <20Å) silicide layer by deposition at room temperature and annealing. This layer is known as the template layer. The procedures involved in the growth of a template layer are exactly those used in SPE. However, since only a few monolayers of metal is deposited the ensuing silicide reaction is affected very much by the metal-Si intermixing at room temperature. The reaction to form disilicide does not necessarily go through the two intermediate silicide phases as in the case of SPE, and the annealing temperature for the disilicide phase is significantly lower than the usual SPE temperature. As a matter of fact, since the extent of the metal-Si intermixing is self-limited, slightly different amounts of deposited metal can lead to significantly different composition profiles for the room temperature deposited films, which, upon annealing, can produce epitaxial silicide layers with very different structures. For instance, the orientation of the template layer may be manipulated in certain cases, such as $NiSi_2$ on Si(111)[14][15] or $CoSi_2$ on Si(100),[16] allowing single crystal orientation to be achieved. Thicker silicide layers are then grown on top of the thin templates using MBE, SPE, or reactive deposition epitaxy (RDE)[8][15]. Appropriate application of the template technique then allows the single crystal epitaxial relationship and the good layer uniformity of the template layers to be preserved in the final thick(er) silicide layers.

II.1 Epitaxial Growth of $NiSi_2$

A few years ago, a variation of the epitaxial orientation as a function of silicide film thickness was discovered in the $NiSi_2$/Si(111) system.[14] It was found that deposition of different amounts (monolayers) of nickel at room temperature could lead to the growth of single crystal $NiSi_2$ layers with either pure type A or type B orientation.[14][17] This relationship, reproduced in Fig. 1, is clearly related to the room temperature Ni-Si intermixing and the kinetics of the silicide reaction.[17] Recent in-situ microscopic studies[18] [19] suggest that intermediate metastable silicide phases may play a role in the determination of epitaxial orientation. With a proper choice of the initial deposition parameters and annealing characteristics,[17] single crystal $NiSi_2$ layers can be grown with very uniform and abrupt interfaces.[20] Deposition on top of the template layers and annealing may then lead to the growth of high quality epitaxial $NiSi_2$ layers with any desired thickness (greater than the thickness of the original template layer).[15]

II.2 Epitaxial Growth of $CoSi_2$

Annealing of deposited cobalt layers on a Si substrate has been a traditional technique of growing epitaxial silicides.[21] [22] [23] [24] [25] Unfortunately, this method leads to

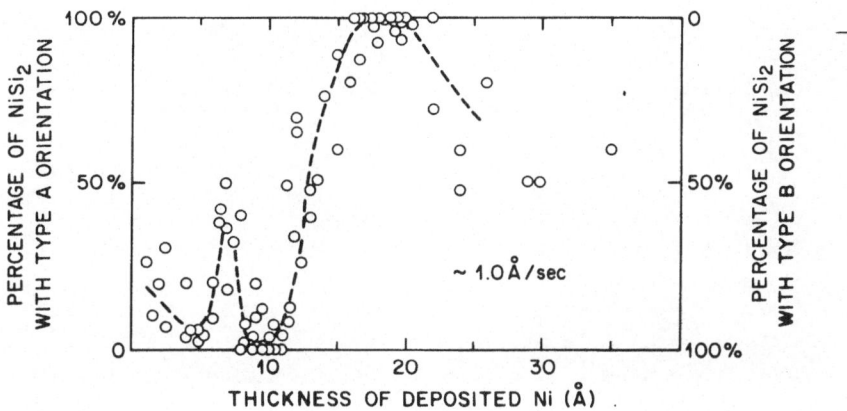

Fig. 1. *Orientation of thin NiSi₂ layers grown on Si(111) by deposition of nickel at room temperature and annealing to ~ 450°C.*

pinhole formation in the reacted CoSi$_2$ layers.[26] [27] If sequential deposition of cobalt and silicon is used,[26][27] or if co-deposition of CoSi$_2$ is used,[28] [29] then pinhole formation may be suppressed during subsequent annealing to form CoSi$_2$. It was speculated recently that diffusion through the CoSi$_2$ lattice may be difficult at the usual CoSi$_2$ reaction temperatures (~400-600°C), and that this may have an important effect on the morphology of thin CoSi$_2$ layers.[30] The formation of pinholes has been shown to be related to this issue as well as the stability of the two surface structures of CoSi$_2$.[30][31]

While the pinhole problem seems to have been solved, the dislocation problem has not. All the CoSi$_2$ films grown by deposition of cobalt and silicon have very high density of dislocations, typically $> 10^{10}$cm^{-2}. A high dislocation density is not restricted to thick CoSi$_2$ films: as films as thin as ~ 14Å have been shown to have similar densities.[32] (See, for instance, Fig. 3.) These dislocations are "grown-in" defects which are not generated to relieve strain from lattice mismatch, although they can relieve strain. Rather, they have to be present at every step (except for those whose heights are multiples of 3 interplanar spacings) of the CoSi$_2$-Si interface because of the type B orientation that the silicide occupies.

II.2.a Co-deposition at Room Temperature It has been known that type B CoSi$_2$ grows at room temperature upon deposition of cobalt onto a clean Si(111) surface.[33] [34] [35] [36] [37] However, this CoSi$_2$ reaction is limited to ~ 5 monolayers (ML) of deposited cobalt. When more than 5ML Co is deposited at room temperature, the low energy electron diffraction (LEED) patterns disappear[38] and other silicide compounds are observed.[34][37] Co-deposition at room temperature results in the growth of ~ 40 Å of type B CoSi$_2$.[39] If co-deposition is continued beyond this thickness, amorphous silicide begins to grow on top of the CoSi$_2$ layer.[39]

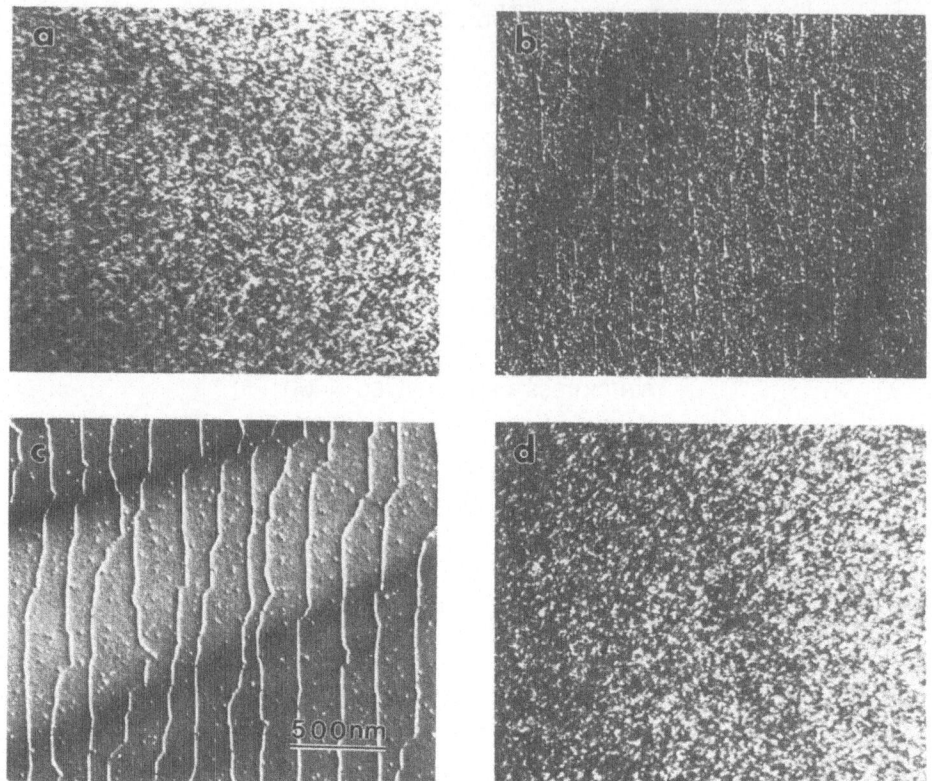

Fig. 2. *Planview dark-field TEM images of four $CoSi_2$ layers grown by co-deposition of ~ 72Å $CoSi_2$ at room temperature. Prior to co-deposition, 1Å, 3Å and 5Å Co was deposited onto clean Si(111) for (b), (c) and (d), respectively. No pre-deposition was used in the growth of layer (a).*

Recently, it was discovered that deposition of a few ML Co prior to co-deposition of $CoSi_2$ led to the growth of high quality epitaxial $CoSi_2$ layers of large thicknesses at room temperature.[38] Planview dark-field ($2\bar{2}0$) TEM images of four $CoSi_2$ layers are shown in Fig.2. These layers were grown by deposition of different amounts of Co, followed by co-deposition of $CoSi_2$ at room temperature. Transmission electron diffraction analyses reveal these layers to be type B oriented $CoSi_2$ except for the layer in Fig.2(a), which is majority type B $CoSi_2$ with faint amorphous rings, in agreement with a previous study.[39] However, if a small amount of cobalt is deposited prior to co-deposition of $CoSi_2$, then single crystal type B $CoSi_2$ layers are grown at room temperature,[38] as shown in Fig. 2(c). Ion channeling studies show that, with an optimum amount of cobalt predeposition (~ 3ML), the quality of the room temperature $CoSi_2$ layers is very high ($\chi_{min} < 4\%$).[38] The crystalline quality of the $CoSi_2$ layers decreases when cobalt predeposition differs from this amount. Furthermore, no dechanneling from the interface is observed for high quality $CoSi_2$ layers grown at room temperature, in sharp contrast to annealed $CoSi_2$ films.[40] [41]

The ~ 2-3Å of cobalt initially deposited on Si(111) apparently reacts to form type B CoSi$_2$ which then serves as template for the subsequent growth of a thicker CoSi$_2$ layer by co-deposition. We have used this technique to grow thick, ~ 300 Å, CoSi$_2$ layers at room temperature and there is no deterioration in either the quality of the observed LEED pattern or the channeling behavior of the layer. There is no correlation of the dislocation density with film thickness. It is therefore expected that much thicker layers of epitaxial CoSi$_2$ can be grown by this technique.

Co-deposition at room temperature, with pre-deposition of cobalt, produces CoSi$_2$ layers with a regular network of line defects as shown in Fig. 2(c). Most of these defects are found to have characters of $1/6<11\bar{2}>$ type dislocations. It is believed that the positions of these defects indicate the locations of steps on the original Si(111) surfaces. It seems that no long range diffusion occurs during the silicide growth procedures at room temperature. Therefore, steps on Si surfaces are preserved at silicide interfaces and are decorated with dislocations due to crystallographic differences. The dislocation densities in CoSi$_2$ layers grown at room temperature are dominated by steps on original Si(111) surfaces. Experiments with substrates of different intentional and unintentional surface misorientations have allowed entirely different networks of dislocations to be observed at the silicide interfaces.[38] This dominating effect of original wafer surface topography on the defect structures of epitaxial silicide films has not been pointed out before.

II.2.b Co-deposition Onto Annealed CoSi$_2$ Templates

From above discussion, it is clear that room temperature is an adequate temperature for MBE growth of high quality CoSi$_2$. However, a prerequisite is the existence of a good quality CoSi$_2$ layer on the surface. In the previous section, this requirement was satisfied by pre-deposition of a few ML of Co. Co-deposition at room temperature has also been performed onto well annealed thin CoSi$_2$ template layers. Shown in Fig.3 are the bright-field TEM images of a variety of thin CoSi$_2$ layers, all with an average thickness of 14Å, grown by room temperature deposition(s) and annealing to ~500°C. (θ_{Co} is the equivalent thickness of Co contained in a co-deposited CoSi$_x$ film. 1 Å is 9×10^{14}cm^{-2} which is ~ 1.15ML on Si(111).) As can be seen in these micrographs, there is a trend of more pinholes when Co-rich layers are deposited. Fig.3 also shows that the more Si-rich the deposited layer is, the more dislocations there are in the annealed CoSi$_2$ layer.

Ultrathin template layers were grown by deposition of ~ 4ÅCo followed by ~ 4Å of Si at room temperature. Annealing to ~ 480°C was then carried out to allow the growth of ~14Å thick type B CoSi$_2$ layers with a low density of pinholes. Line defects in these thin layers are dominated by the initial surface terrace structures, similar to the case of room temperature co-deposition. Co-deposition of thick CoSi$_2$ was then carried out onto these templates. Excellent channeling behavior is found for layers grown at room temperature by this method. An example is shown in Fig.4 which was recorded in the glancing exit geometry. The measured χ_{min} in this 230Å thick layer is ~ 2%.

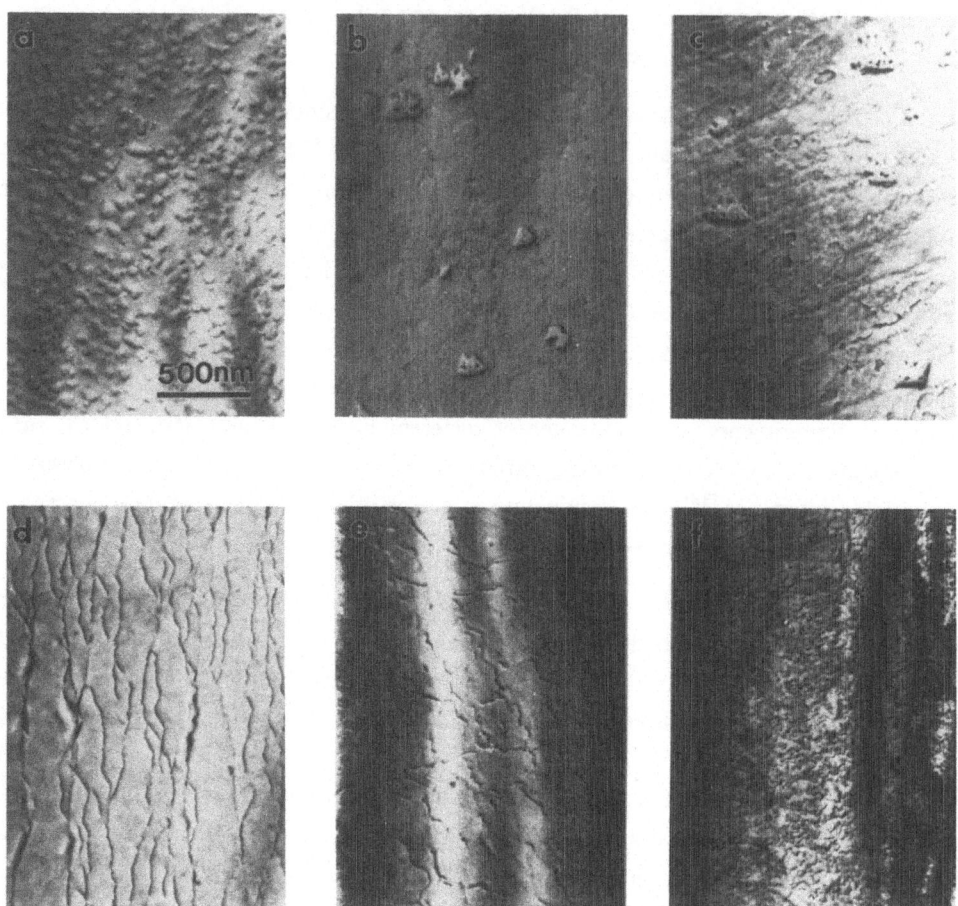

Fig. 3. *Planview bright-field TEM images, taken near the (111) zone axis, of assorted thin CoSi$_2$ layers grown by deposition of cobalt (and silicon) at room temperature and annealing to 500°C. All layers have an average thickness of ~14Å. The depositions used were (a) 4Å Co only, (b) 4Å Co and 4Å Si, (c) 2Å Co and a coevaporated CoSi$_{1.8}$ layer (θ_{Co}=2Å), (d) a coevaporated CoSi$_{1.2}$ layer (θ_{Co}=4Å), (e) a coevaporated CoSi$_{1.2}$ layer (θ_{Co}=2Å) and a coevaporated CoSi$_{1.8}$ layer (θ_{Co}=2Å), (f) a coevaporated CoSi$_2$ layer (θ_{Co}=4Å).*

Plan view dark field TEM images of a ~80 Å thick layer grown at room temperature are shown in Fig.5. Fig.5(b) is a weak beam <2$\bar{2}$0> image showing line defects reminiscent of steps on the original Si(111) surface. The origin of the observed small isolated defects is not clear. A 1/3<$\bar{5}$11> beam, forbidden in Si substrate, was used to form the image in Fig. 5(a). This spot originates from type B oriented $CoSi_2$ and is equivalent to a silicide-related <$\bar{1}$11> diffraction. Very fine dark line defects of high density were observed. After these silicide layers have been annealed to ~ 500°C these defects can

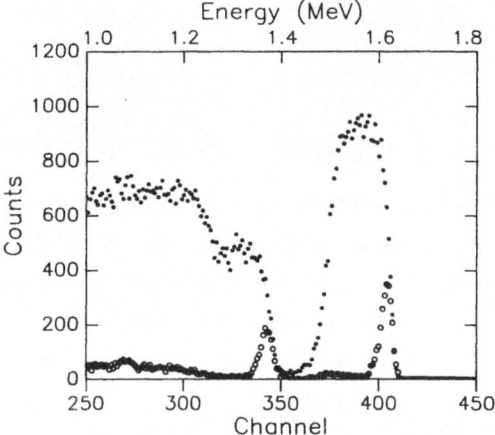

Fig. 4.   2 MeV He channeling and random RBS spectra from a ~ 230Å thick $CoSi_2$ layer grown by co-deposition at room temperature on a thin $CoSi_2$ template which had been annealed to 500°C. A glancing exit angle of ~ 5° was used.

still be observed. This type of defect has not been reported for epitaxial silicide grown on Si(111) and their nature still remains unclear. They are similar in appearance to the 1/4<111> related defects seen in the $NiSi_2$/Si(100) system.[42] A 1/4<11$\bar{1}$> type displacement at the $CoSi_2$/Si(111) interface would bring together silicide regions with different interface atomic structures. So far, these fine line defects have not been seen in fully annealed (>600°C) $CoSi_2$ layers, nor have they been seen in room temperature grown films.

II.2.c Annealing of Room Temperature Films $CoSi_2$ layers grown by co-deposition at room temperature using pre-deposited Co have been annealed to ~ 350-600°C. Generally speaking, more dislocations are generated upon annealing. A detailed description of this study is presented elsewhere.[43] The defect structures in these layers depend on the thickness of the layer as well as on the annealing temperature. A dense dislocation network is invariably found for annealed films with thickness of over ~ 50Å. Strong Moiré fringes are observed in TEM. However, for annealed $CoSi_2$ layers with small thicknesses (< ~ 40 Å), dislocation density and distribution are found to be similar to those found in films grown at room temperature. The terrace structures on the original Si(111) surfaces still dominate the occurrence of the silicide dislocation network. Depending on the

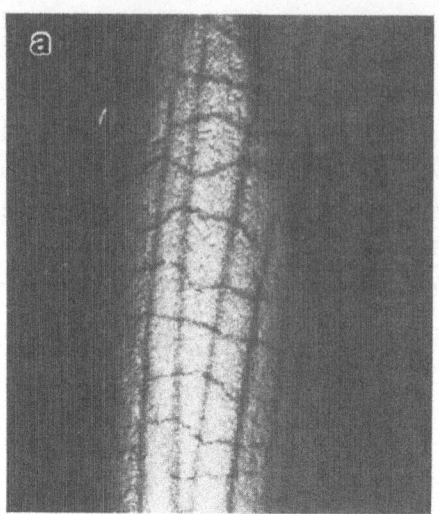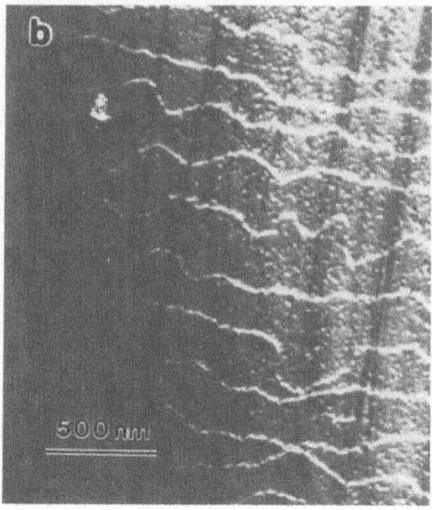

Fig. 5.   Dark-field plan view pictures of a CoSi$_2$ layer grown by co-deposition of CoSi$_2$ at room temperature onto an annealed template layer. The ~14Å thick CoSi$_2$ template had been grown by deposition of ~4ÅCo and ~ 4ÅSi at room temperature followed by annealing to ~ 480°C. (b) is a <2$\bar{2}$0> weak beam image and (a) was taken with a 1/3[$\bar{5}$11] near the [255] pole. This latter diffraction is a type B related <1$\bar{1}$1>.

stoichiometry of the deposition at room temperature, additional dislocations are also introduced. No fine line defects were seen when imaged with silicide diffraction spots.

Shown in Fig.6 are <2$\bar{2}$0> weak beam TEM images of a 25Å thick CoSi$_2$ layer annealed at 600°C. This layer was grown on a (111) wafer with an average terrace width of ~ 1000Å which explains the observed average dislocation separation of the same length. There are three different contrasts of silicide regions when imaged with any <2$\bar{2}$0> diffraction. Contrasts are reversed when -g is used, as shown by comparing Fig.6(c) and (d). Using the three different <2$\bar{2}$0> diffractions at the [111] pole, 120° apart from each other as in Fig. 6(a), (b) and (c), the intensity of most of the regions permutes among strong, medium and weak. There are also regions those contrast remains medium in all three g's. By varying slightly the deposition parameters at room temperature, CoSi$_2$ films annealed at ~500-600°C may contain different proportions of the layers which exhibit this "domain contrasts".[43] An exact explanation of these contrasts is still lacking. However, these observations are consistent with the existence of a slight slip or shear of different CoSi$_2$ regions with respect to the Si crystal. The displacements are along the three <11$\bar{2}$> directions. Those regions which always display medium contrast in weak beam <2$\bar{2}$0> are not displaced. Preliminary results from imaging with the <2$\bar{4}$2> beams and inclined reflections seem to be more consistent with a slip type relaxation at

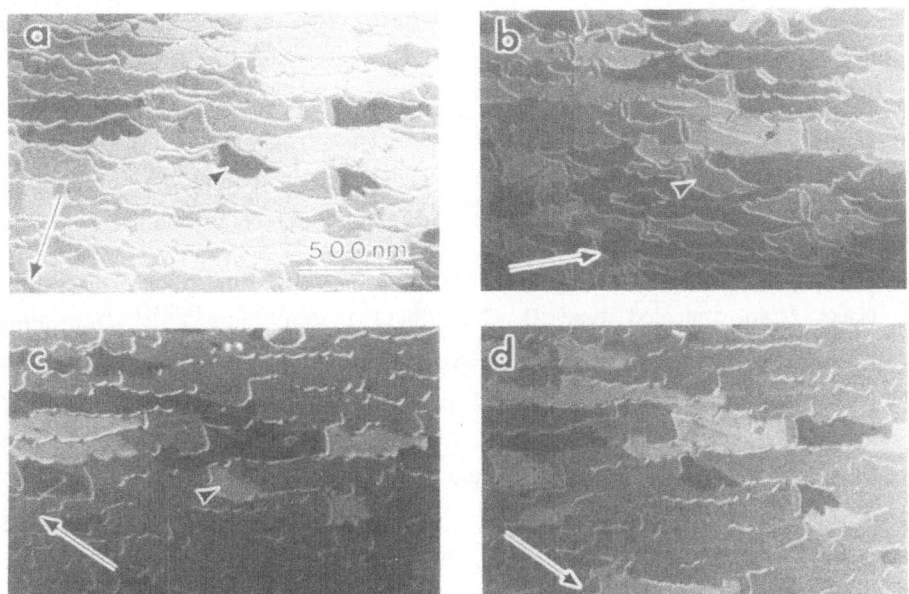

Fig. 6.   *Dark-field <2$\bar{2}$0> TEM images of a 25Å thick CoSi$_2$ layer which had been annealed to 600°C. This layer was originally grown at room temperature by cobalt pre-deposition and co-deposition of CoSi$_2$. The approximate direction of the g vector is indicated on each micrograph. All pictures were taken in the weak beam, with <6$\bar{6}$0> close to Bragg condition.*

the interface. In the next section, we will speculate on a possible relationship between the existence of these domain type contrasts and interface atomic structure.

III. SILICIDE SILICON INTERFACES

III.1 Interface Structure

The atomic structures of epitaxial silicide-Si interfaces have been studied extensively. High resolution electron microscopy (HREM) studies have provided experimental evidence for the atomic structure of epitaxial silicide interfaces.[44] [45] [46] [47] [48] [49] Both type A and type B NiSi$_2$/Si(111) interfaces were found to have the 7-fold model[44][45][46], while NiSi$_2$/Si(100) interface was found to be 6-fold structured.[46][48] These results are in agreement with those from X-ray standing wave (XSW) and medium energy ion scattering (MEIS) studies.[50] [51] [52] [53] The atomic structures of these interfaces are shown in Fig. 6. For the type B CoSi$_2$/Si(111) interface, HREM[47] and XSW[54] [55] both found results which would suggest the 5-fold model. However, the modelling of interface structure from HREM, XSW and MEIS relies on the determination of rigid shifts at the silicide interface, which, for a 5-fold model, are indistinguishable from that at either of two 8-fold models.[40] Two recent theoretical works[56] [57] point to the high interfacial free energy for the 5-fold model in comparison to the 8-fold model.

Recently there have been experimental evidences for more than one quasistable structure for this interface, including HREM images which agree with the 7-fold model.[40] At a type B interface, the boundary between a 7-fold coordinated region and an 8-fold (or 5-fold) coordinated region is characterized by a $1/4<1\bar{1}1>$ type vector. If a step is involved then $1/12[111]$ and $1/12<\bar{5}11>$ are also possible. It is suspected that the fine lines seen in some annealed $CoSi_2$ layers, such as shown in Fig.5, are defects of this nature.

Ion scattering experiments have demonstrated for some time the existence of interface peaks from annealed type B $CoSi_2/Si(111)$ thin films.[40][41] Depending on preparation, $CoSi_2$ layers grown at low temperature ($<500^oC$) may not show this interface peak.[40] No such peak has been observed for either of the two $NiSi_2/Si(111)$ interfaces. The origin of the interface peak is not clear. The high density of dislocations in annealed $CoSi_2$ layers is expected to contribute. We have recently observed a correlation of an interface peak in ion channeling with the existence of domain contrasts from $CoSi_2$ observed in TEM, as shown in Fig. 6.[43] The ion scattering observation also lends support to the notion that these contrasts are due to some lateral displacements. There also seem to be a damage effect by 2MeV He ion beams on both the interface peak and the existence of domain contrasts in TEM. Upon ion bombardment of over $\sim 5\times10^{14}cm^{-2}$, both the interface peak and the domain contrasts disappear.[43] The domain type contrast is most likely related to a particular interface structure. The observation of ion beam induced contrast change casts doubts on the feasibility of studying the contrast-related interface atomic structure by HREM, due to the ion milling involved in TEM sample preparation. It is worth noting that a lateral relaxation has been proposed for the $CoSi_2/Si(111)$ interface from a HREM study of double heterostructures.[49] No lateral displacement has been seen by either XSW or HREM of single $CoSi_2$ epitaxial interface. It is clear that much more work need to be performed to bring about a better understanding of the various structures at a type B $CoSi_2/Si(111)$ interface.

III.2 Schottky Barrier Height

The interfaces between epitaxial silicides and silicon are the only abrupt single crystal metal-semiconductor junctions in existence. They are also the only Schottky junctions where the interface atomic structure has been studied experimentally and theoretically. Therefore, epitaxial silicides are ideal systems for the investigation of SBH formation mechanism. An intriguing dependence of the SBH on the epitaxial orientation has been observed at the epitaxial silicide interfaces. Type A and type B $NiSi_2$ have distinctively different SBH's[58] [59] [60] on Si(111), where epitaxial $NiSi_2/Si(100)$ interface has yet a third different SBH.[61] The initial disagreement on the (111) SBH results[62] appears to have been understood[59][60][63] and resolved. This dependence of SBH on substrate orientation has not been observed for non-epitaxial metal semiconductor systems. In order to understand the difference in SBH's of type A and type B $NiSi_2$, there have been a number of attempts to measure the interface electronic states experimentally. Forward

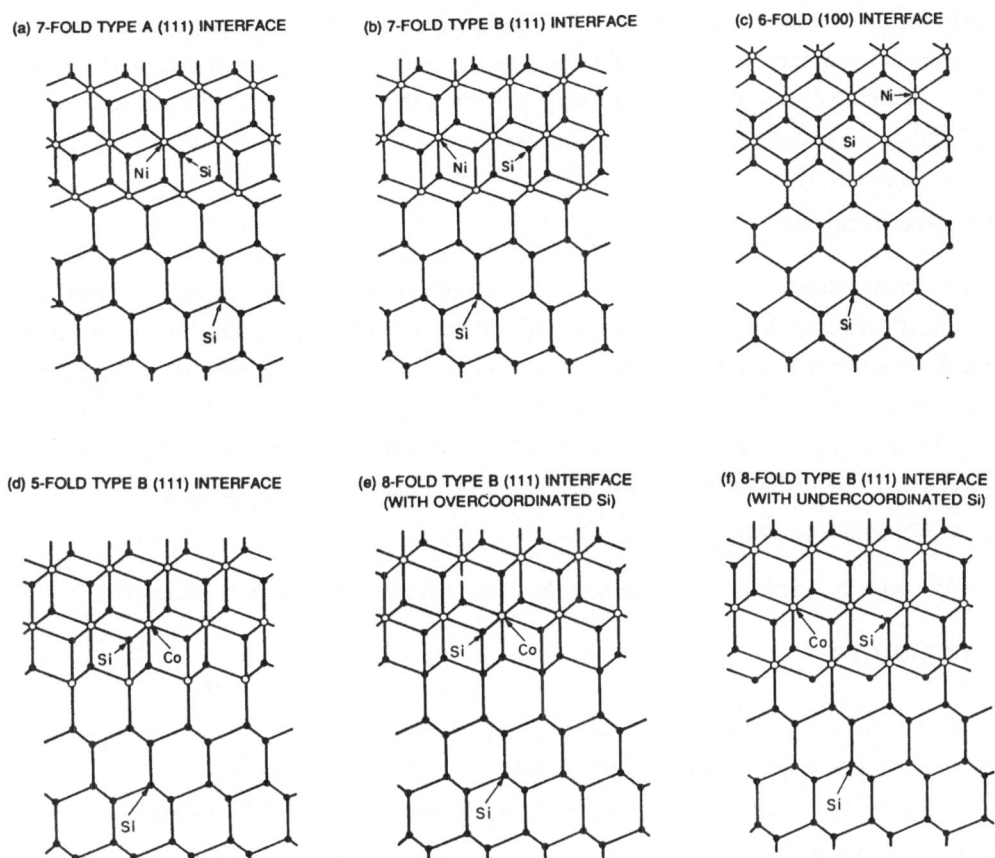

(a) 7-FOLD TYPE A (111) INTERFACE

(b) 7-FOLD TYPE B (111) INTERFACE

(c) 6-FOLD (100) INTERFACE

(d) 5-FOLD TYPE B (111) INTERFACE

(e) 8-FOLD TYPE B (111) INTERFACE (WITH OVERCOORDINATED Si)

(f) 8-FOLD TYPE B (111) INTERFACE (WITH UNDERCOORDINATED Si)

Fig. 7.   Ball and stick models of epitaxial silicide interfaces.

bias capacitance techniques have been used to derive a density of interface states of these Schottky diodes.[64] However, the shortcomings of the forward bias capacitance technique have recently become apparent[65] and results obtained from capacitance measurements are in doubt. Infrared absorption measurements on thin layers of type A and type B $NiSi_2$ have seen no evidence of interface electronic states,[66] in sharp contrast to results from polycrystalline silicide films. These measurements set an upper limit of ~ $10^{14} cm^{-2} eV^{-1}$ for the electronic state density at epitaxial silicide interfaces. There have also been calculations of the electronic structure of epitaxial silicide interfacs.[67] [68]

The SBH of type B $CoSi_2$ on Si(111) shows considerable variation with different preparations. Films grown by room temperature deposition of ~10-50Å thick cobalt and annealing to > $600^\circ C$ usually show a SBH in the range 0.65-0.70eV on n-type Si.[69] [70] [71] However, our recent measurements of thin $CoSi_2$ layers grown by techniques described in this paper have shown SBH's for some layers to be as low as ~ 0.40eV. A detailed analysis of possible correlation of structural characteristics with the observed

SBH does not exist at this time. Preliminary results suggest a possible connection between the presence of the fine line defects, as seen in Fig.5, and the decrease of the SBH. A full account of this relationship will be published.[72] Finally we note a recent calculation suggested the possible dependence of the SBH at type B $CoSi_2$/Si(111) junctions on the interface atomic structure.[73]

IV. CONCLUSIONS

Understanding the origin of the SBH difference at differently-oriented epitaxial silicide interfaces may help solve the old SBH problem. We have briefly reviewed important developments in the fast-moving field of epitaxial silicide. Because of the increasing attention this field has been getting, a lot has been accomplished in the last few years. But the need still exists for epitaxial silicide interfaces with higher structural perfection. We also need to understand the interface atomic and electronic structures better.

V. ACKNOWLEDGEMENTS

We wish to thank D. Eaglesham, J. M. Gibson and D. Loretto for discussions.

REFERENCES

1. K. N. Tu, E. I. Alessandrini, W. K. Chu, H. Krautle and J. W. Mayer, Jpn. J. Appl. Phys., Suppl. 2, Part 1, 669 (1974).

2. S. Saitoh, H. Ishiwara and S. Furukawa, Appl. Phys. Lett. **37**, 203 (1980).

3. K. C. R. Chiu, J. M. Poate, J. E. Rowe, T. T. Sheng and A. G. Cullis, Appl. Phys. Lett. **38**, 988 (1980).

4. J. C. Bean and J. M. Poate, Appl. Phys. Lett. **37**, 634 (1980).

5. S. Saitoh, H. Ishiwara, T. Asano and S. Furukawa, Jpn. J. Appl. Phys. **20**, 1649 (1981).

6. R. T. Tung, J. M. Gibson, J. C. Bean, J. M. Poate and D. C. Jacobson, Appl. Phys. Lett. **40**, 684 (1982).

7. A. Ishizaka and Y. Shiraki, Jpn. J. Appl. Phys. **23**, L499 (1984).

8. Y. C. Kao, M. Tejwani, Y. H. Xie, T. L. Lin and K. L. Wang, J. Vac. Sci. Technol. **B3**, 596 (1985).

9. F. Arnaud D'Avitaya, S. Delage, E. Rosencher and J. Derrien, J. Vac. Sci. Technol, **B3**, 770 (1985).

10. B. D. Hunt, N. Lewis, E. L. Hall, L. G. Turner, L. J. Schowalter, M. Okamoto and S. Hashimoto, Mat. Res. Soc. Symp. Proc. **56**, 151 (1986).

11. J. Henz, M. Ospelt and H. von Känel, Solid State Commun. **63**, 445 (1987).

12. T. L. Lin, R. W. Fathauer, P. J. Grunthaner, and C. d'Anterroches, Appl. Phys. Lett. **52**, 804 (1988).

13. R. T. Tung, J. M. Poate, J. C. Bean, J. M. Gibson and D. C. Jacobson, Thin Solid Films **93**, 77 (1982).

14. R. T. Tung, J. M. Gibson and J. M. Poate, Phys. Rev. Lett. **50**, 429 (1983).

15. R. T. Tung, J. M. Gibson and J. M. Poate, Appl. Phys. Lett. **42**, 888 (1983).

16. S. M. Yalisove, R. T. Tung and J. L. Batstone, MRS Symp. Proc. **106**, in press (1988).

17. R. T. Tung, J. Vac. Sci. Technol. **A 5**, 1840 (1987).

18. P. A. Bennett, B. N. Halawith, and A. P. Johnson, J. Vac. Sci. Technol. **A 5**, 2121 (1987).

19. J. M. Gibson, J. L. Batstone, R. T. Tung and F. C. Unterwald, Phys. Rev. Lett. **60**, 1158 (1988).

20. J. M. Gibson, R. T. Tung and J. M. Poate, MRS Symp. Proc. **14**, 395 (1983).

21. S. Saitoh, H. Ishiwara, T. Asano and S. Furukawa, Jpn. J. Appl. Phys. **20**, 1649 (1981).

22. R. T. Tung, J. M. Gibson, J. C. Bean, J. M. Poate and D. C. Jacobson, Appl. Phys. Lett. **40**, 684 (1982).

23. Y. C. Kao, M. Tejwani, Y. H. Xie, T. L. Lin and K. L. Wang, J. Vac. Sci. Technol. **B3**, 596 (1985).

24. F. Arnaud D'Avitaya, S. Delage, E. Rosencher and J. Derrien, J. Vac. Sci. Technol, **B3**, 770 (1985).

25. J. L. Batstone, J. M. Phillips, and J. M. Gibson, MRS Symp. Proc. **91**, 445 (1987).

26. R. T. Tung, A. F. J. Levi, and J. M. Gibson, Appl. Phys. Lett. **48**, 635 (1986).

27. B. D. Hunt, N. Lewis, L. J. Schowalter, E. L. Hall, and L. G. Turner, Mat. Res. Soc. Symp. Proc. **77**, 351 (1987).

28. T. L. Lin, R. W. Fathauer, P. J. Grunthaner, and C. d'Anterroches, Appl. Phys. Lett. **52**, 804 (1988).

29. J. Henz, M. Ospelt and H. von Känel, Solid State Commun. **63**, 445 (1987).

30. R. T. Tung and J. L. Batstone, Appl. Phys. Lett. **52**, 648 (1988).

31. F. Hellman and R. T. Tung, Phys. Rev. **B 37**, 10786 (1988).

32. R. T. Tung and F. Schrey, Mat. Res. Soc. Symp. Proc. **122**, (1988) in press.

33. C. Pirri, J. C. Peruchetti, G. Gewinner and J. Derrien, Phys. Rev. **B 29**, 3391 (1984).

34. E. Chainet, M. De Crescenzi, J. Derrien, T. T. A. Nguyen and R. C. Cinti, Surface Sci. **168**, 309 (1986).

35. F. Boscherini, J. J. Joyce, M. W. Ruckman and J. H. Weaver, Phys. Rev. **B 35**, 4216 (1987).

36. J. Y. Veuillen, J. Derrien, P. A. Badoz, E. Rosencher and C. d'Anterroches, Appl. Phys. Lett. **51**, 1448 (1987).

37. J. M. Gibson, J. L. Batstone, and R. T. Tung, Appl. Phys. Lett. **51**, 45 (1987).

38. R. T. Tung and F. Schrey, J. Crystal Growth (1988), in press.

39. C. d'Anterroches, H. Nejat Yakupoglu, T. L. Lin, R. W. Fathauer, and P. J. Grunthaner, Appl Phys. Lett. **52**, 434 (1988).

40. R. T. Tung, J. L. Batstone, and S. M. Yalisove, J. Electrochem. Soc. (1988) in press.

41. D. N. Jamieson, G. Bai, Y. C. Kao, C. W. Nieh, M. -A. Nicolet, and K. L. Wang, MRS Symp. Proc. **91**, 479 (1987).

42. J. L. Batstone, J. M. Gibson, R. T. Tung and A. F. J. Levi, Appl. Phys. Lett. **52**, 828 (1988).

43. R. T. Tung, D. Eaglesham and F. Schrey, to be published.

44. D. Cherns, G. R. Anstis, J. L. Hutchison and J. C. H. Spence, Philos. Mag. **A 46**, 849 (1982).

45. H. Föll, Phys. Stat. Sol. (a) **69**, 779 (1982).

46. J. M. Gibson, R. T. Tung and J. M. Poate, MRS Symp. Proc. **14**, 395 (1983).

47. J. M. Gibson, J. C. Bean, J. M. Poate and R. T. Tung, Appl Phys. Lett. **41**, 818 (1982).

48. D. Cherns, C. J. D. Hetherington and C. J. Humphreys, Philos. Mag. **A 49**, 165 (1984).

49. C. d'Anterroches and F. Arnaud d'Avitaya, Thin Solid Films **137**, 351 (1986).

50. E. J. van Loenen, J. W. M. Frenken, J. F. van der Veen and S. Valeri, Phys. Rev. Lett. **54**, 827 (1985).

51. E. Vlieg, A. E. M. J. Fischer, J. F. van der Veen, B. N. Dev and G. Materlik, Surface Sci. **178**, 36 (1986).

52. J. Zegenhagen, M. A. Kayed, K. -G. Huang, W. M. Gibson, J. C. Phillips, L. J. Schowalter and B. D. Hunt, Appl. Phys. **A 44**, 365 (1987).

53. I. K. Robinson, R. T. Tung, and R. Feidenhans'l, Phys. Rev. **B 38**, 3632 (1988).

54. A. E. M. J. Fischer, E. Vlieg, J. F. van der Veen, M. Clausnitzer and G. Materlik, Phys. Rev. **B 36**, 4769 (1987).

55. J. Zegenhagen, K. -G. Huang, B. D. Hunt and L. J. Schowalter, Appl. Phys. Lett. **51**, 1176 (1987).

56. D. R. Hamann, Phys. Rev. Lett. **60**, 313 (1988).

57. P. J. van den Hoek, W. Ravenek and E. J. Baerends, Phys. Rev. Lett. **60**, 1743 (1988).

58. R. T. Tung, Phys. Rev. Lett. **52**, 461 (1984).

59. R. J. Hauenstein, T. E. Schlesinger, T. C. McGill, B. D. Hunt and L. J. Schowalter, Appl. Phys. Lett. **47**, 853 (1985).

60. M. Ospelt, J. Henz, L. Flepp, and H. von Känel, Appl. Phys. Lett. **52**, 227 (1988).

61. A. F. J. Levi, R. T. Tung, J. L. Batstone, J. M. Gibson, M. Anzlowar, and A. Chantre, MRS Symp. Proc. **77**, 271 (1987).

62. M. Liehr, P. E. Schmidt, F. K. LeGoues and P. S. Ho, Phys. Rev. Lett. **54**, 2139 (1985).

63. R. T. Tung, K. K. Ng, J. M. Gibson, and A. F. J. Levi, Phys. Rev. **B 33**, 7077 (1986).

64. P. S. Ho, E. S. Yang, H. L. Evans, and X. Wu, Phys. Rev. Lett. **56**, 177 (1986).

65. J. Werner, A. F. J. Levi, R. T. Tung, M. Anzlowar and M. Pinto, Phys. Rev. Lett. **60**, 53 (1988).

66. Th. Flohr, M. Schulz and R. T. Tung, Appl. Phys. Lett. **51**, 1343 (1987).

67. S. Ossicini and O. Bisi, MRS Symp. Proc. **102**, 315 (1988).

68. G. P. Das, N. E. Christensen and O. K. Anderson, private communication.

69. R. T. Tung, J. Vac. Sci. Technol. **2**, 465 (1984).

70. E. Rosencher, S. Delage and F. Arnaud D'Avitaya, J. Vac. Sci. Technol. **B 3**, 762 (1985).

71. Y. C. Kao, Y. Y. Wu, and K. L. Wang, Proc. 1st Int'l Symp. Si MBE, J. C. Bean ed., The Electrochem. Soc., 1985, p. 261.

72. A. F. J. Levi and R. T. Tung, to be published.

73. N. V. Rees and C. C. Matthai, J. Phys. C **21**, L981 (1988).

THE FRESNEL METHOD FOR THE

CHARACTERISATION OF INTERFACES

W.M.Stobbs and F.M.Ross

Department of Materials Science and Metallurgy
University of Cambridge
Pembroke St
Cambridge CB2 3QZ

INTRODUCTION TO THE PRINCIPLES OF THE METHOD

We describe here the work we have been doing in Cambridge over the last few years on the development and application of the "Fresnel Method" for the study of interfaces. The accuracy to which the shape and magnitude of a local compositional inhomogeneity can be measured using this approach is often startlingly high and our aim now is to encourage others to start to use the approach. While there are still several aspects of the technique which, as we will describe below, can cause difficulties, we have now used it for a sufficient number of different types of materials problems to be confident that the method has a future in compositional analysis at a spatial resolution at, or approaching, the atomic level. Arguably the method is far from new though, as yet, we seem to be alone in making a systematic study of its breadth of application in the analysis of compositional changes at grain and phase boundaries and in man-made layer systems.

The principles behind the method are very well known, as is so often the case for supposedly new approaches generally. The amplitude and phase changes which occur when an electron is elastically scattered by an atom are characteristic of the atomic number. Thus when, as at a relatively discrete interface viewed in projection, there is a compositional irregularity, the form and magnitude of this irregularity causes directly related changes in the elastic scattering. The perhaps more surprising point is that the digital analysis of a rather low resolution and coarse through focal series of images, showing the resultant Fresnel fringe patterns, can yield relatively high resolution data on the form and magnitude of the compositional discontinuity present. Of course it is the local change in the projected scattering potential which is actually measured, not the nature of the elements causing this, so that a low concentration of an element with a large difference in scattering power from that of the matrix can have a similar effect on the Fresnel fringe profiles as a higher concentration of an element with a lower difference. From the outset it must thus be emphasised that the method is powerless unless the element causing the change is identified, even if only qualitatively rather than quantitatively, by a method such as EELS, which (even with the best will in the world) has a much poorer spatial resolution even on a specialised STEM. Accordingly the power of the approach is significantly the greater in cases which involve the change in concentration of effectively only one element. This is, for example, the case at an interface in a GaAs/AlGaAs layer structure when trying to find the compositional abruptness of the boundaries, and it is a very reasonable first approximation when attempting to characterise the local compositional profile of a specific grain boundary segregant although now the effects of changes in the rigid body translation need to be considered as well.

It has been suggested that an analysis technique based on the above principles is much more indirect than, say, EDX or EELS methods which are based on a knowledge of the characteristic energies for core level electronic excitations: this is not so. Of course the form of the near edge structure in an EEL spectrum can yield information on the bonding which can not be obtained from the other methods, but this is not the point. The principle behind using the fact that the elastic scattering factors are characteristic of the element is identical with that of taking the same approach on the inelastic scattering behaviour. By analogy we can distinguish between an apple and a pear as well, or as badly, either by looking at them or by biting them. Which is the more satisfying analysis technique is in this context irrelevant!

In order that the ramifications of our more recent work delineating the limits of the approach can be understood it is first necessary to give a very brief description of the basic experimental and computational routines which are required.

HOW TO APPLY THE METHOD

It will be helpful, as we think through the basic steps in applying the technique, to keep in mind a typical problem, and a good example is the characterisation of the roughly 2.5nm (or less) wide amorphous grain boundaries found in commercial hot pressed ceramics. It was in this area that we first characterised the approach[1], and a much fuller description of the basic method than is presented here is given by Ness et al.[2]. The first point to note is that it is not easy to analyse a single isolated boundary layer which is much wider than this using Fresnel fringe analysis. Here we immediately see the aesthetically pleasing nature of the method which is complementary to the use of conventional EELS: in using EELS, it is layers thinner than this which cause problems. We will deal firstly with the experimental variables in the (near) control of the microscopist.

Experimental method: Remembering now, as will any electron microscopist who has ever adjusted the objective lens astigmatism, that the formation of a good visibility Fresnel fringe system requires the use of illumination conditions as coherent as possible, it will not be surprising that the convergence is kept to a figure in the 10^{-4} to 10^{-5} range when imaging at 100kV. This virtually necessitates the use of a LaB_6 filament but depressingly high magnifications of up to about 1.5×10^5 or more are still needed. This figure is determined by the limitations of drift on the one hand and the resolution required when digitising the through focal image series on the other. As has been analysed elsewhere[2], the appearance of the Fresnel fringes can be a strong function of the applied convergence, but the rather low accuracy to which a convergence of the above magnitude can be measured from the diffraction pattern turns out not to limit the accuracy of the analysis. The microscope we use for this type of work has a Cs of 1.9 mm so that Scherzer defocus is at about 85nm. This will help in the visualisation of the rather coarse steps which are best used in a typical through focal series of about twenty or so plates. Near to Gaussian focus we use steps of about 50nm but at larger defoci the important point is to achieve a large range with an accurately known defocus magnitude so we then use steps as big as about 200nm. For accurate analysis both the defoci and the magnifications have to be calibrated as well as possible, and we find, for example, that the latter can be known consistently with a little care to about 1% by keeping track of the specimen height and focussing current.

The next question that might be reasonably asked by the aspiring Fresnel analyst (if he has not already gone to see his own) is how big an objective aperture should be used. This is not an easy question to answer. It should first be realised that there is no need to use an aperture with anything like the Airy disc resolution implied by the resolution of the data which it is hoped will be obtained. As we will note below, characteristic features in the image series allow the assessment of a profile to a far higher spatial accuracy than the resolution in any given image. Furthermore, when a large objective aperture is used, the sensitivity of finer features of the Fresnel fringe profile to the rapid angular dependence of the phase changes at high defoci can obscure the general trends which actually turn out to be the more useful feature to classify in the analysis as a whole. This suggests the use of a relatively small aperture, and this conclusion is reinforced by the need to obtain accurate measurements of the contrast at various points in the fringe pattern without getting confused by fine scale detail. The larger the aperture, the greater will be the contributions from the generally non-contrast retaining high angle phonon scattered electrons which are the main contributors (with elastic scattering from amorphous contamination) to the background. We tend to use an aperture for most problems with an Airy disc size of 0.63 nm subtending 5.8 mrad.

Arguably the most difficult experimental problem lies in ensuring that the boundary under study is vertical. Thus we immediately arrive at a limitation of the method: it can only be applied to the assessment of a composition profile if this profile has a constant projection through the thickness of the foil. For some features, such as a normal quality interface in an AlGaAs/GaAs heterostructure, any vicinality can be determined by, for example, the careful comparison of 002 dark field images as a function of foil thickness on rotating the specimen about this (the growth) direction[3]. Even so, care has to be taken in assessing the relative potential effects of any remenant tilt, interface steps in the thickness of the foil and a genuine smearing of the composition profile. Under normal circumstances, upper limits can be assessed for the first two effects so that a minimum for the last can be determined[4]. This is not the case for a typical grain boundary of the type we are considering here, but for grain boundary widths of the order of 2nm or so there is no real problem: provided that neither of the grains on either side of the boundary is strongly diffracting, the symmetry of the Fresnel fringe profile allows the boundary to be suitably orientated to within about a degree. If a symmetric fringe profile can not be achieved the boundary is probably not flat. For thinner boundary layers, as in for example the characterisation of the usually sub 0.7 nm SiO_x layer between Si and SiO_2[5,6,7] it can be more difficult to see whether or not the fringes are symmetric and under these circumstances image series have to be taken at a series of tilts over a range of about 5° and the best series then chosen for analysis. Turning to the exciting prospect of applying the method to grain boundary segregation the major problem here turns out to be not the difficulty of orienting the boundary but that when comparing a segregated and unsegregated boundary the rigid body displacement for the two can be very different and this would have to be determined separately[8]; the facetting so characteristic of segregation can also enhance the Fresnel contrast.

Since, to first order, the effect of increased specimen thickness is equivalent to a corresponding change in the forward scattering potential, the accuracy of the method can be no better than the accuracy to which the specimen thickness can be measured. Usually this is best done by the obsrvation of thickness fringes obtained under suitable weak-beam conditions such that the thickness fringe spacing is about 5nm and determined primarily by the deviation parameter. The typical accuracy to which this can be done is about 5% for the specimen thicknesses of about 30nm at which the technique is best applied. Given that there are obvious potential advantages in using thicker foils, the relatively low figure given here needs some explanation. In our earlier investigation of the method as applied to ceramics[2], we suggested that up to thicknesses of perhaps twice the above figure the accuracy did not appear to be limited by the contribution of inelastic scattering (which is hard to calculate) to the background. While this probably remains true in general, an exhaustive characterisation of the thickness dependence of the Fresnel contrast exhibited in the Si/SiO_2 problem suggests that here, at least, thinner foils have to be used for a simple linear relationship of the contrast to the thickness to hold[7,9]. The reason for this will be discussed in more detail below.

Finally it might be noted that while a simple-minded interpretation of the contrast demands that the foil should not be strongly diffracting, if this is impossible as is the case for, for example, platelets of a second phase with a well developed low index habit, then a naive interpretation is no longer applicable but the contrast does remain sensitive (and actually increasingly so) to the lateral discontinuities in the projected potential and can still be compared with simulations, thus permitting compositional analysis. The simulations of the contrast simply now have to done in such a way as to take into account the dynamical nature of the scattering. It is worth noting that the verticality of the interface then precludes the use of conventional Bloch wave programmes so that an atomistic multislice algorithm is, for this type of problem, the more appropriate simulation technique. Since atomistic simulations including interfaces can be demanding in computational time there are advantages in principle in using lower rather than higher accelerating voltages. This possibility has not been examined quantitatively yet but we suspect that, just as for the weak-beam technique, there are more experimental advantages in using higher accelerating voltages than might be considered appropriate theoretically.

Analytic method: The images obtained as described above first have to be digitised. Any modern system might be used but we use a computer controlled SCANDIG densitometer, digitising at 400 pixels/cm on the plate, and ensure that the original magnification is such that the data are acquired at a resolution some three times that in the original micrograph. It is this which requires magnifications in excess of 100k. If the original images prove to be difficult to obtain at the exposure times such magnifications imply, then it is possible to re-photograph the original negatives at higher magnification prior to digitising within the limitations of the emulsion grain size. However in this context it should be noted that there are advantages in using plates which are, by normal standards, substantially under-exposed so as to ensure linearity in the response of the photographic emulsion (this has otherwise to be corrected for). However, re-photographing is not recommended for the accurate measurements of profiles, and further it should be noted that the process of digitisation necessarily reduces the reolution as well as potentially introducing errors due to, for example, imperfect focussing of the densitometer. Such errors have to be assessed and included in the analytic comparison of the modelled simulations with the digitised experimental data. All the image processing we do on the original images is completed using the SEMPER system[10], and this is more than sophisticated enough to allow the appropriate manipulation of aligned windows over the Fresnel fringe system which can then be projected along the direction of the interface to form one-dimensional Fresnel profiles. It is at this stage that judgement is needed in the choice of a suitable length of the fringe system over which to average: the longer this is, the smoother the profile and the more effects due to the Fresnel scattering of superposed contamination can be minimised; the shorter is this length, the more is the control over the important parameter of the specimen thickness at which the profile is to be simulated.

For a very large fraction of the problems we have examined to date it has proved to be perfectly adequate, somewhat to our surprise, to use a continuum model for the scattering behaviour when simulating the profiles to match with the digitised data. This point was in fact checked in the original quantitative analysis applied to amorphous grain boundaries in ceramics[2] and a good qualitative rule is that if the images exhibit any dynamical effects at all in the area of interest (as in this case in the grains on either side of the boundary) then an atomistic multislice approach will have to be applied. In the continuum model the different materials across the boundary are represented in the multislice programme by uniform (as if for amorphous) scattering potentials, V_0, determined from the tabulated electron scattering potentials as a function of the actual structures present in the different regions. Ross[9] has analysed the probable errors associated with the existence or otherwise of changes in bonding effects in using this approach, comparing calculations done using the Doyle and Turner[11] and Radi[12] data sets for the atomic scattering coefficients. Since such errors are both small, when comparing two materials, and in the main systematic, it would appear that they need not limit the accuracies achievable if all that is required is the magnitude of the change in potential, and thence composition; further work in this area is however probably required. It should be noted that when using the continuum model in this simplistic manner the only way amplitude is scattered away from the origin in reciprocal space is through the effects of the shape of the boundary in the periodically repeating model which is sliced in the otherwise standard calculations. While it is clear that dynamical effects will not be modelled properly at all under the continuum approximation, it is nonetheless interesting that the degree of diffuseness of an interface can often be assessed using the simpler model.

Even when using atomistic simulations, particular care has to be taken over the appropriate form of the periodically repeating unit containing the interface to be analysed, and the same is true in the continuum approach. The standard problem is of course that the longer the repeated "unit cell" the poorer is the sampling but the less is the danger of "wrap around". Because of the very large defoci which are of interest it is the latter effects which have to be watched out for with even more vigilance than is usually required. An interesting aspect of the use of the Fresnel method is indeed the degree to which the local contrast of an individual layer in a multilayer is in reality affected by the other layers and there would appear to be ways of using the degree to which it is so affected to obtain, for example, improved values for the layer spacings as well as a better appreciation of the regularity of the system as a whole.

Before proceeding further we should first understand why it is that other apparently more direct approaches to the solution of this type of problem do not have the same potential. After all it is only if there are clear advantages in the use of the Fresnel Method that we should bother to clutter the library with "yet another technique". Here we will limit the discussion to techniques based on the use of TEM.

OTHER COMPETITIVE ANALYTIC METHODS

Why is it, then, that high resolution methods have seen little success in this area of local compositional analysis and, at best, are used to determine the structure once the composition change at the interface has been analysed by some other approach? A major criticism which can be levelled with a certain amount of justification at electron microscopists generally is that too often the micrograph is used only in its analogue form. This is current practice even for the high resolution fraternity, in that while the beautiful images which can be formed are now usually compared with simulations, it is still very rare that authors worry too much about the relative intensities seen from point to point: instead they are heartily relieved if there is a reasonable match of the symmetry and the local pattern. This is well evidenced by the rarity with which the minimum and maximum intensities in even the simulations, let alone the experimental images, are recorded in the literature. The reasons for this are not hard to find: while the coherency of elastic scattering leads to the formation of electron diffraction patterns which can blind one to the frequently higher probability of inelastic scattering, the latter type of process can not be neglected in any realistic attempt to compare the intensities and contrast in an image and simulation. The trouble is, of course, that to make any reasonable sort of job of doing this, the different ways in which all the different types of inelastic scattering might contribute to the image have to be considered and dealt with. This is no mean task, particularly when it is remembered that not only do some inelastic scattering processes allow subsequent elastic scattering to exhibit, to a greater or lesser degree, contast at the atomic level while others do not, but also the relative probabilities for these different processes will change from material to material. It is for these sorts of reasons that the phenomenological theory for the treatment of "absorption" is so successful and yet at the same time necessarily limiting. As soon as we fit an image on this sort of basis we lose the potential to test a structural model, at least to the extent that the uniqueness of the interpretation becomes questionable.

Given the potential which undoubtedly exists for the more quantitative use of transmission electron microscopy through the measurement and matching of the contrast in an image, it is surprising that so little has been done in the above area in the low as well as the high resolution field. We have been aware for a number of years of many of the problems associated with the quantitative interpretation of images, to the extent that while we do a great deal of high resolution microscopy using the Cambridge HREM we seldom rely on its direct interpretation (through comparisons with simulations) alone, but instead seek more indirect methods, of which the Fresnel Method is only one, to obtain the quantitative data we need for the solution of a given materials problem (some of the earlier approaches have been discussed elsewhere[13,14]). We have only recently however begun to attempt to include inelastic scattering processes quantitatively in image formation[15], and have applied the techniques we are developing only, as yet, in preliminary studies of AlGaAs/GaAs interfaces[16,17], and in the analysis of the oxygen ordering problem in $YBa_2Cu_3O_{7-d}$[18,19], in both cases arguably with as much emphasis on the demonstration of the necessity for the type of treatment which was applied as with any real hope for a substantial improvement in the degree of accuracy in model matching which might be achieved. As yet we have applied these approaches to the analysis of Fresnel fringe contrast only fairly qualitatively[7,9] so it is fortunate that, as has been demonstrated, many of the applications of the Fresnel Method are less sensitive to the problems of inelastic scattering than is the high resolution approach[15].

Since we have suggested that it is the effects of inelastic scattering that are generally limiting in the application of high resolution techniques to the compositional characterisation of an interface (and even actually to its local structural assessment), it would now seem to be appropriate to comment briefly on the use of conventional EDX and EELS techniques for this purpose. These methods are of course unrivalled if all that is required is the quantitative characterisation of the <u>nature</u> of a given compositional fluctuation on a relatively coarse scale. In this context the well known problems associated with the production of x-rays from regions far from that examined with the probe make the use of EDX, if extremely convenient, at the minimum subject to the need for considerable interpretative care. On the other hand this is not a problem for EELS methods, though these are apparently doomed to suffer for all time from difficulties in the interpretation (in the main because of multiple inelastic/elastic scattering) and in the subtraction of the background to an edge for anything other than a foil which would be considered thin in high resolution terms.

Even when using a specialist STEM fitted with a LaB_6 or pure field emission filament, the limitations caused synergistically by the need for a small probe and a thin specimen limit either the accuracy and sensitivity of the technique or the smallness of the lateral dimensions of a region which can be analysed. In practice it is really rather rare for a STEM to be used analytically for a region smaller than about 2.5nm across, though this will of course be dependant on the nature of the particular problem examined. Interestingly an, admittedly "in principle", analysis of the relative advantages of using a specialist STEM machine by comparison with a CTEM fitted with a filter for edge loss imaging suggests that for an analysis required over an <u>area</u> rather than at a known <u>point</u> there should be substantial advantages in using the filtered CTEM at <u>any</u> resolution[20]. Whether or not this will be the case awaits the development of filtered CTEMs of higher voltage than the otherwise fascinating Zeiss 902, but in general it would appear to be unlikely that a mixture of reciprocity and the uncertainty principle will not, in fact, make the two approaches comparable. The practical applications of high resolution STEM analysis that have been achieved thus become noteworthy and we are not, for example, aware of any work other than that of Batson et al.[21], on the changes in form of segregation to grain boundaries in polysilicon induced by different thermal treatments, which is of comparable quality in terms of the resolution attained given the retention of analytic accuracy. The other problem in the use of small probe STEM is of course the way in which specimen degradation can occur, an attribute in other applications such as beam writing as now applied even in CTEM[22]. It was this problem of beam damage which was probably the limiting factor in an otherwise unequivocal comparison of high resolution images of dislocation cores in Si with data obtained using a field emission STEM on the presence of oxygen at these defects[23].

The above discussion is not intended to give the impression that the Fresnel method is "better" than EELS: while the former approach yields more easily a superior spatial resolution it nonetheless relies on the use of the latter technique to identify the element whose composition profile is to be quantified. The two methods are obviously best applied (with others if necessary!) in tandem.

Having dealt with what are generally described as the more "direct" approaches we should note, in our comparison here of the Fresnel method with other analytic techniques, that the use of the elastic scattering behaviour of a material for this purpose is also far from new! It is well known, for example, that the "fingerprint" provided by a convergent beam diffraction pattern can often be used to identify an admittedly necessarily fairly large precipitate[24,25]. A comparison too of the relative qualities of the different methods which can be used for the analysis of the Al content of thin layers of $Al_xGa_{1-x}As$ in GaAs is interesting. Not only can fairly abstruse developments of CBED be applied[26], but so too can thickness fringe analyses[27,28,29] (though these probably tend to pay too little attention to variations in the most appropriate Debye-Waller constant, which should be used as a function of the concentration, particularly for III-V systems containing indium) and carefully quantified measurements of the composition sensitive intensity of the 002 beam[30].

It has been argued elsewhere[30] that in this specific application, when measuring the concentration of Al in $Al_xGa_{1-x}As$, it is the last method which is the most accurate but that the Fresnel approach yields the better data on the abruptness of the interfaces present[4]. We should point out, however, that for other III-V systems this is not necessarily the case.

BACKGROUND TO THE FRESNEL METHOD

Before concluding this description of the method with a few examples of its application, it is interesting to examine its pedigree. Certainly the analysis of the form of the Fresnel fringes seen at the edge of a specimen has been attempted for many years and it was recognised as long ago as 1974[31] that this contrast can change as a function of the geometric form of the specimen edge; this realisation is arguably at the heart of its use in the manner we describe here. The early uses of defocus contrast to measure the width of amorphous grain boundary layers[32,33] were of somewhat limited accuracy when compared with later data[34,2] but it has also been recognised for some time, as reviewed by Stobbs[35] that the enhancement of the contrast of small voids resulting from viewing them at an appropriate defocus can allow their recognition down to sizes approaching atomic dimensions. Still more interesting was the measurement by Iijima[36] of the value of the defocus required to enhance the contrast of small pits in the surface of graphite in order to determine their depth. Further related work of interest is that of Rühle et al.[37] who attempted to use changes in the spacings of the Fresnel fringes associated with dislocations on a vertical grain boundary in a ceramic to deduce a value for the scattering potential at the dislocation cores. From our current work we would deduce that the magnitude of a change in potential would be better measured from the magnitude of the Fresnel contrast, while the changes in shape (form) of the contrast with defocus could well be applied in this type of experiment to permit at least a qualitative evaluation of the gradient of the local displacement field. While the use of Fresnel contrast for the enhancement of the visibility of inclined grain boundary dislocations has been demonstrated[38], a quantitative approach on the above lines could well be very interesting. Core displacement fields of grain boundary defects are notoriously difficult to assess and perhaps the most promising method applied to date has been a fairly simplistic "mapping method"[39,40] based on the use of the weak beam technique.

Perhaps the most significant antecedent to the technique as we describe it here was, however, the work of Bursill et al.[41] on the structural and chemical analysis of the infamous platelets in type II diamond. They certainly used the qualitative comparison of the contrast seen in through focus series for different models in attempting to determine which was the more correct. Their work, however, concentrated on higher resolution images than those we have shown to be the more fruitful for chemical analysis and there appears to have been no attempt to use a quantitative approach in which the form of the contrast and the changes in its magnitude with defocus are separately used to determine respectively the form and magnitude of the composition change. This separability is a convenient feature of the developed method, allowing a first order measurement of the width of the inhomogeneity separately from the assessment of the composition change, before the model is refined to evaluate the abruptness of the interfaces.

EXAMPLES OF THE APPLICATION OF THE FRESNEL METHOD

Our aim here, in describing a little of the work we have done using the Fresnel method, is neither to bore the reader with details that can, in the main, be found in the original papers nor simply to demonstrate the breadth of application of the approach, but rather to show how the method is still developing and how different features of a regularly projected inhomogeneity are the better or worse evaluated under different circumstances. We will not dwell on the earlier quantitative application of the approach to the assessment of the composition changes at amorphous grain boundaries[1,2]. We note however that at the time, while we had already developed an approach based on the separation of the measurement of the width of the layer in question from the measurement of the magnitude of its scattering potential relative to that of the matrix (the former from the measurement of the fringe positions and extrapolation to zero defocus and the latter from the assessment of the contrast), we did not appreciate that the data could then be further refined to yield the abruptness of the composition change. This was perhaps because the boundary layers we examined were not particularly flat and we generally found it best to use a moderately diffuse interface model while not attempting to see what changes resulted on modifying it.

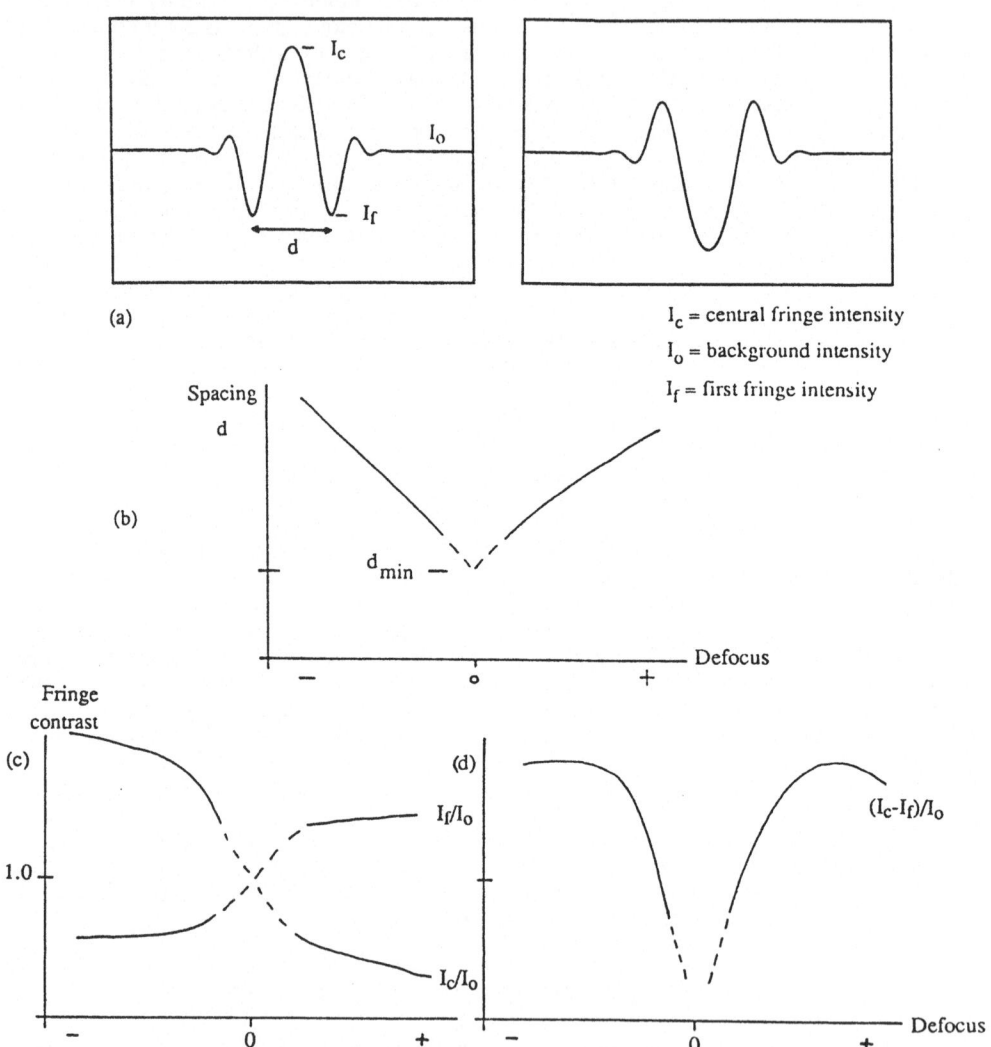

I_c = central fringe intensity
I_o = background intensity
I_f = first fringe intensity

Fig. 1.   The general behaviour of Fresnel fringes from thin layers:
a) The form of the intensity for a region of lower potential than the surrounding matrix underfocus (left) and overfocus (right), with some definitions
b) Schematic diagram of the variation of fringe spacing, d, with defocus. Near focus the contrast is low.
c) Schematic diagram of the variation of fringe contrast with defocus as used by Ness et al.[2].
d) Diagram of contrast variation as is now favoured.

In the light of a particular difficulty we are currently experiencing in determining the importance of incoherent scattering on the contrast, it is interesting that we appear to have obtained in this earlier work consistent data for specimen thicknesses of up to about 30 or 40 nm. It was indeed suggested that thicker rather than thinner specimens should be used in this range since the limit on the accuracy of a compositional measurement was determined to lie in the 5% accuracy range typical of the measurement of a thickness of this magnitude. We are now more dubious on this point and, whereas in earlier work we used the intensity ratios of the central and first fringes to the background (I_c/I_o and I_f/I_o) (see fig.1), we now use the contrast of these features (($I_c-I_f)/I_o$) the better both to minimise the effects of changes in the background and to evaluate ways in which the expected contrast might be reduced as a result of increasing proportions of inelastic scattering as the specimen thickness is increased[7].

The graded composition of the SiO_x layer between Si and SiO_2. We have put a considerable amount of effort into the evaluation of the thickness of the intermediate layer formed in both the wet and dry oxidation of Si. Its form can provide valuable clues on the oxidation mechanism prevailing. The approach we took was to compare high resolution structural images of the overall oxide layer, coated with polysilicon to provide a symmetric scattering potential, with Fresnel contrast image series obtained as described above. The former images yielded a "structural width", the latter a "compositional width". We are currently concerned that it has been reported that prolonged intense electron irradiation can apparently reduce the thickness of an oxide layer of this type [42], but we did not observe

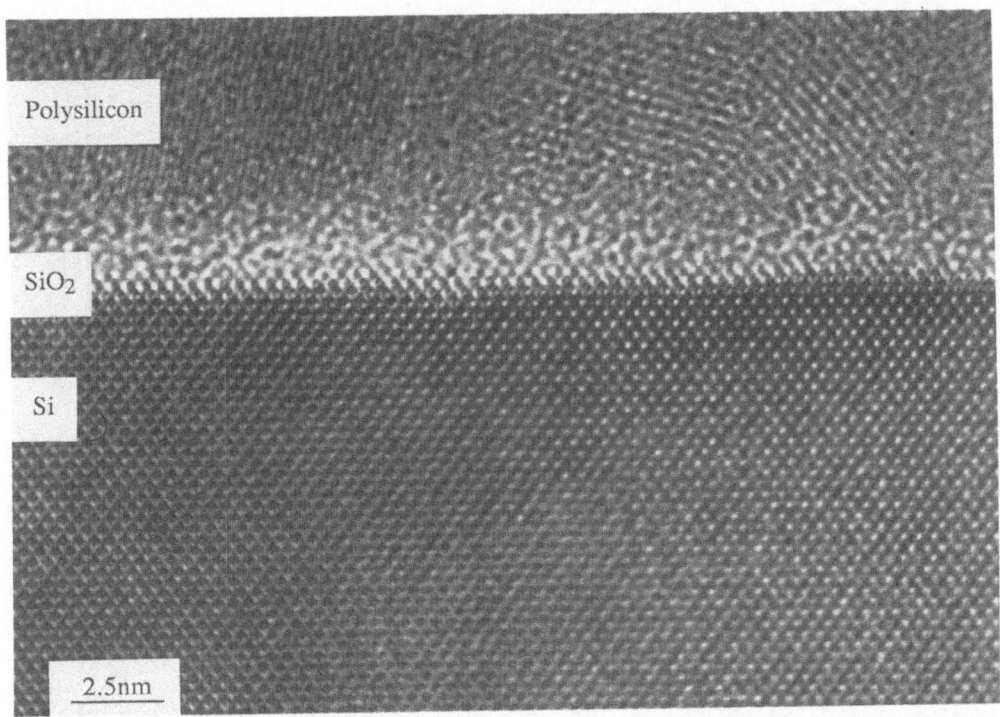

Fig. 2.   High resolution image of a Si/SiO_2/polysilicon interface of the type analysed by the Fresnel method. Note the roughness of the single crystal silicon/SiO_2 interface and the polysilicon grains.

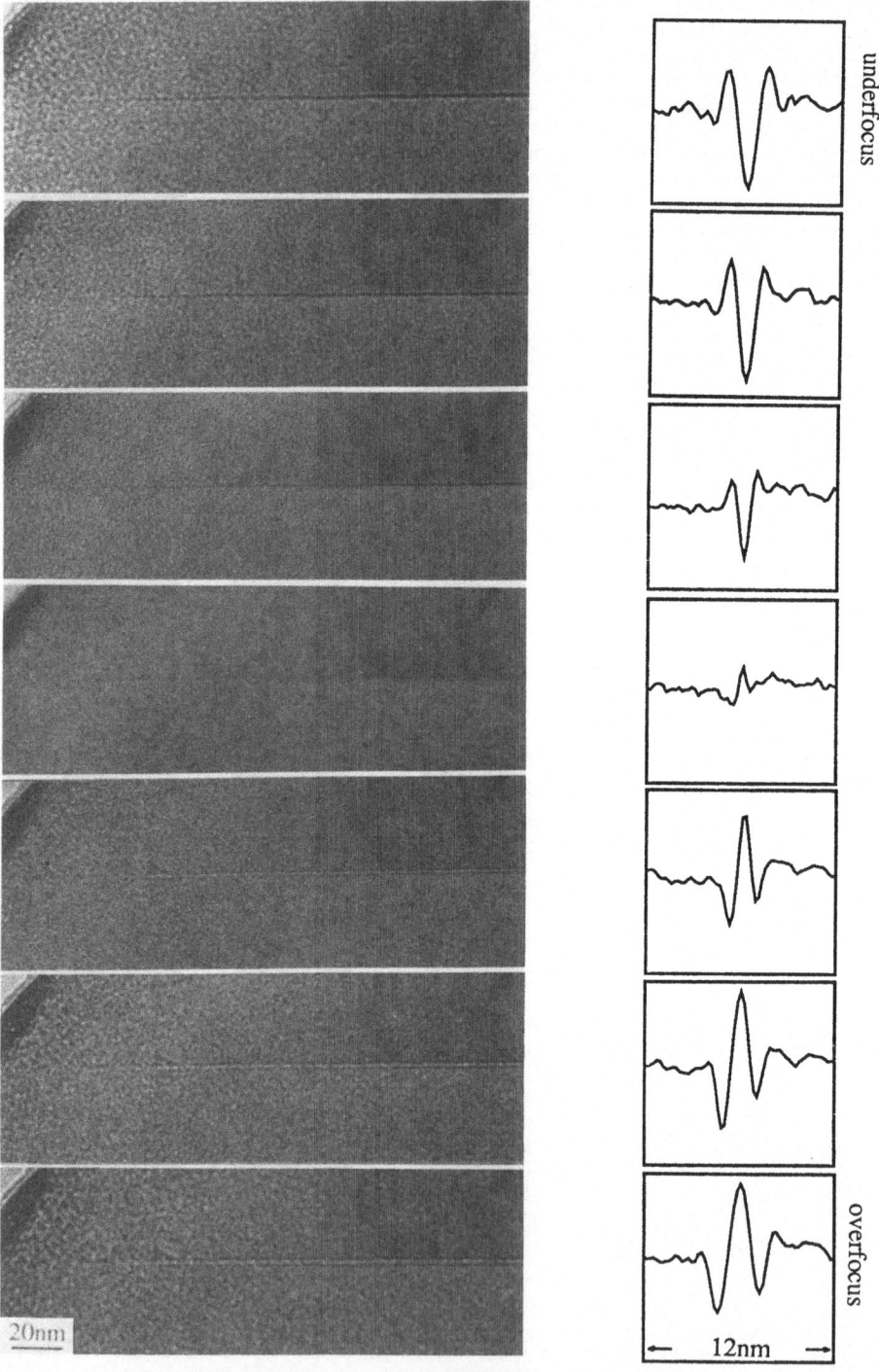

Fig. 3.   Part of a through focal series of an SiO_2 layer on silicon.
            Every fourth member of the series is shown. The single crystal Si is on
            the bottom of each image and the left of each profile. The profiles were
            obtained by averaging over 20nm of the oxide layer, taken from a region
            near the centre of each image at a specimen thickness of about 7.5nm,
            along the direction of the interfaces. The original defocus steps were
            nominally 50nm.

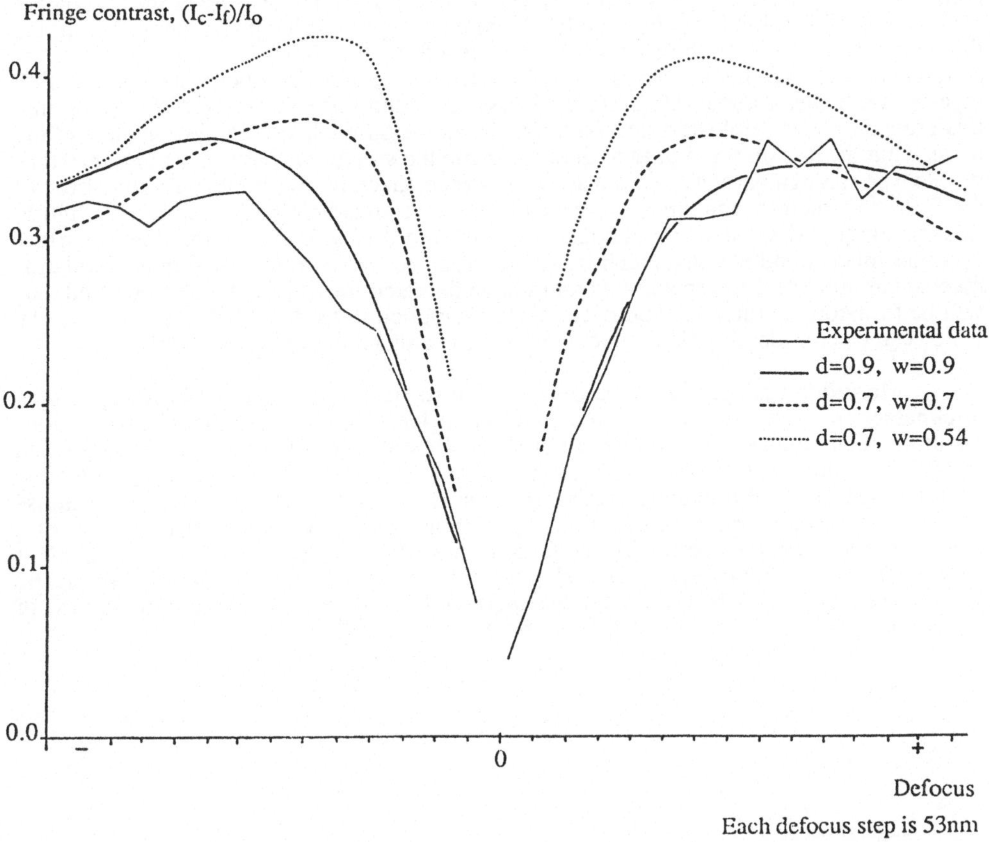

Fringe contrast, $(I_c-I_f)/I_o$

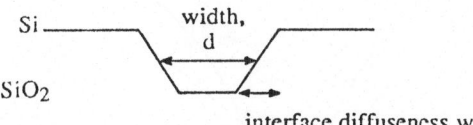

Experimental data
——— d=0.9, w=0.9
- - - - d=0.7, w=0.7
·········· d=0.7, w=0.54

0.4

0.3

0.2

0.1

0.0

−

0

+

Defocus

Each defocus step is 53nm

Si

width,
d

SiO$_2$

interface diffuseness, w

Fig. 4.   Graph showing contrast values measured from the data set of fig. 3
together with predictions from simulations for the oxide widths and
interface diffuseness values as indicated. The best fitting simulation has
rather broad interfaces.

ε

193

such an effect. Summaries of our results have already been reported[5,6], and we show here only a single data set for a thin oxide layer as an example of the overall approach. A high resolution image is shown in fig.2, as is part of a lower resolution through focal series together with its digitised profiles in fig.3. While the compositional and structural thicknesses of the layer could be compared as a function of the thickness of the oxide, so providing useful information on probable changes in the oxidation mechanism as the process develops, the interesting point was that it proved possible (once the thickness and composition change had been fitted) to refine the model to gain a measure of the <u>abruptness</u> of the compositional change. Essentially the more abrupt this change is, the more rapid is the variation observed in the Fresnel contrast as a function of defocus. This is shown for different models and the data set in fig.4. We were thence able to demonstrate that the SiO_x layer was in general about 0.5 nm in thickness, the impressive thing about this being that this proved to be possible despite a comparable, and additional, structural roughness of the underlying Si. It is only too easy to underestimate the structural roughness of an interface of this type (though particular care was, for example, taken in examining very thin areas of the foil, the structural roughness observed in these regions being assumed in the slightly thicker regions where it was much less obvious) and it is well known that the Si surface becomes much smoother on annealing. However, since we were interested in the oxidation mechanism to anneal the specimen would have defeated the object. Much improved data will be forthcoming once the approach has been applied to oxidised MBE grown material which can be considerably flatter than the wafers examined in our current work.

More depressingly we have been unable to fit the <u>contrast</u> levels for specimen thicknesses of more than about 20nm (without at least rather questionable assumptions about the relative levels of contrast retained in different types of inelastic scattering), and equally intriguingly found the contrast to be <u>reduced</u> when using a <u>smaller</u> objective aperture (see fig.5). While these observations have cast into doubt our earlier assertions[2] that thicker (<40nm) rather than thinner specimens are better for the measurement of a layer's composition, the aperture dependence of the effect suggests that the problem might be specific to the specimens examined and might be associated with the diffuse elastic scattering caused either by the amorphous oxide or by the inherent structural roughness of the interface. We are currently evaluating these propositions[9].

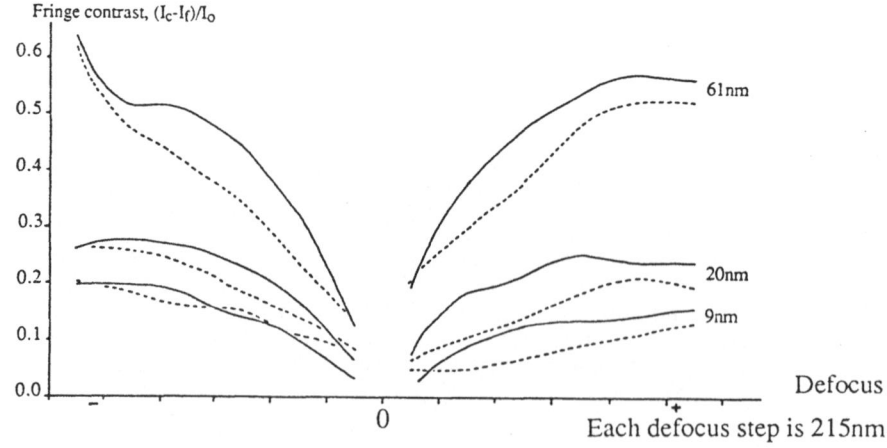

Fig. 5. Comparative contrast data for a small and large objective aperture showing how with the latter the contrast is increased. The solid lines show contrast values measured using a 5.8mrad aperture at the specimen thicknesses indicated, the dotted lines corresponding values for a 1.9mrad aperture.

Cu/NiPd multilayers. The origin of the anomalous properties of metal multilayers has been of interest for several years. The problem has been examined quantitatively using electron microscopy, to our knowledge, in only one instance[43,44] in which, for an {001} Cu/NiPd superlattice, it was demonstrated that as the wavelength of the layering is reduced there is a change in the magnitude of the epitaxial strains. Put in readily understandable terms, this requires at the least that the material compliances are radically altered by the presence of the layering below a given wavelength. The effect can be understood qualitatively in terms of the probable way in which the Brillouin zone boundaries introduced by the presence of the layering might affect the electron distribution of the alloy to introduce, in turn, a degree of tetragonal symmetry. We are currently examining the Si/Ge system to see whether or not the same effect is seen there, though the effects on a semiconductor band structure would be expected to be smaller than they could be in a metal.

This evaluation of the Cu/NiPd system required the careful comparison of high resolution images with simulations but, for these simulations, it was necessary to evaluate the interdiffusion between the layers. This proved to be possible to an accuracy approaching an atomic spacing by the comparison of coarse, small aperture size, Fresnel defocus series with simulations[43]. The interesting point in our discussion here is that the approach taken was somewhat different to that applied above in that now, because we were examining a multilayer, repeating features of the contrast, as a function of the defocus for any given wavelength, proved to be a sensitive function of the abruptness of the compositional changes at the boundaries.

There are related applications of the method in the examination of spinodal decomposition, provided, that is, that the waveform of the spinodal is sufficiently well behaved and of a short enough wavelength. The approach has been attempted, without success, in this laboratory for a fairly long wavelength CuMnAl alloy for which it instead proved to be much easier simply to measure the dark field intensity profiles in a long extinction distance reflection[45]. This failure is indicative of the the way the whole approach is really best applied to relatively fine and discrete interface problems.

GaAs/Al$_x$Ga$_{1-x}$As interface smoothness. Relatively smoother layers than those which arise when a Si wafer is oxidised can be evaluated rather more easily by the Fresnel technique. This has been demonstrated for MBE grown layers of varying thicknesses composed of supposedly pure AlAs in GaAs[4]. We remain intrigued that the compositional diffuseness of the growth proved to exceed the apparent roughness which is directly associated with the vicinity of the layering. However here we note that the change in scattering potential is in this instance rather small, and isolated layers with x less than about 0.5 could probably not be evaluated in this way. However the amplification of the contrast caused by examining a multilayer, as noted for Cu/NiPd, could well be useful in this context and we are currently evaluating this point.

W/Si multilayers. From the above discussion one would be forgiven for assuming that the gross difference in the scattering potential of W and Si would make the evaluation of the local roughness of the layering for this system relatively easy by the Fresnel method. After all it is precisely this difference, but for x-rays, which is exploited in the use of such a system as a sychrotron mirror. In fact systems of this type are causing considerable difficulty. This is not just because they are fairly difficult to thin well edge-on, nor because of the fact that (given the amorphous nature of the Si and the fine polycrystalline form of the W) it is very difficult to measure the thickness of the TEM specimen examined. The real problem is that the difference in scattering potential is so large that, even for fairly diffuse layering, the form of the contrast changes substantially with the specimen thickness in the range of thicknesses normally used for compositional assessment. An example of a Fresnel image pair of such a multilayer, showing this effect, is given in fig.6 together with (fig.7) a first order set of simulations as a function of specimen thickness and defocus demonstrating how the contrast tends to repeat. The work described is still under evaluation[46]. It should be noted that the presence of the superlattice again strengthens the contrast and thus exacerbates the effect described, but we nonetheless believe that this "superlattice reinforcement" will allow us to use the data quantitatively.

"Omega" precipitates in Al-Cu-Mg-Ag alloys. The structure of the {111} precipitates which can form in Al-Cu alloys containing also small amounts of Mg and Ag has been readily confirmed as being monoclinic rather than hexagonal using conventional selected area diffraction and high resolution electron microscopy methods[47]. However it remains interesting to determine how the Ag and Mg get incorporated into the structure and inhibit the formation of the usual {100} θ' precipitates seen on ageing the binary alloy. Since conventional high resolution image simulation[47] proved inadequately sensitive in this respect we have tried using the Fresnel Method. At first we supposed that the major difficulty in this application of the technique would lie in the grossly different scattering factors of Mg and Ag. However, while our initial experimental work[48] on the problem demonstrated that the precipitates, partially because of their very flat {111} interfaces, exhibit very strong Fresnel effects, it quickly became clear that the characteristics of the contrast could not even be approximated using simulations based on the continuum model which works so well in the majority of the other problems to which the approach has been applied. We have since demonstrated that atomistic calculations do predict the way that at different thicknesses the contrast can reverse and yet often not do so through focus[9]. Equally, that both Mg and Ag are involved precludes, in this instance, a unique solution to the problem of how they might be incorporated into the precipitates. Examples of experimental profiles and their matched simulations are shown in fig. 8 to demonstrate the importance of the dynamical nature of the scattering by the matrix in this instance. The precipitates have to be imaged with the Al{111} row systematically excited and the small magnitude of the reciprocal lattice vector of these reflections makes their dynamical behaviour dominate the Fresnel behaviour.

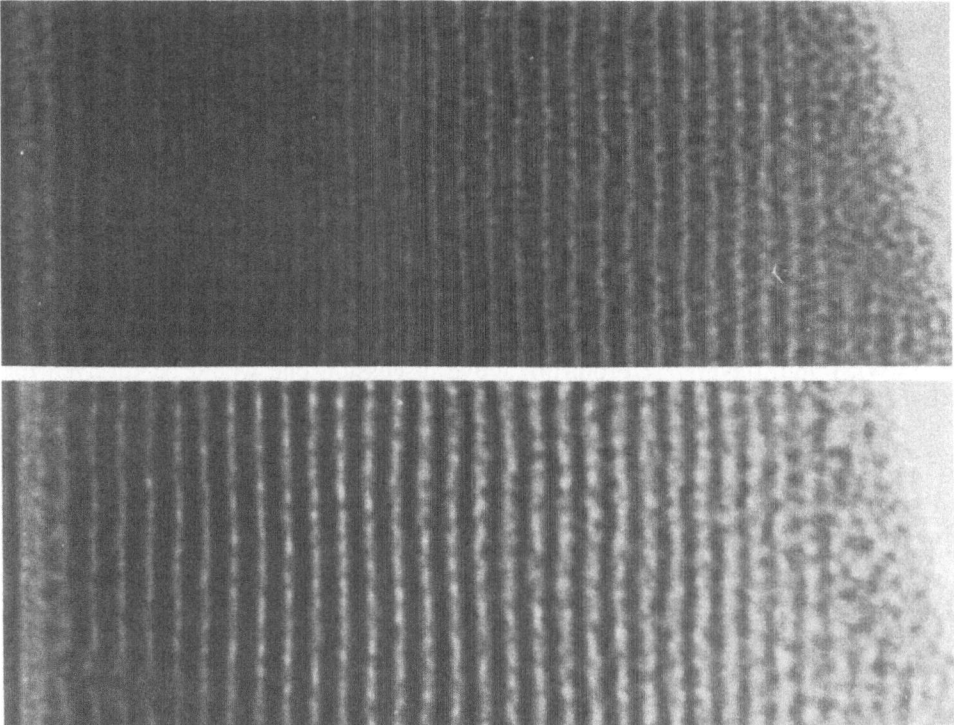

Fig. 6.   A pair of images at different defoci of a W/Si multilayer showing the way the character of the contrast can change with specimen thickness (courtesy of W. C. Shih). In this multilayer, the wavelength is 2.3nm and the W layers are much narrower than the Si layers.

Thickness

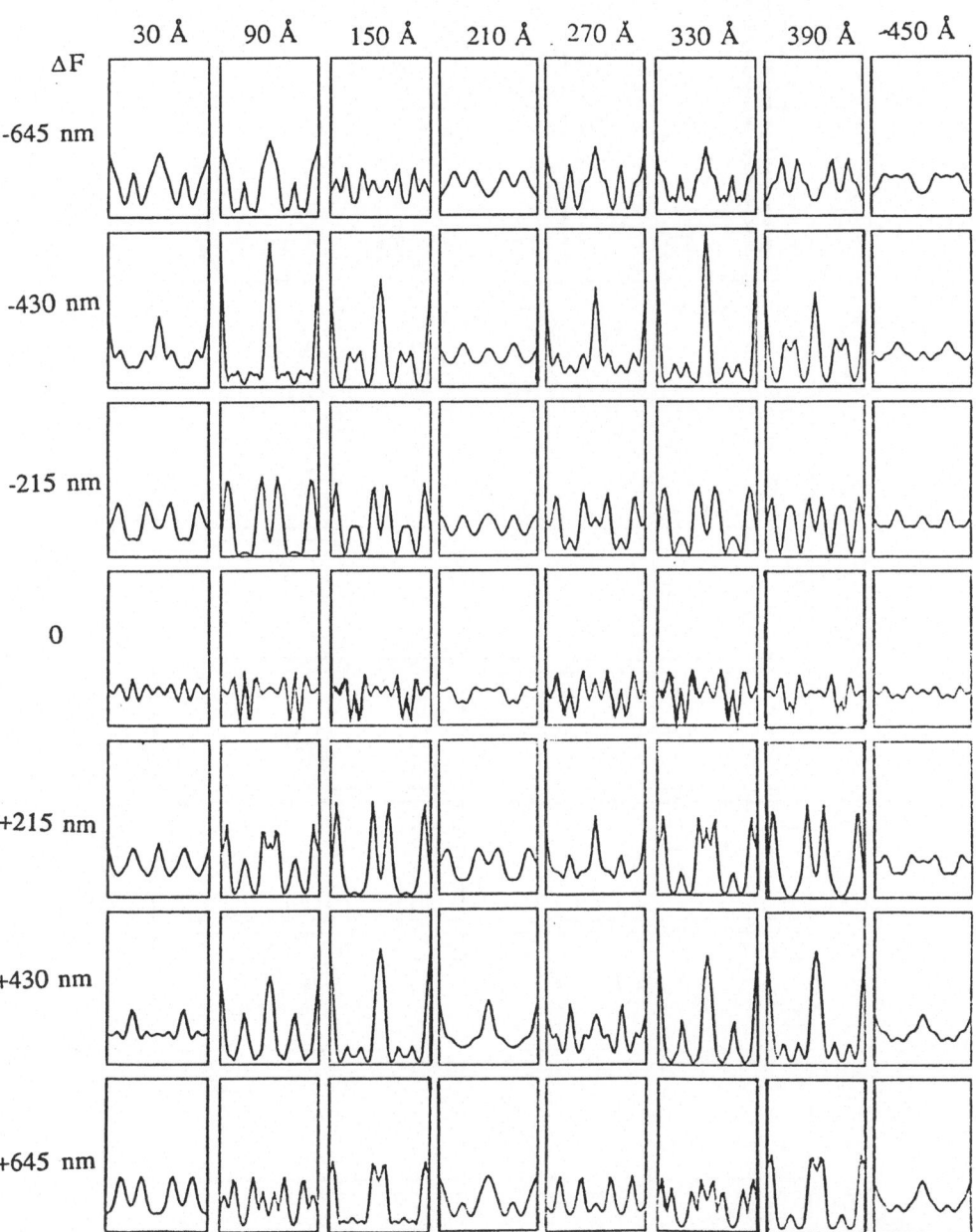

Fig. 7.   Examples of contrast simulations as a function of thickness and defocus for a W/Si multilayer. Two unit cells of the structure are shown in each simulation, for which the wavelength was 2.5nm with the W layer thickness 0.36nm. The aperture limited resolution was taken to be 0.6nm. It should be noted that not only is the contrast now a variable function of the specimen thickness but it can be shown that the contrast also changes strongly with the multilayer wavelength (courtesy of W. C. Shih).

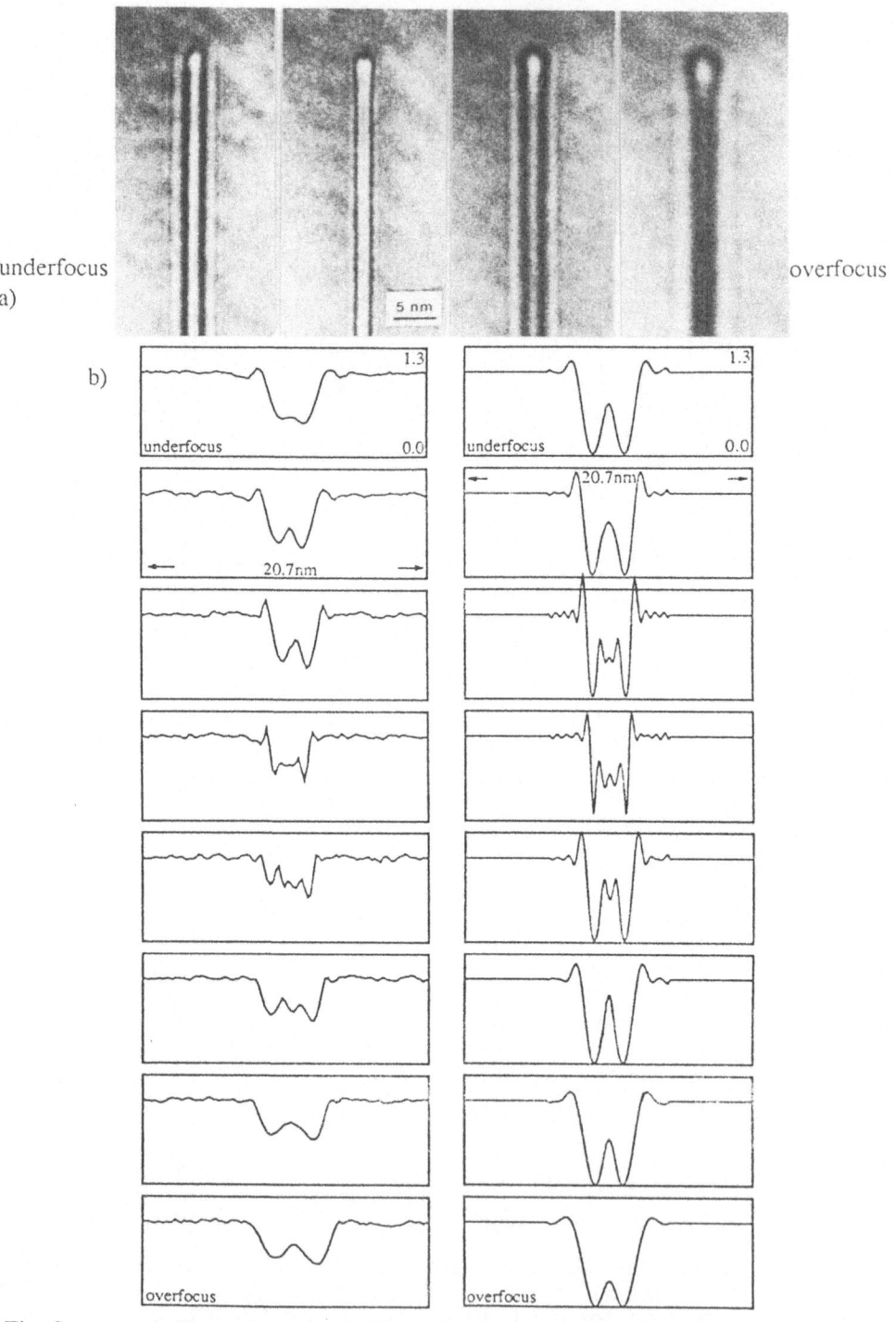

underfocus
a)

overfocus

b)

Fig. 8. a) Examples of images of the Ag containing {111} platelets in the Al alloy at different defoci, together with b) an experimental profile set and its matched simulations. The defocus step between images is 215nm. Note the differences in the contrast values. The Fresnel contrast is, for this situation, strongly affected by the 111 matrix reflections so that the simulations have to be atomistic.

The example serves as a warning in two ways. Firstly, as was noted in the introduction, the relative magnitudes of the changes in concentration of two elements are unlikely to be unequivocally determined using this method alone. Secondly the continuum model can be grossly inadequate and care has to be taken in general in choosing the simulation model needed for any given problem. On the more positive side, when Fresnel effects are weak they can be enhanced, whether in bright or dark field images, by putting the foil into a Bragg condition and this was the basis of the approach which we used rather early on in trying to assess whether or not there is segregation to twin boundaries in copper[8].

Grain boundary segregation. A further piece of work currently being completed in this laboratory and which has as yet not been published concerns the assessment of grain boundary segregation by the Fresnel method. One of the systems that is being examined is Fe/B[49]. While it has been demonstrated, using a parallel recording EELS system[50], that there is indeed extensive segregation of B to the grain boundaries, quite fascinatingly they exhibit remarkably weak Fresnel contrast even when this contrast is enhanced by putting one of the grains into a Bragg condition. It is interesting, but as yet rather dangerous, to speculate that this <u>low</u> contrast and thus <u>weakening</u> of the discontinuity of the scattering potential, which is normally associated with a grain boundary due to the rigid body displacement there (the effects of which are readily normally observed[8]), could be itself associated with the well known grain boundary <u>strengthening</u> which B can induce in this material.

CONCLUSION

While there is currently considerable activity in the application and the development of the Fresnel Method in this laboratory, and a number of short papers have already been published or are in press on individual aspects of the approach, this is the first opportunity we have had to discuss the method more generally. As well as describing how to use the technique we have, in briefly noting a number of the current problems to which it is being applied, delineated its strengths and weaknesses. It certainly does not have universal application to the analysis of even a uniformly projected inhomogeneity but, if used sensibly and with care, the way in which it is complementary to the use of EELS suggests, at the minimum, that it should be still further developed. Essentially, the finer the localised composition change, the more easily the approach is applied: while EELS is virtually powerless at the sub 1.5nm level, it is in precisely this size range that composition profiling can be contemplated using the Fresnel approach.

ACKNOWLEDGEMENTS

We are grateful to Prof. D. Hull for the provision of laboratory facilities and to both the SERC and a number of industries for support including STC(F.M.R), GEC, Philips and BT. We particularly thank those of our colleagues who have both contributed to this work and allowed us to discuss both unreported and published data. These include C.S.Baxter, C.B.Boothroyd, E.G.Bithell (nee Britton), K.Sato and W.C.Shih.

REFERENCES

1. J. N. Ness, W. M. Stobbs and T. F. Page, The detemination of the mean inner potential of grain boundary films in WC-Co composites by Fresnel techniques, in: <u>Inst. Phys. Conf. Ser. 75</u>, G. J. Tatlock, ed., Adam Hilger, Bristol, p. 523 (1985).
2. J. N. Ness, W. M. Stobbs and T. F. Page, A TEM Fresnel diffraction based method for characterising thin grain boundary and interfacial films, <u>Philos. Mag. A</u> 54:679 (1986).
3. K. B Alexander, C. B. Boothroyd, E. G. Britton, F. M. Ross, C. S. Baxter and

W. M. Stobbs, Methods for the assessment of layer orientation, interface step structure and chemical composition in GaAs/AlGaAs multilayers, in: Inst. Phys. Conf. Ser. 78, A. G. Cullis, ed., Adam Hilger, Bristol, p. 195 (1987).

4. F. M. Ross, E. G. Britton, W. M. Stobbs, The application of Fresnel fringe contrast analysis to the measurement of composition profiles in GaAs/(AlGa)As heterostructures, in: EMAG '87 Analytical Electron Microscopy, G. W. Lorimer, ed., Inst. Metals, London, p. 205 (1988).

5. F. M. Ross and W. M. Stobbs, Interface aanalysis using elastic scattering in the Transmission electron microscope: Application to the oxidation of silicon, Surf. and Interface Anal., 12:35 (1988).

6. F. M. Ross and W. M. Stobbs, Study of composition changes across the Si/SiO$_x$ interface using Fresnel fringe contrast analysis, in: M. R. S. Proc. 105, G. Lucovsky and S. T. Pantelides, eds., M. R. S. Publications, Pittsburgh (1988).

7. W. M. Stobbs and F. M. Ross, The use of the Fresnel method for the study of localised composition changes at interfaces, in: EMAG '87 Analytical Electron Microscopy, G. W. Lorimer, ed., Inst. Metals, London, p. 165 (1988).

8. C. B. Boothroyd, A. P. Crawley and W. M. Stobbs, The measurement of rigid body displacements using Fresnel fringe intensity methods, Philos. Mag. A 54:633 (1986).

9. F. M. Ross, The development and application of the Fresnel method, Ph.D. Thesis, Cambridge (1988).

10. W. O. Saxton, T. J. Pitt and M. Horner, Digital image processing: the SEMPER system, Ultramicrosc., 4:343 (1979).

11. P. A. Doyle and P. S. Turner, Relastivistic Hartree-Fock x-ray and electron scattering factors, Acta. Crystallogr. A 24:390 (1968).

12. G. Radi, Complex lattice potentials in electron diffraction calculated for a number of crystals, Acta. Crystallogr. A 26:41 (1970).

13. D. J. Smith, V. E. Cosslet and W. M. Stobbs, Atomic resolution with the electron microscope, Interdisc. Sci. Rev., 6:155 (1981).

14. W. M. Stobbs, High resolution: direct or indirect?, Ultramicrosc., 9:221 (1982).

15. W. M. Stobbs and W. O. Saxton, Quantitative high resolution transmission electron microscopy: the need for energy filtering and the advantages of energy-loss imaging, J. Microsc., 151:171 (1988).

16. C. B. Boothroyd and W. M. Stobbs, The effects of contributions from energy loss electrons to "centre stop" high resolution images of (AlGa)As/GaAs interfaces, in: Inst. Phys. Conf. Ser. 90, L. M. Brown, ed., Institute of Physics, Bristol, p. 237 (1987).

17. C. B. Boothroyd and W. M. Stobbs, The contribution of inelastically scattered electrons to high resolution images of (AlGa)As/GaAs heterostructures, Ultramicrosc., in press (1988).

18. M. J. Hÿtch and W. M. Stobbs, The effects of single electron and plasmon scattering on [100] and [010] images of YBa$_2$Cu$_3$O$_{7-\delta}$, in: Inst. Phys. Conf. Ser. 93, P. J. Goodhew and H. G. Dickinson, eds., Institute of Physics, Bristol, 2:347 (1988).

19. M. J. Hÿtch and W. M. Stobbs, The relative effects of the Debye Waller factor and inelastic scattering on high resolution imaging of [100] and [010] orientations of YBa$_2$Cu$_3$O$_{7-\delta}$, in: Proc. 46th Annual Meeting of EMSA, G. W. Bailey, ed., San Francisco Press, San Francisco, p. 958 (1988)

20. S. H. Stobbs and W. M. Stobbs, Relative advantages and disadvantages of TEM and STEM for energy loss imaging, in: EMAG '87 Analytical Electron Microscopy, G. W. Lorimer, ed., Inst. Metals, London, p.111 (1988).

21. P. E. Batson, C. R. M. Grovenor, D. A. Smith and C. Wong, in: Proc. 41st Annual Meeting of EMSA, G. W. Bailey, ed., p.154 (1983).

22. R. W. Devenish, D. J. Eaglesham, D. M. Maher and C. J. Humphreys, Nanometre scale lithography in the CTEM, in: Inst. Phys. Conf. Ser. 93, P. J. Goodhew and H. G. Dickinson, eds., Institute of Physics, Bristol, 2:391 (1988).

23. A. Bourret and C. Colliex, Combined HREM and STEM microanalysis of decorated dislocation cores, Ultramicrosc., 9:183 (1982)

24. CBED of Alloy Phases, J. Steeds and J. Mansfield, eds., Adam Hilger Ltd., Bristol (1984)

25. Convergent Beam Electron Diffraction, M. Tanaka and T. Terauchi, JEOL Ltd., Tokyo (1985)

26. P. Spellward, A new CBED method of composition determination in ternary semiconductors, in: Inst. Phys. Conf. Ser. 93, P. J. Goodhew and H. G. Dickinson, eds., Institute of Physics, Bristol, 2:31 (1988).

27. H. Kakibayashi and F. Nagata, Composition dependence of equal thickness fringes in an electron microscope image of GaAs/AlGaAs multilayer, Jap. J. Appl. Phys., 24:L905 (1985).

28. H. Kakibayashi and F. Nagata, Simulation studies of a composition analysis by thickness fringe in an electron microscope image of GaAs/AlGaAs superstructure, Jap. J. Appl. Phys., 25:1644 (1986).

29. D. J. Eaglesham, C. J. D. Hetherington and C. J. Humphreys, Compositional studies of semiconductor alloys by bright field alactron microscope imaging of wedged crystals, in: M. R. S. Proc. 77, J. D. Dow and I. K. Schuller, eds., M. R. S. Publications, Pittsburgh, p. 473 (1987).

30. E. G. Bithell and W. M. Stobbs, Composition measurements in the GaAs/(Al,Ga)As system using dark field T. E. M. contrast, Philos. Mag., in press, (1989).

31. K. Fukushima, H. Kawakatsu and A. Fukami, Fresnel fringes in electron microscope images, J. Phys. D, 7:257 (1974).

32. D. R. Clarke, On the detection of thin intergranular flms in electron microscopy, Ultramicrosc., 4:33 (1979).

33. N. W. Jepps, T. F. Page and W. M. Stobbs, A method for the TEM characterisation of grain boundary films in ceramics, in: Inst. Phys. Conf. Ser. 61, M. J. Goringe, ed., Adam Hilger, Bristol, p. 453 (1981).

34. M. Rühle, E. Bischoff and O. David, The structure of grain boundaries in ceramics, Ultramicrosc., 14:37 (1984)

35. W. M. Stobbs, Electron microscopical techniques for the observation of cavities, J. Microsc., 116:3 (1979).

36. S. Iijima, High resolution electron microscopy of phase objects: Observation of small holes and steps on graphite crystals, Optik, 47:437 (1977).

37. M. Rühle and S. L. Sass, The detection of the change in mean inner potential at dislocations in grain boundaries in NiO, Philos. Mag. A, 49:759 (1984).

38. C. B. Boothroyd and W. M. Stobbs, Fresnel effects for grain boundary dislocations, Philos. Mag. A, L5:49 (1984).

39. P. E. Donovan and W. M. Stobbs, A method for the mapping of localised displacement fields in boundaries, J. Microsc., 130:361 (1983).

40. P. E. Donovan and W. M. Stobbs, A computational assessment of a method for the mapping of localised displacement fields at boundaries, Ultramicrosc., 23:119 (1987).

41. L. A. Bursill, J. C. Barry and P. R. Hudson,Fresnel diffraction at {100} platelets in diamond: An attempt at defect structure analysis by high resolution by high resolutionphase contrast microscopy, Philos. Mag. A, 37:789 (1978).

42. H. Oppolzer, Electron microscopy of semiconductor devices and materials, in: Inst. Phys. Conf. Ser. 93, P. J. Goodhew and H. G. Dickinson, eds., Institute of Physics, Bristol, 2:73 (1988).

43. C. S. Baxter and W. M. Stobbs, The structural characterisation of multilayered Cu/NiPd films at the atomic level, in: Inst. Phys. Conf. Ser. 78, G. J. Tatlock, ed., Adam Hilger, Bristol, p. 387 (1985).

44. C. S. Baxter and W. M. Stobbs, A "phase transition" in fcc Cu/NiPd multilayers characterised by high resolution lattice imaging, Nature, 322:814 (1986).

45. K. Sato and W. M. Stobbs, Quantitative dark field image analysis of spinodal decomposition in $Cu_{3-x}Mn_xAl$ alloys, in: Inst. Phys. Conf. Ser. 90, L. M. Brown, ed., Institute of Physics, Bristol, p. 253 (1988).

46. W-C. Shih, private communication.

47. K. M. Knowles and W. M. Stobbs, The structure of {111} age hardening precipitates in Al-Cu-Mg-Ag alloys, Acta Crystallog. B, 44:207 (1988).
48. K. M. Knowles, F. M. Ross and W. M. Stobbs, Precipitate formation in Al-Cu-Mg-Ag alloys, in: EMAG '87 Analytical Electron Microscopy, G. W. Lorimer, ed., Inst. Metals, London, p. 55 (1988).
49. K. Sato, private communication.
50. A. J. Bourdillon, W. M. Stobbs, K. Page, R. Home, C. J. Wilson, B. A. Ambrose, L. J. Turner and G. P. Tebby, A dual parallel and serial detection spectrometer for EELS, in: Inst. Phys. Conf. Ser. 78, G. J. Tatlock, ed., Adam Hilger, Bristol, p. 161 '1985).

STRAINS AND MISFIT DISLOCATIONS AT INTERFACES

C.J. Humphreys*, D.J. Eaglesham*, D.M. Maher†,
H.L. Fraser‡ and I. Salisbury*

*Department of Materials Science and Engineering, University of
Liverpool, P.O. Box 147, Liverpool L69 3BX, England
†AT&T Bell Laboratories, Murray Hill, New Jersey 07974, U.S.A.
‡Department of Materials Science and Engineering, University of Illinois
Urbana, Illinois 61801, U.S.A.

INTRODUCTION

In recent years there have been great advances in the heteroepitaxial growth of non-lattice-matched epilayers and strained-layer superlattices (SLSs). The role of lattice strain in these structures is extremely important. Not only does strain exert a large influence on band gaps, band offsets, effective masses and mobilities, but strain can be used deliberately to "fine-tune" these device properties. Hence it is essential to be able to measure local strains in order to understand and quantify the physical properties of the material. In this paper we will illustrate the use of Convergent Beam Electron Diffraction (CBED) for the measurement of local strain, and we will describe the use of a new technique, Convergent Beam Imaging (CBIM), for detecting, mapping and measuring small crystalline distortions.

As is well known, in very thin strained epilayers, the epilayer-substrate strain is initially accommodated elastically, but at sufficiently large epilayer thicknesses misfit dislocations occur at or near the substrate-epilayer interface. These dislocations, and particularly the threading dislocations connecting the misfit dislocations to the growth surface, can seriously affect the electrical properties of the epilayer and it is therefore important to minimise their density. The process by which misfit dislocations are first introduced when the substrate is dislocation free has been the subject of debate for a number of years. In this paper we will describe a new internal dislocation source we have called the diamond defect: a single diamond defect can act as a regenerative source of misfit dislocations which propagate to lie in an orthogonal array at the interface.

MEASURING LOCAL STRAINS BY CBED

It is well known that Higher-Order Lane Zone (HOLZ) lines in the bright-field disc of CBED patterns can provide accurate measurements of lattice parameters[1] to within about 1 part in 10^4, with about 40 Å spatial resolution. This has been used by the authors to detect and measure local strains in Si/Ge_xSi_{1-x} SLSs, and other materials[2,3,4].

We shall illustrate the application of CBED with reference to investigations of a model Si/Ge_xSi_{1-x} strained-layer structure (with growth direction [100]) which is shown in fig.1. The structure was grown by molecular-beam epitaxy: for details of the growth conditions see refs 2 and 5. (001) cross-sections of this Si/Ge_xSi_{1-x} SLS were used and [001] zone-axis CBED patterns recorded. This orientation has the great advantage that deviations from cubic symmetry are immediately visually apparent in the CBED patterns.

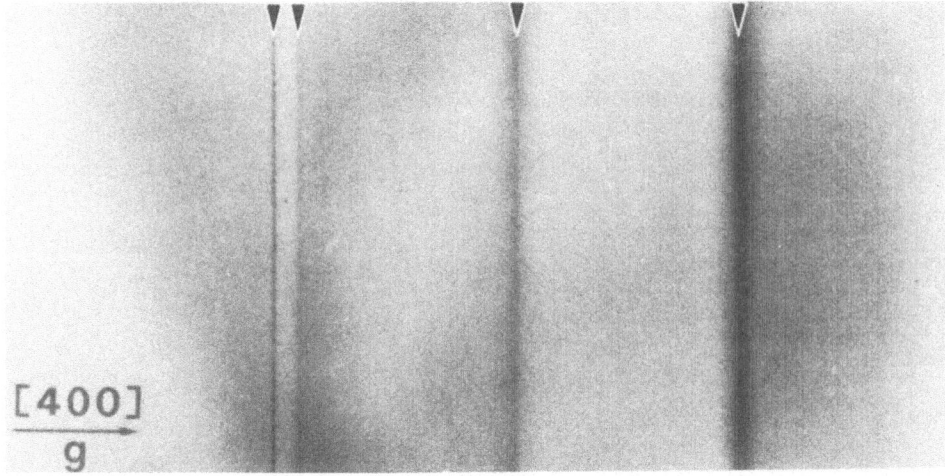

$[400]$

g

Fig. 1. Bright-field cross-sectional image of a Si/Ge_xSi_{1-x} strained-layer structure which shows from left to right the following: Si(100) substrate; Si buffer 0.1 μm thick; $Ge_{0.05}Si_{0.95}$ alloy 1 μm thick; Si buffer 1 μm thick; $Ge_{0.10}Si_{0.90}$ alloy 1 μm thick. The electron beam direction is approximately [011] and the crystal growth direction is [100] which is parallel to the [400] g vector used for imaging. Each interface is identified by arrowheads.

Fig. 2 shows a typical CBED pattern from the Si substrate, from which it is obvious that the pattern symmetry is 4mm (i.e. a fourfold axis, namely [001], with two independent sets of mirror planes), as expected for a cubic crystal. Fig. 3 shows a pattern from a Ge_xSi_{1-x} epitaxial layer, where x is at 5%. It is clear that the material is not cubic, and the pattern has symmetry 2mm, which is consistent with a tetragonal structure. However, detailed computer simulation shows that the HOLZ pattern observed in fig. 3 cannot be accounted for by a tetragonal distortion along the [100] growth direction. If variable values not only of a_{100} (growth direction) but also of a_{001} (to allow for surface relaxation) are considered, then excellent computer matches to experiment are obtained. Hence the effects of surface relaxation are to give a structure which is, in general, orthorhombic. The experimental values of the distortion thus obtained lie between those expected for a bulk crystal and a fully relaxed crystal[4].

DETECTING MONOCLINIC FORMS OF Ge_xSi_{1-x}

Fig.3 was recorded from a region of $Ge_{0.05}Si_{0.95}$ away from the $Si/Ge_{0.05}Si_{0.95}$ interface. CBED patterns recorded closer to the interface show a breakdown of the mirror planes present in fig. 3, implying a monoclinic structure. The patterns from 10% Ge-Si are even clearer in their loss of mirror symmetry, see fig.4, and in this case the break in mirror symmetry is observed independent of the distance from the heterointerface.

There are two possible sources for the symmetry breaking exhibited in fig.4. First, the substrate orientation may not be precisely (100): vicinal (100) substrates off-cut towards, say, either (011) or (010) should give monoclinic epilayers. Second, if the cross-sectional sample deviates from a perfect (001) orientation this may cause symmetry breaking since the strain relaxation occurs along the specimen normal: this latter effect appears to dominate in our case since some residual symmetry breaking is apparent from a detailed examination of CBED patterns from the Si substrate, close to the interface.

The above results may be of considerable significance since they demonstrate that materials which in their bulk form may be, say, cubic (e.g. bulk Ge_xSi_{1-x} alloy) may become tetragonal, orthorhombic or monoclinic under "strain engineering" deliberately using surface relaxation effects. The band structure of these new forms may be markedly different from the band structure of the cubic form, which may give rise to new electronic properties. In addition, surface relaxation effects will inevitably be important in thin film devices, and CBED techniques will therefore be important in the characterisation of these materials.

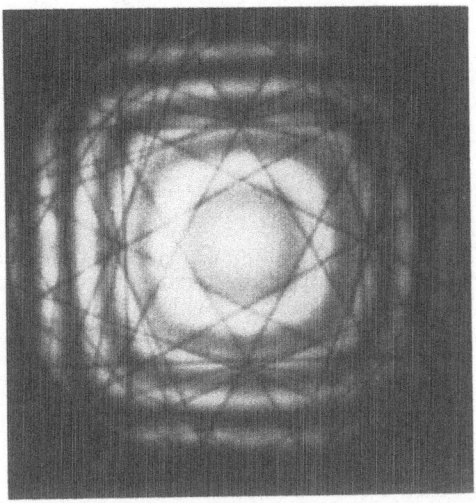

Fig.2. Bright-field disc of an [001] CBED pattern from the Si substrate in a Si-Ge$_x$Si$_{1-x}$ heterostructure, showing 4-fold symmetry consistent with the undistorted cubic structure.

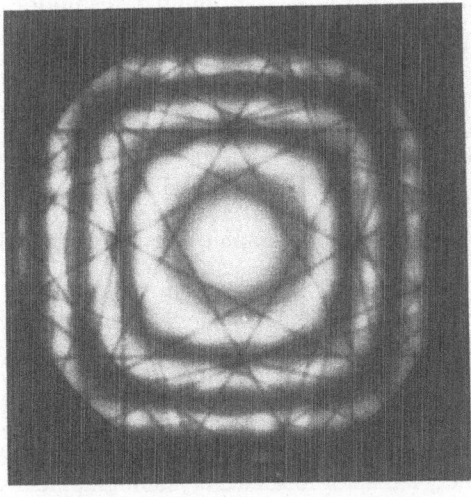

Fig. 3. [001] CBED bright-field disc from a Ge$_{0.05}$Si$_{0.95}$ epitaxial layer (on Si); the 4-fold symmetry is clearly broken. Simulations show that this pattern can only come from an epilayer which has relaxed into an orthorhombic structure.

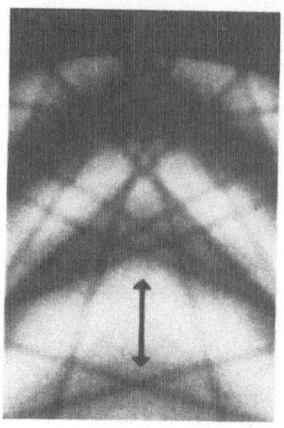 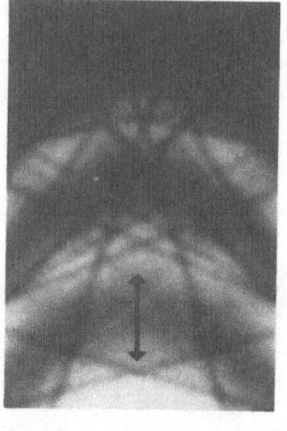 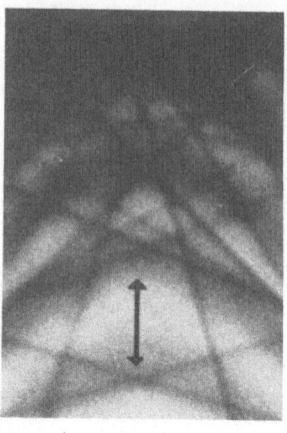

a) ORTHORHOMBIC   b) MONOCLINIC   c) MONOCLINIC

Fig. 4.   Details of [001] CBED bright-field disc from two $Ge_{0.05}Si_{0.95}$ epitaxial layers (one orthorhombic, one monoclinic) and one $Ge_{0.1}Si_{0.9}$ (more highly monoclinic) layer illustrating the broken 2mm symmetry characteristic of monoclinic distortion: (a) orthorhombic; (b) monoclinic; (c) monoclinic.

CONVERGENT BEAM IMAGING (CBIM)

CBIM is a new transmission electron microscopy imaging technique for detecting, mapping and measuring small crystalline distortions. The technique is described in detail in 6 and some applications are given in 7. Whereas CBED patterns are formed in the diffraction plane, convergent beam images are formed in the image plane of the microscope, using a convergent defocussed probe, and a map of HOLZ lines is superimposed on the normal bright-field image. Strains, lattice parameter variations and structural distortions are revealed as displacements of the HOLZ lines. The image has its normal resolution (about 5 Å), the superimposed diffraction information has an angular resolution of ~10^{-4} rad, and this diffraction information comes from regions of the specimen defined approximately by the cross-over size of the electron probe, broadened by beam spreading.

A convergent-beam image of the strained-layer structure is shown in fig.5, where it can be seen clearly that significant curvature of particular HOLZ lines occurs as these lines cross a Si/Ge_xSi_{1-x} interface. The HOLZ pattern is parallel to the [013] zone axis on the Si side of the interface; however, thin film effects have allowed the tetragonally distorted $Ge_{0.05}Si_{0.95}$ layer to relax at the interface in the [011] surface normal direction, and this relaxation is accompanied by a slowly varying crystallographic rotation of the [013] zone axis about the plane of the interface.

A portion of the convergent-beam image of fig.5 appears in fig.6. A comparison of the positions of intersection of the <14 4 2> and <13 5 1> types of HOLZ lines marked with braces in fig.6, with CBED patterns of HOLZ lines from the individual layers of Si and $Ge_{0.05}Si_{0.95}$[2, 7], shows that the crossing positions are identical in CBIM and CBED. Hence CBIM spatially resolves the lattice parameter variations between $Ge_{0.05}Si_{0.95}$ and Si. Moreover, the convergent-beam image reveals information which is not obtainable directly from a CBED pattern, namely a map of localised crystallographic distortions superimposed on the image (see, for example, the disappearance and curvature of HOLZ lines near the $Ge_{0.05}Si_{0.95}$/Si interface (i.e. at D and C, respectively, in fig.6)). Analysis of these CBIM effects shows that they arise from surface relaxation of the tetragonal strain in the thin Ge_xSi_{1-x} epitaxial layers. The disappearance of HOLZ lines is attributed to lattice plane

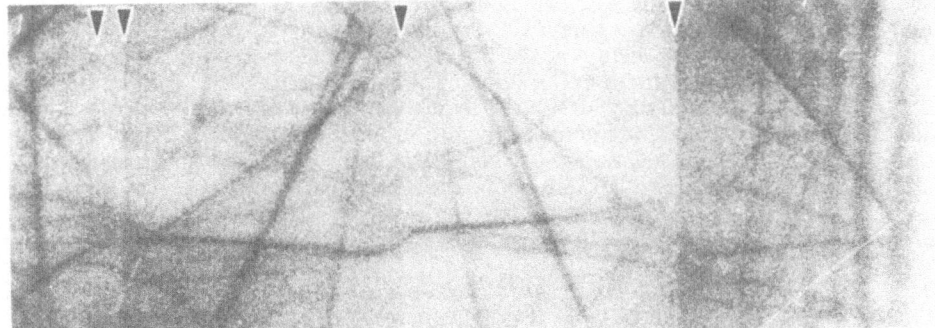

Fig.5.   Bright-field convergent-beam image of the structure shown in fig. 1. The positions of the four interfaces are identified by arrowheads; the electron beam direction is approximately [013] and the electron probe diameter at specimen cross-over is about 5 nm.

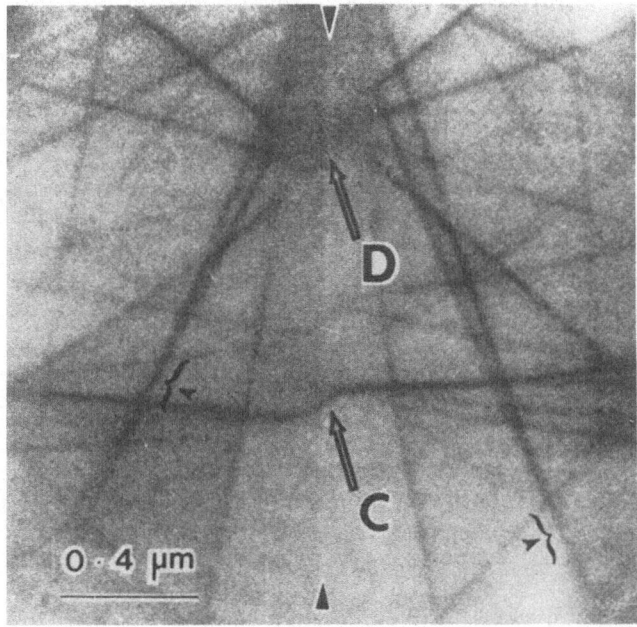

Fig. 6.   Convergent-beam image of the region across the $Ge_{0.05}Si_{0.95}$ alloy and Si buffer (i.e. a portion of fig. 5). The alloy-buffer interface is marked by arrowheads. Braces mark the intersections of the <14 4 2> and <13 5 1> types of HOLZ lines whose crossing positions are changed with respect to the interface. D corresponds to regions where lattice bending causes HOLZ lines to disappear and C corresponds to regions where crystallographic rotations cause HOLZ lines to curve.

bending at an interface and the curvature of HOLZ lines is a consequence of very small orientation differences across an interface. With regard to the second effect, and once again with reference to fig.6, the [013] HOLZ pattern is approximately on axis at the $Ge_{0.05}Si_{0.95}$/Si interface (i.e. [013] is nearly parallel to the electron beam direction); however, thin film effects have allowed the tetragonally distorted $Ge_{0.05}Si_{0.95}$ layer to relax in the [001] direction and this relaxation is accompanied by a slowly varying crystallographic rotation of the [013] zone axis about the 'plane' of the interface. From the convergent-beam image which is shown in fig.6, this rotation is estimated to be about 10^{-3} rad. Furthermore, the slowly varying curvature of the HOLZ lines which run nearly perpendicular to the $Ge_{0.05}Si_{0.95}$/Si interface maps the rate of change in projected crystal symmetry across the interface. This oscillatory behaviour of the HOLZ lines in CBIM is consistent with crystallographic rotations of the [013] zone axis in a thin Ge_xSi_{1-x} strained-layer structure owing to the surface relaxation effects that we have described for a single interface. Therefore CBIM provides direct experimental evidence of thin-crystal elastic relaxation effects[8, 9].

COMPOSITIONAL MODULATIONS ('BANDING') IN EPITAXIAL LAYERS

During the initial course of our work on GeSi/Si[2], it was observed that cross-sectional transmission electron microscopy (x-TEM) images of epilayers (either ~5 or ~10at% Ge) exhibit periodic bands of image contrast which are perpendicular to the growth direction (see Fig.7). These contrast features are similar to those reported by several authors for a number of alloy systems (e.g. $Ga_xIn_{1-x}As$[10], $Al_xIn_{1-x}As$[10], $Al_xGa_{1-x}As$[11,12] and Ge_xSi_{1-x}[13,14]) which are grown by MBE[10,12,13], MOCVD[11] and CVD[14], so that the banding phenomenon is quite widespread. Alavi et al.[10] concluded that in their case the bands correspond to compositional modulations caused by variations in the flux profiles of the group III elements, and they were able to correlate the band periodicity with the rotational speed of the substrate during growth. In the present case of MBE grown Si/Ge_xSi_{1-x} heteroepitaxial layers, banding contrast was observed even without substrate rotation, although rotation makes the observed effect quite periodic. In order to estimate the degree of inhomogeneity, we note that modulations in composition imply that the lattice parameters in adjacent bands of material will be different thus giving rise to local strains. We have shown that images such as fig.7 are dominated by strain contrast and not by structure factor contrast. Considerations of diffraction contrast theory and elasticity theory give upper and lower limits for the composition of modulations in fig.7 of ±1at% and ±0.25 at %Ge respectively[15]. This small inhomogeneity may be explained by minor instabilities in either the flux or the substrate temperature.

THE CRITICAL THICKNESS CONCEPT IN STRAINED EPITAXIAL LAYERS

It is widely believed that beyond a critical thickness, h_c, a strained epilayer will no longer grow coherently and misfit dislocations will be incorporated at the epilayer/substrate interface to relax the lattice mismatch strain. This topic is of considerable technological importance because of the effect of misfit, and particularly threading, dislocations upon electronic properties of devices.

Van der Merwe[16] argued that as a thin epitaxial layer grew coherently upon a substrate with different lattice parameter a critical thickness, h_c, would be reached at which it was energetically favourable to accommodate the lattice misfit using an array of dislocations rather than by increasing the elastic strain in the epilayer. This is clearly an equilibrium argument which does not take into account either the dislocation introduction mechanisms or any energy barriers to nucleating the misfit dislocations.

Matthews[17] and Matthews et al[18] provided a model for the introduction of misfit dislocations, based on the existence of dislocations already in the substrate and threading up to the substrate/epilayer interface. According to their theory, the critical thickness occurs when the epilayer stress becomes sufficient to cause the existing threading dislocations in the substrate to bend over at the interface and form misfit dislocations. This model is also an equilibrium model and it leads to a similar expression for h_c.

Both models[16,17] provide an adequate description of the behaviour of many systems (e.g. 19). However it is evident that they cannot adequately explain h_c for the growth of epilayers on dislocation free substrates since they ignore the problem of dislocation nucleation. There have been many reports (e.g. ref. 20) of experimental determinations of h_c for epilayer growth on low dislocation density semiconductor substrates in which the observed critical thickness is far greater than that predicted by the equilibrium theories[16,17]. This implies that the kinetics of dislocation nucleation and propagation are central to our understanding of epitaxial semiconductor systems. Before studying this in detail it is necessary to take a closer look at the experimental determination of critical thickness since, as Fritz[21] has argued, the apparent critical thickness must depend strongly on the experimental technique used.

As an example of a strained layer system, the GeSi/Si(100) system will be considered (Ge has a lattice parameter about 4% larger than that of Si). For high lattice parameter mismatch (>2%), the misfit dislocations are an orthogonal array of mainly edge type dislocations whereas at low mismatch (<2%) an orthogonal array of 60° dislocations is formed (Kvam et al.[22]), see Fig.8. Eaglesham et al[23] have performed a detailed study of coherency breakdown in low mismatch GeSi/Si(100) using X-ray topography to probe the critical thickness (X-ray topography is of course much more sensitive than electron microscopy to detecting low densities of dislocations. The minimum dislocation density detectable using electron microscopy is about 10^5 dislocations cm^{-2} whereas X-ray topography can detect a single dislocation in a specimen). Finite dislocation densities (in excess of 10^3 cm^{-2}) were found for an epilayer thickness a factor of 4 less than the accepted critical thickness for this lattice mismatch. This result demonstrates that in a low-mismatched system the critical thickness h_c is not easily defined experimentally, since for a given epilayer thickness the dislocation density increases continuously with increasing Ge content. There is not an abrupt change from no dislocations to some dislocations at a particular critical thickness: at very low dislocation density some regions of the specimen will have zero dislocations whereas other regions of the same specimen normally have a finite dislocation density. We conclude that, at least in low mismatched systems, there is no sharply defined critical thickness, and that misfit dislocations may exist at epilayer thicknesses substantially below the critical thickness reported in the literature.

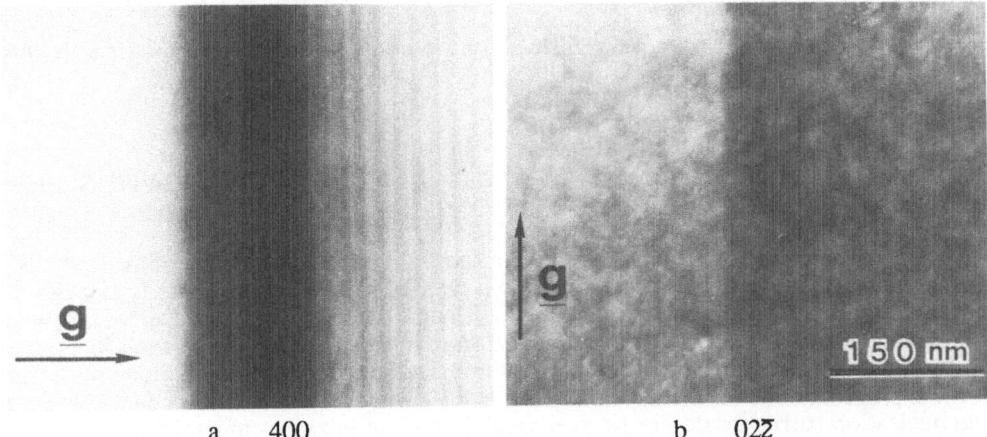

a   400   b   02$\bar{2}$

Fig. 7.   Bright-field, (001) x-TEM images of the Si/Ge$_{0.1}$Si$_{0.9}$ layers. The images were recorded approximately at the Bragg position and close to the [001] zone-axis orientation. When g (=[400]) is parallel to the [100] growth direction banding is observed in the epilayer (a) and when g (=[040]) lies in the (100) growth plane no (or very weak) banding is observed in the epilayer (b). The marked difference in contrast between the two images cannot be associated with variations in structure factor, so the image contrast (i.e. banding) in Fig. 7a can now be unambiguously attributed to local variations in strain. Upward drawn arrowheads mark the heterointerface.

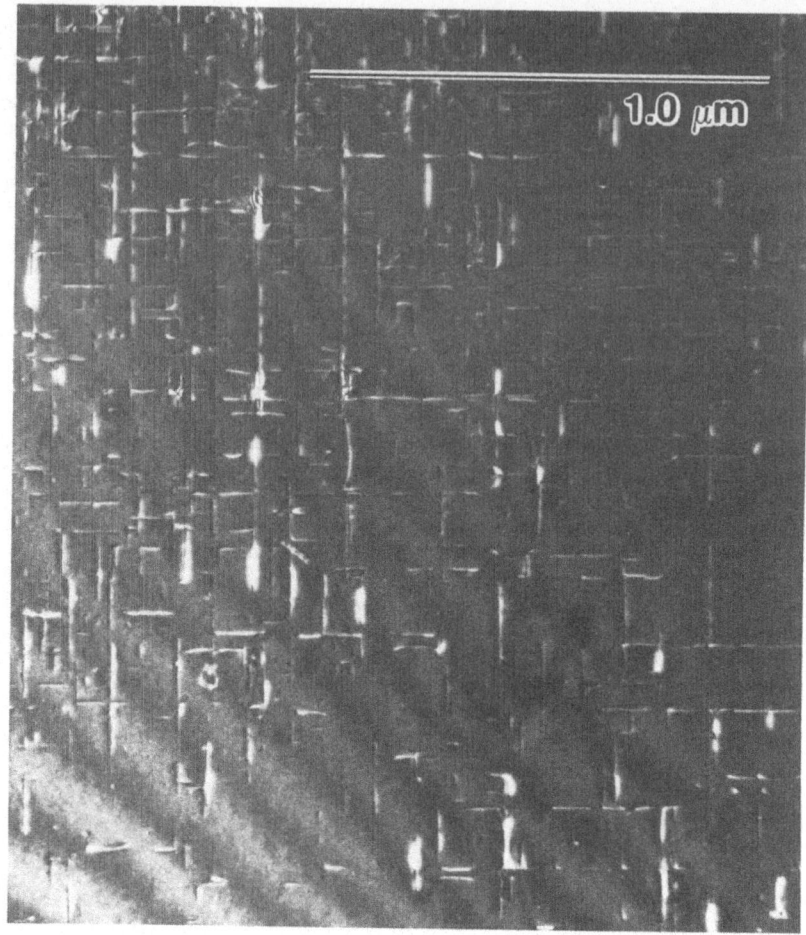

Fig. 8   An orthogonal array of 60° dislocations in a low mismatch GeSi/Si(100) strained layer system.

THE INTRODUCTION OF MISFIT DISLOCATIONS IN DISLOCATION FREE SYSTEMS: THEORETICAL CONSIDERATIONS

For epilayer growth on a dislocation free substrate, what is the source of the first misfit dislocations? Frank[24] and Hirth[25] have shown that the lowest energy route is through the nucleation and propagation of a dislocation half-loop from the growth surface. Matthews et al[18] have considered in detail dislocation half-loop nucleation and propagation in strained epilayers and have given expressions for the critical radius a dislocation half loop must have for it to propagate, and the corresponding activation energy required. It was concluded[18] that the nucleation barrier could not be overcome (at typical growth temperatures) for misfits below about 2% for <u>any</u> epilayer thickness. Eaglesham et al[26] have re-examined these calculations using a higher value of this dislocation core parameter (probably appropriate for dislocations in semiconductors) and calculate that the nucleation energy for a critical-radius half-loop is significantly higher than that calculated by Matthews: the new value is about 100eV at 2% misfit, and it increases to about 1000eV as the misfit tends to zero. Eaglesham et al suggest that half-loop nucleation at the growth surface is not a realistic mechanism for strains below about 5% for any epilayer thickness. The very large nucleation energies required contrast with the experimental nucleation barrier of 0.7eV measured by Hull et al[27] to produce the observed temperature dependence of dislocation densities in 1.26% misfit GeSi/Si(100).

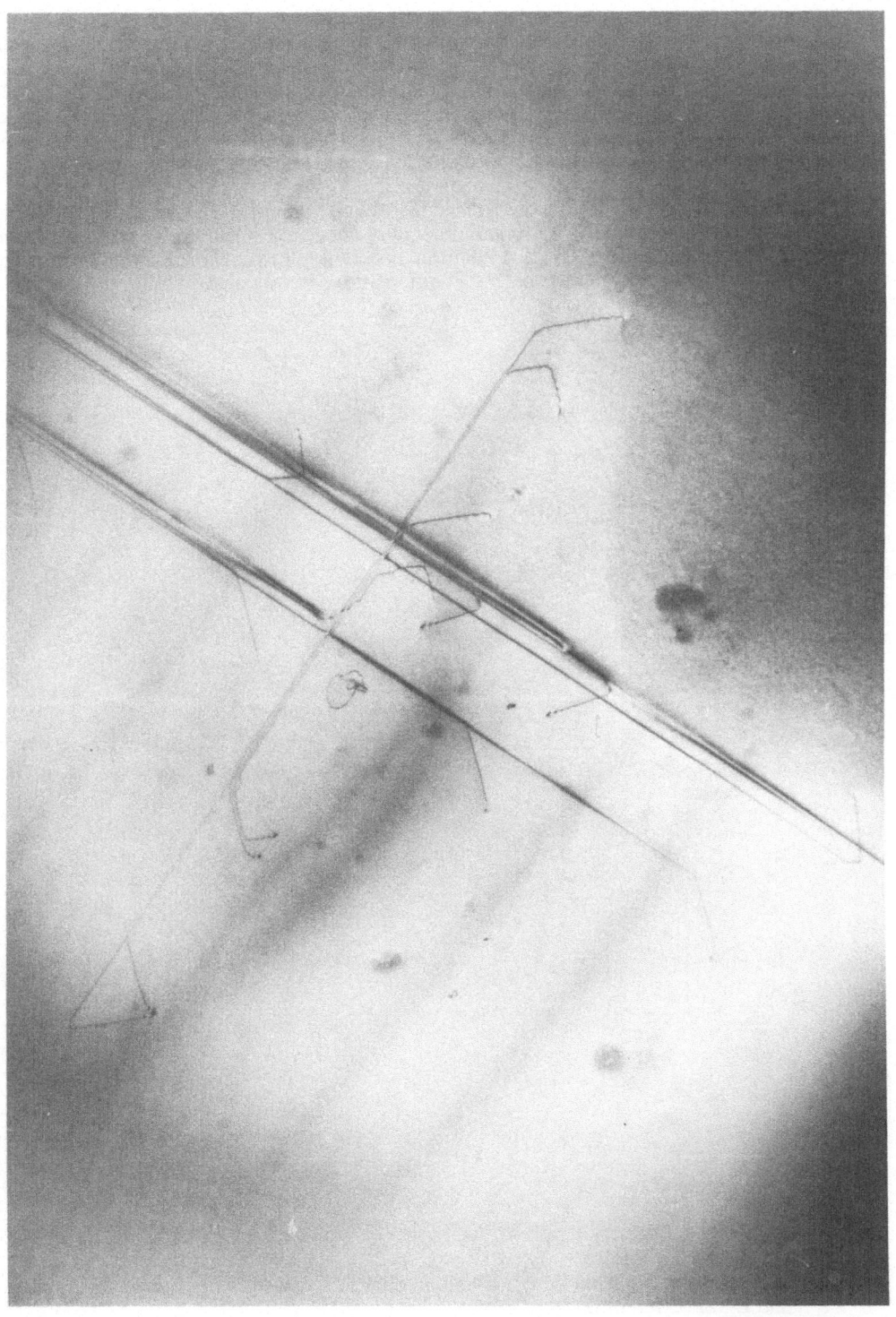

Fig.9   A bunch of misfit dislocations apparently arising from a single defect.

A NEW DISLOCATION SOURCE IN STRAINED EPILAYERS

From the above discussion an interesting problem arises. The experimental evidence from X-ray topography[23] and electron microscopy[27] is that it is rather easy to nucleate misfit dislocations in low mismatch strained epilayers grown on low dislocation density substrates. The theoretical calculations[26] however show that homogeneous nucleation of misfit dislocations should not be possible at any epilayer thickness for lattice mismatches of less than about 5%. It therefore seems possible that a new type of dislocation source may be operating and we have performed a detailed search for this.

The introduction of misfit dislocations in low misfit GeSi on Si(100) was studied using epilayers which were grown by MBE on deliberately unrotated substrates to provide graded compositions across the layers. Thus in addition to studying a critical thickness transition for epilayers of different thickness at a fixed composition, it was also possible to study the

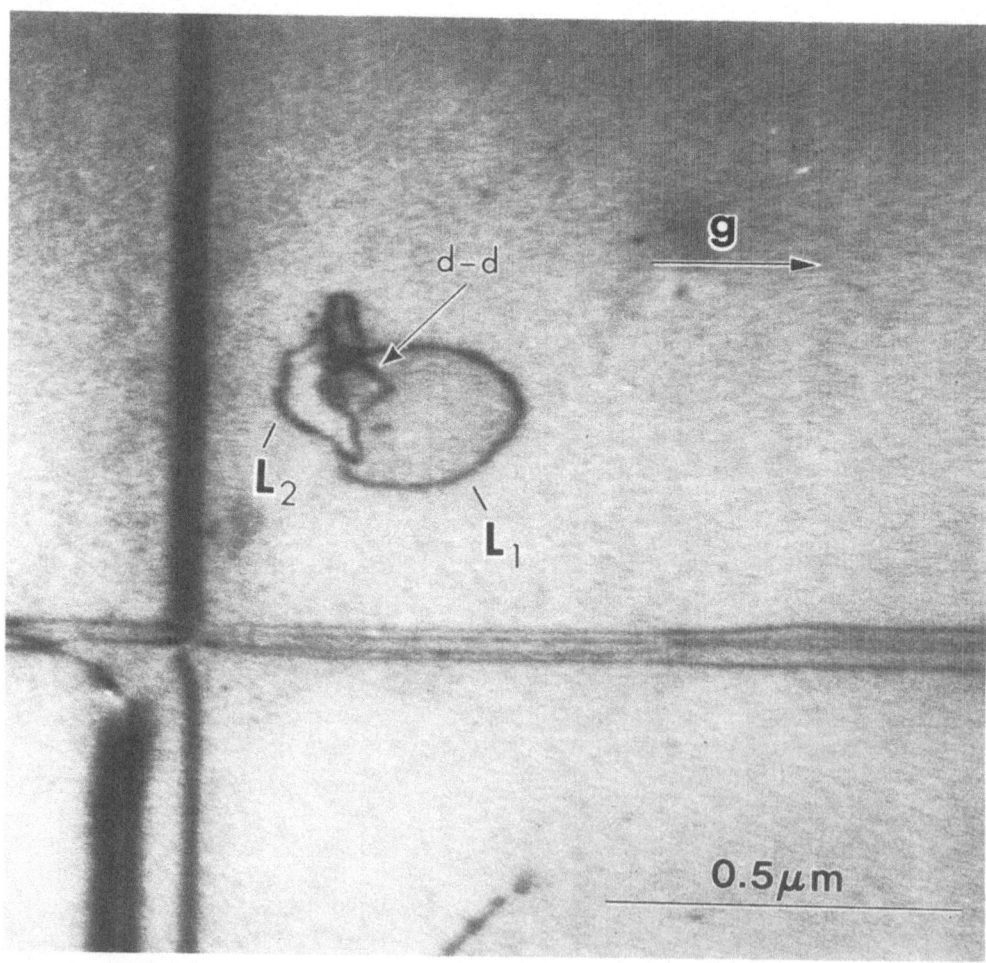

Fig.10   A detail from Fig.9 showing a diamond defect, d-d, generating two dislocations, L_1 and L_2, of different Burgers vector.

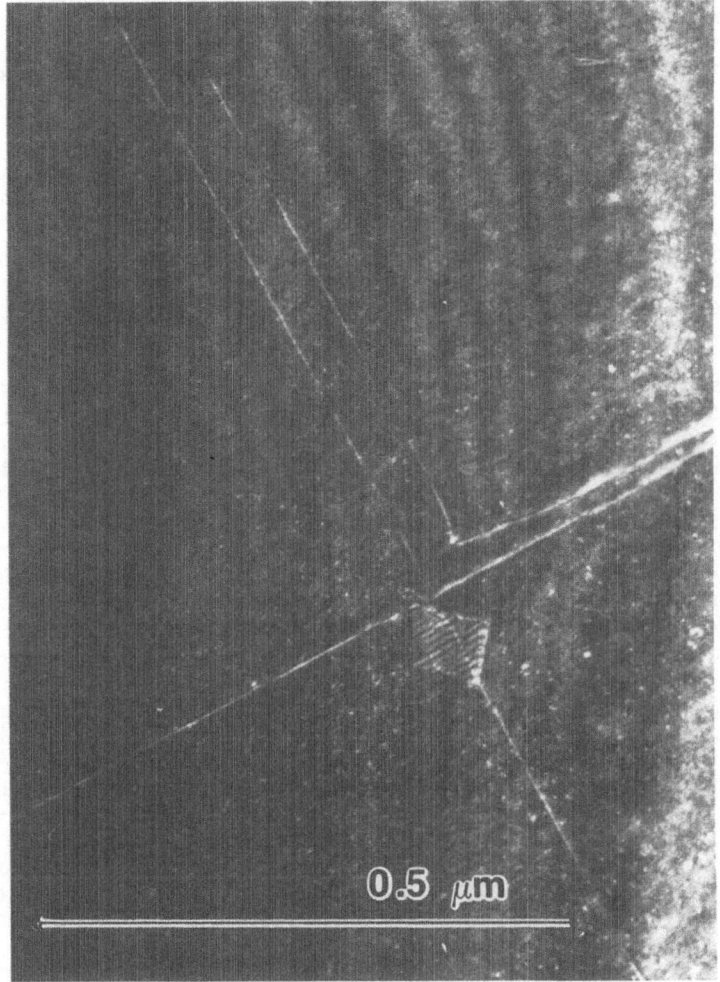

Fig. 11 A weak-beam image of a diamond shaped defect showing its faulted nature.

same transition at a fixed thickness as a function of composition. Epilayers of nominal 20% Ge composition (0.8% lattice mismatch) were grown in bands of different thickness, and the source and substrate geometry gave a composition difference of typically at ±4 % across the unrotated wafer. Further details are given in Eaglesham et al[26, 28]. The specimens were studied by strong-beam and weak-beam diffraction contrast in plan view and by HREM in cross-section.

At low misfit, misfit dislocations are observed in an orthogonal array (along <110>). The dislocations are mainly 60° in character and very long (10-100 μm). The 60° dislocations are not evenly spaced but arranged in bunches[22]. Stereo microscopy shows that the dislocations in a band often lie on the same inclined {111} plane. In addition, although a single bunch often consists of dislocations of identical 60° Burgers vector, frequently bunches are observed containing parallel 60° dislocations with different Burgers vectors (e.g. a/2 [110] and a/2 [$\bar{1}$01]) fig. 9.

The above observations suggest that the bunches of dislocations arise from a single source, capable of operating repetitively and producing dislocations of different Burgers vector. All known regenerative sources (Frank-Read, double cross-slip and vacancy disc) produce coplanar dislocations having the same Burgers vector. The source required to explain the present observations therefore has unusual properties.

Most of the 60° dislocations observed in our specimens are so long (~50 μm) that few have their entire length located in the thin region of the foil. However some short dislocations were observed: the interfacial misfit segment has 60° character and the two threading segments connecting this to the surface are usually screws, although 60° and edge segments are also common. This geometry initially suggests homogeneous half-loop nucleation at the surface: the 60° misfit segment gliding down an inclined {111} plane to the interface, and elongating by the outward glide of the screw or 60° epithreading end segments. However, as argued above, homogeneous nucleation is unlikely at low misfits.

Detailed study of GeSi/Si(100) epilayers from several different wafers revealed, in addition to the dislocation microstructure, a small number of diamond-shaped planar faults (Eaglesham et al[26,28]) fig.10. These defects were typically 20 to 200 nm in diameter and the number varied widely from 10^9 cm^{-3} to 10^{12} cm^{-3}. Stereomicroscopy and weak beam analysis (fig.11) have shown that these diamond shaped defects lie on {111} with inclined <110> edges, have a displacement vector of a/6<114> and are interstitial in character. Faulted loops of similar displacement have been reported following ion implantation (Salisbury[29]). The latter had the form of six sided polyhedra with edges comprising the three <110>'s to be found in the {111} habit plane and were considerably elongated along the <110> perpendicular to the Burgers vector. It is this edge which is missing in the diamond shaped defects studied so far, and the reason for this difference is not, as yet, clear.

The morphology of the diamond defects that have been analysed may be generalised as follows: a defect lying on (111) in an epitaxial layer with an [001] normal will have edges parallel to [10$\bar{1}$] and [0$\bar{1}$1] but not [1$\bar{1}$0] and will have an interstitial Burgers vector of a/6[114]. The "missing" <110> edge in the diamond defect is the one perpendicular to the growth direction. The Burgers vector is also perpendicular to this "missing" edge and is a <114> which gives a displacement for the fault which is close to edge (i.e., for a (111) fault the displacement will be parallel to [114] rather than [11$\bar{4}$]). This gives a unique Burgers vector for each fault plane. No (111) faults with a/6[141] or a/6[411] displacements have, for example, yet been found.

The presence of small a/6<114> diamond defects might, at first sight, appear surprising and some account of why these, rather than lower energy a/3<111> edge faults, precipitate is necessary. Since an interstitial a/6<114> defect contains an intrinsic stacking fault (Salisbury[29]) there will be a difference in fault energy between the two systems. While no information is yet available concerning fault energies in the alloys used here, it is worth noting that in silicon this difference would not favour the intrinsically faulted defect[31].

If the defects arise as the result of the aggregation of interstitials then the nucleation of the non-edge defect may be favoured since it may precipitate between the widely spaced partial {111} planes. The half planes are alternately a/4<111> and a/12<111> apart and an a/3<111> fault comprises two widely spaced half planes, a/4<111> apart, precipitated between lattice planes separated by a/12<111>. Three bonds must be broken for each interstitial pair precipitated. Inserting a closely spaced pair of interstitial half planes between widely spaced matrix {111} planes requires the breaking of only one bond for each atom pair precipitated and gives the observed a/6<114> displacement[29].

On a simple $\underline{b}^2$ basis the a/6<114> dislocation has rather less than 20% more line energy than the a/3<111> but this may be reduced by dissociation. It has been suggested that in unstrained silicon[29] the edges of the a/6[114] defect described above would dissociate to give a stair-rod and a Shockley partial thus:

[10$\bar{1}$] edge : a/6[114] → a/3[011] + a/6[1$\bar{1}$2]

[0$\bar{1}$1] edge : a/6[114] → a/3[101] + a/6[$\bar{1}$12]

The combined energy of these defects is only about 6% greater than that of an a/3<111> dislocation. It is clear that the strain in the epitaxial layer promotes different dissociations around the diamond defect in order to give rise to the observed misfit dislocations and further work is needed to achieve a full understanding of this system.

The significance of the diamond defect lies in its association with dislocations. Diamond defects were observed to be associated with all complete dislocation systems studied in this material. The number of diamond defects is almost certainly too low for this association to be coincidental, suggesting that this defect may act as a source. A source mechanism has been suggested on the basis of a possible dissociation of the defect, which allows the defect to emit perfect dislocations with more than one Burgers vector. It seems probable that the diamond defect is a new regenerative source of misfit dislocations in the low-misfit GeSi/Si(100) system.

References

1. P.J. Jones, G.M. Rackham and J.W. Steeds, Proc. Roy. Soc. (London), A354:197 (1977).
2. H.L. Fraser, D.M. Maher, C.J. Humphreys, C.J.D. Hetherington, R.V. Knoell and J.C. Bean, in: Microscopy of Semiconducting Materials 1985, Inst. Phys. Conf. Ser. 76, Eds. A.G. Cullis and D.B. Holt (Inst. Phys., London-Bristol) 307 (1985).
3. D.M. Maher, H.L. Fraser, C.J. Humphreys, R.V. Knoell, R.D. Field, J.B. Woodhouse and J.C. Bean, in: Electron Microscopy and Analysis 1985, Inst. Phys. Conf. Ser. 78, Ed. G.J. Tatlock (Inst. Phys., London-Bristol) 49 (1986).
4. D.M. Maher, H.L. Fraser, C.J. Humphreys, R.V. Knoell and J.C. Bean, Appl. Phys. Letters 50:574 (1987).
5. J.C. Bean, Science, 230:127 (1985).
6. C.J. Humphreys, D.M. Maher, H.L. Fraser and D.J. Eaglesham, Phil. Mag., 58:787 (1988).
7. C.J. Humphreys, D.J. Eaglesham, D.M. Maher and H.L. Fraser, Ultramicroscopy, 26:13 (1988).
8. M.M.J. Treacy, J.M. Gibson, and A. Howie, , Phil. Mag.A, 51:389 (1985).
9. J.M.Gibson, R. Hull, J.C. Bean, and M.M.J. Treacy, Appl. Phys. Lett., 46:649 (1985).
10. K. Alavi, P.M. Petroff, W.R. Wagner and A.Y. Cho, J. Vac. Sci. Technol. B1(2):146 (1983)
11. K.-H. Kuesters, B.C. de Cooman, J.R. Shealey and C.B. Carter, J. Cryst. Growth, 71:514 (1985).
12. J.M. Gibson, private communication.
13. J.M. Baribeau, D.C. Houghton, D.J. Lockwood and T.E. Jackman, in Semiconductor Based Heterostructures: Interfacial Structures and Stability, edited by M.L. Gree et al. (TMS, Warrendale, PA, 1986) 185.
14. J.F. Mansfield, D.M. Lee and G.A. Rozgonyi, in Microscopy of Semiconducting Materials 1987, edited by A.G. Cullis and P.D. Augustus (IOP Publishing Ltd, Bristol), Inst. Phys. Conf. Ser. 87, 169 (1987).
15. H.L. Fraser, D.M. Maher, R.V. Knoell, D.J. Eaglesham, C.J. Humphreys and J.C. Bean, J. Vac. Sci. Technol. (1989) in press.
16. J.H. Van der Merwe, J. Appl. Phys., 34:123 (1963).
17. J.W. Matthews, J. Vac. Sci. Technol., 12:126 (1975).
18. J.W. Matthews, A.E. Blakeslee and S. Mader, Thin Solid Films, 33:253 (1976).
19. Y. Kuk, L.C. Feldman and P.J. Silverman, Phys. Rev. Lett., 50:511 (1983).
20. R. People and J.C. Bean, Appl. Phys. Lett., 47:327 (1985).
21. I.J. Fritz, Appl. Phys. Lett., 51:1080 (1987).
22. E.P. Kvam, D.J. Eaglesham, D.M. Maher, C.J. Humphreys, J.C. Bean, G.S. Green and B.K. Tanner, Mat. Res. Soc. Symp. Proc. 104:623 (1988).
23. D.J. Eaglesham, E.P. Kvam, D.M. Maher, C.J. Humphreys, G.S. Green, B.K. Tanner and J.C. Bean, Appl. Phys. Lett. 53:2083 (1988).
24. F.C. Frank, Symposium on Plastic Deformation of Crystalline Solids, Carnegic Inst. of Technology, Pittsburgh, 89 (1950).

25. J.D. Hirth, in Relation Between Structure and Strength in Metals and Alloys, HMSO: London, 218 (1963).

26. D.J. Eaglesham, E.P. Kvam, D.M. Maher, C.J. Humphreys and J.C. Bean, Phil. Mag., 1989 (in press).

27. R. Hull, J.C. Bean, D.J. Warder and R.E. Leibenguth, Appl. Phys. Lett., 52:1605 (1988).

28. D.J. Eaglesham, D.M. Maher, E.P. Kvam, J.C. Bean and C.J. Humphreys, Phys. Rev. Lett. (1989) in press.

29. I.G. Salisbury, Acta Metall., 30:27 (1982).

30. W. Hagen and H. Strunk, Appl. Phys. 17:28 (1978).

31. A. Gomez, D.J.H. Cockayne, P.B. Hirsch and V. Vitek, Phil. Mag. A 31:105 (1975).

TEM AND STEM OBSERVATIONS OF COMPOSITION VARIATIONS IN III-V SEMICONDUCTORS

Frank Glas

Centre National d'Etudes des Télécommunications
196, avenue Henri Ravéra
92220 Bagneux, France

INTRODUCTION

In first approximation, the quaternary $A_xB_{1-x}C_yD_{1-y}$ III-V semiconducting alloys have the same sphalerite structure[1] as their 'constituent binaries' AC, AD, BC and BD; their lattice parameter a and their band gap energy vary continuously with the compositions x and y. These materials are thus attractive for the fabrication of optoelectronic devices, because a suitable choice of these in principle independent compositions usually allows both the epitaxy of a thin alloy layer on a bulk binary substrate and the subsequent obtaining of a device emitting or detecting light at a given wavelength. Conversely, any inhomogeneity in the alloy is likely to induce local variations of its structural and electronic properties. Such composition variations are either introduced intentionally to obtain novel effects, for instance in superlattices, or unintentionally. In the latter case, they are often caused by changes in the growth conditions of the layer: this may happen in Liquid Phase Epitaxy (LPE) when the liquid bath changes composition as growth proceeds, or in Chemical Vapor Deposition[2], because of instabilities in the growth process; the composition then varies only in the growth direction.

However, inhomogeneities of a more fundamental origin (with isoconcentration surfaces not necessarily planes parallel to the growth front of the layer) may exist even in samples grown under temporally uniform conditions. This is expected to be the case if the homogeneous alloy is thermodynamically unstable against disproportionation. Surprisingly, most III-V alloys are now generally believed to be partially immiscible. Early investigations showed that the restricted available portions of their phase diagrams are described rather satisfactorily by a regular solution model[1,3]. In this model, the enthalpy of mixing of a ternary alloy $A_xB_{1-x}C$ is $\Omega x(1-x)$, where Ω is the 'interaction parameter'[3]; the alloy is immiscible under some critical temperature T_c if the interaction parameter is positive. Similarly, the quaternary alloys are immiscible if the interaction parameters relative to the pairs of constituent binaries are positive. For the III-V alloys, the Ω's are all found stricly positive provided the constituent binaries are not latticed-matched[4]. This predictable immiscibility was in apparent contradiction with the existence under T_c of lattice-matched layers with well defined emission wavelengths, and was not commented upon until the first experiments of Hénoc et al.[5] revealed that composition inhomogeneities indeed exist in some III-V alloys.

In this paper, we will first review the Transmission Electron Microscopy (TEM) and Scanning Transmission Electron Microscopy (STEM) microanalysis experiments demonstrating that, in a range of average composition and growth conditions, $In_xGa_{1-x}As_yP_{1-y}$ layers display very specific composition modulations with components parallel to the substrate surface and a characteristic coarse scale of about 100 nm. The complexity of this phenomenon, happening during growth and subsequently frozen, but clearly related to the predicted immiscibility, will then be discussed. However, these often confirmed data leave open the question of the homogeneity of the alloy on a smaller scale. Thus, the TEM study of the fine scale contrast (~10 nm) universally observed in alloys whith lattice-mismatched constituent binaries will then be reviewed and its strain nature proven; its often admitted relation with smaller scale composition modulations will be critically discussed, in relation with the recent microscopical thermodynamic models of the III-V alloys, which, although they rightly insist on the existence of strains at the atomic level, will be shown not to describe suitably disordered materials.

In a ternary $A_xB_{1-x}C$ alloy, we call *mixed* the sublattice occupied by A and B; both the sublattices of a quaternary alloy are mixed. We qualify as *disordered* a model alloy where the occupation probabilities of the different sites of the mixed sublattices are uncorrelated. We call *intrinsic* the value $a(x,y)$ of the lattice parameter of the alloy in its bulk homogeneous stress-free form; it varies linearly with x and y (Vegard's law).

EXPERIMENTAL STUDY OF THE QUASIPERIODIC COMPOSITION MODULATIONS

In this section we recall that characteristic composition modulations exist in lattice-matched $In_xGa_{1-x}As_yP_{1-y}$ layers epitaxially grown by LPE on (001) oriented InP substrates. The experimental evidence is given for layers of average composition x=0.72, y=0.60 grown at temperatures T_g between 620 and 650°C. The micrographs were taken in a Vacuum Generators HB5 STEM at an energy E_0=100 keV, and are interpreted in the usual TEM terms; X-ray spectra were recorded in the same instrument with a Kevex Si:Li detector. For a Bragg reflection **g** of modulus g, we denote by F_g and ξ_g respectively the structure factor and the extinction distance, and by $w=g\xi_g\Delta\theta$ the deviation parameter, if $\Delta\theta$ is the angle between the electron beam and the exact Bragg incidence[6].

The quasiperiodic contrast

The study[7] of numerous 'plan view' specimens thinned from the substrate side either mechano-chemically with a solution of bromine in methanol, or by Ar⁺ ion bombardment, confirms and expands the first experiments of Hénoc et al.[5]:

(a) The Bright Field (BF) and Dark Field (DF) (Fig. 1 a,b,c) two-beam images, taken at or near the exact Bragg position for reflection **g**, display contrast elements roughly parallel to the directions [100] and [010] normal to the growth direction, repeated respectively along the directions **u**=[010] and [100] about every 100-200 nm; hence the term 'quasiperiodic' (QP).

(b) Both contrast directions appear for **g** of 220 type (Fig. 1 a); only the direction **u** colinear to **g** appears for **g** of 400 type (Fig. 1 b). The quasiperiod is the same in both types of images.

(c) DF images show one sharp black/white (bw) transition per quasiperiod (the 'whiteness' of a pixel grows with the number of electrons contributing to it); this transition is reversed to wb if **g** is changed in -**g** (Fig. 1 a,c). In a given image and for a given repeat direction **u**, these sharp transitions are always in the same sense, such that **g.u**>0 if **u** is chosen from black to white[8].

(d) BF images are less contrasted. Two black bands flanking a whiter one correspond to the most pronounced transitions of the DF images.

(e) In images formed with other reflections than 220 and 400, the

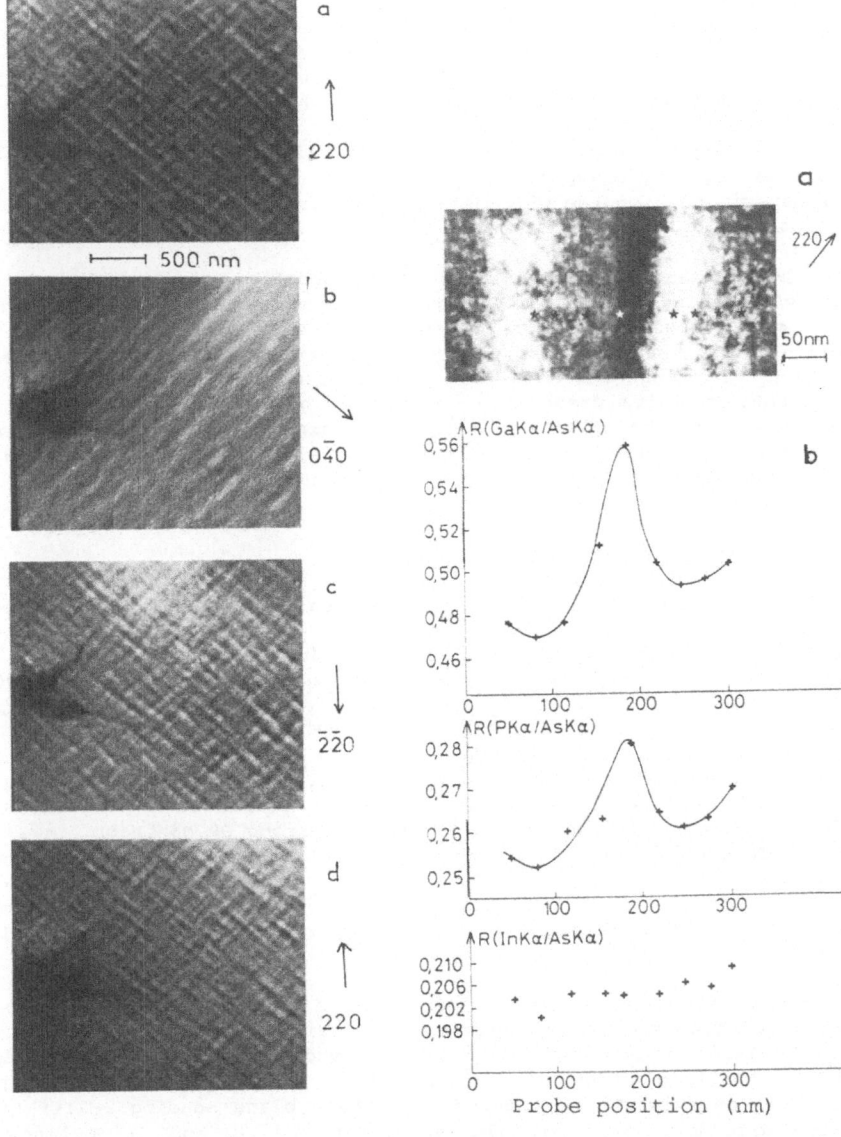

Figure 1. STEM two-beam Dark Field micrographs of the same area of an $In_xGa_{1-x}As_yP_{1-y}$ specimen ($x \approx 0.72$, $y \approx 0.60$).
(a) $\mathbf{g}=2\overline{2}0$ ($w_0 \approx 0$); (b) $\mathbf{g}=0\overline{4}0$ ($w_0 \approx 0$);
(c) $\mathbf{g}=\overline{2}\overline{2}0$ ($w_0 \approx 0$); (d) $\mathbf{g}=220$ ($w_0 \approx 1$).

Figure 2. (a) STEM Dark Field micrograph of a zone of an $In_xGa_{1-x}As_yP_{1-y}$ specimen showing a quasiperiodic contrast element;

(b) measurement by X-ray microanalysis, at the points indicated in (a), of the ratios of the count numbers for the Ga$K\alpha$, P$K\alpha$ and In$K\alpha$ lines to the count number for the As$K\alpha$ line.

contrast keeps the same local quasiperiod and:
- a contrast repeated along **u** is seen only if **g.u**≠0
- the contrast amplitude decreases rapidly as g increases
- the images **g**=200 show only a weak contrast.

(f) When increasing |w|, the DF contrast weakens but neither shifts nor changes quasiperiod (Fig. 1 d), and finally vanishes.

(g) The contrast varies with the specimen thickness t. For 220 DF images, it is weak for $t<0.75\xi_g$ and around $t=(n+1/2)\xi_g$, and strong around $t=n\xi_g$ (n integer).

(h) In a given specimen, the contrast amplitude varies; one of the two directions may locally disappear.

(i) Superimposed on the QP contrast is a finer granular contrast (Fig. 1 a-d), which will be discussed later.

The QP contrast cannot be induced by specimen thickness variations, since it would then be identical in **g** and **-g** images; it is not the contrast of any common extended defect, either tridimensional (precipitates of a well-defined second phase), bidimensional (stacking fault) or monodimensional (dislocation). Although few detailed studies of the QP contrast exist[7,8], many workers[9-13] confirmed its presence in a wide range of samples, which will be detailed later. On the other hand, only the experiments carried out in our group[5,7,9,10] showed, by using direct microanalytical techniques, its association with QP composition modulations. These experiments are now summarized.

The quasiperiodic composition modulations

Series of X-ray spectra were recorded with a stationary ~1 nm diameter STEM probe, which was moved between spectra across QP contrast elements by steps of typically 5-20 nm. The spatial resolution of the method was of a few nm in the zones analyzed, whose thicknesses were of the order of 100 nm. R(A/B) will denote the ratio of the numbers of photons of lines A and B recorded in a given spectra. All the profiles (Fig. 2) show that:

(a') $R(GaK\alpha/AsK\alpha)$ varies in phase with the QP contrast, with extrema at the bw and wb transitions; the sharp bw transitions (c) correspond to maxima. Large contrast amplitudes correspond to large composition variations. ±5% variations are commonly recorded in zones with strong QP contrast.

(b') $R(PK\alpha/AsK\alpha)$ varies in phase with $R(GaK\alpha/AsK\alpha)$, with a smaller amplitude.

(c') $R(InK\alpha/AsK\alpha)$ varies little, without correlation with the previous ratios, and is often constant within the statistical accuracy of the measurements.

We retained only experiments where the film was thin enough so that absorption and fluorescence effects were negligible[7], except for the strongly absorbed PK line. We checked that the observed variations were not due to spurious channelling effects[7,9], which had to be considered since the QP contrast will be shown to be induced by lattice plane bending. Cliff-Lorimer k-factors[14] were measured and calculated[7] for the Ga and In K lines with respect to the AsK line, giving: $(1-x)/y=(0.89\pm0.02)R(GaK\alpha/AsK\alpha)$ and $x/y=(6.1\pm0.6)R(InK\alpha/AsK\alpha)$, this larger uncertainty being caused by the apparent variation between experiments of the Si:Li detector efficiency at high photon energy. x and y were thus measured with an absolute precision of about 5%; the accuracy of the *relative* variation of concentration ratios in a given zone was much better, being only limited by the statistics.

In conclusion, the samples of average composition x=0.72, y=0.60 grown by LPE at 620-650°C exhibit composition modulations. In both the imaging and the microanalysis experiments described above, the beam direction **B** was nearly parallel (to a few degrees) to the growth direction [001], along which the information was thus integrated. Assuming nothing about the composition distribution in the depth of the sample, the Ga to As concentration ratio must vary by at least ±5% in the zones with strong QP contrast (a'). If the concentrations are assumed not to vary along [001], we measured the actual modulations (possibly broadened by the limited spatial resolution of the microanalysis), which are then in particular such that the In to As ratio is nearly constant (c'). For a stress-free alloy with x/y constant, $\Delta a/a \approx 2 \times 10^{-2} \Delta[(1-x)/y]/[(1-x)/y]$[7]; the recorded modulations thus correspond to large (up to several 10^{-3}) *intrinsic* lattice parameter variations. In a thin layer with composition variations inducing intrinsic lattice parameter variations, a more complex strain field must obviously exist.

The relation between the contrast and the geometry of the composition modulations

Contrast and composition modulations have the same quasiperiod; if the contrast is absent (see below), the specimen is homogeneous at the spatial resolution of our measurements. The contrast is thus obviously due to composition variations, but two extreme mechanisms can be considered, whether the contrast is dominated by the variations of the composition-dependent structure factor or by the strain field induced by the composition variation. We show that this second mechanism indeed dominates. To discuss the experimental micrographs, we use the two-beam and column (Fig. 3) approximations[6], whereby, for a crystal oriented near Bragg position $\mathbf{g}$, the intensities of the transmitted and diffracted waves at depth Z along the beam direction are respectively the squares of the modules of the quantities ϕ_0 and ϕ_g governed by the Howie-Whelan equations:

$$\frac{d\phi_0}{dZ} = -\frac{\pi}{\xi'_0}\phi_0 + \pi\left(\frac{i}{\xi_g} - \frac{1}{\xi'_g}\right)\phi_g \qquad (1a)$$

$$\frac{d\phi_g}{dZ} = \pi\left(\frac{i}{\xi_g} - \frac{1}{\xi'_g}\right)\phi_0 + \left[-\frac{\pi}{\xi'_0} + 2\pi i\left(\frac{w_0}{\xi_g} + \beta'_g\right)\right]\phi_g \qquad (1b)$$

ξ'_0 and ξ'_g are the absorption distances[6] (for measured values, see Glas[7]), w_0 is an average deviation parameter corresponding to the global disorientation of the specimen from the Bragg position, and $\beta'_g \approx \mathbf{g}.(d\mathbf{R}/dZ)$, where $\mathbf{R}$ is the local strain with respect to a crystal uniformly disoriented of w_0, measures the local tilt of the $\mathbf{g}$ planes. Neglecting the possible changes in absorption distances, it is useful to discuss separately the two mechanisms mentioned above (which obviously coexist), namely the effects of the variations of structure factor (appearing in ξ_g[6]) and of β'_g. No distinction will be made between the column direction and [001], and thus between the planes of the layer and of the micrographs. It is worth considering consecutively if the images may be explained by supposing that F_g or β'_g vary only between columns, or if they must also vary in the depth of the thinned specimen.

Hypothesis (I): column uniformity. At the exit ($Z=t$) of each column where ξ_g, ξ'_0, ξ'_g and β'_g are uniform, one has:

$$|\phi_g(t)|^2 = \frac{1}{2\sqrt{1+w^2}}\exp(-2\pi t/\xi'_0)\,[\cosh(2\pi t/\xi_g\xi'_g s') - \cos(2\pi t s')] \qquad (2)$$

where $w = w_0 + \xi_g\beta'_g$ and $s' = (1+w^2)^{1/2}/\xi_g$.

Thus, if only the disorientation of the $\mathbf{g}$ planes varied between uniform columns (this would be a simple approximation if, for instance, intrinsic lattice parameter gradients along [001], of alternated signs, were distributed quasiperiodically in the plane of the specimen; see Fig. 3 a), it

221

would be possible, by tilting the specimen (varying w_0), to bring successively each column to the Bragg position $w=0$; this is contradicted by result (f). We would also get (if $\xi_g = \xi_{-g}$) the same DF images with g and $-g$ for $w_0=0$, since $\beta'_g = -\beta'_{-g}$ and since (2) is symmetrical in β'_g; this is ruled out by (c).

On the other hand, it is easily shown[7] from (2) that, if only ξ_g varies between columns inside each of which it is uniform, one has at all thicknesses:

$$d|\phi_g|^2/|\phi_g|^2 \leq M |d\xi_g/\xi_g|$$ (3)

where M depends on the reflection and on w. For $g=220$ and $w=0$, we calculated[7] that $M\sim 6$. From the definition of ξ_g[8], one finds[8], for an undistorted cubic crystal of lattice parameter a:

$$\frac{d\xi_g}{\xi_g} \approx -\frac{dF_g}{F_g} + 3\frac{da}{a}$$ (4)

For the variations of F_g, two cases should be considered. Either the inhomogeneous alloy is disordered (see the introduction), and the contrast should then be the same for all equivalent sphalerite reflections (e.g. 220 and 220 or 400 and 040), since their structure factors only depend then on the local composition[7]; this is not the case (b,c). Otherwise the alloy is partially or totally ordered, and equivalent sphalerite reflections might produce different images; however, we never observed any tridimensional ordering in our samples[7], and the effect expected on the strong reflections used here (220, 400) is also too small to account for the observed contrast, since, for $h+k+l=4n$, F_{hkl} is only affected by the small atomic displacements induced by ordering[7]. On the other hand, from (4), the variations of a in a stress-free alloy where $(1-x)/y$ varies by about 10% would produce a contrast of less than 3%, much lower than those observed; moreover, the contrast would again be the same for equivalent sphalerite reflections.

Thus, the QP contrast cannot be interpreted by supposing that the parameters that govern it are uniform through the specimen depth.

Hypothesis (II): non uniform columns. Again the hypothesis of a contrast dominated by the variations of ξ_g can be discarded, since then, after (1), the same images could be obtained with equivalent g vectors. This is also confirmed by the very weak contrast observed using the reflections whose structure factor is most sensitive to composition variations, such as 200 (e). Thus β'_g must vary in the depth of the specimen. Again, two mechanisms

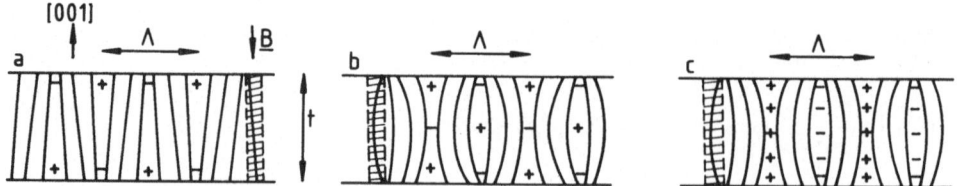

Figure 3. Schematic of three hypotheses for the distortion of the reflecting planes in a thinned specimen with contrast of quasiperiod ∧. + and −: regions of large and small intrinsic lattice parameter. Dashed areas: columns . (a) no lattice plane bending; (b) bending induced by composition variation in the depth of the specimen; (c) composition uniform in depth and bending induced by relaxation at the free surfaces (model of Treacy et al.[9]).

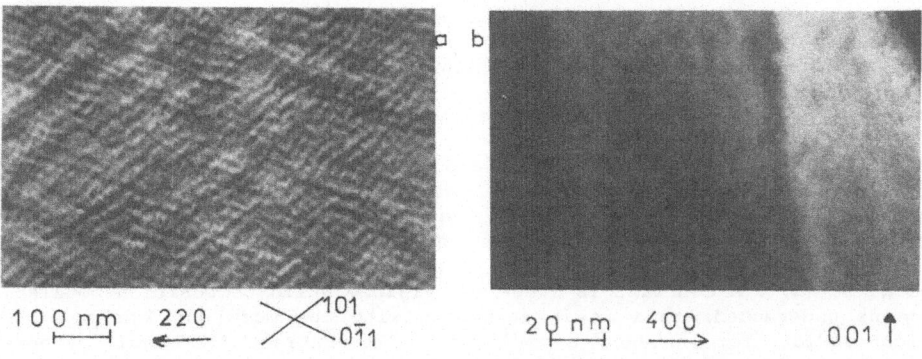

Figure 4. (a) 220 STEM Dark Field image of a plan view $In_xGa_{1-x}As_yP_{1-y}$ specimen tilted through a large angle (beam close to the [111] direction), showing the damping of the QP contrast and the subsidiary fringes. (b) 400 STEM Dark Field image of a cross-sectional specimen showing contrast elements approximately parallel to the growth direction [001].

can be considered: either composition variations along the growth direction produce a strain field (Fig. 3 b), or the composition is constant in this direction (Fig. 3 c). Using the simple model of a sinusoidal composition modulation in a direction normal to [001], Treacy et al.[*] proved, by inserting into (1) the corresponding strain field, provided by their solution of the linear isotropic elasticity, that the bending of the lattice planes induced by the free surfaces of the thinned specimen (Fig. 3 c), could explain the characteristics and the magnitude of the contrast of the plan-view micrographs. This demonstrates elegantly that, along [001], the composition may be uniform and the lattice plane bending non uniform, leading to the observation of both large composition modulations and contrast.

Further experiments confirm the plausibility of this model. First, in two-beam images taken on specimens tilted so that the beam direction **B** is no longer parallel to [001], bands of contrast subsist along the projections in the new image plane of the original [100] type directions, repeated along the projections **u′** of the original directions **u** by the projection of the quasiperiod; furthermore, subsidiary fringes appear[7,13] (Fig. 4 a), but only if **u′**.[001]$\neq$0. Again, QP contrast and subsidiary fringes are only visible if **g.u′**$\neq$0. Images simulations using (1) and the strain field calculated by Treacy et al.[*] indeed show[7] that fringes should appear in tilted specimens for w$\neq$0, but no quantitative comparison with the experiments has been made. Interestingly, the occurrence of fringes does not imply composition discontinuities and related phase jumps of the beam. Second, micrographs of cross-sectional specimens obtained with **B** parallel to [010] display coarse bands of contrast parallel to [001] for **g**=400 (Fig. 4 b), but not for **g**=004[12]. Both the fringes and the cross-sectional experiments are at least qualitatively consistent with a composition roughly constant along [001] over distances of several 100 nm.

THERMODYNAMICS AND KINETICS OF THE QUASIPERIODIC COMPOSITION MODULATIONS

Domain of existence of the quasiperiodic composition modulations

We observed QP contrast and composition modulations in many $In_xGa_{1-x}As_yP_{1-y}$ layers grown by LPE on (001) InP. The average lattice mismatch at T_g

estimated from room temperature X-ray double-diffraction was never more than a few 10^{-4}; recall that for alloys lattice-matched to InP, $1-x\approx0.47y$. The emission by photoluminescence of light of a well-defined wavelength was attributed to carrier recombination in the regions of small gap only[5]. In plan-view specimens, the contrast elements are always roughly parallel to [100] and [010]; although no systematic contrast measurements were performed, contrast and composition modulation amplitude were found to vary in the same sense. A particularly sharp contrast, which could be due to coherent lamellar precipitates lying on the (100) type planes, is sometimes observed[9], accompanying the largest composition modulations measured (up to 25% for $(1-x)/y$); such sharp features were later observed by Mahajan et al.[11] and Cherns et al.[13]. A contrast is sometimes visible while composition modulations remains undetected; this is in agreement with the model of Treacy et al.[9], which predicts for instance[7] a comfortable 20% contrast for hardly detectable variations of $(1-x)/y$ of ±1%. The quasiperiod ranges between 80 and 250 nm, but usually lies between 100 and 150 nm; its dispersions in and among samples are of the same order. In all the analyzed specimens with an average x lying between 0.67 and 0.72, the modulations keep x/y constant. The ternary lattice-matched $In_{0.53}Ga_{0.47}As$ grown at sufficiently low temperature (see below) also exhibits QP modulations[10], but, as expected, such that the sum of the atomic concentration ratios Ga/As and In/As remains equal to 1. The amplitude of the modulations recorded in various specimens are summarized in Fig. 5. To our knowledge, no proper QP modulations were ever observed in any III-V alloy other than $In_xGa_{1-x}As_yP_{1-y}$.

Fig. 6 indicates, together with the results of other groups[11-13], the average compositions and LPE growth temperatures T_g for which we observed QP composition modulations. A domain of existence, and in particular a composition dependent critical growth temperature, under which the layers systematically exhibit QP modulations, clearly appear.

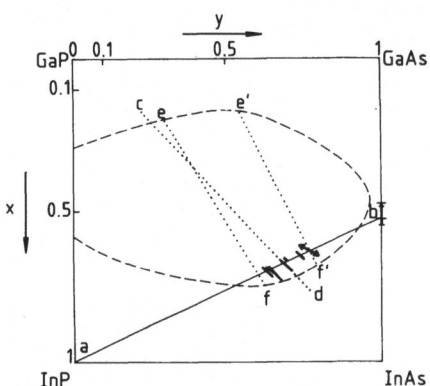 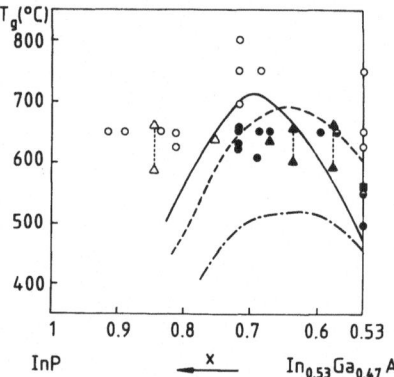

Figure 5. Composition modulations in various $In_xGa_{1-x}As_yP_{1-y}$ layers grown by LPE, shown in the composition diagram (each point represents an alloy composition). Thick segments: our measurements of the composition excursion across some QP contrast elements. Arrowed segment: result of Cherns et al.[13]. ab: alloys lattice matched to InP. cd: experimental tie-line[17]. Dashed line: calculated spinodal domain at 650°C, with tie-lines ef, e'f'[15].

Figure 6. Presence (filled symbols) and absence (empty symbols) of the coarse quasiperiodic contrast in $In_xGa_{1-x}As_yP_{1-y}$ layers grown on (001) InP by LPE $(1-x\approx0.47y)$, as a function of their average In content and of their growth temperature. o,●: our results. Δ,▲: others[11-13]. ■: MBE specimen[12]. Dashed and dashed-dotted lines: spinodal gap calculated with Ω's differing by 15%[4,15]. Full line: calculated miscibility gap[4].

Several epitaxial layers were submitted to various thermal treatments[10]:
- three layers with x=0.72 were grown at T_g=650°C: one was kept 30 hours at T_g, one slowly cooled, spending several hours between 650 and 630°C, and the last one was brought to room temperature as soon as the growth ended; the QP modulations were analogous in all layers.
- a layer of the same composition grown at 750°C, and thus without QP modulations (Fig. 6), was annealed at 650°C: no QP modulations appeared, although they exist systematically if growth is carried out at this temperature (Fig. 6).

Discussion

To discuss the possible origin of the observed QP composition modulations, and also from an historical point of view, it is useful to recall briefly the thermodynamic models of de Crémoux[15] and Stringfellow[4]. In the simple case of a bulk homogeneous ternary $A_xB_{1-x}C$ alloy, treated as a 'pseudo-binary' $(AC)_x(BC)_{1-x}$ disordered compound, the molar 'chemical' free enthalpy of mixing is simply, with R the gas constant:

$$\Delta G_m^c(x) = \Omega x(1-x) + RT[x\ln x + (1-x)\ln(1-x)] \qquad (5)$$

As seen in the introduction, these models predict for Ω>0 the occurence of a miscibility gap, and in particular of a critical temperature $T_c=\Omega/2R$; only above T_c is any alloy's composition stable. Inside the miscibility gap exists a spinodal gap, for which the first stages of the decomposition of an initially homogeneous alloy should produce smooth composition modulations rather than distinct phases[16]. This analysis can be extended to quaternary alloys. The striking fact is that these models lead to miscibility gaps which closely ressemble the domain of existence of the QP composition modulations, provided the temperature considered is T_g (Fig. 6), although it is also clear from Fig. 6 that slight changes in the experimental values of the Ω's lead to miscibility or spinodal gaps differing significantly. Moreover, the directions of the composition diagram corresponding to the observed modulations are nearly the decomposition directions ('tie-lines') predicted by the models (Fig. 5). In addition, several characteristics of the QP modulations are strongly reminiscent of spinodal decomposition. First, with the exception of the abovementioned possible lamellar precipitates and of some tridimensional coherent precipitates[7] found in $In_xGa_{1-x}P$ layers with x≈0.5, we always observed modulations continuous to the resolution of the STEM microanalysis. Second, following Cahn[16], an elastic contribution ΔG_m^e must be added to ΔG_m for alloys where composition variations induce intrinsic lattice parameter variations, when the decomposition preserves the coherency of the crystal lattice. Then, for a sinusoidal modulation in direction u, of any wavelength:

$$\Delta G_m^e = \sigma(u)(\Delta a/a)^2 \qquad (6)$$

where $\Delta a/a$ is the amplitude of the induced intrinsic lattice parameter modulation; $\sigma(u)$>0 depends on the elastic constants[16]; for the III-V compounds, it is found minimum for u of [100] type, and modulations in these directions thus minimize the added elastic energy.

These remarkable similarities probably explain that the QP modulations are often taken for the product of a spinodal decomposition. However, a closer examination reveals important differences:
(1) The spinodal description of Cahn[16] applies to a bulk alloy prepared homogeneous, which starts decomposing when quenched under its critical temperature; in metallic alloys, the decomposition morphology, and in

particular the modulation amplitude and its wavelength, are sensitive to annealing treatments[16]. This is not the case for the QP modulations, which we have recalled to be totally unaffected by any thermal treatment following the actual growth of the layer: our experiments prove that the modulations do not happen by solid state diffusion in the layer once it is grown; they must thus appear during the growth of the layer itself.

(2) The elastic energy ΔG_e^a makes decomposition energetically unfavourable, thus reducing the extension of the miscibility gap[16]. Stringfellow[4] showed that, for most III-V alloys, including $In_xGa_{1-x}As_yP_{1-y}$, this was indeed sufficient to suppress any tendency to disproportionate ($T_c\approx0$).

(3) The fact that we are dealing with a thin layer of the material grown on a substrate matters: Quillec et al.[17] showed that when growth is carried out in conditions giving rise to QP modulations on InP, but on a strongly mismatched GaP substrate ($\Delta a/a\approx7\%$), incoherent phases of distinct compositions, close to those predicted by de Crémoux and Stringfellow, appear (Fig. 5). That only smooth QP modulations occur for the InP substrate must be related to the 'lattice pulling' effect, whereby, for *miscible* III-V alloys, the presence of a substrate energetically favours the growth of the compounds most closely lattice-matched to it[18]. This effect has been extended in a 'substrate stabilization' effect, whereby the substrate renders metastable a small composition range of homogeneous *immiscible* alloys, around those exactly lattice-matched to this substrate[15]; this is usually described by a substrate orientation-dependent elastic energy, formally analogous to ΔG_e^a given by (6), where $\Delta a/a$ is now the layer/substrate mismatch. Such an effect was invoked[15] to justify the possibility of growing layers, believed to be homogeneous before the discovery of the QP modulations, inside the miscibility gap.

Any explanation of the QP modulations must thus recognize both the specificity of the layer/substrate system, and that they appear during growth and are subsequently frozen. However, the unique but important observation by Norman et al.[12] of QP modulations in an $In_xGa_{1-x}As$ layer grown by Molecular Beam Epitaxy (MBE) on InP (Fig. 6), forbids us invoking the peculiarities of the LPE growth. Moreover, we showed[7] that the observed quasiperiod and the growth velocity are too small and the solute diffusion coefficients in the liquid bath too large to allow hypothetical stationary QP concentration modulations in the LPE bath parallel to the growth front, as encountered in eutectic solidification, to exist. A satisfactory treatment of the difficult problem of the growth of many-component immiscible alloys has yet to be given. The simple models mentioned above are probably inadequate: first, following the treatment by Cahn[16] of *metallic* alloys, they assume that the chemical enthalpy of mixing is a function of the composition only; Extended X-ray Absorption Fine Structure (EXAFS) experiments[19,20] and more recent models[21,22], which will be discussed later, imply on the contrary that, for the *covalent* III-V alloys, the strain state of the material is of paramount importance. Second, we showed recently[23] that the treatments of the elastic energy used until now do not apply to a modulated layer, but either to a bulk modulated crystal (Stringfellow[4], following Cahn[16]) or to an homogeneous mismatched epitaxial layer (de Crémoux[15]). We gave an exact analytical calculation of the elastic energy of an epitaxial layer compositionnally modulated in directions parallel to the substrate; we showed that, provided the modulation period and the layer thickness are comparable, the elastic energy was considerably reduced with respect to the bulk alloy case, because of elastic relaxation at the free surface and at the layer/substrate interface: the stabilization by the elastic energy is much less pronounced, and T_c *higher* than previously calculated[4,15], but still lower than the usual LPE growth temperatures[23]. The strain at the surface of such a layer was also calculated, and it was suggested that, since dilated regions are probably sites of preferential incorporation of the atoms of large covalent radius, this could explain why, once a QP modulation has appeared, it might reproduce as the layer grows, thus maintaining the composition roughly constant along some distance in the growth direction[23].

The results reported above amply show that the coarse QP contrast is due to composition modulations, whose development mechanism is however not yet entirely clear. This contrast has up to now been observed only in layers of the InGaAsP system, in a precisely determined range of average compositions and growth temperatures (Fig. 6). However, as already mentioned (i), the micrographs of the layers with QP modulations also display a finer granular contrast. There is considerable confusion in the literature about this contrast, which, following the analysis of the coarse QP contrast, has often been attributed *without any proof* to composition modulations, and even to 'spinodal' ones. It is thus worth summarizing our detailed study of this contrast[7,24] and discussing its possible origin and its implications for the validity of the recently proposed 'microscopical' thermodynamic models[21,22] of the III-V alloys.

Domain of existence and characteristics of the fine contrast

In the plan-view micrographs of $In_xGa_{1-x}As_yP_{1-y}$ layers grown on (001) oriented substrates, the fine contrast (Fig. 7), apparently first reported by Roberts et al.[25], exists *whatever the growth method and conditions*, and thus irrespective of the presence of the coarse QP contrast. We also observed it in the GaAsSb and InGaAlAs systems, but never in the binary III-V compounds or in the $Ga_xAl_{1-x}As$ alloys (Fig. 7 b). From our observations and many others[11,12,25-29], we conclude that it is present in all the two-beam plan-view micrographs of any (001) epitaxial layer of any ternary or quaternary III-V alloy whose constituent binaries *are not lattice-matched*. We discuss its characteristics from DF STEM micrographs of mechanochemically thinned $In_xGa_{1-x}As$ layers without QP modulations, epitaxially grown by LPE or MBE on (001) InP (x=0.53 on average); we show (Fig. 7 c-g) zones where an accidental cleavage on a (202) type plane has produced 45° wedges[7], in order to demonstrate the effect of the variation of the specimen thickness t on the contrast (at a distance d from the edge, t=d). We call w_0 the deviation parameter averaged on distances large compared with the characteristic scale of the contrast, which it is useful to distinguish from its local value w, since the fine contrast will be shown to be of strain nature.

(i) In g=220-type images (Fig. 7 a), the contrast is rather isotropic in the plane; for w_0=0, the repeat distance or 'size' of the contrast is of the order of 10-15 nm. In g=400-type images (Fig. 7 c-e), the contrast consists of elements elongating in the direction normal to g, but on distances rarely exceeding three times their separation. The contrast is very weak in g=200-type images. It decreases if g increases.

(ii) For g=400 and w_0=0, the contrast is very weak for $t \leq 0.75\xi_{400}$, but remains visible up to thicknesses of several hundreds nm (Fig. 7 c-e).

(iii) If $|w_0|$ increases, the contrast becomes visible for smaller t (Fig. 7 f).

(iv) If g is changed to $-g$ for w_0=0, there is either inversion of the contrast (i.e. exchange between maxima and minima), or no evident correlation (Fig. 7 c,d).

(v) For a given g, the contrast is inverted if w_0 is changed in $-w_0$, except maybe for $t \approx n\xi_g$ (low diffracted intensity)[24].

(vi) It is most often impossible to establish any contrast correlation between micrographs taken with different values of w_0. If $|w_0|$ increases, the characteristic scale of the contrast diminishes (Fig. 7 e,f); for g=400, the elements remain normal to g and fringes with spacing down to 2 nm can be observed. An elongated contrast is still visible in the weak beam micrographs (Fig. 7 g).

(vii) For w_0=0 and w_0=0.75[24], the contrast is maximum for t equal to the 'effective extinction distance' $\xi'_g = \xi_g/(1+w^2)^{1/2}$.

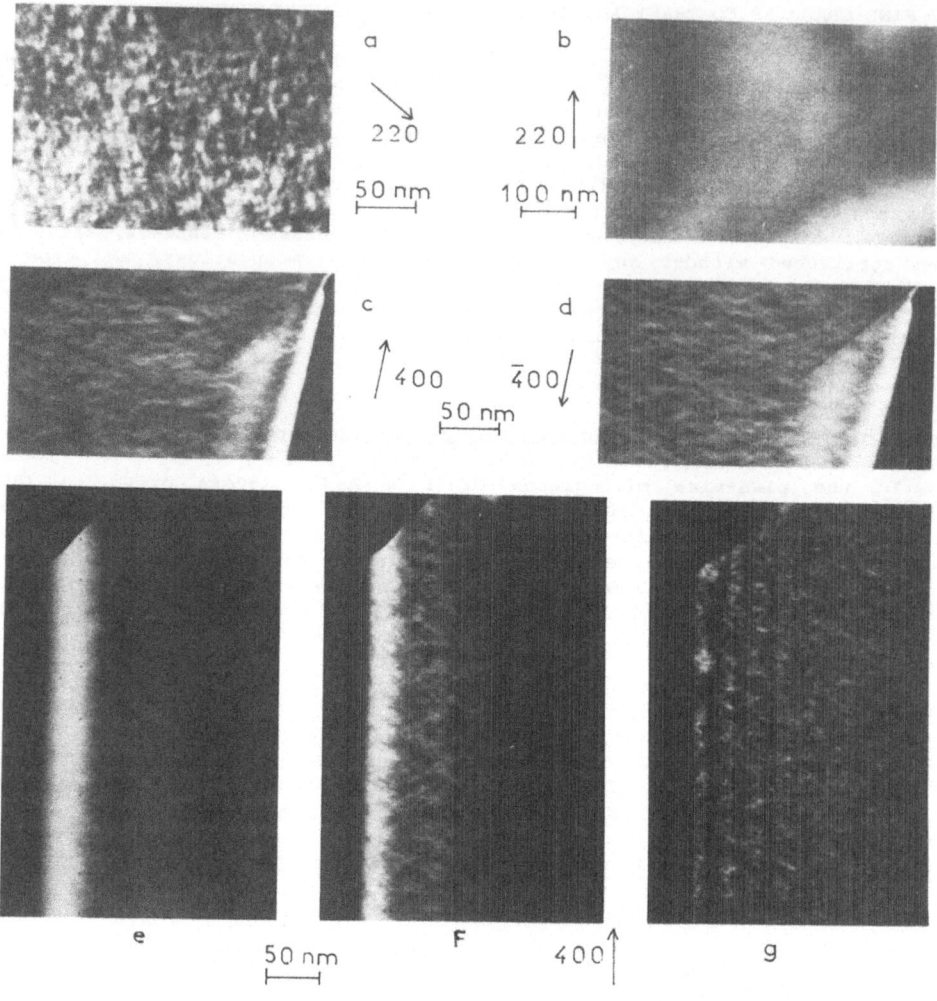

Figure 7. The granular contrast in STEM Dark Field images.
    (a) $In_{0.72}Ga_{0.28}As_{0.6}P_{0.4}$, $\mathbf{g}$=220, $w_0 \approx 0$;
    (b) the contrast is absent from $Ga_xAl_{1-x}As$;
    (c) $In_{0.53}Ga_{0.47}As$, $\mathbf{g}$=400, $w_0 \approx 0$;
    (d) same zone as (c), $\mathbf{g}=\bar{4}00$, $w_0 \approx 0$;
    (e) $In_{0.53}Ga_{0.47}As$, $\mathbf{g}$=400, $w_0 \approx 0$;
    (f) same zone as (e), $\mathbf{g}$=400, $w_0 \approx 1$;
    (g) same zone as (e), $\mathbf{g}$=400, $w_0 \approx 4$ (weak beam).

Discussion of the mechanism of formation of the fine contrast

As in the case of the coarse QP contrast, the fine contrast is neither due to thickness variations, which would imply $|\phi_g(t)|^2 = |\phi_{-g}(t)|^2$ for $w_0=0$, in contradiction to (iv), nor to variations of w or of ξ_g between columns where these parameters would be uniform, because of (i) and because $\mathbf{g}$=400 and $\mathbf{g}$=040 images display contrasts elongated in perpendicular directions.

Contrary to what is often assumed, the contrast is also not the 'direct' image of hypothetical tridimensional domains, which would be visible because of a structure factor different from that of their environment. Such a difference might be of compositional origin, but again the contrast would then be the same for equivalent sphalerite reflections and larger for $g=200$ than for $g=400$[7], which is not (i); different natures or degrees of atomic order might also exist between these domains, or between them and a disordered matrix, but again the effect would be at most a few % on the diffracted intensities for reflections 220 and 400[7]. The most obvious argument against the 'domain image' hypothesis remains however the dramatic change in contrast scale observed when increasing $|w_0|$ (which is not due to small thickness variations, as is common in weak beam imaging, since the contrast elements remain normal to g of 400 type (vi)), and the consequent impossibility to correlate features in images taken at different $|w_0|$; this is also the fundamental difference between the fine and QP contrasts.

The fine contrast is thus also a strain contrast, with a lattice plane bending varying in the depth of the specimen. Since the layer thickness is much larger than the scale of the contrast, the mechanism of relaxation at the free surfaces proposed by Treacy et al.[8] to explain the coarse QP contrast is unlikely to be significant in the present case. Discussing his two-beam g micrographs taken with $w_0=0$, Gowers[26] proposed a simple model based on two hypotheses:

(H1) There exists a displacement field R whose component along g is $R_g(X,Y,Z) = R_g^* \sin[(2\pi Z/L) + \theta(X,Y)]$: it oscillates in the depth of the layer over a distance L, and in its plane XY over distances equal to the size of the contrast (through a modulation of the phase θ).

(H2) R is due to composition modulations *with the same geometry* (H2a), which induce, supposing the structure remains locally cubic, a modulation of the lattice parameter (H2b).

Bearing in mind that R is not a proper solution of the equations of elasticity, (H1) accounts for most of the characteristics of the fine contrast. By calculating β'_g from (H1) and solving (1) for $w_0=0$, Gowers[26] obtained a contrast reaching several 10% for strains of the order of 2% (and thus, assuming (H2), for plausible variations of x of 30%), provided L is of the order of ξ_g. Extending these calculations to $w_0 \neq 0$, we studied[7,24]:

- the visibility of the contrast: it is maximum for $t = n\xi_g$, in agreement with (vii); it is weak for $t \leq \xi_g$ if $w_0=0$ but increases with $|w_0|$ for a given t, in agreement with (ii) and (iii).

- the symmetry of the contrast: it is inverted if g is changed to $-g$ for $w_0=0$, as suggested by (iv). Its behaviour when w_0 is changed to $-w_0$ is complex, depending on t, ξ_g and w_0.

(H1) thus appears compatible with our observations, except (vi): in Gowers' model, the contrast periodicity does not change with w_0. (H2) implies further that the size of the contrast elements should not change when g is rotated, in contradiction to (i). This suggests the replacement in (H1) of the displacement field R by a sum of Fourier components in different directions and with different wavelengths[7]. (vi) would then be analog to a weak beam observation of an *isolated* defect, where, by increasing $|w_0|$, one images Fourier components of shorter wavelengths of its strain field. In the present case however, no isolated strain centre would be identifiable and the strain field would oscillate through the whole specimen. The widely admitted hypothesis (H2a), although not disproved, is on the other hand highly questionable; there is, in particular, no reason to assume composition modulations on the 10 nm contrast scale observed for $w_0=0$, since this scale changes with w_0. As usual, the strain field is imaged, not its origin. Neither we nor Mahajan et al.[11] observed the diffraction satellites, corresponding to a ~10 nm direct space period, reported by Norman and Booker[12]. A detailed study of the fine contrast of the cross-sectional images, where elongated features seem to appear sometimes even for $g=220$, would be worthwile. If composition modulations actually caused the fine contrast, they would again appear during growth itself, since the contrast was also unaffected by our annealing experiments. We now suggest a possible origin of the fine contrast in composition *fluctuations* at the atomic scale rather than in proper composition *modulations*.

A possible origin of the fine contrast and its implications

To clarify this discussion, first recall that composition modulations or clustering occur if the probability of finding identical atoms on neighbouring sites of the same sublattice is larger than in the fully disordered alloy. However, *even in a disordered alloy*, the number of atoms of a given element in different regions having a small fixed volume is not constant, but follows a binomial distribution[7]. Second, some EXAFS experiments[19,20] proved that in $In_xGa_{1-x}As$ alloys, the nearest neighbour (III-As) distances are not those encountered in an hypothetical sphalerite crystal of parameter a(x) (virtual crystal[1] VC), but nearly retain the values they take in the corresponding constituent binary; at least some atoms must thus be considerably displaced from the perfect VC sites. These experiments support the use of the notion of covalent radius[1] in the III-V alloys. Although our electron channelling experiments[30] show that the As sublattice is more distorted than the mixed III sublattice, a correct interpretation[31] of the EXAFS results indicates that the latter is also likely to be considerably distorted. In quaternary compounds, both sublattices must obviously be strained. We thus propose that the static atomic displacements necessary to accommodate at best the different covalent radii of *all* the atoms of the alloy, together with the statistical *fluctuations* in the distributions of these atoms at the microscopical scale (which disappear only in ordered alloys), might cause the fine contrast, through a strain field possessing a large spectrum of wavelengths. Some authors claimed that non microscopical measurements (e.g. of phonon spectra[32] or of carrier mobility[33]) support the existence of proper clustering, but the evidence given is very indirect and similar measurements were interpreted by other authors in terms of purely statistical fluctuations[34].

To conclude, let us briefly discuss the recently proposed microscopical models of the III-V alloys. They aim to calculate the thermodynamic functions of a ternary $A_xB_{1-x}C$ alloy by evaluating the energies of its various possible atomic configurations, including the near bond length conservation revealed by EXAFS. This evaluation relies either on a phenomenological microscopic elasticity model[22] or on 'first principles' electronic structure calculations[21]. In both cases, the energy of an elementary tetrahedral cell is calculated, assuming that only the C atoms are displaced from the VC sites. Consequently, an extension to *macroscopic* crystals can at best describe *ordered* alloys, and these models must simulate disordered alloys by the simple juxtaposition of non-interacting elementary cells, without allowing for the mixed lattice relaxation. It is thus not surprising if ordering[21], or a tendency of the disordered alloy so described to possess more A-B first neighbour pairs than the perfectly disordered alloy[22], is predicted. Ordering has now been clearly observed in many III-V layers[35], but can by no means be considered as a universal feature, and depends in particular strongly on the growth conditions. This is in sharp contrast with the constant presence of the fine scale contrast in the images of layers of III-V alloys having mismatched constituent binaries. Whatever its origin (truly compositional or only statistical), the microscopic strain field revealed by this contrast should be considered when discussing the physical properties of the non-ordered III-V alloys.

CONCLUSION

We reviewed the study by TEM and microanalysis of two clearly distinct classes of phenomena affecting the epitaxial layers of the III-V ternary and quaternary alloys. First, coarse composition modulations are present in some $In_xGa_{1-x}As_yP_{1-y}$ layers in directions parallel to the substrate. The modulations and the strain field they induce always have quasiperiods of the order of 150 nm. They develop during growth itself, only in some well defined conditions. Second, a much smaller scale strain field with a large wavelength spectrum exists, on the contrary, in all the layers of the III-V alloys having lattice-mismatched binary constituents; it induces a contrast of characteristic size 2-20 nm in the TEM images. We suggested that it might not be due, as usually assumed, to proper composition modulations or clustering, but to mere statistical fluctuations in the distributions of atoms having different covalent radii. Both phenomena remain unaffected by any annealing treatment following growth; their influence on the electronic properties of the alloys is not yet clear. The apparent inevitability of the fine scale strain field should however be borne in mind when discussing the microscopical properties of these alloys.

ACKNOWLEDGMENTS

We thank Drs. H. Launois, P. Hénoc, M. Quillec and M. M. J. Treacy for many fruitful discussions, S. Slempkès for the growth of numerous samples and Dr. C. C. Gray for a critical reading of the manuscript.

REFERENCES

1. J. C. Phillips, "Bonds and Bands in Semiconductors," Academic Press, New York (1973).
2. S. K. Maksimov and E. N. Nagdaev, Self-modulation of the composition of GaAsP epitaxial films, Sov. Phys. Dokl. 24:297 (1979).
3. G. B. Stringfellow, Calculation of ternary and quaternary III-V phase diagrams, J. Cryst. Growth 27:21 (1974).
4. G. B. Stringfellow, Spinodal decomposition and clustering in III-V alloys, J. Electron. Mat. 11:903 (1982).
5. P. Hénoc, A. Izrael, M. Quillec and H. Launois, Composition modulation in liquid phase epitaxial $In_xGa_{1-x}As_yP_{1-y}$ layers lattice matched to InP substrates, Appl. Phys. Lett. 40:963 (1982).
6. P. Hirsch, A. Howie, R. B. Nicholson, D. W. Pashley and M. J. Whelan, "Electron Microscopy of thin crystals," R. E. Krieger, Malabar (1977).
7. F. Glas, "Démixtion et ordre local dans les composés semiconducteurs III-V: étude par microscopie électronique et microanalyse des couches épitaxiées d'alliages InGaAsP," Thèse de Doctorat d'Etat, Université Paris XI (1986). Copies available from the author.
8. M. M. J. Treacy, J. M. Gibson and A. Howie, On elastic relaxation and long wavelength microstructures in spinodally decomposed $In_xGa_{1-x}As_yP_{1-y}$ epitaxial layers, Phil. Mag. A 51:389 (1985).
9. F. Glas, M. M. J. Treacy, M. Quillec and H. Launois, Interface spinodal decomposition in LPE $In_xGa_{1-x}As_yP_{1-y}$ lattice matched to InP, J. de Physique 43:C5-11 (1982).
10. H. Launois, M. Quillec, F. Glas and M. J. Treacy, Interface spinodal decomposition in LPE $In_xGa_{1-x}As_yP_{1-y}$ lattice-matched to InP, in: "GaAs and Related Compounds 1982," Inst. Phys. Conf. Ser. No 65, G. E. Stillman, ed., The Institute of Physics, London (1983).
11. S. Mahajan, B. V. Dutt, H. Temkin, R. J. Cava and W. A. Bonner, Spinodal decomposition in InGaAsP epitaxial layers, J. Cryst. Growth 68:589 (1984).
12. A. G. Norman and G. R. Booker, TEM and TED studies of alloy clustering in GaInAsP, GaInAs and GaInP epitaxial layers, in: "Microscopy of Semiconducting Materials 1985", Inst. Phys. Conf. Ser. No 76, A. G. Cullis and D. B. Holt, eds., Adam Hilger, Bristol (1985).

13. D. Cherns, P. D. Greene, A. Hainsworth and A. R. Preston, Phase separation in GaInAsP epitaxial layers, in: "Microscopy of Semiconducting Materials 1987", Inst. Phys. Conf. Ser. No 87, A. G. Cullis and P. D. Augustus, eds., Institute of Physics, Bristol (1987).

14. G. W. Lorimer, Quantitative X-ray microanalysis of thin specimens, in: "Quantitative Electron Microscopy," J. N. Chapman and A. J. Craven, eds., Scottish Universities Summer School in Physics, Edinburgh (1984).

15. B. de Crémoux, Instability criteria in ternary and quaternary III-V epitaxial solid solutions, J. de Physique 43:C5-19 (1982).

16. J. W. Cahn, Spinodal decomposition, Trans. Met. Soc. AIME 242:166.

17. M. Quillec, C. Daguet, J.-L. Benchimol and H. Launois, $In_xGa_{1-x}As_yP_{1-y}$ alloy stabilization by the InP substrate inside an unstable region in liquid phase epitaxy, Appl. Phys. Lett. 40:325 (1982).

18. G. B. Stringfellow, The importance of lattice mismatch in the growth of $Ga_xIn_{1-x}P$ epitaxial crystals J. Appl. Phys. 43:3455 (1972).

19. J. Bellessa, C. Gors, P. Launois, M. Quillec and H. Launois, Extended x-ray absorption fine structures study of short range order in $In_xGa_{1-x}As$ and $Ga_xAl_{1-x}As$ alloys, in: "GaAs and related compounds 1982," Inst. Phys. Conf. Ser. No 65, G. E. Stillman, ed., The Institute of Physics , London (1983).

20. J. C. Mikkelsen and J. B. Boyce, Extended x-ray-absorption fine-structure study of $Ga_xIn_{1-x}As$ random solid solutions, Phys. Rev. B 28:7130 (1983).

21. G. P. Srivastava, J. L. Martins and A. Zunger, Atomic structure and ordering in semiconductor alloys, Phys. Rev. B 31:2561 (1985).

22. P. Letardi, N. Motta and A. Balzarotti, Atomic bonding and thermodynamic properties of pseudo-binary semiconducting alloys, J. Phys. C 20:2853 (1987).

23. F. Glas, Elastic state and thermodynamical properties of inhomogeneous epitaxial layers: Application to immiscible III-V alloys, J. Appl. Phys. 62:3201 (1987).

24. F. Glas, P. Hénoc and H. Launois, TEM and STEM study of the microstructure of ternary and quaternary III-V epitaxial layers, in: "Microscopy of Semiconducting Materials 1985", Inst. Phys. Conf. Ser. No 76, A. G. Cullis and D. B. Holt, eds., Adam Hilger, Bristol (1985).

25. J. S. Roberts, G. B. Scott and J. P. Gowers, Structural and photoluminescent properties of $Ga_xIn_{1-x}P$ (x~0.5) grown on GaAs by molecular beam epitaxy, J. Appl. Phys. 52:4018 (1981).

26. J. P. Gowers, TEM image contrast from clustering in Ga-In containing III-V alloys, Appl. Phys A 31:23 (1983).

27. S. N. G. Chu, S. Nakahara, K. E. Strege and W. D. Johnston, Surface layer spinodal decomposition in $In_{1-x}Ga_xAs_yP_{1-y}$ and $In_xGa_{1-x}As$ grown by hydride transport vapor-phase epitaxy, J. Appl. Phys. 57:4610 (1985).

28. O. Ueda, S. Isozumi and S. Komiya, Composition-modulated structures in InGaAsP and InGaP liquid phase epitaxial layers grown on (001) GaAs substrates, Jap. J. Appl. Phys. 23:L241 (1984).

29. T. H. Chiu, W. T. Tsang, S. N. G. Chu, J. Shah and J. A. Ditzenberger, Molecular beam epitaxy of $GaSb_{0.5}As_{0.5}$ and $Al_xGa_{1-x}Sb_yAs_{1-y}$ lattice matched to InP, Appl. Phys. Lett. 46:408 (1985).

30. F. Glas and P. Hénoc, Study of static atomic displacements by channelled-electron-beam-induced x-ray emission: Application to $In_{0.53}Ga_{0.47}As$ alloys, Phil. Mag. A 56:311 (1987).

31. M. Podgórny, M. T. Czyżyk, A. Balzarotti, P. Letardi, N. Motta, A. Kisiel and M. Zimnal-Starnawska, Crystallographic structure of ternary semiconducting alloys, Solid State Comm. 55:413 (1985).

32. S. Yamazaki, A. Ushirokawa and T. Katoda, Effect of clusters on long-wavelength optical phonons in $Ga_{1-x}In_xAs$, J. Appl. Phys. 51:3722 (1980).

33. P. Blood and A. D. C. Grassie, Influence of clustering on the mobility of III-V semiconductor alloys, J. Appl. Phys. 56:1866 (1984).

34. J. H. Marsh, Effects of compositional clustering on electron transport in $In_{0.53}Ga_{0.47}As$, Appl. Phys. Lett. 41:732 (1982).

35. A. G. Norman, this volume.

TRANSMISSION ELECTRON MICROSCOPY AND TRANSMISSION ELECTRON DIFFRACTION

STUDIES OF ATOMIC ORDERING IN GROUP III-V COMPOUND SEMICONDUCTOR ALLOYS

Andrew G. Norman

Department of Metallurgy and Science of Materials
University of Oxford, Parks Road, Oxford OX1 3PH, UK

INTRODUCTION

Ternary and quaternary Group III-V compound semiconductor alloys e.g. $Ga_xIn_{1-x}As$, $Al_xIn_{1-x}As$, $Ga_xIn_{1-x}As_yP_{1-y}$ etc. are important for a wide range of optoelectronic and microwave devices. For these devices the alloys are usually required in the form of thin epitaxial layers grown on binary compound substrates such as InP or GaAs. A variety of growth techniques are used to produce these epitaxial layers such as liquid phase epitaxy (LPE), vapour phase epitaxy (VPE), molecular beam epitaxy (MBE) and organometallic vapour phase epitaxy (OMVPE).

These ternary and quaternary III-V compound semiconductor alloys are substitutional solid solutions which possess the zinc-blende crystal structure. The zinc-blende crystal structure can be thought of as two interpenetrating fcc sublattices, one composed of Group III atoms and the other composed of Group V atoms, that are displaced with respect to each other by $a_0\sqrt{3}/4$ along the <111> direction where a_0 is the lattice parameter. It has long been thought that these ternary and quaternary III-V alloys form as disordered, metastable phases i.e. with the Group III and Group V atoms arranged at random on their respective sub-lattices. However, recent theoretical work and experimental results indicate that atomic ordering can occur in these alloys with the Group III or Group V atoms forming ordered arrangements on their respective mixed atom sublattices.

The interaction parameter Ω and enthalpy of mixing $\Delta H(mix)$ of ternary and quaternary III-V compound semiconductor alloys have been estimated from liquidus and solidus data[1-3] or calculated, e.g. using the delta lattice parameter (DLP) model[3], and it has been found that Ω, $\Delta H(mix) > 0$. Phase diagram calculations for these alloy systems, using for example the Regular Solution Approximation[4,5] or DLP model[6-10], have hence predicted the existence of miscibility gaps in many cases at low temperatures and also the possibility that some of these alloy systems may be unstable to phase segregation by spinodal decomposition. Miscibility gaps have been experimentally observed for some alloy systems[11-17] and the occurrence of spinodal decomposition in epitaxial layers of a few of these alloys has also been reported[18-29]. Atomic ordering in these alloys was not predicted from the above mentioned thermodynamic calculations since one would expect Ω, $\Delta H(mix) < 0$ for

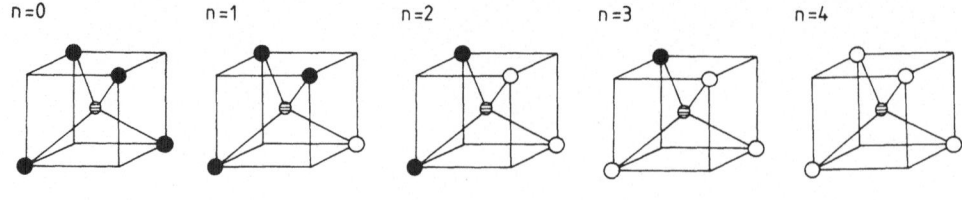

●–A O–B ◉–C

Fig.1. The five different tetrahedral units of four nearest neighbour A and B cation atoms surrounding the central anion C atom, denoted n = 0, 1, 2, 3 and 4, possible in a ternary III–V alloy $A_xB_{1-x}C$ e.g. $Ga_xIn_{1-x}P$.

alloys which might show a tendency for atomic ordering and the formation of superlattice structures at low temperatures. However, recent first principles local-density total energy minimization calculations, performed by Srivastava et al.[30] for bulk $Ga_xIn_{1-x}P$ alloys, have indicated that the thermodynamically stable low temperature ground state for ternary III–V compound semiconductor alloys might be as ordered intermediate phases.

A ternary III–V alloy $A_xB_{1-x}C$ e.g. $Ga_xIn_{1-x}P$ can be thought of as being composed of a mixture of different tetrahedral units comprising of the C anion atom surrounded by the four nearest neighbour cation atoms. Five different tetrahedral units are possible denoted by n = 0,1,2,3 and 4 corresponding to A_4C, A_3BC, A_2B_2C, AB_3C and B_4C as shown in Fig.1. A random ternary $A_xB_{1-x}C$ alloy is composed of a random statistical mixture of these tetrahedral units whilst an ordered intermediate phase consists of a coherent, periodic arrangement of one or more of the possible tetrahedral units. Extended X-ray absorption fine structure (EXAFS) studies on $Ga_xIn_{1-x}As$ alloys[31-33] have indicated that the Group III cation atoms, Ga and In, are very nearly distributed on their ideal fcc sublattice sites, with only a very small broadening in this distribution. The EXAFS results also indicated that the Ga–As and In–As bond lengths are only deformed slightly from their ideal binary compound values across the entire composition range of the alloy i.e. the virtual crystal approximation (VCA) does not hold at the atomic structure level for these alloys. The two different bond lengths in the alloy are thus accommodated almost entirely by displacements of the As anion atoms away from their ideal VCA fcc sublattice sites accompanied by bond angle

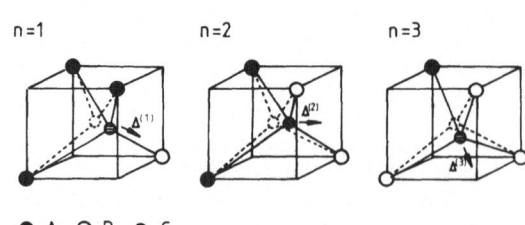

●–A O–B ◉–C

Fig.2. The nature of the displacements Δ of the C anion atoms for n = 1, 2 and 3 tetrahedral units in an $A_xB_{1-x}C$ alloy. The A and B cation atoms are assumed to be on their VCA sites.

distortions away from the ideal tetrahedral angle of 109·5°. The nature of the displacements Δ of the C anion atoms for n = 1, 2 and 3 tetrahedral units in a $A_xB_{1-x}C$ alloy are shown in Fig.2.

Srivastava et al.[30], using a model suggested from the EXAFS results[31-33] but with the cation atoms assumed to be on their ideal fcc sites, calculated the equilibrium bond length deformations and changes in total energies for both ordered intermediate phases and for a randomly disordered alloy model for $Ga_xIn_{1-x}P$ in the bulk form using the self consistent local-density pseudopotential total-energy minimization method. The ordered intermediate phases considered for these calculations were the conventional zinc-blende structures composed of all n = 0 or n = 4 tetrahedral units, the Chalcopyrite $CuFeS_2$-type structure and simple tetragonal (CuAu I-type cation sublattice) structure which are composed entirely of n = 2 tetrahedral units and the Luzonite Cu_3AsS_4-type (Cu$_3$Au-type cation sublattice) structure and Famatinite Cu_3SbS_4-type (Al$_3$Ti-type cation sublattice) structure which are composed entirely of n = 1 or n = 3 type tetrahedral units. These structures are illustrated in Fig.3(a) together with the trigonal (CuPt-type cation sublattice) structure composed of equal numbers of n = 1 and n = 3 tetrahedral units and which was not investigated by Srivastava et al.[30]. The results of the calculations indicated that, contrary to what is expected from the Regular Solution model, the ordered intermediate phases could be the thermodynamically stable low-temperature ground state of the ternary $Ga_xIn_{1-x}P$ III-V compound semiconductor alloy, whereas the disordered phase for $Ga_xIn_{1-x}P$ was shown to be metastable. It was also shown that despite the stability of the ordered phases the substitutionally random alloy would have $\Delta H(mix) > 0$ as a result of the dominance of strain effects over chemical bonding effects. It was concluded that the stability of the ordered phases arose from the fact that they are strain reducing, being better able to accommodate two dissimilar bond lengths in a coherent fashion, with less strain than in a disordered alloy.

Mbaye et al.[34][35] used a simple valence force field method and harmonic elasticity theory to investigate the relative stability of the disordered $Ga_xIn_{1-x}P$ alloy and ordered intermediate phases $Ga_nIn_{4-n}P_4$ (n = 0-4) in both the bulk and epitaxial layer form. The results indicated that the availability of structural degrees of freedom in the ordered intermediate phases could lead to their energetic stabilisation when grown epitaxially even though they may be unstable in the bulk form. It was also shown that the existence of substrate induced strain in epitaxial materials could preferentially stabilise one ordered intermediate phase over another, even if they were equally stable or unstable in the bulk form.

The first experimental observation of atomic ordering in a ternary III-V compound semiconductor alloy was reported by Kuan et al.[36]. These authors observed by transmission electron diffraction (TED) simple tetragonal (CuAu I-type cation sublattice) ordering in OMVPE and MBE $Al_xGa_{1-x}As$ layers grown on (110) GaAs substrates. Kuan et al.[37] have also reported identical simple tetragonal ordering in MBE $Ga_xIn_{1-x}As$ layers grown on (110) InP substrates. Famatinite Cu_3SbS_4-type ordering (Al$_3$Ti-type cation sublattice) was observed using TED and high resolution electron microscopy by Nakayama and Fujita[38] in LPE $Ga_xIn_{1-x}As$ layers grown on (001) InP substrates. Jen et al.[39][40] reported the existence of a mixture of simple tetragonal and Chalcopyrite $CuFeS_2$-type ordering in OMVPE $GaAs_ySb_{1-y}$ layers grown on (001) InP substrates. Murgatroyd et al.[41-43] obtained the first evidence of trigonal (CuPt-type anion sublattice) ordering in a ternary III-V compound semiconductor alloy layer. The trigonal ordering was observed by TED in MBE

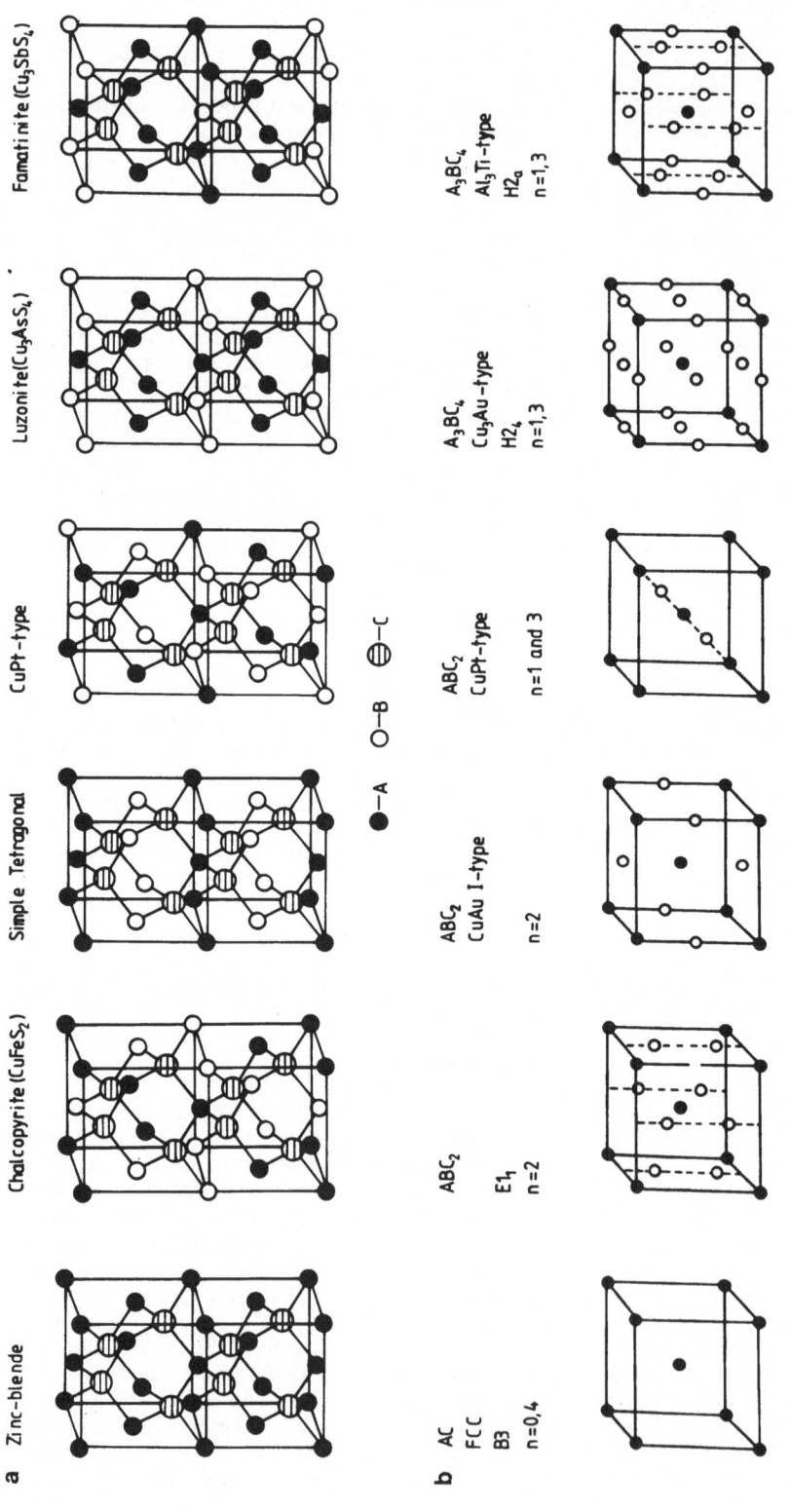

Fig.3. (a) Five possible ordered structures and the zinc-blende structure (AC) for a ternary III-V compound semiconductor alloy $A_x B_{1-x} C$ e.g. $Ga_x In_{1-x} As$. The ideal composition, cation sublattice, Strukturbericht designation and the component tetrahedral units n are given below each structure. (b) Distribution of superlattice spots in reciprocal space corresponding to the structures shown in Fig.3(a).

GaAs$_y$Sb$_{1-y}$ layers grown on (001) GaAs and InP substrates. Identical trigonal ordering in MBE GaAs$_y$Sb$_{1-y}$ layers grown on (001) InP and GaAs substrates has also been reported by Ihm et al.[44][45]. Trigonal (CuPt-type cation sublattice) ordering has also been observed in OMVPE Al$_x$In$_{1-x}$As[46][47] and Ga$_x$In$_{1-x}$As[47] layers grown on (001) InP substrates, vapour levitation epitaxy (VLE) Ga$_x$In$_{1-x}$As and Ga$_x$In$_{1-x}$As$_y$P$_{1-y}$ layers grown on (001) InP substrates[48][49] and more recently in OMVPE Ga$_x$In$_{1-x}$P layers grown on (001) GaAs substrates[50-58].

The occurrence of atomic ordering in epitaxial layers of ternary and quaternary III-V semiconductor alloys may have significant effects on their optical, electrical and structural properties. For instance the band gap energy of OMVPE Ga$_{0.5}$In$_{0.5}$P layers which exhibit trigonal ordering has been measured to be 50-90meV lower than that of random alloy layers of the same composition[50][56-60].

This paper will describe the use of electron microscopy to investigate atomic ordering in ternary and quaternary III-V compound semiconductor alloy layers. Examples will be given using results obtained by the author from OMVPE Ga$_x$Al$_y$In$_{1-x-y}$As epitaxial layers grown on (001) InP substrates.

ELECTRON DIFFRACTION

Transmission electron diffraction (TED) may be used to determine if atomic ordering has occurred in an alloy, to identify the structure of the ordered phases present and also to estimate the degree of long range order.

Determination of the occurrence of atomic ordering

In a disordered ternary III-V semiconductor alloy A$_x^{III}$B$_{1-x}^{III}$C^V e.g. Ga$_x$In$_{1-x}$As the A and B atoms are distributed at random on the Group III atom sublattice. Atomic ordering of the alloy occurs if the A e.g. Ga atoms arrange themselves in an orderly, periodic manner on one set of atomic sites of the Group III sublattice and the B e.g. In atoms do likewise on another set. The alloy is then said to be ordered or to possess a superlattice structure.

In an ordered alloy the distance between equivalent lattice planes may become double or another multiple of that in the random alloy. Since the A e.g. Ga and B e.g. In atoms have different atomic scattering amplitudes then extra diffraction spots may become allowed for the ordered alloy, known as superlattice spots, which are normally forbidden for the zinc-blende crystal structure of the random alloy. The occurrence of atomic ordering in these alloys may thus be determined by the appearance of superlattice spots in TED patterns obtained from the alloys.

Identification of the structure of ordered phases

The structure of ordered phases present in an alloy may be identi-fied by determining the distribution of superlattice spots in reciprocal space. In Fig.3(a) are shown five possible ordered structures and the zinc-blende crystal structure (AC) for a ternary A$_x$B$_{1-x}$C III-V alloy e.g. Ga$_x$In$_{1-x}$As. Below, in Fig.3(b) are shown the corresponding distributions in reciprocal space of the superlattice and fundamental diffraction spots for these possible structures. It can be seen that each of the ordered structures has a characteristic, fingerprint, distribution of super-lattice spots in reciprocal space. And so, by obtaining TED patterns

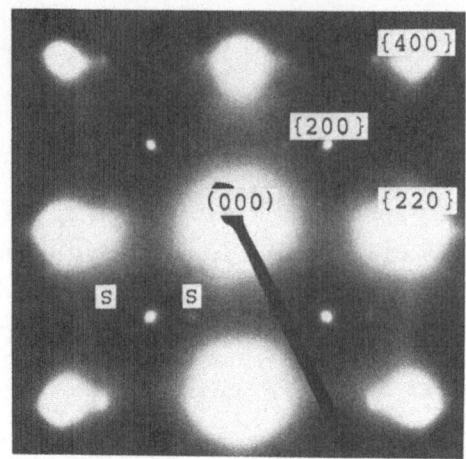

Fig.4. [001] pole TED pattern obtained from an AP-OMVPE $Al_xIn_{1-x}As$ layer (T_g=600°C). All of the fundamental spots are seen to be associated with pairs of very weak extra spots e.g. S aligned along one of the <110> directions at a spacing slightly less than ¼g220.

from several different orientations of the ordered layers, one can map out the distribution of superlattice spots in reciprocal space and identify the structure of the ordered phases present.

As an example we will consider the results obtained[46][47] from a detailed TED investigation of an atmospheric pressure (AP-) OMVPE $Al_xIn_{1-x}As$ (x ~ 0.5) layer, growth temperature (T_g) 600°C, grown close to lattice match on an (001) InP substrate. In Fig.4 is shown an [001] pole TED pattern obtained from a plan-view TEM sample of this layer. The fundamental diffraction spots expected for the zinc-blende structure i.e. {200}, {220}, {400} etc. are visible together with pairs of very weak extra spots, e.g. those marked S, which are associated with all of the fundamental diffraction spots including the 000 transmitted spot. These pairs of extra spots are aligned along one of the <110> directions and are situated at a distance of close to, but not exactly, ¼g220 from the fundamental diffraction spots. The [001] plan-view sample was then tilted out along the two orthogonal 220 Kikuchi bands to reach the four <112> poles at a tilt of ~ 35° from the [001] pole. The two <112> pole TED patterns obtained by tilting along the {220} Kikuchi band lying parallel to the pairs of extra spots visible in the [001] pole TED pattern of Fig.4 were as shown in Fig.5(a). The fundamental spots expected for the zinc-blende structure are present together with strong, sharp superlattice spots at ½{111} and ½{311} positions which are normally forbidden for the zinc-blende structure. No pairs of weak extra spots associated with the fundamental spots were visible in the TED patterns obtained from these two <112> poles. The two <112> pole TED patterns obtained after tilting along the orthogonal {220} Kikuchi band from the [001] pole were as shown in Fig.5(b). At these two poles only the fundamental spots expected for the zinc-blende structure were observed with no superlattice spots visible at ½{111} or ½{311}. Very weak pairs of extra spots e.g. those marked S, were however visibly

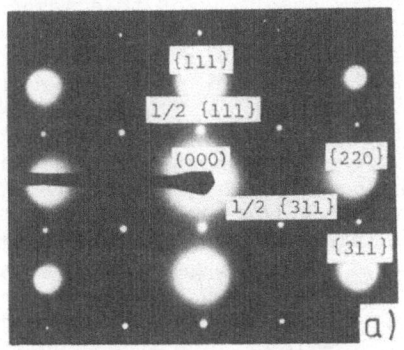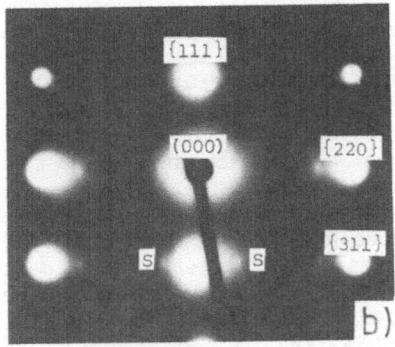

Fig.5. <112> pole TED patterns obtained from AP-OMVPE $Al_xIn_{1-x}As$ layer (T_g=600°C).

(a) <1$\bar{1}$2> pole obtained by tilting from the [001] pole along the {220} Kikuchi band running parallel to the pairs of weak extra spots present at the [001] pole. Strong sharp superlattice spots present at ½{111} and ½{311} positions.

(b) <112> pole obtained by tilting along the orthogonal {220} Kikuchi band from the [001] pole. No superlattice spots present. Very weak pairs of extra spots present associated with the fundamental spots e.g. S aligned along the <110> direction at a spacing of ∼ ¼g220.

associated with the fundamental diffraction spots at a distance of nearly ± ¼g220 along the <110> direction, similar to those observed previously at the [001] pole in Fig.4.

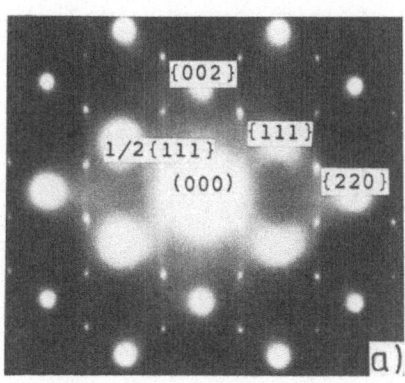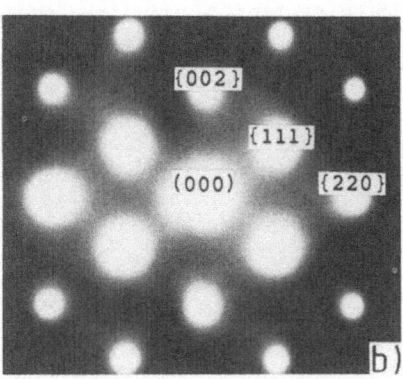

Fig.6. TED patterns obtained from orthogonal <110> cross-section samples of AP-OMVPE $Al_xIn_{1-x}As$ layer (T_g=600°C).

(a) <110> pole TED pattern containing strong superlattice spots at ½{111} positions. The ½{111} superlattice spots are connected together in the [001] growth direction by wavy lines of diffuse intensity.

(b) Orthogonal <110> pole TED pattern which shows only the fundamental zinc-blende diffraction spots.

Two orthogonal <110> cross-section TEM specimens of this layer were then prepared and examined by TED. The TED pattern obtained from one, shown in Fig.6(a), contained the fundamental zinc-blende spots but also showed strong superlattice spots at ½{111} positions which are normally forbidden for the zinc-blende structure. In addition the ½{111} superlattice spots were connected together in the [001] growth direction by faint wavy lines of diffuse intensity. These faint lines of diffuse intensity, visible in Fig.6(a), correspond to wavy rods of diffuse intensity in reciprocal space which run along the [001] direction. The intersection of these rods of diffuse intensity with the Ewald sphere gives rise to the very faint pairs of extra spots associated with the fundamental spots in the [001] pole TED pattern of Fig.4 and the two <112> pole TED patterns as in Fig.5(b). TED patterns obtained from the orthogonal <110> cross-section TEM specimen contained only the fundamental zinc-blende diffraction spots as shown in Fig.6(b).

All of the superlattice spots visible in these TED patterns can be explained by the existence of separate regions in the $Al_xIn_{1-x}As$ layer ordered on two of the four possible sets of {111} planes i.e. two variants of the trigonal (CuPt-type cation sublattice) ordered structure being present. It has been determined[47] that the two variants of the trigonal ordered structure present correspond to ordering on ($\bar{1}1\bar{1}$) and ($1\bar{1}\bar{1}$) planes in the layer which share the [110] direction as a common direction at the (001) growth surface. A [110] projection of an $Al_{0.5}In_{0.5}As$ crystal perfectly ordered on ($\bar{1}1\bar{1}$) planes is shown in Fig.7. It is believed that the ordering occurs at the surface of the growing layer and that the occurrence of only two out of the four possible variants of the trigonal ordered structure is related to the non equivalence of the [110] and [$\bar{1}$10] directions at the (001) surface of the polar zinc-blende crystal.

The origin of the faint wavy [001] rods of diffuse intensity in reciprocal space is less certain. These rods of diffuse intensity may arise from an abrupt breakdown of the ordering occurring in the [001] growth direction[43], by the presence of thin ordered platelets lying

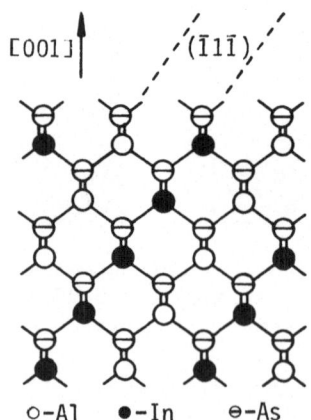

o—Al   ●—In   ⊖—As

Fig.7. [110] projection of an $Al_{0.5}In_{0.5}As$ crystal perfectly ordered on ($\bar{1}1\bar{1}$) planes.

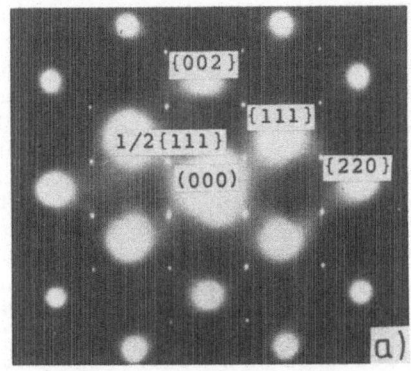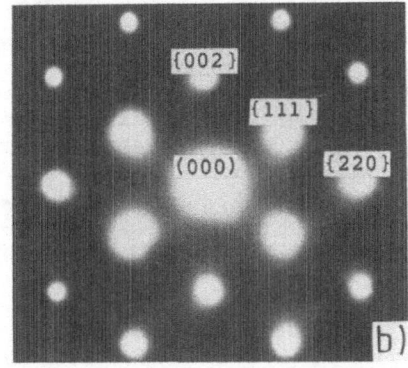

Fig.8. TED patterns obtained from orthogonal <110> cross-section samples of an AP-OMVPE $Ga_xIn_{1-x}As$ layer (T_g=600°C) which shows evidence of trigonal ordering.

(a) <110> pole TED pattern containing strong superlattice spots at ½{111} positions which are connected together in the [001] growth direction by wavy lines of diffuse intensity.

(b) Orthogonal <110> TED pattern which contains only the fundamental zinc-blende diffraction spots.

nearly on the (001) plane[47][51] or from the occurrence of an array of antiphase domain boundaries (APBs) or order twin boundaries (OTBs) lying on (001) planes[47][53][55-57]. The waviness of these rods of diffuse intensity may arise from lattice distortions associated with APBs and OTBs[56] or the boundary between an ordered region and the disordered matrix[51].

Identical trigonal ordering was also observed in AP-OMVPE $Ga_xIn_{1-x}As$ (x ~ 0.5) layers (T_g = 600°C) grown close to lattice match on (001) InP substrates[47] as can be seen from the TED patterns taken from orthogonal <110> cross-section TEM specimens shown in Fig.8.

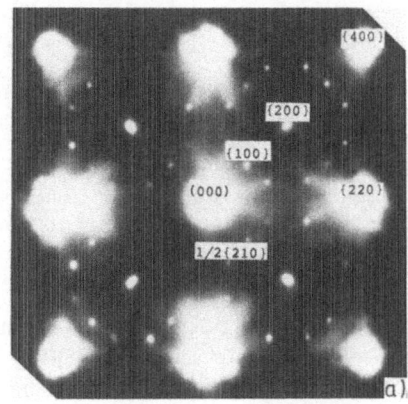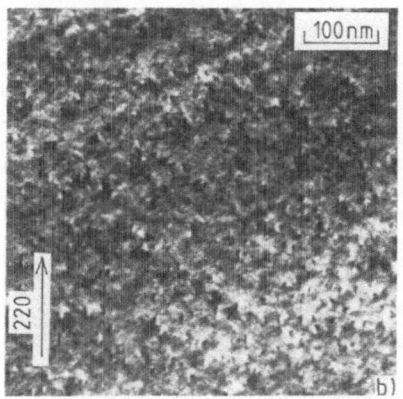

Fig.9. (a) [001] pole TED pattern of AP-OMVPE $Al_xIn_{1-x}As$ layer (T_g=650°C) containing superlattice spots at {100} and ½{210} positions.

(b) g[220]DF micrograph of layer in (a) showing evidence of small precipitates e.g. area X.

241

In samples which contain several variants of different ordered structures some problems may be encountered in interpreting the TED patterns obtained. As an example consider the [001] pole TED pattern of Fig.9(a) which was obtained from an AP-OMVPE $Al_xIn_{1-x}As$ (x ~ 0.5) layer (T_g = 650°C) grown on an (001) InP substrate. The TED pattern contains the fundamental zinc-blende spots plus superlattice spots at {100}, $\frac{1}{2}${210} etc. positions. Such patterns were obtained from regions of the layer that appeared to contain small precipitates as can be seen in the g[220] dark field micrograph of Fig.9(b) e.g. area marked X. This type of [001] pole TED pattern could be generated by the presence in the layer of two variants of the Famatinite Cu_3SbS_4 type (Al_3Ti-type cation sublattice) ordered structure as proposed by Nakayama and Fujita[38] to explain similar TED patterns obtained from LPE $Ga_xIn_{1-x}As$ layers. However, the identical [001] pole TED pattern could also arise from the existence in the layer of a mixture of two variants of the simple tetragonal ordered structure (CuAu I-type cation sublattice) and two variants of the Chalcopyrite $CuFeS_2$-type ordered structure as proposed by Jen et al.[39] to explain identical TED patterns obtained from OMVPE $GaAs_ySb_{1-y}$ layers. To distinguish between these two possibilities the use of dark field TEM or high resolution electron microscopy (HREM) may be required.

Estimation of degree of long range order

The intensity of superlattice beams is related to the degree of long range order in the crystal. In the kinematic theory of diffraction the intensity I_S of the superlattice beams obtained from e.g. a ternary $A_x^{III}B_{1-x}^{III}C^V$ semiconductor alloy which exhibits long range order is given simply by[61]:

$$I_S = |F|^2 \propto S^2(f_A - f_B)^2$$

where F is the structure factor, f_A, f_B are the atomic scattering amplitudes of A, B atoms and S is the long range order parameter defined by

$$S = \frac{r_A - x}{1-x}$$

and r_A is the fraction of A sites occupied by the 'right' atoms i.e. A atoms and x is the fraction of A atoms in the alloy. For perfect long range order S = 1 and in a random alloy S = 0. The kinematic theory works well for X-ray diffraction where a measurement of the integrated intensity ratio of a superlattice and fundamental reflection can be used relatively easily to determine the degree of long range order in the crystal. However, a quantitative measurement of the degree of long range order in a crystal using electron diffraction is not so straightforward since multiple scattering between beams can lead to significant changes in their relative intensities from the kinematic values.

In order to make a quantitative measurement of S using electron diffraction the thickness and orientation of the crystal must be accurately known. The measured ratio of intensities of the superlattice and fundamental beams then need to be compared with the ratios of intensities measured from samples of the same thickness and orientation but of known degree of order[62] (e.g. as previously measured by X-ray diffraction) or alternatively with ratios of intensities calculated using the dynamical theory of electron diffraction, e.g. using a multislice method, which takes into account the effect of multiple scattering between beams[37].

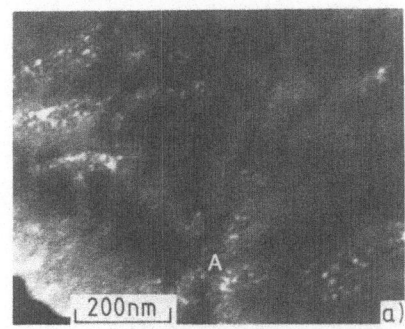 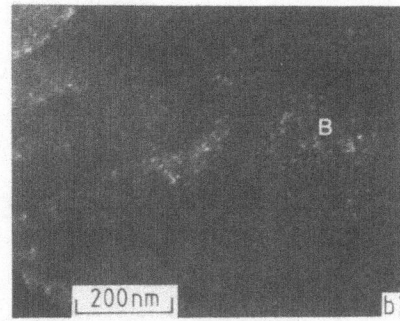

Fig.10. Superlattice spot dark field micrographs taken of the same area
of a TEM plan-view specimen of an AP-OMVPE $Al_xIn_{1-x}As$ layer
(T_g=600°C) which had been tilted out to a <112> pole containing
strong ½{111} and ½{311} superlattice spots.

(a) ½{111}DF micrograph showing
ordered regions e.g. A
containing 10-20nm size
"microdomains" of material
ordered on one set of {111}
planes.

(b) ½{311}DF micrograph showing
ordered regions e.g. B
containing 10-20nm size
"microdomains" of material
ordered on the other set of
{111} planes.

TEM DARK FIELD TECHNIQUES

Dark field TEM micrographs taken with superlattice spots may be used
to reveal ordered regions in a random alloy matrix, to see variations in
the degree of order and to image antiphase domain boundaries (APBs) in
long range ordered alloys.

Imaging ordered regions and variations in the degree of ordering

Regions of ordered material present in a random alloy matrix may be
revealed by taking dark field (DF) TEM micrographs using superlattice
spots. The ordered regions contributing to the intensity of the superlattice spot will appear bright against the dark background intensity of
the random alloy. The contrast observed for the ordered regions in the
dark field images will be related to their degree of atomic ordering.

Two superlattice spot dark field images taken from the same area of
a plan-view sample of an AP-OMVPE $Al_xIn_{1-x}As$ (x ~ 0·5) layer (T_g = 600°C)
are shown in Fig.10. This layer contained ordered regions of two
variants of the trigonal (CuPt-type cation sublattice) ordered structure
i.e. ordering on two sets of {111} planes[46][47]. The micrographs were
taken after tilting the sample out to a <112> pole which contained strong
superlattice spots at ½{111} and ½{311} positions as shown in Fig.5(a).
At this pole the ½{111} superlattice spots arise from the regions present
of one variant of the trigonal structure whereas the ½{311} spots arise
from the regions of the other variant. The ½{111}DF micrograph of
Fig.10(a) shows ordered regions of one variant, e.g. area A, consisting
of large numbers of bright spots, each spot corresponding to a 10-20nm
size "microdomain" of material ordered on one set of {111} planes. The
½{311}DF micrograph of Fig.10(b) shows ordered regions of the other
variant, e.g. area B, which also contain large numbers of bright spots
corresponding to 10-20nm size "microdomains" of material ordered on the
other set of {111} planes. The darker regions in between the "microdomains" correspond either to unordered material or much less ordered
material. It can be seen from these two micrographs that the ordering on
the two sets of {111} planes occurs in different regions of the layer and

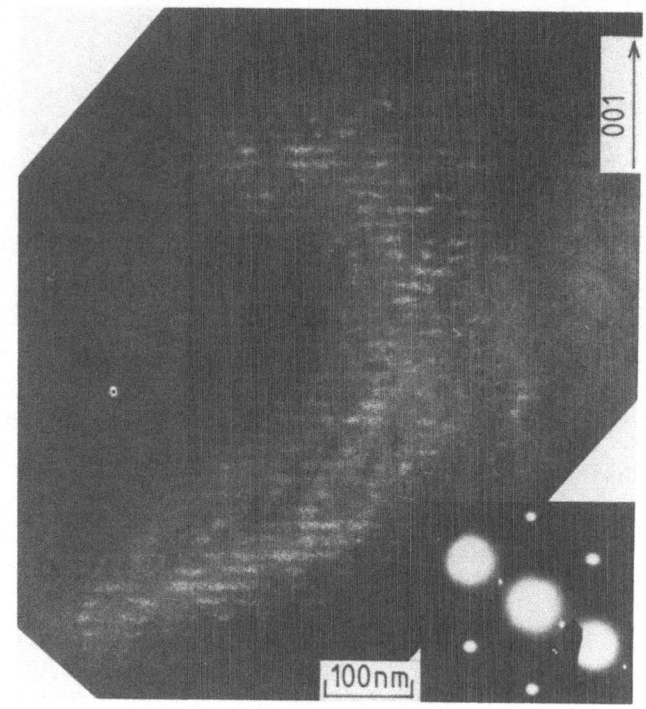

Fig.11.   ½{111}DF micrograph taken from a [110]
cross-section specimen of an AP-OMVPE
$Ga_xIn_{1-x}As$ layer (T_g=600°C). A periodic
variation in the degree of order is
visible along the [001] growth direction. Inset is the diffraction pattern
for this micrograph with the superlattice spot used marked with the beam
stop.

that the degree of order varies appreciably in these regions.

Another example is shown in Fig.11 which is a ½{111}DF micrograph
taken from a [110] cross-section specimen of an AP-OMVPE $Ga_xIn_{1-x}As$
(x ~ 0·5) layer (T_g = 600°C). This layer also contained ordered regions
of two variants of the trigonal (CuPt-type cation sublattice) ordered
structure and possessed strong ½{111} superlattice spots at the [110]
pole as shown in Fig.8(a)[47]. Inset on the micrograph is the diffraction
pattern for this image with the superlattice spot used indicated by the
beam stop. Quite a large region of material ordered on one set of {111}
planes is visible with a fairly sharp boundary on the left hand side.
Within this ordered region there appears to be quite large variations in
the degree of order both parallel to and perpendicular to the [001]
growth direction of the layer. In particular a regular variation in the
degree of order is visible in the [001] growth direction of the layer.
This regular variation has a period of ~ 19nm and may have been caused by
a periodic variation in the growth temperature and/or composition of the
growing layer.

Imaging antiphase domain boundaries

An antiphase domain boundary (APB) separates two ordered domains in
which the ordered atoms in their preferred sites are out of step with

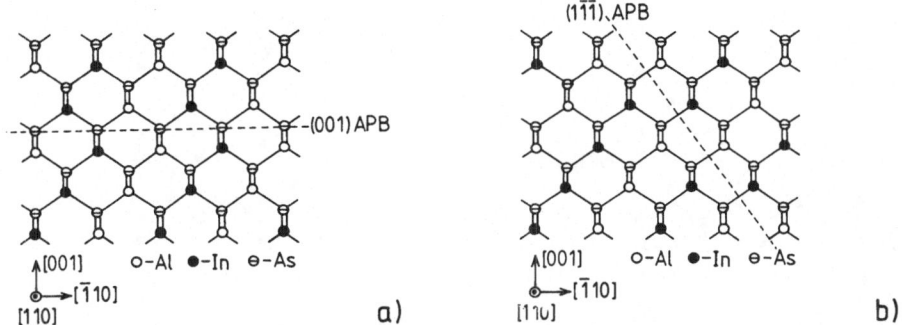

Fig.12. $[110]$ projections of APBs in an $Al_{0.5}In_{0.5}As$ alloy trigonally ordered on $(\bar{1}1\bar{1})$ planes.

(a) (001) APB   (b) $(1\bar{1}\bar{1})$APB

each other. Fig.12 shows $[110]$ projections of (001) and $(1\bar{1}\bar{1})$ APBs in an $Al_{0.5}In_{0.5}As$ alloy trigonally ordered on $(\bar{1}1\bar{1})$ planes. It can be seen that on one side of the APB the Al atoms are on one set of preferred sites, α sites, of the Group III atom sublattice but are on another set, β sites, on the other side of the APB. For each APB a displacement vector R can be defined which corresponds to the vector required to shift, within a single domain, atoms from the α sites to the β sites. For the (001) APB in Fig.12(a) the value of R is $\frac{1}{2}[\bar{1}10]$ and for the $(1\bar{1}\bar{1})$ APB in Fig.12(b) R is $\frac{1}{2}[101]$. The visibility of an APB for a certain reflection g is governed by the value of the phase factor $\alpha = 2\pi g \cdot R$[63]. The displacement vector R is a lattice vector in the disordered alloy and hence for fundamental reflections α is an integral multiple of 2π and an APB will normally be invisible. However, for certain superlattice reflections α will be an odd multiple of π and the APB will become visible. In the case of the APBs shown in Fig.12 they will be visible if $\frac{1}{2}(\bar{1}1\bar{1})$ reflections are used. If such a superlattice reflection is used on an APB which is inclined to the plane of the TEM sample the APB will exhibit fringe type contrast characteristic of a stacking fault[63]. However, the fringe spacing observed may be quite large and only one or two fringes may be visible. This is because the structure factor F for a superlattice reflection is proportional to the difference of the two atomic scattering amplitudes involved and hence may be quite small in comparison with F of a fundamental reflection. The fringe spacing observed is proportional to the extinction distance of the superlattice reflection which is inversely proportional to F and hence can be quite large. One can increase the number of fringes observed at an APB by using weak beam techniques. APBs in highly trigonally ordered OMVPE $Ga_xIn_{1-x}P$ alloys have been imaged by McKernan et al.[53][55].

Although APBs should normally be invisible in fundamental reflections they may become visible in ordered alloys where the difference in atomic size is large. At an APB atoms have the wrong kinds of nearest neighbour atoms (in a ternary III-V alloy wrong nearest neighbour atoms on the mixed atom sublattice) and this may cause extra atomic displacements at the APB, in addition to the displacement vector R, in alloys where a large difference in atomic size exists. These extra atomic displacements at the APB may then give rise to displacement contrast in fundamental reflection images[62].

In addition to APBs in alloys which undergo trigonal (CuPt-type cation sublattice) ordering, other types of boundary may exist between the different variants of trigonal ordering. In Fig.13 are shown $[110]$

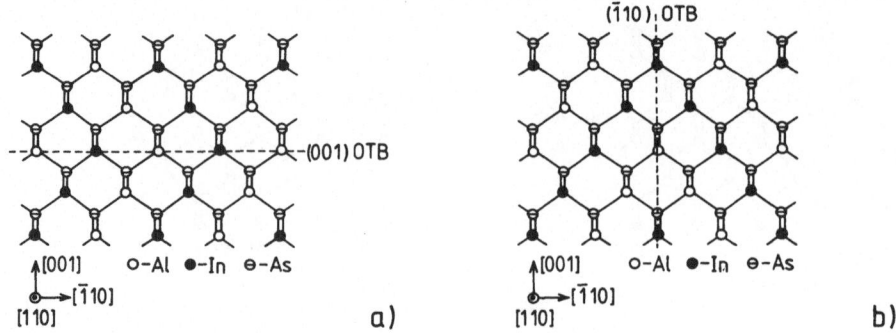

Fig.13. [110] projections of OTBs in an Al$_{0.5}$In$_{0.5}$As alloy trigonally
ordered on ($\bar{1}1\bar{1}$) and ($1\bar{1}\bar{1}$) planes.
(a) (001) OTB.   (b) ($\bar{1}10$) OTB.

projections of two examples of this type of boundary, referred to as
order twin boundaries (OTBs), in an Al$_{0.5}$In$_{0.5}$As layer trigonally ordered
on ($\bar{1}1\bar{1}$) and ($1\bar{1}\bar{1}$) planes. Such boundaries may be revealed by taking
dark field micrographs of the same area using the different $\frac{1}{2}(\bar{1}1\bar{1})$ and
$\frac{1}{2}(1\bar{1}\bar{1})$ superlattice spots or by using high resolution electron microscopy
(HREM) if the boundary plane lies parallel to the electron beam.

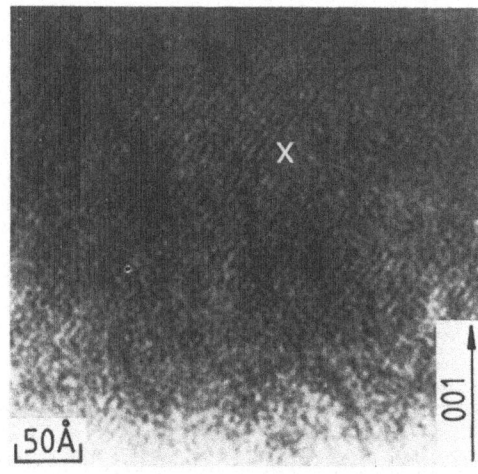

Fig.14. [110] cross-section HREM image
of a trigonally ordered
AP-OMVPE Al$_x$In$_{1-x}$As layer
(T$_g$=600°C) taken at the [110]
pole which showed strong $\frac{1}{2}\{111\}$
superlattice spots. The micro-
graph was taken with a
JEOL 200CX using an objective
aperture which included only
the central 000 beam and the
four closest $\frac{1}{2}\{111\}$ superlattice beams. The ordered
regions, e.g. X, show $\{111\}$
oriented fringes of spacing
~6·78Å i.e. double the $\{111\}$
plane spacing of Al$_x$In$_{1-x}$As
lattice matched to InP.

High resolution electron microscopy (HREM) may be used to image small ordered regions in a disordered matrix, to image APBs and OTBs if their boundary plane lies parallel to the electron beam and to help identify the structure of ordered phases present in alloys.

Imaging of ordered regions, APBs and OTBs

In Fig.14 is shown a HREM image taken from a $[110]$ cross-section specimen of an (001) AP-OMVPE $Al_xIn_{1-x}As$ (x ~ 0·5) layer (T_g = 600°C) which exhibited ordered regions of two variants of the trigonal (CuPt-type cation sublattice) ordered structure. The TED pattern at this pole contained strong $\frac{1}{2}\{111\}$ superlattice spots as shown in Fig.6(a). This image was taken using a JEOL 200CX at 200kV using a $0·2A^{-1}$ objective aperture which just included the central 000 beam and the four closest $\frac{1}{2}\{111\}$ superlattice beams. The ordered regions e.g. area X are revealed as areas which show $\{111\}$ oriented fringes of spacing ~ 6·78A which is double the normal $\{111\}$ plane spacing for $Al_xIn_{1-x}As$ lattice matched to InP. These fringes arise at certain values of specimen thickness and defocus due to interference between the central 000 beam and the super-lattice beams. In such images it should be possible to identify OTBs etc.

In Fig.15 is shown another HREM lattice image taken from the same $[110]$ cross-section sample as Fig.14. The image was taken with a JEOL 200CX HREM (extended Scherzer resolution 2·37A at -660A defocus) at 200kV with a $0·4A^{-1}$ objective aperture which allows all beams up to and including the two $\{002\}$ fundamental beams to pass through. In the

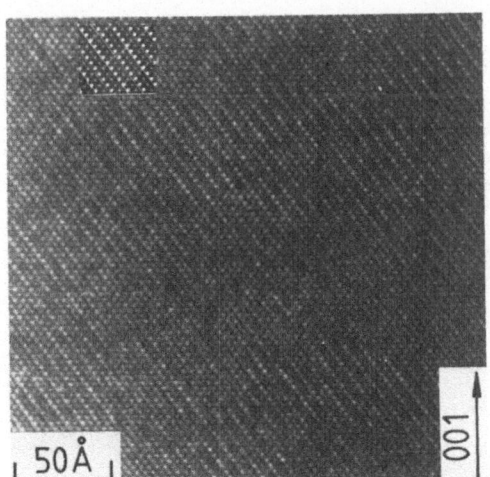

Thickness 125Å, defocus -660Å

0   5   10   25   50   75   100

% degree of ordering ⟶

50 Å

001

Fig.15. HREM lattice image of the same sample as Fig.14 taken at the same $[110]$ pole with the JEOL 200CX but using a $0·4A^{-1}$ objective aperture which allowed through all beams up to and including the two $\{002\}$ fundamental beams. A doubling in periodicity of $\{111\}$ lattice fringes is visible in the ordered regions. Beside the experimental image are shown some computer simulated images of an $Al_{0.5}In_{0.5}As$ crystal ordered on one set of $\{111\}$ planes as a function of degree of ordering for a microscope defocus of -660A and specimen thickness of 125A. Inset on the experimental lattice image is the computer simulated image for a 5% degree of order under the above conditions.

ordered regions a doubling in periodicity of the {111} lattice fringes is visible. This doubling in periodicity of the {111} lattice fringes arises at certain values of specimen thickness and microscope defocus due to the presence of the superlattice beams and their interference with the other beams. The HREM image contrast observed can be interpreted with the aid of multislice image simulation calculations and the results of some of these calculations for a trigonally ordered $Al_{0.5}In_{0.5}As$ alloy are shown in Fig.15 beside the experimental lattice image. These calculations were performed by Mr R E Mallard using a 256 X 256 fast Fourier transform programme developed by Drs M A O'Keefe and W G Waddington. An extended unit cell of the bulk composition $Al_{0.5}In_{0.5}As$ with the degree of ordering on one set of {111} planes varying from 0 to 100% was used as the basis for these calculations. Fourier coefficients were generated out to $6A^{-1}$ and multislice calculations were performed using 614 beams out to $2.8A^{-1}$. The input parameters describing the microscope performance were $C_s = 1.2mm$, objective aperture size = $0.4A^{-1}$, beam divergence = $0.8mrad$ and Gaussian defocus spread = $80A$. The results of these calculations indicated that the HREM image contrast could be sensitive to quite small degrees of ordering under certain imaging conditions for this alloy system. For thin crystal, < 75A, very weak contrast effects were predicted, even for quite high degrees of ordering. Inset on the experimental HREM image is the simulated image for 5% degree of ordering at Scherzer defocus (-660A) and a specimen thickness of 125A.

Using HREM it should be possible to image APBs and OTBs if they lie parallel or nearly parallel to the electron beam. An HREM image of a possible APB in trigonally ordered OMVPE $Ga_{0.5}In_{0.5}P$ has been reported by Ueda et al.[51].

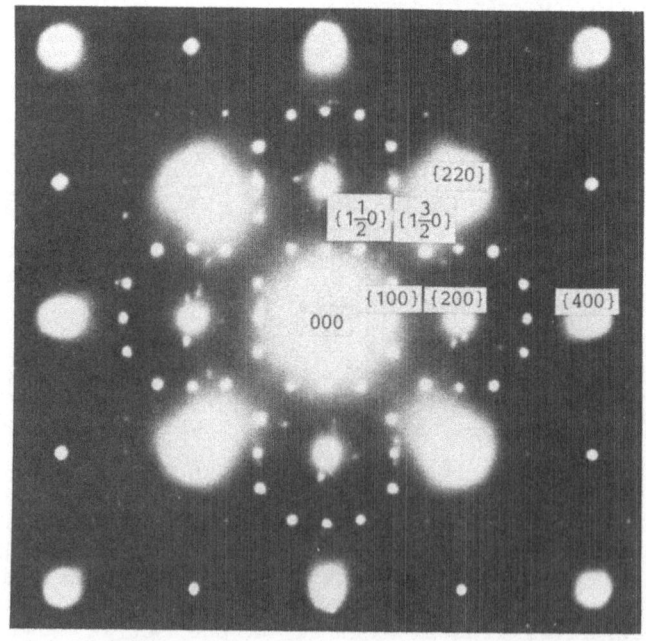

Fig.16. [001] pole TED pattern obtained from an OMVPE $Ga_xAl_yIn_{1-x-y}As$ layer ($T_g=680°C$) which contains superlattice spots at {100} and ½{210} positions.

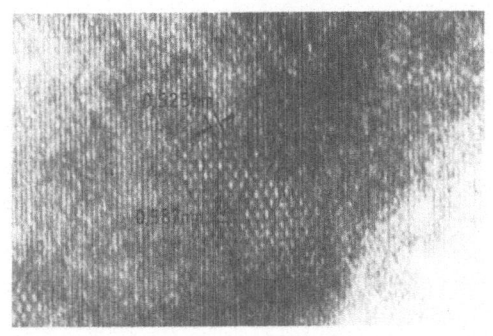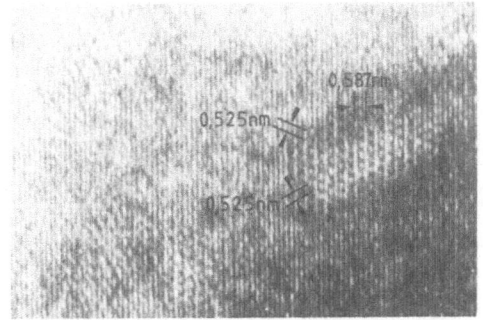

Fig.17. Slightly off [001] pole HREM images of same $Ga_xAl_yIn_{1-x-y}As$ layer as Fig.16 taken with a JEOL 200CX using an objective aperture including all beams up to the four {002} fundamental beams. Small ordered regions are visible which contain extra fringes of spacing 0·525nm and 0·587nm superimposed on the fundamental lattice fringes and which correspond to both the ½{210} and {100} superlattice spots of Fig.16.

Identification of the structure of ordered phases

In Fig.16 is shown an [001] pole TED pattern obtained from an OMVPE $Ga_xAl_yIn_{1-x-y}As$ layer (T_g = 680°C) grown close to lattice match on (001) InP. The TED pattern contains superlattice spots at {100} and ½{210} positions which could arise from the presence of two variants of the Famatinite type structure[38] or a mixture of two variants of the simple tetragonal and two variants of the Chalcopyrite type ordered structures[39]. In Fig.17 are shown HREM images taken close to this pole using a JEOL 200CX HREM at 200kV using an objective aperture size of $0·4A^{-1}$ which just includes all beams out to the four {002} fundamental diffracted beams. Small ordered regions are visible which contain extra fringes of spacing 0·525nm and 0·587nm, corresponding to both the ½{210} and {100} superlattice spots, superimposed on the fundamental lattice fringes. This indicates that the domains of ordered material are probably two variants of the Famatinite type ordered structure and not a mixture of simple tetragonal and Chalcopyrite type ordered phases. Similar results were obtained by Nakayama and Fujita[38] for LPE $Ga_xIn_{1-x}As$ alloy layers. Care however must be taken that the images obtained are not of several ordered domains overlapping in the beam direction since this may lead to misleading results[64].

CONCLUSION

Electron microscopy has been shown to be a very valuable technique for the study of atomic ordering in ternary and quaternary III-V compound semiconductor alloys.

ACKNOWLEDGEMENTS

The author would like to acknowledge Mr R. E. Mallard, University of Oxford, for the multislice image simulations, the SERC and UK Department of Trade and Industry for supporting this work under a Joint Opto-electronics Research Scheme and Plessey Research (Caswell) Ltd. for provision of samples.

REFERENCES

1. M. B. Panish and M. Ilegems, Phase Equilibria in Ternary III-V Systems, in: "Progress in Solid State Chemistry", H. Reiss and J. O. McCaldin, ed., Pergamon, New York 7:39 (1972).
2. L. M. Foster and J.F. Woods, Thermodynamic Analysis of III-V Alloy Semiconductor Phase Diagrams, J. Electrochem. Soc. 118:1175 (1971).
3. G. B. Stringfellow, Calculation of Ternary and Quaternary III-V Phase Diagrams, J. Cryst. Growth 27:21 (1974).
4. K. Onabe, Unstable Regions in III-V Quaternary Solid Solutions Composition Plane Calculated with Strictly Regular Solution Approximation, Jpn. J. Appl. Phys. 21:L323 (1982).
5. K. Onabe, Immiscibility Analysis for III-V Quaternary Solid Solutions, NEC Research and Development 72:1 (1984).
6. B. de Cremoux, P. Hirtz and J. Ricciardi, On the Presence of a Solid Immiscibility Domain in the GaInAsP Phase Diagram, Int. Symp. GaAs and Related Cpds., Vienna 1980, Inst. Phys. Conf. Ser. 56:115 (1981).
7. B. de Cremoux, Instability Criteria in Ternary and Quaternary III-V Epitaxial Solid Solutions, J. de Physique 43 (12, Suppl.C5):C5-19 (1982).
8. G. B. Stringfellow, Miscibility Gaps in Quaternary III-V Alloys, J. Cryst. Growth 58:194 (1982).
9. G. B. Stringfellow, Spinodal Decomposition and Clustering in III-V Alloys, J. Electron. Mater. 11:903 (1982).
10. G. B. Stringfellow, Immiscibility and Spinodal Decomposition in III-V Alloys, J. Cryst. Growth 65:454 (1983).
11. E. K. Müller and J. L. Richards, Miscibility of III-V Semiconductors Studied by Flash Evaporation, J. Appl. Phys. 35:1233 (1964).
12. M. F. Gratton, R. G. Goodchild, L. Y. Juravel and J. C. Woolley, Miscibility Gap in the $GaAs_ySb_{1-y}$ System, J. Electron. Mater. 8:25 (1979).
13. K. Nakajima, K. Osamura, K. Yasuda and Y. Murakami, The Pseudo-Quaternary Phase Diagram of the Ga-In-As-Sb System, J. Cryst. Growth 41:87 (1977).
14. R. E. Nahory, M. A. Pollack, E. D. Beebe, J. C. DeWinter and M. Ilegems, The Liquid Phase Epitaxy of $Al_xGa_{1-x}As_{1-y}Sb_y$ and the Importance of Strain Effects near the Miscibility Gap, J. Electrochem. Soc. 125:1053 (1978).
15. J. R. Pessetto and G. B. Stringfellow, $Al_xGa_{1-x}As_ySb_{1-y}$ Phase Diagram, J. Cryst. Growth 62:1 (1983).
16. M. Quillec, C. Daguet, J. L. Benchimol and H. Launois, $In_xGa_{1-x}As_yP_{1-y}$ Alloy Stabilisation by the InP Substrate Inside an Unstable Region in Liquid Phase Epitaxy, Appl. Phys. Lett. 40:325 (1982).
17. A. J. SpringThorpe, An Experimental Investigation of the GaAs-InAs-GaP-InP Pseudo-Quaternary Phase Diagram at 780°C, Paper presented at the 163rd ECS Meeting, Abs. No. 329, San Francisco (May 1983).
18. P. Hénoc, A. Izrael, M. Quillec and H. Launois, Composition Modulation in Liquid Phase Epitaxial $In_xGa_{1-x}As_yP_{1-y}$ Layers Lattice Matched to InP Substrates, Appl. Phys. Lett. 40:963 (1982).
19. F. Glas, M. J. Treacy, M. Quillec and H. Launois, Interface Spinodal Decomposition in LPE $In_xGa_{1-x}As_yP_{1-y}$ Lattice Matched to InP, J. de Physique 43(12, Suppl.C5):C5-11 (1982).
20. H. Launois, M. Quillec, F. Glas and M. J. Treacy, Interface Spinodal Decomposition in LPE $In_xGa_{1-x}As_yP_{1-y}$ Lattice-Matched to InP, Int. Symp. GaAs and Related Cpds., Albuquerque 1982, Inst. Phys. Conf. Ser. 65:537 (1983).

21. J. P. Gowers, TEM Image Contrast from Clustering in Ga-In Containing III-V Alloys, Appl. Phys. A 31:23 (1983).

22. S. Mahajan, B. V. Dutt, H. Temkin, R. J. Cava and W. A. Bonner, Spinodal Decomposition in InGaAsP Epitaxial Layers, J. Cryst. Growth 68:589 (1984).

23. O. Ueda, S. Isozumi and S. Komiya, Composition-Modulated Structures in InGaAsP and InGaP Liquid Phase Epitaxial Layers Grown on (001) GaAs Substrates, Jpn. J. Appl. Phys. 23:L241 (1984).

24. J. H. Chiu, W. T. Tsang, S. N. G. Chu, J. Shah and J. A. Ditzenberger, Molecular Beam Epitaxy of $GaSb_{0.5}As_{0.5}$ and $Al_xGa_{1-x}Sb_yAs_{1-y}$ Lattice Matched to InP, Appl. Phys. Lett. 46:408 (1985).

25. A. G. Norman and G. R. Booker, Transmission Electron Microscope and Transmission Electron Diffraction Observations of Alloy Clustering in Liquid-Phase Epitaxial (001) GaInAsP Layers, J. Appl. Phys. 57:4715 (1985).

26. S. N. G. Chu, S. Nakahara, K. E. Strege and W. D. Johnston, Jr., Surface Layer Spinodal Decomposition in $In_{1-x}Ga_xAs_yP_{1-y}$ and $In_{1-x}Ga_xAs$ Grown by Hydride Transport Vapour-Phase Epitaxy, J. Appl. Phys. 57:4610 (1985).

27. F. Glas, P. Hénoc and H. Launois, TEM and STEM Study of the Microstructure of Ternary and Quaternary III-V Epitaxial Layers, Microsc. Semicond. Mater. Conf., Oxford 1985, Inst. Phys. Conf. Ser. 76:251 (1985).

28. A. G. Norman and G. R. Booker, TEM and TED Studies of Alloy Clustering in GaInAsP, GaInAs and GaInP Epitaxial Layers, Microsc. Semicond. Mater. Conf., Oxford 1985, Inst. Phys. Conf. Ser. 76:257 (1985).

29. D. Cherns, P. D. Greene, A. Hainsworth and A. R. Preston, Phase Separation in GaInAsP Epitaxial Layers, Microsc. Semicond. Mater. Conf., Oxford 1987, Inst. Phys. Conf. Ser. 87:83 (1987).

30. G. P. Srivastava, J. L. Martins and A. Zunger, Atomic Structure and Ordering in Semiconductor Alloys, Phys. Rev. B 31:2561 (1985).

31. J. C. Mikkelsen, Jr. and J. B. Boyce, Atomic-Scale Structure of Random Solid Solutions: Extended X-ray-Absorption Fine-Structure Study of $Ga_{1-x}In_xAs$, Phys. Rev. Lett. 49:1412 (1982).

32. J. Bellessa, C. Gors, P. Launois, M. Quillec and H. Launois, Extended X-ray Absorption Fine Structures Study of Short Range Order in $In_xGa_{1-x}As$ and $Ga_xAl_{1-x}As$ Alloys, Int. Symp. GaAs and Related Cpds., Albuquerque 1982, Inst. Phys. Conf. Ser. 65:529 (1983).

33. J. C. Mikkelsen, Jr. and J. B. Boyce, Extended X-ray Absorption Fine-Structure Study of $Ga_{1-x}In_xAs$ Random Solid Solutions, Phys. Rev. B 28:7130 (1983).

34. A. A. Mbaye, A. Zunger and D. M. Wood, Structural Stability and Selectivity of Thin Epitaxial Semiconductors, Appl. Phys. Lett. 49:782 (1986).

35. A. A. Mbaye, D. M. Wood and A. Zunger, Stability of Bulk and Pseudomorphic Epitaxial Semiconductors and Their Alloys, Phys. Rev. B 37:3008 (1988).

36. T. S. Kuan, T. F. Kuech, W. I. Wang and E. L. Wilkie, Long-Range Order in $Al_xGa_{1-x}As$, Phys. Rev. Lett. 54:201 (1985).

37. T. S. Kuan, W. I. Wang and E. L. Wilkie, Long-Range Order in $In_xG_{1-x}As$, Appl. Phys. Lett. 51:51 (1987).

38. H. Nakayama and H. Fujita, Direct Observation of an Ordered Phase in a Disordered $In_{1-x}Ga_xAs$ Alloy, Int. Symp. GaAs. and Related Cpds., Karuizawa 1985, Inst. Phys. Conf. Ser. 79:289 (1986).

39. H. R. Jen, M. J. Cherng and G. B. Stringfellow, Ordered Structures in $GaAs_{0.5}Sb_{0.5}$ Alloys Grown by Organometallic Vapour Phase Epitaxy, Appl. Phys. Lett. 48:1603 (1986).

40. H. R. Jen, M. J. Jou, Y. T. Cherng and G. B. Stringfellow, The Kinetic Aspects of Ordering in $GaAs_{1-x}Sb_x$ Grown by Organometallic Vapour Phase Epitaxy, J. Cryst. Growth 85:175 (1987).

41. I. J. Murgatroyd, A. G. Norman and G. R. Booker, Atomic Ordering in $GaAs_{0.5}Sb_{0.5}$, Paper presented at the 1986 MRS Spring Meeting, Abs. No.B5.2, Palo Alto USA (April 1986).

42. I. J. Murgatroyd, A. G. Norman, G. R. Booker and T. M. Kerr, Lattice Imaging of Long Range Order in $GaAs_{0.5}Sb_{0.5}$ Grown by Molecular Beam Epitaxy, Proc. XIth Int. Cong. on Electron Microscopy, Kyoto, Japan 1986, 1497 (1986).

43. I. J. Murgatroyd, "D. Phil. Thesis", University of Oxford (1987).

44. Y. E. Ihm, N. Otsuka, J. Klem and H. Morkoc, Ordering in $GaAs_{1-x}Sb_x$ Grown by Molecular Beam Epitaxy, Appl. Phys. Lett. 51:2013 (1987).

45. Y. E. Ihm, N. Otsuka, Y. Hirotsu, J. Klem and H. Morkoc, Transmission Electron Microscope Study of an Ordered Structure in $GaAs_{0.5}Sb_{0.5}$ Grown by Molecular Beam Epitaxy, Paper presented at the 1987 MRS Fall Meeting, Abs. No. C8.11, Boston (Dec. 1987).

46. A. G. Norman, R. E. Mallard, I. J. Murgatroyd, G. R. Booker, A. H. Moore and M. D. Scott, TED, TEM and HREM Studies of Atomic Ordering in $Al_xIn_{1-x}As$ (x ~ 0.5) Epitaxial Layers Grown by Organometallic Vapour Phase Epitaxy, Microsc. Semicond. Mater. Conf. Oxford April 1987, Inst. Phys. Conf. Ser. 87:77 (1987).

47. A. G. Norman, "D. Phil. Thesis", University of Oxford (1987).

48. M. A. Shahid, S. Mahajan, D. E. Laughlin and H. M. Cox, Atomic Ordering in $Ga_{0.47}In_{0.53}As$ and $Ga_xIn_{1-x}As_yP_{1-y}$ Alloy Semiconductors, Phys. Rev. Lett. 58:2567 (1987).

49. M. A. Shahid and S. Mahajan, Long-Range Atomic Order in $Ga_xIn_{1-x}As_yP_{1-y}$ Epitaxial Layers [(x,y) = (0.47,1), (0.37,0.82), (0.34,0.71) and (0.27,0.64)], Phys. Rev. B 38:1344 (1988).

50. A. Gomyo, T. Suzuki, K. Kobayashi, S. Kawata, I. Hino and T. Yuasa, Evidence for the Existence of an Ordered State in $Ga_{0.5}In_{0.5}P$ Grown by Metalorganic Vapour Phase Epitaxy and its Relation to Band-gap Energy, Appl. Phys. Lett. 50:673 (1987).

51. O. Ueda, M. Takikawa, J. Komeno and I. Umebu, Atomic Structure of Ordered InGaP Crystals Grown on (001) GaAs Substrates by Metalorganic Chemical Vapour Deposition, Jpn. J. Appl. Phys. 26:L1824 (1987).

52. J. P. Goral, M. M. Al-Jassim, J. M. Olson and A. Kibbler, TEM and TED Studies of Ordering in GaInP, Paper presented at the 1987 MRS Fall Meeting, Abs. No. C8.10, Boston (Dec. 1987).

53. S. McKernan, B. C. De Cooman, C. B. Carter, D. P. Bour and J. R. Shealy, TEM Studies of Ordering in MOCVD-Grown (GaIn)P on GaAs, Paper presented at the 1987 MRS Fall Meeting, Abs. No. E8.43, Boston (Dec. 1987).

54. P. Bellon, J. P. Chevalier, G. P. Martin, E. Dupont-Nivet, C. Thiebaut and J. P. André, Chemical Ordering in $Ga_xIn_{1-x}P$ Semiconductor Alloy Grown by Metalorganic Vapour Phase Epitaxy, Appl. Phys. Lett. 52:567 (1988).

55. S. McKernan, B. C. De Cooman, C. B. Carter, D. P. Bour and J. R. Shealy, Direct Observation of Ordering in (GaIn)P, J. Mater. Res. 3:406 (1988).

56. A. Gomyo, T. Suzuki and S. Iijima, Observation of Strong Ordering in $Ga_xIn_{1-x}P$ Alloy Semiconductors, Phys. Rev. Lett. 60:2645 (1988).

57. M. Kondow, H. Kakibayashi and S. Minagawa, Ordered Structure in OMVPE-Grown $Ga_{0.5}In_{0.5}P$, J. Cryst. Growth 88:291 (1988).

58. M. Kondow, H. Kakibayashi, S. Minagawa, Y. Inoue, T. Nishino and Y. Hamakawa, Influence of Growth Temperature on Crystalline Structure in $Ga_{0.5}In_{0.5}P$ grown by Organometallic Vapour Phase Epitaxy, Appl. Phys. Lett. 53:2053 (1988).

59. F. P. Dabkowski, P. Gavrilovic, K. Meehan, W. Stutius, J. E. Williams, M. A. Shahid and S. Mahajan, Disordering of the Ordered Structure in Metalorganic Chemical Vapour Deposition Grown $Ga_{0.5}In_{0.5}P$ on (001) GaAs substrates by Zinc Diffusion, Appl. Phys. Lett. 52:2142 (1988).

60. M. Kondow and S. Minagawa, Study on Photoluminescence and Raman Scattering of GaInP and AlInP Grown by Organometallic Vapour-Phase Epitaxy, J. Appl. Phys. 64:793 (1988).

61. B. D. Cullity, "Elements of X-ray Diffraction", Addison-Wesley, Reading Massachusetts (1956).

62. M. H. Loretto, "Electron Beam Analysis of Materials", Chapman and Hall, London (1984).

63. P. B. Hirsch, A. Howie, R. B. Nicholson, D. W. Pashley and M. J. Whelan, "Electron Microscopy of Thin Crystals", Krieger, New York (1965).

64. W. M. Stobbs, Private communication (1988).

ELASTIC RELAXATION AND TEM IMAGE CONTRASTS

IN THIN COMPOSITION–MODULATED SEMICONDUCTOR CRYSTALS

Michael M. J. Treacy

Exxon Research & Engineering Company
Clinton Township, Route 22E
Annandale, New Jersey 08801

INTRODUCTION

Strong image contrasts can arise in transmission electron micrographs from remarkably small strain gradients in thinned crystals. Shear strains with amplitudes as small as 10^{-4} can produce detectable contrasts under optimum imaging conditions [1], much more than would be predicted on the basis of the perturbed projected potential alone. Strong dynamical scattering effects, stimulated by the bending of diffracting lattice planes, are primarily responsible for these strong contrasts. Internal shear strains (ie lattice bending) can result from stresses associated with crystal defects, such as dislocations, point defects, coherent interfaces, planar defects, inclusions, compositional inhomogeneities, surfaces, surface steps and surface irregularities. Temperature gradients, due to uneven electron beam heating, can also generate internal stresses. Although it is possible to fabricate semiconductor materials which are essentially free of structural defects, most operational semiconductors contain dopants and interfaces. Atomic radii of dopant atoms are generally not identical to that of the host lattice, thus static disorder is introduced into the lattice. Molecular beam epitaxy permits the microfabrication of semiconductor materials which have coherent strain fields deliberately introduced, such as strained layer superlattices [2]. If structural details of such materials are to be interpreted accurately from electron micrographs, it is important that the imaging and structural artifacts caused by internal stresses be thoroughly understood.

Of particular importance is elastic relaxation, which occurs when materials containing defects or composition modulations are thinned. This is an insidious artifact which causes the crystal lattice to bend near the specimen surfaces. Furthermore, the form of the bending depends on specimen thickness. Relaxation is most pronounced in those Fourier components of the stress field which are comparable to the specimen thickness, and is thus prevalent in longer wavelength superlattice and quasi–periodic structures. When relaxation dominates, specimen properties measured directly from TEM images, such as unit cell dimensions, will not reflect the properties of either the stressed bulk or the fully relaxed materials.

There are several excellent discussions in the literature which analyze the structures, and associated TEM contrasts, from dislocations [3; 4], precipitates (Ashby–Brown contrasts) [5] and stacking faults [6; 7]. It is not intended to review these well–documented areas in this article. Instead, the emphasis is on elastic relaxation in composition–modulated materials, in particular the long wavelength modulations found in strained layer superlattices and spinodally decomposed $In_xGa_{1-x}As_yP_{1-y}$ alloys. It is important to realise, however, that strain contrasts are not necessarily an impediment to correct interpretation of micrographs. When their origins are recognized and understood, strain contrasts can render valuable information about the material under study.

STRAIN CONTRAST MECHANISMS

The physical mechanisms underlying strain contrasts are best understood within the context of two–beam dynamical theory [4]. Dynamical theory has had much success in explaining the contrasts from stacking faults [4; 7], inclusions [5] and dislocations [6]. Here, for simplicity, we follow the two–beam column approximation Bloch wave description presented in Hirsch, Howie, Nicholson, Pashley & Whelan (HHNPW) [4].

The two–beam electron wavefield in a thin crystal can be written in terms of the Bloch wave functions $b^{(i)}(\mathbf{k}^{(i)}, \mathbf{r})$,

$$\psi(\mathbf{r}) = \psi^{(1)} b^{(1)}(\mathbf{k}^{(1)}, \mathbf{r}) + \psi^{(2)} b^{(2)}(\mathbf{k}^{(2)}, \mathbf{r}) \qquad \ldots (1)$$

The $\psi^{(i)}$ are the Bloch wave excitation amplitudes, and, ignoring absorption for the moment, the Bloch waves themselves are described by

$$b^{(1)}(\mathbf{k}^{(1)}, \mathbf{r}) = \frac{1}{\sqrt{2}}\left\{\left(1 + \frac{w}{\sqrt{1 + w^2}}\right)^{1/2} - \left(1 - \frac{w}{\sqrt{1 + w^2}}\right)^{1/2}\exp(2\pi i \mathbf{g}.\mathbf{r})\right\}\exp(2\pi i \mathbf{k}^{(1)}.\mathbf{r})$$

$$\ldots (2a)$$

$$b^{(2)}(\mathbf{k}^{(2)}, \mathbf{r}) = \frac{1}{\sqrt{2}}\left\{\left(1 - \frac{w}{\sqrt{1 + w^2}}\right)^{1/2} + \left(1 + \frac{w}{\sqrt{1 + w^2}}\right)^{1/2}\exp(2\pi i \mathbf{g}.\mathbf{r})\right\}\exp(2\pi i \mathbf{k}^{(2)}.\mathbf{r})$$

$$\ldots (2b)$$

The z components of the wavevectors $\mathbf{k}^{(i)}$ are given by

$$k_z^{(1)} = K_z + \left(w - \sqrt{1 + w^2}\right)/2\xi_g \qquad \ldots (3a)$$

$$k_z^{(2)} = K_z + \left(w + \sqrt{1 + w^2}\right)/2\xi_g \qquad \ldots (3b)$$

and the x and y components are the same as those of the incident beam wavevector $\mathbf{K}$. K_z is the z component of $\mathbf{K}$ as modified by the average crystal potential. As usual, w is the deviation parameter, representing the error from the exact Bragg condition (which is at $w = 0$), and ξ_g is the extinction distance of the operating diffraction vector $\mathbf{g}$. The equations describing the coupling between the amplitudes $\psi^{(1)}$ and $\psi^{(2)}$ are [4]

$$\frac{d\psi^{(1)}}{dz} = -\frac{\pi i}{\sqrt{1 + w^2}}\frac{d}{dz}(\mathbf{g}.\mathbf{R}(z))\left\{\left(w - \sqrt{1 + w^2}\right)\psi^{(1)} + \exp(2\pi i \Delta k\, z)\,\psi^{(2)}\right\} \quad \ldots (4a)$$

$$\frac{d\psi^{(2)}}{dz} = \frac{\pi i}{\sqrt{1 + w^2}}\frac{d}{dz}(\mathbf{g}.\mathbf{R}(z))\left\{\left(w + \sqrt{1 + w^2}\right)\psi^{(2)} - \exp(-2\pi i \Delta k\, z)\psi^{(1)}\right\} \quad \ldots (4b)$$

where Δk is equal to $\sqrt{(1 + w^2)}/\xi_g$.

The coupling strength, therefore, is governed by the gradient along z of the quantity $\mathbf{g}.\mathbf{R}(z)$, where $\mathbf{R}(z)$ is the local atomic displacement at depth z. This gradient term can be replaced by the sum $\mathbf{g}.d\mathbf{R}/dz + \mathbf{R}.d\mathbf{g}/dz$. The term $d\mathbf{R}/dz$ represents the local rotation of the diffraction planes, and usually dominates over the term $\mathbf{R}.d\mathbf{g}/dz$. Thus the coupling of the Bloch wave amplitudes tends also to be dominated by the bending of the diffraction planes, rather than by rigid body linear displacement terms. As we shall see later, elastic relaxation near the foil surfaces will ensure that even nominally uniform, one dimensional modulations within the plane of the foil, will also be accompanied by significant lattice bending.

The first terms within the curly brackets of equation 4 represent the intraband transitions. As shown by HHNPW, these terms can be removed by transforming to new variables

$$\psi^{'(1)} = \psi^{(1)} \exp\left(-\pi i \mathbf{g}.\mathbf{R}\left[1 - w / \sqrt{1 + w^2}\right]\right) \qquad \ldots (5a)$$

$$\psi^{'(2)} = \psi^{(2)} \exp\left(-\pi i \mathbf{g}.\mathbf{R}\left[1 + w / \sqrt{1 + w^2}\right]\right) \qquad \ldots (5b)$$

This transformation is equivalent to changing the z components of the wavevectors such that the Bloch waves tend to follow the average tilting of the reflecting lattice planes. Thus intraband scattering tends to modify the relative phases of the Bloch waves, but not their amplitudes. In terms of the new variables $\psi^{'(i)}$ equation 4 becomes

$$\frac{d\psi^{'(1)}}{dz} = -\frac{\pi i}{\sqrt{1 + w^2}} \frac{d}{dz}(\mathbf{g}.\mathbf{R}) \exp(2\pi i \Delta k z) \psi^{'(2)} \qquad \ldots (6a)$$

$$\frac{d\psi^{'(2)}}{dz} = -\frac{\pi i}{\sqrt{1 + w^2}} \frac{d}{dz}(\mathbf{g}.\mathbf{R}) \exp(-2\pi i \Delta k z) \psi^{'(1)} \qquad \ldots (6b)$$

These equations describe purely interband scattering in terms of the modified Bloch wave amplitudes $\psi^{'(i)}$. It follows immediately from equation 6, that, in the limit of weak interband scattering, the strength of the coupling between Bloch wave amplitudes is given by a Fourier transform. In other words, the interband scattering is strongest for those Fourier components of the bending term $d(\mathbf{g}.\mathbf{R})/dz$ (which will be dominated by the Fourier coefficients of $d\mathbf{R}/dz$) which are equal to $\Delta k = \sqrt{(1 + w^2)}/\xi_g$. Interband scattering is not necessarily strongest at the exact Bragg condition, $w = 0$. If the strongest Fourier component has characteristic wavelength less than ξ_g, strongest contrast from interband scattering may be found at some non–zero value of w (ie. at a weak beam condition). If the dominant Fourier components have wavelength $\geq \xi_g$, then the strongest interband scattering occurs at the exact Bragg condition. Of course if the predominant Fourier components are much larger than ξ_g, then interband scattering will be weak overall, and intraband scattering may dominate.

In the absence of any absorption, intensity modulations in bright field and dark field, under two–beam conditions, should be complementary, but of equal magnitude. Experimentally, it is found that dark field contrasts tend to be stronger, and are asymmetric relative to the strain modulation symmetry. Furthermore, strain contrasts are strongest for thicknesses exceeding several extinction distances. These effects are principally due to anomalous absorption which affects the relative Bloch wave amplitudes. For simplicity, the absorption terms have not been included in the above treatment, but they play a major role in contrast generation in thick specimens. When absorption occurs, the Bloch wave on branch i of the dispersion surface decays exponentially with depth z by a factor $\exp(-2\pi i q^{(i)} z)$, where the $q^{(i)}$ are given by

$$q^{(1)} = \frac{1}{2}\left(\frac{1}{\xi_0'} - \frac{1}{\xi_g' \sqrt{1 + w^2}}\right)$$

$$\qquad \ldots (7)$$

$$q^{(2)} = \frac{1}{2}\left(\frac{1}{\xi_0'} + \frac{1}{\xi_g' \sqrt{1 + w^2}}\right)$$

The two Bloch waves are not absorbed at the same rate, Bloch wave 2, which peaks in intensity on the reflecting planes, being attenuated more rapidly than Bloch wave 1, which peaks between the atomic planes. Interband scattering, however, allows the Bloch waves to exchange energy. The more strongly scattered Bloch wave 2 can be replenished by interband scattering from the less strongly absorbed Bloch wave 1, thus helping to maintain a high scattering rate. Since the sign of $\mathbf{g}.\mathbf{R}$ determines both the diffracted amplitude, and the Bloch wave coupling strength, anomalous absorption is also responsible for the asymmetry of contrasts in dark field relative to bright field.

The importance of lattice bending, or shear strain, in determining image contrasts can be seen in the following examples of composition–modulated materials. In some instances, the contrast due to relaxation of small lattice mismatches overwhelms the structure factor contrasts due to the composition modulation itself.

COMPOSITION AND STRUCTURE MODULATIONS

Compositional and structural inhomogeneities in crystalline alloys generally cause internal stresses due to the accompanying changes in unit cell dimensions. Inhomogeneities are quite common in mixed systems where complex phase diagrams can occur (for a review see ref. [8]). It is common for phase segregation to occur, where extreme composition fluctuations develop such that a discontinuous phase, or particle, precipitates. The precipitate may be structurally incoherent with the host lattice, or it may maintain a coherent interface if the structural differences are not too large, and if the particle is small enough to allow elastic accommodation of the misfit. However, under certain conditions [8], spinodal decomposition may occur, where the solid solution decomposes continuously, with no discrete nucleation event, into quasi–sinusoidal composition waves.

In the light of the emphasis placed in the previous section on the role of lattice bending in producing image contrasts, it is easy to see how composition modulations along the beam direction can introduce pronounced dR/dz terms, since the lattice parameter will change concomitantly with the composition fluctuations. However, it is not so obvious that modulations perpendicular to the beam direction can also introduce significant dR/dz terms, through the agency of elastic relaxation, near the upper and lower surfaces of the thin foil. The spinodal decomposition which occurs in $In_xGa_{1-x}As_yP_{1-y}$ alloys provides an excellent example with which to illustrate how such lattice bending, induced by elastic relaxation, can have pronounced impact on image contrasts.

Spinodal Decomposition in $In_xGa_{1-x}As_yP_{1-y}$

Hénoc *et al.* [9] originally demonstrated that, over a certain composition range, 220 dark field images of $In_xGa_{1-x}As_yP_{1-y}$, grown by LPE on [001] InP at 650°C, displayed a long period "basket weave" or "tweed" pattern of periodicity ~100 to 200 nm along the <100> directions. Figure 1 shows STEM images of a typical "tweed" pattern in an

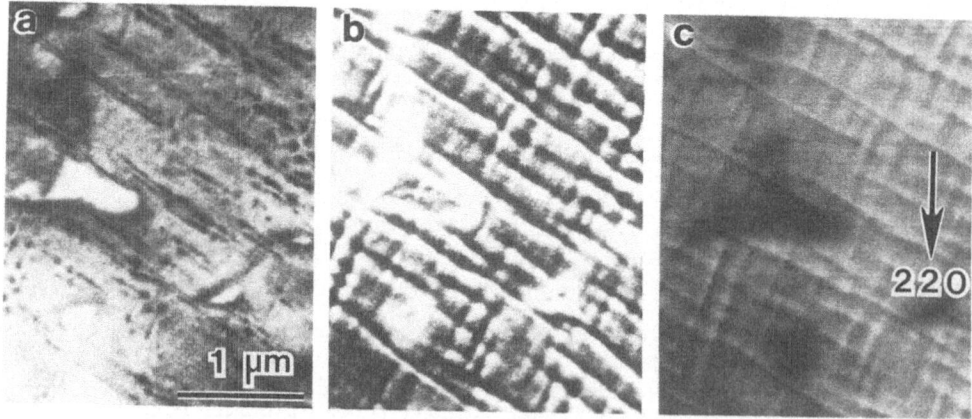

Figure 1. STEM images of a spinodally decomposed $In_{0.72}Ga_{0.28}As_{0.63}P_{0.37}$ sample grown by LPE on [001] InP. The crystal is aligned close to [001] and is in a strong 220 two–beam diffraction condition. a) Bright field. Note the weak, symmetrical long–period contrast features running diagonally on the micrograph. b) 220 dark field image. Contrast features are stronger than in bright field, and are asymmetrical. c) High angle annular detector (HAAD) image. Contrast is complementary to that in dark field .

$In_{0.72}Ga_{0.28}As_{0.63}P_{0.37}$ sample, taken with the crystal aligned in strong 220 two–beam condition. Tilting experiments [10], and cross–section specimens [11], confirm that, for a thin enough foil, the quasi–periodic modulation directions are essentially perpendicular to the growth direction, and thus lie within the plane of the foil. Cherns et al. [11], however, have shown that the amplitude of the modulation varies with position relative to the InP/InGaAsP interface, resolving into platelet precipitates away from the interface. This result supports the notion that the lattice matching at the interface tends, in the initial stages of growth, to stabilize the alloy against exsolution. X–ray microanalysis confirms that the material is attempting to decompose into GaP–enriched and InAs–enriched regions, consistent with theoretical predictions [12; 13; 14]. The amplitude of the observed contrasts are found to correlate with the composition modulation amplitude as determined by X–ray microanalysis [1; 10].

A fine scale "speckle" is also visible in these images (this is more clearly seen in figure 4). The behaviour of this contrast is consistent with a short wavelength lattice modulation, presumably associated with a short wavelength composition modulation (clustering)[15; 16]. Recent thermodynamic calculations [17] show that, at the atomic level, In–P and Ga–As bonds are favoured in $In_xGa_{1-x}As_yP_{1-y}$ materials. Interestingly, this is in contrast to the GaP and InAs enrichments found at larger scales in the spinodal decomposition. (For a more detailed discussion of solid phase instabilities in $In_xGa_{1-x}As_yP_{1-y}$ alloys, see the article by F. Glas in this volume.)

The role of lattice bending in generating the long period "tweed" contrast is revealed by detailed comparison of the three figures shown in figure 1. The "tweed" contrast is strongest in the dark field image, figure 1b, and shows regions of pronounced black–white contrasts. The bright field image, figure 1a, shows weaker symmetrical contrasts, with a bright line at the sharp boundary delineating the black–white regions seen in dark field. The high angle annular detector (HAAD) image, figure 1c, also exhibits asymmetric contrast features, but the contrast is complementary to that seen in the dark field image. The (HAAD) image contrasts disappear when the crystal is tilted away from strong diffraction conditions. This result shows that the anomalous absorption is a function of position [18], and confirms that the diffracting planes are bent. For a composition modulation that is travelling strictly within the plane of the foil, perpendicular to the beam direction, such bending can arise through the agency of elastic relaxation at the foil surfaces. If we model the unit cell modulation by

$$a_x = a_y = a_z = a_0 \{1 + \varepsilon_0 \sin(\alpha x)\} \qquad \ldots (8)$$

where ε_0 is the strain modulation amplitude, and $\alpha = 2\pi/\Lambda$, where Λ is the modulation wavelength, then, for a cubic isotropic material, the bending term as a function of depth z within the foil is [1]

$$\frac{dR_x}{dz} = 2\varepsilon_0 \frac{1+\nu}{1-\nu} \left\{ \frac{(\alpha t/2)\cosh(\alpha t/2)\cosh(\alpha z) - (\alpha z)\sinh(\alpha z)\sinh(\alpha t/2) - (1-2\nu)\sinh(\alpha t/2)\cosh(\alpha z)}{\sinh(\alpha t) + \alpha t} - \frac{1}{2} \right\} \cos(\alpha x)$$
$$\ldots (9)$$

Here, ν is Poisson's ratio and $\alpha = 2\pi/\Lambda$. The foil distortion is sketched as a function of t/Λ in figure 2 for $\varepsilon_0 = 0.1$, and $\nu = 0.33$. For the thinnest foils, where $t << \Lambda$, there is negligible bending since the x–z shear stress components are essentially fully relaxed. For thick foils the bending is confined to within a distance of approximately Λ of the upper and lower surfaces. Material near the center layers exhibits the same tetragonal distortion as the bulk material, with the tetragonal axis along the modulation direction, x, and strain amplitude $\varepsilon_0(1 + \nu)/(1 - \nu)$ along y and z. The bending amplitude at the surfaces is $2(1 + \nu)\varepsilon_0$, but does not decrease monotonically to zero with increasing depth. Instead, it swings to a smaller negative value at a depth $\sim\Lambda/2\pi$ before decreasing monotonically. It is important to note that it is only the thicker specimens, where $t >> \Lambda$, that contain the same tetragonal distortion as the bulk material. In the limit $t/\Lambda \to 0$, the axis of the tetragonal distortion is along y and the strain amplitude along x and z is reduced to $\varepsilon_0(1 + \nu)$. For the intermediate values, particularly $t/\Lambda \approx 1$, the whole crystal is bent and, in general, the distortion is monoclinic.

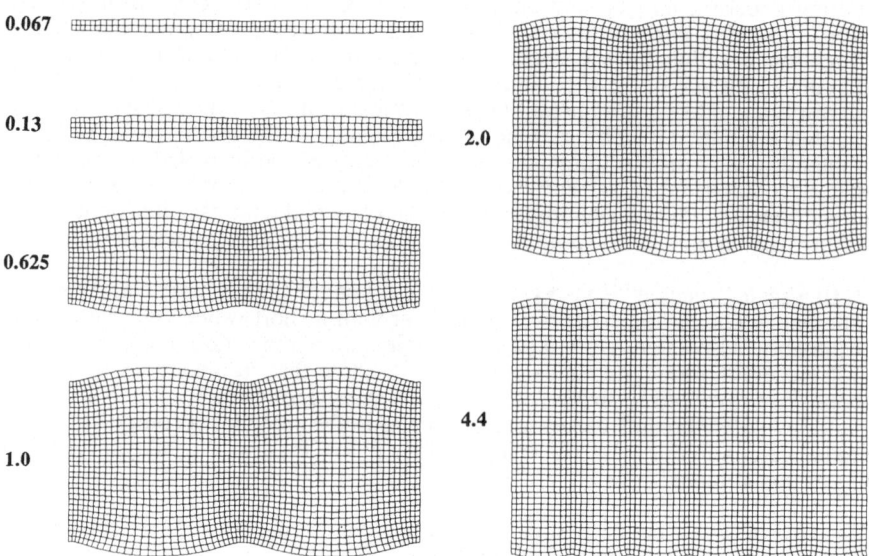

Figure 2.   Cross sectional views illustrating the elastic relaxation of a sinusoidal dilatation wave, $a_x = a_y = a_z = a_0\{1 + \varepsilon_0\sin(2\pi x/\Lambda)\}$, in a thin foil as a function of foil thickness t, expressed as t/Λ. The calculations are for $\varepsilon_0 = 0.1$.

The contrast calculated from two–beam theory gives good qualitative agreement with images of $In_{0.72}Ga_{0.28}As_{0.63}P_{0.37}$ for a strain amplitude of the order of $\varepsilon_0 \approx 10^{-3}$ and $\Lambda \approx 200$ nm. Figure 3 shows the two–beam, column approximation bright and dark field computed contrasts for $\varepsilon_0 = 10^{-3}$, and $\nu = 0.33$. For comparison, the accompanying distortion is added (sketched in exaggerated form, with $\varepsilon_0 = 0.1$). In agreement with experiment, dark field contrast is stronger than bright field and dark field contrasts are asymmetric about the maxima and minima in lattice parameter. It is a useful rule of thumb to note that, in dark field, when crossing from an image region of dark intensity to a region of bright intensity in the same direction as **g**, a minimum in unit cell dimension is traversed. This has been confirmed in the $In_{0.72}Ga_{0.28}As_{0.63}P_{0.37}$ case with X–ray microanalysis in the STEM [19]. Calculations show that, in this material, structure factor contrasts are negligible.

The sensitivity of image contrast to the amplitude of the predominant Fourier coefficients can be seen when comparing the $2\bar{2}0$ strong beam and weak beam images shown in figures 4a and 4b. The long period contrast (where $\Lambda > \xi_{220}$) diminishes under weak beam conditions, since the amplitude of Δk^{-1} decreases to a value less than ξ_{220} with increasing w. Conversely, the short period "speckle" contrast sharpens up, since the interband coupling terms are now better attuned to the shorter wavelengths. The magnitude of the operating Bragg reflection, **g**, also plays a significant role, as can be seen on comparing the $0\bar{4}0$ and $0\bar{2}0$ dark field images in Figure 4. The amplitude of dR_x/dz is, of course, identical in both images, however, the **g** vector is half the magnitude in $0\bar{2}0$ compared with $0\bar{4}0$. Although the extinction distance of $0\bar{2}0$ is nearly twice as long as $0\bar{4}0$ ($\xi_{400} \approx 85$ nm, $\xi_{200} \approx 145$ nm), and is comparable to the modulation wavelength of ~ 200 nm, contrast is still significantly weaker in the $0\bar{2}0$ image compared with the $0\bar{4}0$ image.

A gradation in modulation amplitude with depth, of the form noted by Cherns *et al.* [11], will give rise to similar contrasts to those observed for elastic relaxation. However, the rule of thumb will be different; a column of material which has the smaller lattice parameter

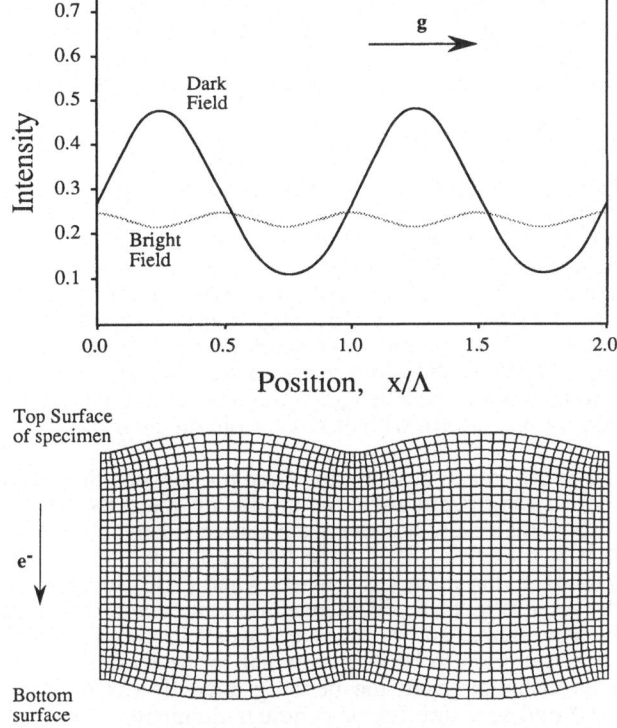

Figure 3.   Contrasts calculated from the two–beam column approximation for a sinusoidal dilatation wave, as a function of position x/Λ. Bright field contrasts
are symmetrical about the maxima and minima of the dilatation wave,
whereas the dark field contrasts are asymmetric and stronger. The asymmetry in dark field is such that when the intensity goes from black to white
in the same direction as **g**, a minimum in lattice parameter is crossed.

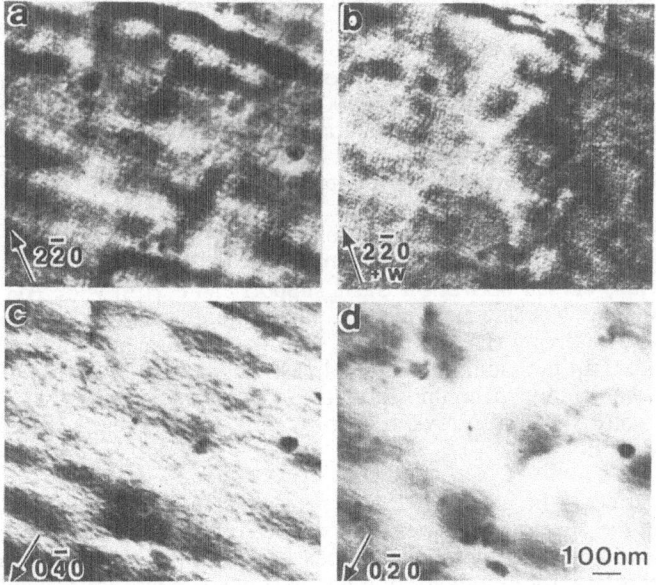

Figure 4.   Spinodally decomposed $In_{0.72}Ga_{0.28}As_{0.63}P_{0.37}$. a). $2\bar{2}0$ (strong beam) dark
field. b) $2\bar{2}0$ weak beam. c) $0\bar{4}0$ dark field. d) $0\bar{2}0$ dark field.

at the electron beam entrance surface will generate a black–white contrast vector parallel to **g**. However, unlike the contribution from relaxation, at a given region in the specimen, the sign of this vector should reverse if the specimen is turned upside down. This effect might provide an indirect method for detecting composition uniformity along the beam direction.

Strained Layer Superlattices and Interfaces

Strained layer superlattices are also subject to relaxation on thinning [20; 21]. Since these structures are man–made, there is more potential variability in the relative lattice mismatch between layers and the abruptness of the interfaces. Furthermore, since the individual layers can be made from widely disparate materials, structure factor contrasts can also be important. The strain relaxation field for superlattices can be modelled in exactly the same way as for the sinusoidal case by Fourier decomposing the superlattice strain modulation and applying the relaxation independently to each Fourier component [20; 22]. It follows that, at any given specimen thickness, the longer wavelength Fourier components will tend to relax more relative to the shorter wavelength components, and that the extent of the relaxation will not necessarily be uniform with distance from the interface.

Due to the large difference in scattering strength between Si and Ge, Ge_xSi_{1-x}/Si superlattices exhibit both strong strain and structure factor contrasts [20; 23; 24]. In the case of Al_xGa_{1-x}As/GaAs III–V materials, however, the lattice mismatch between the GaAs and AlAs end–members is small ($\sim 1.3 \times 10^{-3}$; AlAs has the smaller unit cell constant) and structure factor contrast tends to dominate, particularly when {200} imaging conditions are used (the {200} structure factor reflects the difference in atomic scattering factors of the constituent III–type and V–type atoms, and is thus very weak in GaAs, but relatively strong in AlAs). Of course, if **g** is chosen to be perpendicular to the modulation direction, such that d(**g**.**R**)/dz = 0, the contribution from the bending terms is essentially eliminated (under two–beam conditions) and structure factor contrasts dominate. It is typically observed in Al_xGa_{1-x}As/GaAs materials, imaged near the [01$\bar{1}$] axis, that the interface boundaries are less well–defined in 022 images, perpendicular to the modulation direction, than in 400 images, even though the structure factors are similar. This is due, in part, to the strain contribution sharpening up the interface contrasts under 400 conditions. The breakdown of the column approximation will also play a role in determining interface contrasts. To correctly model contrasts near abrupt interfaces, the Takagi equations should be used, as they do not rely on the column approximation [25].

Figure 5 shows 200 and 400 dark field micrographs of an $Al_{0.3}Ga_{0.7}$As/GaAs superlattice with layer widths of 90 and 10 nm respectively, to give an overall wavelength of 100 nm. The relative lattice mismatch between the layers is $\sim 4 \times 10^{-4}$. Structure factor contrasts predominate, particularly in the 200 image. However, faint, but sharp, contrast lines are visible at the interfaces in some regions of the 400 image. Interface contrasts are also enhanced under weak beam conditions [23]. Such contrasts are not purely the result of elastic relaxation. Calculations [26] verify that dynamical coupling effects across the interface (ie. the breakdown of the column approximation) contribute to image contrasts.

In strained layer superlattices, relaxation contrasts are most pronounced in the vicinity of a single interface where the effective value of Λ is large. Figure 6 shows an interface in a thick (~ 200 nm) crystal between a GaAs support and a 2μm wide $Al_{0.3}Ga_{0.7}$As layer. Shown are the 200 and $\bar{2}$00 dark field images, parallel (and anti–parallel) to the modulation direction, with accompanying HAAD images. The area is near a hole in the foil and thus the strain is also relaxing in the vicinity of the hole as well as at the upper and lower surfaces. As in the case of the spinodal decomposition, the contrast reverses sign with **g**, and the high angle annular detector signal also reverses sign with **g** but exhibits the opposite contrast to that seen in 200 dark field.

Convergent beam imaging (CBIM) experiments show that, at a distance t from an isolated interface, the specimen reaches 10% of the fully relaxed value of $\varepsilon_0(1 + v)$ [27]. This is in excellent agreement with calculations based on the elastic relaxation model [1]. (This result corrects an error of a factor of 6 which appears in previous calculations [20].)

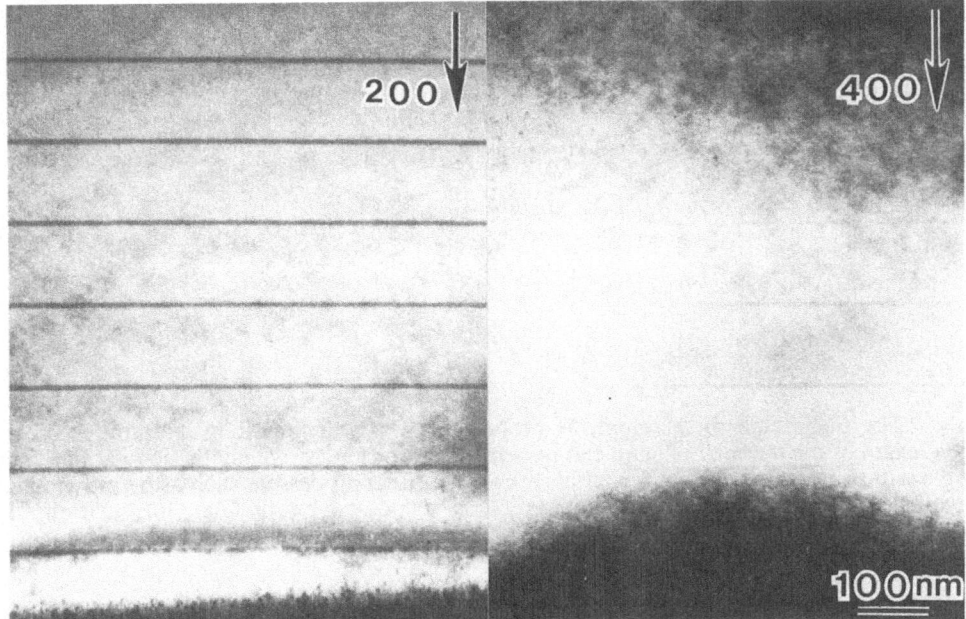

Figure 5. TEM images of an $Al_{0.3}Ga_{0.7}As$/GaAs superlattice with layer widths of 90 and 10 nm respectively, to give an overall wavelength of 100 nm. a) 200 dark field. b) 400 dark field. Structure factor contrasts dominate in the 200 image. The lattice mismatch is too weak for strain contrasts to dominate, although they are still detectable.

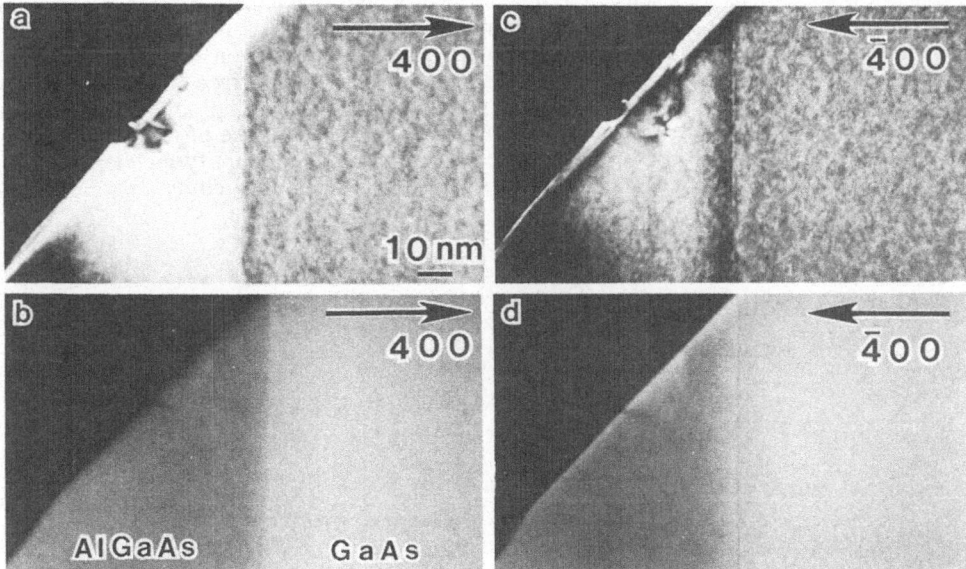

Figure 6. Interface in a thick crystal between GaAs and $Al_{0.3}Ga_{0.7}As$. a) 200 dark field. b) $\bar{2}$00 dark field. c) 200 HAAD image. d) $\bar{2}$00 HAAD image. Note the weak black–white contrasts at the interface which reverse sign with **g**. Contrasts in the HAAD images are complementary to the dark field images. These contrasts arise in part from relaxation and from dynamical scattering effects at the interface.

Surface Ripple in Superlattices

Even though surface relaxation will have negligible effect on bulk properties, the surfaces perpendicular to the modulation direction will always be rippled due to the ever–present relaxation. If the layer widths are a and b, and the intrinsic cell constants are a_A and a_B respectively, the surface ripple is given by the Fourier series

$$R_{zz} = \frac{2(1+\nu)}{\pi^2} \varepsilon_0 \Lambda \sum_{m=1}^{\infty} \left\{ \frac{1}{m^2} \sin\left(\frac{m\pi a}{\Lambda}\right) \cos\left(\frac{2m\pi x}{\Lambda}\right) \right\} \qquad \ldots (10)$$

where, the origin is centered in layer A, and here

$$\varepsilon_0 = \frac{(a+b)(a_A - a_B)}{(a\,a_A + b\,a_B)} \; ; \qquad \Lambda = a+b$$

The magnitude of the ripple is proportional to both the strain amplitude and the wavelength of the modulation, and can be significant for long wavelength modulations. This ripple will be important if such materials are to be further processed, such as by growing epilayers perpendicular to the modulation direction. As pointed out by Glas [10], such rippling may play a role in the evolution of the LPE–grown spinodally–decomposed $In_{0.72}Ga_{0.28}As_{0.63}P_{0.37}$ as the epilayer thickness increases.

Evidence for surface ripple in $Al_xGa_{1-x}As/GaAs$ has been found by Yamamoto [28] using reflection electron microscopy. However, the ripple amplitude estimated from image contrasts ($\sim 10^{-2}$ nm) is somewhat larger than that predicted by equation 10 ($\sim 2 \times 10^{-3}$ nm).

Steps at interfaces

Elastic relaxation as a phenomenon does not occur exclusively when materials are thinned. Relaxation can also occur around steps at interfaces. This relaxation is present in the bulk material, and is a potential source of strong localized image contrasts, particularly for plan view specimens. In a sense, the relaxation around a step can be likened to that at an aneurysm, where material which is under compression at one side of an interface is presented with an opportunity to intrude into the material under tension on the other side, and thereby relieve some of the strain energy. The strain around an interface step can be calculated by superimposing the strain field from a platelet precipitate in a homogeneous material with the tetragonal distortion from the bulk superlattice. The outcome of this superimposition is sketched in figure 7. It is clear that the relaxation tends to amplify the step's contribution to the interface roughness, since it also bends the lattice in its vicinity.

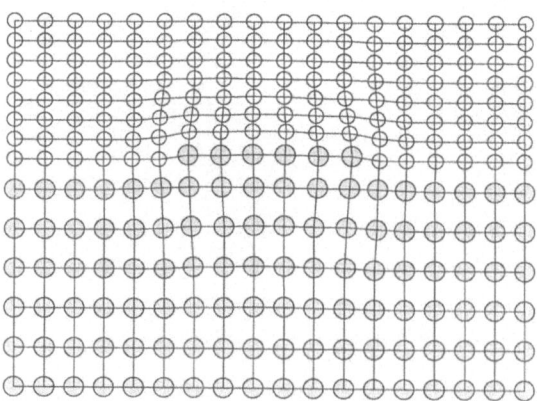

Figure 7.   Sketch of the strain field around a step at a coherent interface between two lattice mismatched layers. This form of relaxation does not arise from specimen thinning but is inherent in the interface structure.

Relaxation around interface steps may have been responsible for the peculiar image features observed by Vincent *et al.* [29] in bend contours associated with superlattice diffraction spots, from superlattices oriented in 'plan view'. Strong relaxation contrasts will appear in the superlattice reflections because these alone are sensitive to the pronounced dR_z/dx bending parallel to the interfaces (see figure 7). The principal lattice reflections, being perpendicular to the foil normal, are insensitive to these components of the bending.

SUMMARY

The microscopist should beware that not all specimen strain fields, detected through their image contrasts, are necessarily inherent to the original material. Apart from bending and buckling introduced by the sample holder, and uneven specimen heating due to the incident beam, the specimen thinning process itself can relax internal stresses associated with crystal defects and interfaces. The extent of relaxation is most pronounced for those Fourier components of the strain field along the beam direction, whose wavelength is comparable to, or greater than, the specimen thickness. When relaxation occurs, structural details measured in the micrograph are not necessarily representative of either the bulk or the unstressed material. With improved modelling of elastic relaxation, TEM strain contrasts might provide a convenient method of analyzing the spatial variation in local elastic constants of composition–modulated materials.

ACKNOWLEDGMENTS

The author would like to thank his friends and colleagues, J. M. Gibson, S. B. Rice, A. J. Jacobson, J. M. Newsam, T. Moustakas, H. Launois, F. Glas and A. Howie, for their help and encouragement, and for many stimulating discussions over the years.

REFERENCES

[1] M. M. J. Treacy, J. M. Gibson & A. Howie, On Elastic Relaxation and Long Wavelength Microstructures in Spinodally Decomposed $In_xGa_{1-x}As_yP_{1-y}$ Epitaxial Layers, Phil. Mag. 51:389 (1985).

[2] K. Ploog, Microscopical structuring of solids by molecular beam Epitaxy – Spatially Resolved Materials Synthesis, Angew. Chemie, 27:593 (1988).

[3] H. Hashimoto & M. Mannani, On The Contrast Of The Electron Microscopic Image Due To An Edge Dislocation, Acta Cryst., 13: 363 (1960).

[4] P. B. Hirsch, A. Howie, R. B. Nicholson, D. W. Pashley and M. J. Whelan, "Electron Microscopy of Thin Crystals," Krieger, New York (1977).

[5] M. F. Ashby & L. M. Brown, Diffraction Contrast From Spherically Symmetrical Coherency Strains, Phil. Mag. 8:1083 (1963a); On Diffraction Contrast From Inclusions, Phil. Mag. 8:1649 (1963b).

[6] D. J. H. Cockayne, I. L. F. Ray & M. J. Whelan, Investigations Of Dislocation Strain Fields Using Weak Beams, Phil. Mag. 20:1265 (1969).

[7] W. M. Stobbs & C. H. Sworn, The Weak Beam Technique As Applied To The Determination Of The Stacking Fault Energy Of Copper, Phil. Mag. 24:1365 (1971).

[8] A. Putnis and J. D. C. McConnell, "Principles Of Mineral Behaviour," Elsevier, New York (1980).

[9] P. Hénoc, A. Izrael, M. Quillec & H. Launois, Composition Modulation In $In_xGa_{1-x}As_yP_{1-y}$ LPE Layers Lattice Matched To InP Substrates, Appl. Phys. Letts., 40:963 (1980).

[10] F. Glas, Démixtion et ordre local dans les composés semiconducteurs III–V: étude par microscopie électronique et microanalyse des couches épitaxiées d'alliages InGaAsP. Thesis, No 3212, Université de Paris–sud, Orsay (1986): Also, see article by Glas in this proceedings

[11] D. Cherns, P. D. Greene, A. Hainsworth & A. R. Preston, Phase Separation in InGaAsP Epitaxial Layers, in: "Microscopy of Semiconductor Materials", eds. A. G. Cullis & P. D. Augustus, Inst. Phys. conf. Ser. No. 87, p83, The Institute of Physics, London–Bristol (1987).

[12] B. de Cremoux, P. Hirtz & J. Ricciardi, On The Presence Of A Solid Immiscibility Domain In The GaInAsP Phase Diagram, in: "Gallium Arsenide And related Compounds" H. W. Thim, ed., Inst. Phys. Conf. Ser. No 56, p 115, The Institute of Physics, London (1980).

[13] B. de Cremoux, Instability criteria in ternary and quaternary III–V epitaxial solid solutions, J. Phys., Paris, 43:C5–19 (1982).

[14] G. B. Stringfellow, Miscibility gaps in quaternary III/V alloys, J. Crystal Growth, 58:194 (1982).

[15] J. P. Gowers, TEM image contrast from clustering in Ga–In containing III–V alloys, Appl. Phys. A., 31:23 (1983).

[16] F. Glas & P. Hénoc, Study of static atomic displacements by channelled–electron–beam–induced X–ray emission: Application to $In_{0.53}Ga_{0.47}As$ alloys., Phil. Mag., 56:311, (1987).

[17] M. Ichimura & A. Sasaki, Bond statistics and their influence on materials properties of III–V quaternary alloys of type $(AB)^{III} (CD)^{V}$, J. Electronic Mats., 17:305 (1988).

[18] M. M. J. Treacy & J. M. Gibson, On the detection of point defects in crystals using high–angle diffuse scattering in the STEM, Inst. Phys. Conf. Ser. No. 61, p 263 The Institute of Physics, London (1982).

[19] F. Glas, M. M. J. Treacy, M. Quillec, & H. Launois, Interface spinodal decomposition in $In_xGa_{1-x}As_yP_{1-y}$ lattice matched to InP, J. Phys., Paris, 43:C5–11 (1982).

[20] J. M. Gibson, R. Hull, J. C. Bean & M. M. J. Treacy, Elastic relaxation in transmission electron microscopy of strained–layer superlattices, Appl. Phys. Letts., 46:649 (1985).

[21] G. C. Weatherly, D. D. Perovic & D. C. Houghton, Elastic relaxation effects in strained layer Si–Ge superlattices, in: "Microscopy of Semiconductor Materials", eds A. G. Cullis & P. D. Augustus, Inst. Phys. Conf. Ser. No. 87, p237, The Institute of Physics, London–Bristol (1987).

[22] J. M. Gibson & M. M. J. Treacy, The effect of elastic relaxation on the local structure of lattice–modulated thin films, Ultramicroscopy, 14:345 (1984).

[23] S. McKernan, B. C. De Cooman, J. R. Conner, S. R. Summerfelt & C. B. Carter, Electron Microscope Imaging of II–V Compound Superlattices, in: "Microscopy of Semiconductor Materials", eds A. G. Cullis & P. D. Augustus, Inst. Phys. conf. Ser. No. 87, p201 The Institute of Physics, London–Bristol (1987).

[24] U. Bangert & P. Charsley, Diffraction contrast of tilted interfaces in $Ga_{0.7}Al_{0.3}As/$GaAs heterostructures, in: "Microscopy of Semiconductor Materials", Inst. Phys. Conf. Ser. No. 87, p89, The Institute of Physics, London (1987).

[25] A. Howie & Z. S. Basinski, Approximations of the dynamical theory of diffraction contrast, Phil. Mag., 17:1039 (1968).

[26] J. M. Gibson, private communication, (1987).

[27] C. J. Humphreys, D. J. Eaglesham, D. M. Maher & H. L. Fraser, CBED and CBIM from semiconductors and Superconductors, Ultramicroscopy, 26:13 (1988).

[28] N. Yamamoto, REM of GaAs/Al_xGa_{1-x}As superlattice, in "Proceedings of the 11th International Congress on Electron Microscopy", eds. T. Inura, S. Maruse & T. Suzuki, Japanese Society of Electron Microscopy, Vol II:1481(1986).

[29] R. Vincent, D. Cherns, S. J. Bailey & H. Morkoç, Structure of AlGaAs/GaAs multilayers imaged in superlattice reflections, Phil. Mag. Letts., 56, No1:1 (1987).

SURFACE AND THIN FILM GROWTH STUDIED BY REFLECTION HIGH ENERGY ELECTRON DIFFRACTION

P.J. Dobson

Department of Engineering Science, University of Oxford
Parks Road
Oxford   OX1 3PJ

1. INTRODUCTION

Reflection High Energy Electron Diffraction (RHEED) continues to play an important role in surface research. It is used routinely to monitor the growth of films and epitaxial layers, particularly during molecular beam epitaxy (MBE) and it may still provide a means of providing detailed and accurate information about surface reconstruction. The increasing use of reflection electron microscopy also provides some impetus to obtain a more detailed description of electron scattering and diffraction from surfaces. In this short review I will place emphasis on the description of the most significant features in RHEED patterns from semiconductor surfaces and, in particular, describe some of the most significant features of rocking curves. Finally, I will examine the phenomenon of variations and oscillations of the intensity of RHEED patterns during epitaxial growth.

2. FORMATION OF RHEED PATTERNS

In common with all other diffraction techniques, the most convenient starting point is to use the Ewald construction to describe the main features in diffraction patterns. In the case of RHEED, first of all we have to consider what form the reciprocal lattice should take. This is not straightforward, since electrons of energy 10-100 keV have rather restricted mean free paths [1,2] and, at the low angles of incidence which are used, the sampled depth is only a few atomic layers. If the diffraction was restricted to contributions from the top layer only, then for a regular flat crystal surface the reciprocal lattice would consist of an array of rods whose spacing is inversely related to the inter-row spacing of atoms [3]. We shall use this representation, but we will treat the rods as being modulated at the "bulk" reciprocal lattice points to allow for the effects of finite penetration of the electron beam into the underlying crystal layers. The Ewald construction for a reciprocal lattice of rods is shown in fig. 1 [2] and it will give rise to a set of beams lying on an arc defined by the zero order Laue zone. Each zone will contribute an arc of beams as illustrated in fig. 2 for the case of a (2x4) reciprocal lattice of the GaAs (001) surface. For the [1$\bar{1}$0] beam direction there are three fraction order Laue zones i.e.: $\frac{1}{4}, \frac{2}{4}, \frac{3}{4}$ between the zero order and first (bulk) zone. These Laue zones provide a convenient way of obtaining a plan view projection of the reciprocal lattice rods and has formed the basis of a unique design of RHEED

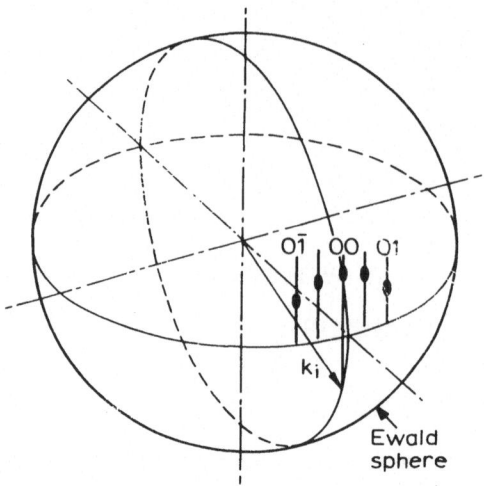

Fig.1 Ewald construction showing the intersection of the Ewald sphere with a set of reciprocal lattice rods. Note that these points of intersection lie on an arc known as a Laue zone.

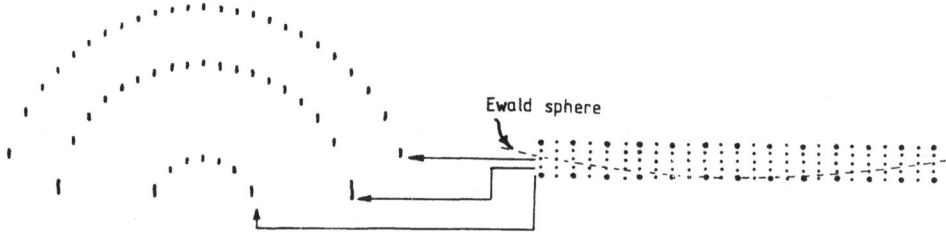

Fig.2 Schematic diagram of a RHEED pattern for a GaAs (001) 2x4 surface along the [110] direction, showing the zero, 1/4 and 1/2 order Laue zones and their relation to the reciprocal lattice section on the right.

apparatus by Ino[4]. Generally, any RHEED equipment can be used to display these high order Laue zones if the "camera length" i.e: the sample to fluorescent screen distance, is made sufficiently short. This will result in some loss of resolution of the detail perpendicular to the reciprocal lattice rods, but could provide useful information about the symmetry of the surface unit cell and, as we will now describe, disorder effects.

Disorder manifests itself in several ways in RHEED. Firstly, any amorphous or polycrystalline material will give patterns consisting of diffuse or sharp semicircular rings (see for example the books and reviews by Thomson and Cochrane, [5] Pinsker, [6] Vainshtein [7] and Bauer [8]). These are well known effects and can be easily interpreted, the polycrystalline rings being simply electron diffraction Debye-Scherrer patterns.

In MBE, there is a feature in RHEED patterns which is strongly indicative of one-dimensional disorder, namely elongated streaks. Such streaks frequently extend all the way between the zero order and adjacent Laue zones. These streaks result from an intersection of a sheet in reciprocal space and the Ewald sphere. The origin of the sheet in reciprocal space is some one-dimensional arrangement in real space. There are several possible origins of this one dimensional disorder, ranging from steps [9-11] rows of atoms [13] or anti-phase boundaries [14,15]. The latter, in particular, is very likely to occur on reconstructed semiconductors since adjacent unit cells may be an integral fraction out of phase with each other in terms of dimer bond formation and re-arrangement [12,14]. These anti-phase boundary effects will give sheets in reciprocal space which pass through the $\frac{1}{2}$ order features for the [110] azimuth (fig.3). The sheet nature of the reciprocal space features becomes particularly apparent for other azimuths where the plane of incidence lies at an angle to the reciprocal lattice sheet, resulting in streaks which are curved [12].

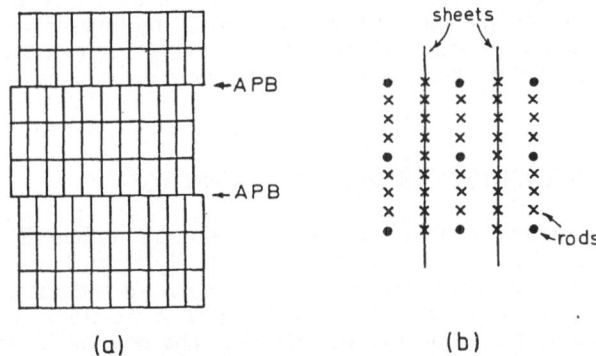

(a)   (b)

Fig.3   (a) Real space representation of one-dimensional disorder arising from anti-phase boundaries (APB) between 2x4 units.

(b) Section of reciprocal space for the 2x4 reconstruction showing sheets in reciprocal space arising from the APBs passing through the 1/2 order rods.

It must be emphasised that statements attributing the presence of long well defined streaks to flat well-ordered surfaces, which have often been made in publications about MBE growth, are incorrect. Long streaks are indicative of disorder and more effort needs to be made in establishing the nature of the disorder i.e: steps, rows of atoms or anti-phase boundaries, and of quantifying this disorder.

The topic of diffraction from regular stepped surfaces has been dealt with at length for low energy electron diffraction (LEED) by Henzler [16]. The reciprocal lattice construction which he uses can be directly applied to RHEED and is basically a convolution of reciprocal lattice rods from the geometric "average" surface and the rods from the low index terraces. Pukite et al. [17] have demonstrated how the degree of misorientation can be determined from the resulting diffraction features. Surprisingly, little use has been made of the ability of RHEED to determine the step distribution during growth by MBE. This is most definitely within the capabilities of the technique, because as we will see in a later section the RHEED intensity is very sensitive to the presence of steps. The change of _shape_ of certain diffraction features should tell us about the change of step distributions.

One other type of feature is often seen in RHEED patterns during thin film growth and that is the quasi-transmission spot pattern. This occurs when growth is three dimensional and the electron beam penetrates the asperities of the three dimensional islands or growth structures. Sometimes it is possible to infer the size of the islands from the diffraction broadening of the spots. It is also often possible to see additional features due to stacking faults and twins [18,19]. The interpretation of such features follows that of conventional transmission electron diffraction and is described by Hirsch et al [20]. In the limit of three dimensional island growth, when islands are large (~ μm across) there could be additional inclined streaked features from the sides of the islands if they have a well developed facet structure [21].

In summary, it can be said that a simple visual inspection of RHEED patterns can yield a great deal of morphological and structural information. It is also possible to obtain the in-plane lattice spacings to a higher accuracy by measuring the spacing between features in the lowest order Laue zone parallel to the shadow edge, and indeed pseudomorphic growth and the strain in thin layers has been determined using RHEED [22].

3. QUANTITIVE DESCRIPTION OF RHEED INTENSITIES

In the diffraction pattern from a clean, flat well order surface (if such a thing exists!) the most prominent features are the short steaks lying on Laue zone arcs as illustrated in fig.1. The intensity of three features can be related to the structure factors for the surface and hence to the geometric arrangement of the atoms in the surface layers. This is the long term objective of RHEED. The relationship between the intensity and different surface structure models is not obvious and much work remains to be done before confident surface structure models can be ascribed.

3.1 Pseudo-kinematic Approach

If the intensity of a particular beam I_{HK} is measured as the angle of incidence is changed over a wide range (say from $0°$ to $5°$) then the integrated intensity $\int I_{HK} \, d\theta \cong F_{HK} F^*_{HK}$ where we have used the two dimensional rotation [23] to index a particular reciprocal lattice rod and F_{HK} is the two dimensional structure factor. Strictly this relationship is only true if there is no strong coupling (dynamical interaction) between beams, and such procedures have produced controversy when applied to low energy electron diffraction. Woodruffe [24] has demonstrated how this method breaks down for LEED. However, this approach is undoubtedly useful as a first step in surface structure determination and it has been successfully applied by Ino [25]. In the most recent variant of the technique [26] the intensity data is taken from a long time exposure photographic recording of the diffraction pattern which is taken while the angle of incidence is varied continuously, and a variable shaped annular aperture is used to allow only the Laue zone features to be recorded. Ino has successfully applied the technique to describe the atom positions for Si(111) 7x7 and 5x5 absorption structures. Despite the doubts raised about the validity of the procedure if strong dynamic coupling effects are present, this approach should be taken seriously in helping to define possible surface models for a more detailed dynamical scattering treatment.

3.2 Dynamical Scattering

The dynamical description of RHEED intensities can be performed in several ways. The early attempts [27,28] were based on Bethe's n-beam dynamical theory in which the scattering potential is expanded as a three-dimensional Fourier series. This does not appear to be a very convenient way of dealing with reflection diffraction although it is satisfactory for high energy transmission electron diffraction. The reason for this is connected with the boundary conditions, particularly when the surface structure differs from the bulk. This problem can be overcome by treating the crystal as a set of two dimensional gratings as was originally attempted by Boersch et al. [29] for the transmission case. More recently, Maksym and Beeby [30-32] have developed a method which is based on Fourier expansions only in the two dimensions parallel to the surface. In this approach, the geometric arrangement in the layers can be varied and the Schrodinger equation can be solved by integrating a set of coupled equations. The procedure which Maksym and Beeby use has been described in detail [30-34], and the outline of their method is as follows.

The two-dimensional potential is computed from tabulated data for scattering factors e.g. those of Doyle and Turner [35]. Transfer matrices which describe the scattering by the individual layers are then produced by integration of the Schrodinger equation. The transfer matrices are then converted into scattering matrices which relate the amplitudes of the waves entering and leaving the layers. The diffracted beam amplitudes are obtained by combining the scattering matrices using the layer doubling algorithm of LEED theory. In common with most other approaches to (high energy) electron diffraction, only the elastic intensities are computed, allowance for inelastic effects being made by the choice of a suitable optical potential.

This approach has met with some success in comparisons with experimental data for Mg(001) [36] and Si(001) 2x1 and (1x1) H stabilized surfaces [37]. More recently, a large number of possible reconstruction models of the 2x4 GaAs (001) surface have been examined by this method [38].

Some doubts have been expressed regarding the ability of the method adopted by Maksym and Beeby to handle large numbers of evanescent waves such as may occur on reconstructed surfaces. This led Tong and co-workers [39,40] to develop their invariant-imbedding method. In this method, the ratio of the wave function and its first derivative - called the R-matrix - is solved by a recursion formula. This is essentially a layer-by-layer approach with the R matrices being solved for individual layers and combinations of layers. Tong claims good convergence and stability properties for this method and the agreement between theory and experiment for GaAs (110) is quite impressive [39].

Whichever method is adopted, the first objective should be to construct a reasonable model based on any additional information about the surface e.g. from photoemission or scanning tunneling microscopy etc... Then, the two-dimensional structure factors should be calculated and compared roughly with the experimental intensities, particularly of the fractional order beams. This can eliminate many models and will save expensive time consuming computations.

4. SEMI-QUANTITATIVE DESCRIPTION OF ROCKING CURVES FROM A FLAT SURFACE

In this section we will show how we can give a phenomenological description of the main features in a rocking curve. Any full dynamical treatment will, or should, be able to account for the same features. We can describe a rocking curve from a flat surface in terms of azimuthally independent features which result from primary Bragg scattering by the crystal planes parallel to the surface and other features due to secondary Bragg scattering (resonances) and surface resonances which are strongly dependent on the beam azimuth. All of these features appear at angles which require some allowance to be made of the refraction of the electron beam by the crystal potential. Here, we will consider three main origins of structure in the rocking curve, all of which can be identified without recourse to major theoretical calculations. The features are those arising from primary Bragg scattering, secondary Bragg scattering (often referred to as double diffraction) and surface resonance/beam emergence scattering.

Primary Bragg scattering will give maxima for the allowed (hkl) reflections from an (hkl) surface. For example, for the (001) GaAs surface we expect strong reflections for the 004 and 008 conditions and fairly weak reflections for the 002 and 006 conditions. The incident angle for these conditions is found by estimating the Bragg angle for each reflection <u>inside</u> the solid θ_{in} and then applying the refraction condition for θ_o, the angle outside of the solid i.e.

$$\cos \theta_o = \left(1 + \frac{V_o}{E}\right)^{1/2} \cos \theta_{in} \qquad (1)$$

where V_o is the inner potential and E is the energy of the electron beam. This will give the angular position of the centroid of the reflected beam. In practice, the reflection has an angular width which is related to the particular Fourier potential V_{hkl} for that reflection. The angular limits can be obtained from

$$\cos \theta_o = \left(1 + \frac{V_o \pm V_{hkl}}{E}\right)^{1/2} \cos \theta_{in} \qquad (2)$$

The refraction effects will often completely suppress some low angle reflections, i.e. prevent beams from escaping, and will give rise to strong asymmetry of low angle reflections. Finally, we should note that there should not be any azimuthal dependence for these primary Bragg features from planes which are parallel to the crystal surface.

Secondary Bragg scattering gives rise to maxima in the specular beam when other beams lying outside the plane of incidence are excited. This is sometimes referred to as "double diffraction", and is the condition referred to by Miyake and Hayakawa [41] as the "second kind of intensity anomaly'. Again, we consider the situation which exists inside the "solid" in order to define the angles θ_{in} for such a condition and then apply the refraction condition to estimate the external angles of observation θ_o. Of course, this condition will be strongly azimuth dependent. Taking (001) GaAs as an example, we will expect a strong secondary Bragg resonance to occur when the 115 beams are excited if the incident beam lies in a plane directed along the <110> azimuths. We can further estimate that at an incident beam energy of 12.5 kV this will occur when $\theta_{in} = 2.98°$. Using realistic values for the refractive inner potential, [42] $\theta_o = 2.33°$ for this 115 secondary Bragg condition. Now, any deviation from the precise <110> azimuth will profoundly change the situation i.e. the beams will be out of resonance, no coupling between the 115 and the specular beam will occur and the maximum will be absent. Estimation of the range of incident polar or azimuthal angles over which the condition occurs is not so simple since the condition is now a three or four beam condition and more Fourier potential terms are involved than in equation 2. As has already been stated, this condition is the one referred to as the "second kind of intensity anomaly" by Miyake and Hayakawa [41] and it is recognised by the condition when the specular beam crosses the appropriate inclined hkl Kikuchi lines. For the example above, it occurs when the specular beam crosses the 115 Kikuchi line. The Kikuchi line merely provides an additional geometric indicator of the precise condition of resonance. As noted by Miyake and Hayakawa, the specular beam often shows an order of magnitude increase in its intensity when the condition is fulfilled.

The third source of structure in the specular beam is when there is strong coupling to a surface related beam. Here, we think of the two-dimensionality of the surface giving rise to a reciprocal lattice of rods. When the Ewald sphere is tangential to a rod, a surface wave is said to be excited [43,44]. This is strictly the condition for beam emergence. However, at an incident angle just lower than necessary for beam emergence there will still be a surface wave excited in the surface region of the solid, since the Ewald condition will be met by electrons which have entered the surface and have a correspondingly larger wave-vector than electrons outside of the solid. Hence there will be coupling between this surface wave and the specular beam, leading to a maximum of intensity in the latter. This effect can be predicted from a knowledge of the 2-D cell symmetry and some inner potential correction. This correction is not straightforward however. In order to define the correction, we need to be able to estimate the two-dimensional Fourier components of the potential V_{HK} and for this, we need the details about the actual surface crystallographic cell. This is where the true surface crystallographic information enters in to the rocking curves. We can summarise by saying that the reconstruction symmetry can tell us at what incident angles the surface resonance effects will occur, but the width or shape of these features tell us about the crystallographic detail within the reconstructed unit cells.

We can see the significance of the surface resonance contributions by comparing the rocking curves from the orthogonal [$\bar{1}$10] and [110] azimuths of the (001) GaAs surface which has a (2x4) arsenic stabilized reconstruction [45] fig.4. The incident beam along the [$\bar{1}$10] azimuth excites 1/4 order beams, whilst along the [110] azimuth only 1/2 order beams will be excited. Therefore, for the [$\bar{1}$10] azimuth there will be twice as many resonance/beam emergence conditions when the polar angle (i.e. incident angle) is varied, corresponding to each set of 1/4 order beams. At first sight, one might expect this to give much more structure in the [$\bar{1}$10] rocking curve relative to that for the [110]. However the 2-D Fourier coefficients will give each beam emergence condition a finite angular width, and this gives overlap of the features associated with each 1/4 order condition and thereby smooths out the rocking curves for the [$\bar{1}$10] azimuth.

We can also see the rationale behind the large differences in rocking curves which exist for different reconstructions when observed along one particular azimuth. In fig.5 we compare the rocking curves for the c(4x4), (2x4) and (3x1) reconstructions for the GaAs (001) surface.

It would have been interesting to compare the arsenic rich (2x4) [$\bar{1}$10] rocking curve with the gallium rich (4x2) [110] rocking curve since both show 1/4 order reconstruction features. However, so far, it has not been possible to obtain rocking curve data from the gallium rich (4x2) surface since it is difficult to maintain stability for the long recording times required. Faster recording methods for obtaining rocking curves are highly desirable.

We note that in a recent publication of results for the (110) cleavage surface of GaAs, Jamison et al [46] also emphasise the fact that surface resonant features tend to dominate rocking curves.

5. INTENSITY VARIATIONS IN RHEED DURING EPITAXIAL GROWTH

When epitaxial growth is initiated, oscillations of the intensity of diffracted beams can be observed [47-62] figure 6. This is a widely reported phenomenon and has been seen for III-V, II-VI [52,53] and group IV [54-56] semiconductors and for metal epitaxy [57,58]. Furthermore, oscillations of the intensity of the diffuse background, the secondary electron emission [59] or the sample current [12,60] have also been observed.

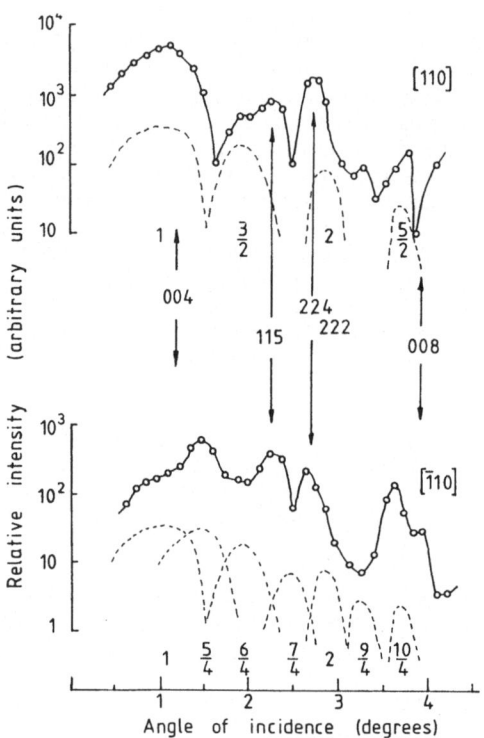

Fig.4 Specular beam rocking curves for the two orthogonal [110] and [1̄10] azimuths for the GaAs (001) 2x4 surface. The 004 and 008 Bragg reflection angles and the secondary Bragg conditions corresponding to the 115 and 224/222 excitations are indicated. The primary beam energy = 12.5 keV, and an inner potential of 13.2 eV has been applied.

The dashed curves represent the effects of beam emergence/surface resonance on the rocking curve. Each feature is labelled according to the associated emergent beam, e.g. $\frac{7}{4}$ refers to the excitation of the $0, \frac{7}{4}$ beam.

Cohen and co-workers originally attempted to explain the effect in terms of a two level interference model [49,61,62] and they tried to establish the conditions for the angle of incidence where the beams from adjacent terraces were in-phase or out-of-phase. Their model enjoyed widespread support, but it is certainly inadequate to explain most of the features in time dependent RHEED from growing surfaces. In particular it cannot explain the strong dependence on beam azimuth and the fact that for some angles of incidence <u>increases</u> in RHEED intensity occur. The two level interference model can also not help to explain the changes of diffuse background and secondary emission.

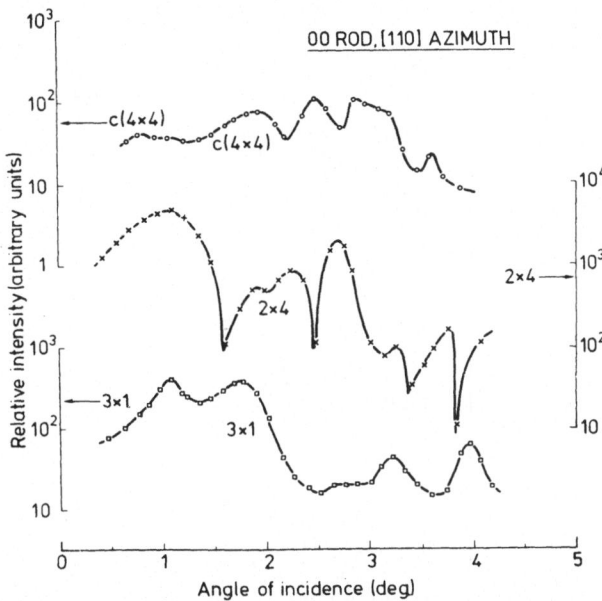

Fig.5   Comparison of the 00 beam rocking curves in the [110] azimuth for three differently reconstructed GaAs (001) surfaces. Primary beam energy = 12.5. The very different character of these curves reflects the importance of the surface resonance conditions.

Most of these effects can however be explained by a step-edge scattering model developed by Dobson and co-workers [12,50,51, 63,64]. In this model the main point is that the de Broglie wavelength for the incident electrons is ~0.1 Å, whereas the step heights are ~3Å, so steps will strongly scatter electrons, increasing the diffuse background and reducing the specular elastic intensity. Similarly, steps will change the effective absorption of the incident electrons and therefore influence the current flowing into the sample and the secondary emitted flux. Details of the azimuthal and polar angle dependence can also be understood by careful consideration of the specular scattered intensity from a surface. Here we need to recall the information contained in the

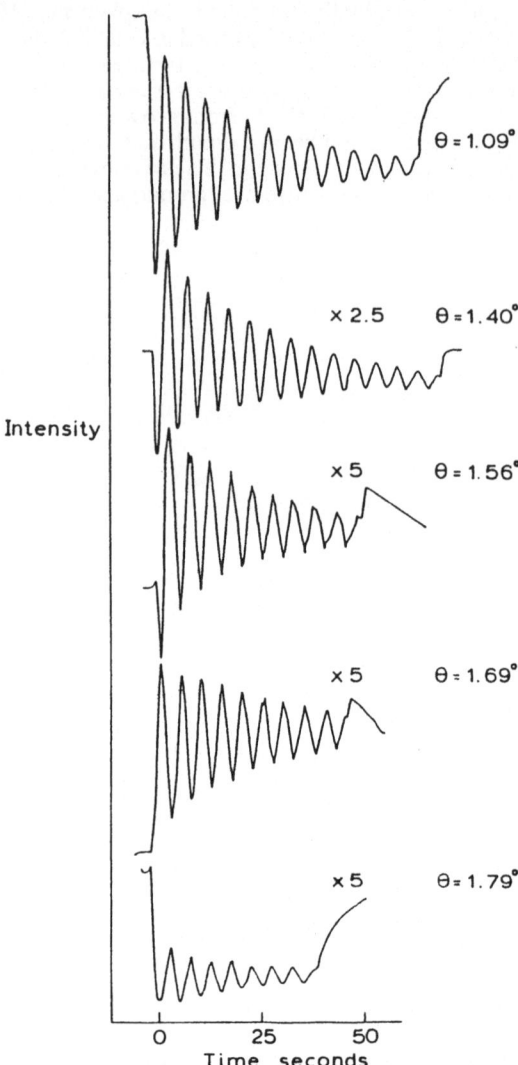

Fig.6 RHEED intensity oscillation in the specular beam observed at different angles of incidence for the [110] azimuth of a GaAs (001) 2x4 surface. Primary beam energy = 12.5 keV.

rocking curves referred to in the previous section. The rocking curve gives the angular variation of intensity from a flat surface. Now, for semiconductors, when growth is initiated, two important changes can occur. Firstly, the surface reconstruction might change due to a different surface stoichiometry (e.g. for GaAs (001) the (2x4) arsenic stable surface may tend towards the (3x1) less arsenic rich surface because of the increased gallium supply.) Secondly, two dimensional growth will give an increase in the step density at the surface and this step density will oscillate with time, being minimum at integers of a mono-molecular layer.

The effect of reconstruction changes should have a dramatic effect on the specular intensity since, as we have shown above, different reconstructions give markedly different rocking curves. Even a small change of surface composition will have a significant effect on the surface structure factor and hence the intensity of the specular and other diffracted beams. Now, if the surface stoichiometry varied periodically this could alone account for RHEED intensity oscillations. In general, for III-V materials I do not believe this to be the case. Only for the special case of migration enhanced epitaxy where the surface composition is varied significantly by alternately closing off the supply of group III or group V flux is this likely to periodically influence the RHEED. This has been beautifully demonstrated by Horikoshi [65] who showed that during a half cycle of RHEED intensity oscillation the reconstruction changes from (2x4) via (3x1) to (4x2).

In conventional MBE, the change of composition when the As/Ga surface population is changed by opening or closing the gallium shutter does manifest itself by giving an abrupt change in the intensity at the initiation or cessation of growth. Briones et al [66] were the first to draw attention to this effect and they noted that the first period of oscillation depended on the growth conditions, in particular on the arsenic overpressure. We had noted a marked dependence of the initial behaviour with diffraction condition [50]. These two apparently paradoxical views can be accommodated since the measured diffracted intensity is both composition and angle of incidence dependent. One other piece of evidence which strongly supports the mechanism for surface compositional changes of intensity is provided by the results of our study of deposition on a stepped surface at different temperatures [63]. In this experiment we still observed large changes at the initiation and cessation of growth, even when the growth did not introduce changes of step density.

More generally in order to explain the oscillatory intensity behaviour we have to look at the second origin of intensity changes, namely the changing step edge density during growth. Just prior to growth, the surface will have some step distribution which is determined by the misorientation of the crystal from a perfect low index plane, local variations in temperature and supersaturation across the surface etc.... When growth starts, the step edge density may increase, particularly if nucleation of two dimensional islands or growth centres occurs on the flat terrace regions. This will lead to a reduction of the specular reflection and other diffracted beam intensities, and an increase in the level of diffuse scattering from topographical disorder. If observations are performed at an angle of incidence and azimuth such that the diffracted intensity from the flat surface is high, (e.g. at 1.09° in fig.6) then the RHEED intensity (for specular and diffracted beams) will be reduced, reaching a minimum when the step density is at its maximum i.e. at approximately half a mono-molecular layer. On the other hand, if the observations performed at angles such that the diffracted intensity from the flat surface is low (i.e. at, or close to a minimum of the rocking curve) then diffuse scattering may start to dominate and the measured intensity will increase and reach a maximum when the step density is highest (e.g. at $\theta=1.69°$ in fig.6). If the measured intensity owes its origin to either a reduction of specular scattering or an increase in the topographical diffuse scattering we can anticipate that some interesting effects will occur when the two contributions are similar. This is illustrated schematically in fig. 7a and will give oscillations at twice the frequency of the corresponding mono-molecular growth rate. This situation has been observed in practice and depends critically, as expected, on the angle of observation (fig. 7b).

I should emphasise that this situation is very different to that reported by Sakamoto et al [67] for Si(001) growth for which double frequency oscillations in the 00 beam result from a dynamic coupling (in diffraction theory sense) between the 1/2 order beams originating from the (2x1) and (1x2) reconstructed domains and the 00 specular beam.

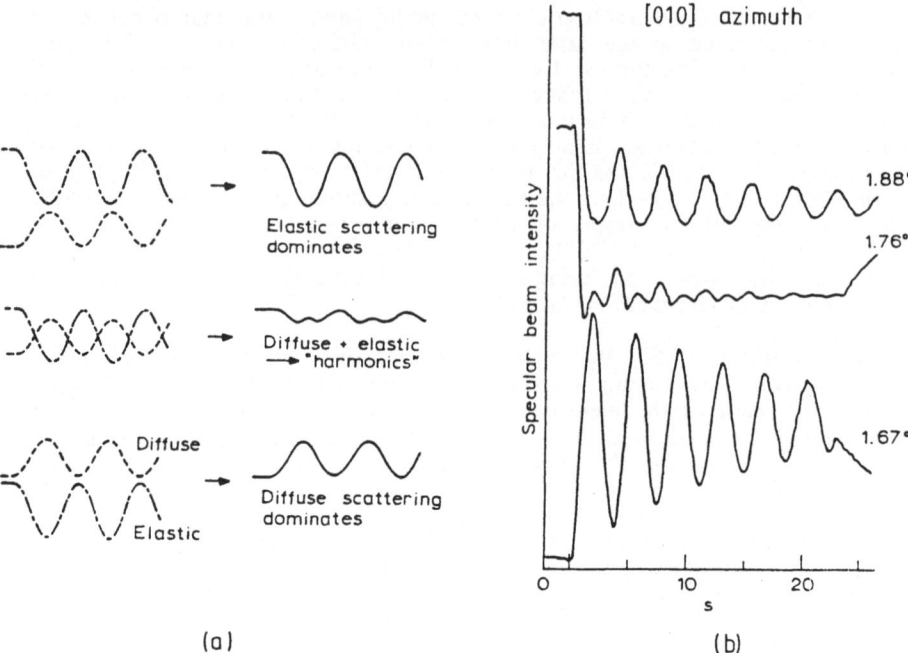

[010] azimuth

1.88°

1.76°

1.67°

Specular beam intensity

0   10   20
                s

(a)   (b)

Fig.7   (a) Schematic diagram showing how the relative contributions of the elastic
         specular scattering and the diffuse scattering intensities affect the shape of the
         observed oscillations. When the contributions are approximately the same,
         "harmonics" may occur.

         (b) The experimental evidence supporting the model. Note the very high
         sensitivity to the diffraction condition. The data at 1.67° corresponds to the
         minimum in the rocking curve for this azimuth. Primary beam energy = 12.5
         keV.

        Finally we should summarise the situation regarding the oscillations of RHEED
intensity, by saying that they mainly result from fluctuations in the step-edge density
and as such they can be used to measure the growth rate. If the conditions chosen for
observations are optimum i.e. a high specular intensity for the initial "flat" surface, then
subsequent maxima correspond to mono-molecular layer completion. The accuracy of
such a measurement will be affected by the changes to the specular intensity resulting
from surface reconstruction which can give a transient initial behaviour and some time
variation of the first period of oscillation. As growth proceeds there will also be some
statistical error in correlating the point of maximum intensity with the completion of an
integral number of mono-molecular layers. I would therefore suggest that RHEED
intensity oscillations should <u>not</u> be relied on as a method of defining the thickness of
quantum wells to better than ± 1 atomic layer.

6. FUTURE TRENDS

        In most applications of semiconductor layers grown by MBE it is necessary   to
achieve uniform growth over a large area of the substrate slice and this necessitates

substrate rotation and really rules out the use of RHEED for real-time monitoring of the growth process. This can be overcome by the use of "gated" RHEED observations i.e. observation of the pattern only at a specific azimuthal angle during the substrate rotation, or by the use of a stationary "monitor slice". The sensitivity of RHEED to surface conditions and the mode of growth will always ensure its use as the technique of choice to monitor growth by MBE and related techniques. There are perhaps two main areas which will be usefully exploited viz: the temporal recording aspect and the spectroscopic or analytical aspect.

The temporal aspect of RHEED has hardly been exploited at present. Our group [68] and others [69,70] have looked at the various time constants associated with the recovery of the diffraction intensity following cessation of growth. The time resolution was typically > 0.1s. The capability exists to greatly improve on this and pico-second resolution has been demonstrated [71]. We can expect to learn a great deal about surface processes by studying transient RHEED intensities in the millisecond to picosecond range. This type of study will become even more important if pulsed laser beams are used to stimulate or enhance the growth process.

RHEED is essentially a structural probe. It has already been successfully combined with X-ray fluorescence emission [72-75] as a method for surface composition measurement. We might also ask what other spectroscopic technique could be combined with RHEED which would be useful for advanced semiconductor growth studies. An answer might be to use the incident electron beam and the secondary emitted electrons as "contacts" for photocurrent spectroscopy. This technique can be easily incorporated in any MBE growth chamber by illuminating the sample area which is probed by the RHEED beam with chopped light from a monochromator. The synchronously detected secondary electron emission current will then be recorded as the wavelength of the light from the monochromator is varied. Since electron transport in the surface layers is involved in the secondary emission, this procedure should give a spectrum which resembles a photocurrent spectrum i.e. an optical absorption spectrum. Such an in-situ, contactless technique will have tremendous application in MBE since it will enable the alloy composition and effective band-gap of quantum wells and superlattices to be measured in the growth chamber.

7. CONCLUSIONS

RHEED from a semiconductor surface during growth is capable of yielding a great deal of information. A full description of the atomic arrangement within the complex reconstructed unit cells is still not straightforward and will require further work, probably in conjunction with other surface techniques. However, a detailed semi-quantitive understanding of both the diffraction patterns and rocking curves now exists which enables us to identify certain types of disorder and to identify certain types of disorder and to identify the optimum conditions for making use of time dependent changes of RHEED intensity. These changes of intensity can be related to periodic changes in step density and hence growth rate, and to surface compositional changes of reconstruction. Future studies should explore the time dependences of RHEED on shorter time scales and investigate the possibilities of combining RHEED with optical spectroscopic techniques so that the electronic band structure of layers can be determined in real time within the growth chamber.

Acknowledgements

Much of this work was performed when the author was at Philips Research Laboratories and it is a pleasure to acknowledge many useful contributions from my colleagues and in particular B.A. Joyce, J.H. Neave, J. Zhang, R.K. Larsen, P. Fewster, J. Gowers, B. Bolger and J. Aarts.

REFERENCES

1. A. Howie, "Electron Diffraction (1927-1977)" Eds., P.J. Dobson, J.B. Pendry and C.J. Humphreys. IOP Conf. Series No 41 p.1 (1978).
2. P.J. Dobson, "Surfaces and Interface Characterisation by Electron Optical Methods", Eds., A. Howie and V. Valdre, Plenum Press (1989), in press.
3. E. Bauer, "Techniques of Metals Research", Ed., R.F. Bunshah, Interscience - Wiley, New York, Vol.2, Ch.15, (1969).
4. S. Ino, Japan. J. Appl. Phys., 16:891, (1977).
5. G.P. Thomson and W. Cochrane, "Theory and Practice of Electron Diffraction", MacMillan, London (1939).
6. Z.G. Pinsker, "Electron Diffraction", Butterworths, London (1953).
7. B.K. Vainshtein, "Structure and Analysis by Electron Diffraction", Pergammon Press/MacMillan, New York, (1964).
8. E. Bauer, "Elektronenbeugung" Verlag Moderne Industrie, Munchen (1958).
9. F. Hottier, J.B. Theeten, A. Masson and J.L. Domange, Surface Sci., 65:563 (1977).
10. R.H. Milne, Surface Sci., 122:474 (1982).
11. P.R. Pukite, P.I. Cohen and S. Batra, Proc. of NATO-ARW on Reflection High Energy Electron Diffraction and Reflection Electron Imaging of Surfaces. Eds., P.K. Larsen and P.J. Dobson, Plenum Press, New York (1988) p.427.
12. J.H. Neave, B.A. Joyce, P.J. Dobson and N. Norton, Appl Phys., A31:1 (1983).
13. R.L. Gerlach and T.N. Rhodin, Surface Sci., 10:446 (1968).
14. P.J. Dobson, J.H. Neave and B.A. Joyce, Surface Sci., 119:L339 (1982).
15. T. Kawamura, M. Hasebe and P.J. Dobson, J. Phys Soc. Japan, 54:3675 (1985).
16. M. Henzler, Appl. Phys., 9:11 (1976).
17. P.R. Pukite, J.M. Van Hove and P.I. Cohen, Appl. Phys. Lett., 44:456 (1984).
18. D.W. Pashley, Adv. in Phys. 5:173 (1956).
19. D.W. Pashley, Phil. Mag., 4:316 (1959).
20. P.B. Hirsch, A. Howie, R.B. Nicholson, D.W. Pashley and M.J. Whelan, "Electron Microscopy of Thin Crystals", Butterworths, London (1965).
21. G.W. Simmons, D.F. Mitchell and K.R. Lawless, Surface Sci., 8:130 (1967).
22. G.N. Burland and P.J. Dobson, Thin Solid Films, 75:383 (1981).
23. E.A. Wood, J. Appl. Phys., 35:1306 (1964).
24. D.P. Woodruffe and T.A. Delchar, "Modern Techniques of Surface Science", Cambridge Univ. Press (1986), p.46.
25. S. Ino, Japanese J. Appl. Phys., 19:1277 (1980).
26. S. Ino, Proc. of NATO - ARW on Reflection High Energy Electron Diffraction and Reflection Electron Imaging of Surfaces. Eds. P.K. Larsen and P.J. Dobson, Plenum Press, New York (1988) p.3.
27. R. Collela and J.F. Menadue, Acta Cryst., A28:16 (1972).
28. K. Britze and G. Meyer - Ehmsen, Surface Sci., 77:131 (1978).
29. H. Boersch, G. Jeschke and H. Raith, Z. Physik., 181:436 (1964).
30. P.A. Maksym and J.L. Beeby, Surface Sci., 110:423 (1981).
31. P.A. Maksym and J.L. Beeby, Surface Sci., 140:70 (1984).
32. P.A. Maksym, Surface Sci., 149:157 (1985).
33. M.G. Knibb and P.A. Maksym, Proc. of NATO-ARW on Reflection High Energy Electron Diffraction and Reflection Electron Imaging of Surfaces. Eds. P.K. Larsen and P.J. Dobson, Plenum Press, New York (1988) p.43.
34. J.L. Beeby ibid p.29.
35. P.A. Doyle and P.S. Turner, Acta Cryst., A24:390 (1968).
36. P.A. Maksym, Proc. NATO-ARW on Thin film Growth Techniques for Low Dimensional Structures, Eds. R.F.C. Farrow, P.J. Dobson and J.H. Neave, Plenum Press, New York (1987), p.95.

37. J.V. Ashby, N. Norton and P.A. Maksym, Surface Sci., 175:604 (1986).
38. M.G. Knibb and P.A. Maksym, Appl. Phys. A46:25, (1988).
39. S.Y. Tong, T.C. Zhas, H.C. Poon, K.D. Jamison, D.N. Zhow and P.I. Cohen, Phys. Lett., 128:447 (1988).
40. S.Y. Tong, T.C. Zhao and H.C. Poon., Proc. NATO-ARW on Reflection High Energy Electron Diffraction and Reflection Electron Imaging of Surfaces. Eds. P.K. Larsen and P.J. Dobson, Plenum Press, New York (1988) p.63.
41. S. Miyake and K. Hayakawa, Acta Cryst., A26:60 (1970).
42. J.M. Zuo, J.C.H. Spence and M. O'Keefe, Phys. Rev.Lett., 61:353 (1988).
43. A. Ichimiya, K. Kambe and G. Lehmpfuhl, J. Phys.Soc.Jap., 49:684 (1980).
44. G. Lehmpfuhl and W.C.T. Dowell, Acta Cryst., A42:569 (1986).
45. P.K. Larsen, P.J. Dobson, J.H. Neave, B.A. Joyce, B. Bolger and J. Zhang, Surface Sci., 169:176 (1986).
46. K.D. Jamison, D.N. Zhou, P.I. Cohen, T.C. Zhao and S.Y. Tong, J.Vac.Sci.Technol., A6:611 (1988).
47. J.J. Harris, B.A. Joyce and P.J. Dobson, Surface Sci., 103:L90 (1981); ibid 108:L444 (1981).
48. C.E.C. Wood, Surface Sci., 108:L441 (1981).
49. J.M. Van Hove, C.S. Lent, P.R. Pukite and P.I. Cohen, J. Vac Sci.Technol., B1:741 (1983).
50. P.J. Dobson, B.A. Joyce, J.H. Neave and J. Zhang, J.Cryst.Growth, 81:1 (1987).
51. B.A. Joyce, P.J. Dobson, J.H. Neave, K. Woodbridge, J. Zhang, P.K. Larsen and B. Bolger, Surface Sci., 168:423 (1986).
52. R.L. Gunshor, L.A. Kolodziejski, M.R. Melloch, M. Vaziri, C. Choi and N. Otsuka, Appl.Phys.Lett., 50:200 (1987).
53. T. Yao, H. Taneda and M. Funaki, Japanese J. Appl.Phys., 25:L952 (1986).
54. T. Sakamoto, K. Sakamoto, S. Nagao, G. Hashiguchi, K. Kuniyoshi and Y. Bando, Proc. NATO-ARW on Thin Film Growth Techniques for Low Dimensional Structures. Eds. R.F.C. Farrow, P.J. Dobson and J.H. Neave, Plenum Press, New York (1987), 225.
55. J. Aarts, W.M. Gerits and P.K. Larsen, Appl.Phys.Lett., 48:931 (1986).
56. J. Aarts and P.K. Larsen, Proc. NATO-ARW on Reflection High Energy Electron Diffraction and Reflection Electron Imaging of Surfaces. Eds. P.K. Larsen and P.J. Dobson, Plenum Press, New York (1988), 449.
57. C. Koziol, G. Lilienkamp and E. Bauer, Appl.Phys.Lett., 51:901 (1987).
58. S.T. Purcell, B. Heinrich and A.S. Arrott, Phys.Rev., B35:6458 (1987).
59. L.P. Erickson, M.O. Longerbone, R.C. Youngman and B.E. Dies, J.Cryst.Growth., 81:55 (1987).
60. P.J. Dobson, N. Norton, J.H. Neave and B.A. Joyce, Vacuum, 33:593 (1983).
61. C.S. Lent and P.I. Cohen, Surface Sci., 139:121 (1984).
62. P.R. Pukite, C.S. Lent and P.I. Cohen, Surface Sci., 161-39 (1985).
63. J.H. Neave, P.J. Dobson, B.A. Joyce and J. Zhang, Appl.Phys.Lett., 47:400 (1985).
64. B.A. Joyce, J.H. Neave, J. Zhang, P.J. Dobson, P. Dawson, K.J. Moore and C.T. Foxon, Proc. NATO-ARW on Thin Film Growth Techniques for Low Dimensional Structures, Eds. R.F.C. Farrow, P.J. Dobson and J.H. Neave, Plenum Press, New York (1987), 19.
65. Y. Horikoshi, M. Kawashima and H. Yamaguchi, Japanese J.Appl.Phys., 27:169 (1988).
66. F. Briones, D. Golmayo, L. Gonzalez and J.L. de Miguel, Japanese J.Appl.Phys., 24:L478 (1985).
67. T. Sakamoto, T. Kawamura and G. Hashiguchi, Appl.Phys.Lett., 48:1612 (1986).
68. J.H. Neave, B.A. Joyce and P.J. Dobson, Appl. Phys., A34:179 (1984).
69. B.F. Lewis, F.J. Grunthaner, A. Madhukar, T.C. Lee and F. Fernandez., J.Vac.Sci.Technol., B3:1317 (1985).

70. F-Y. Juang, P.K. Bhattacharya and J. Singh, Appl.Phys.Lett., 48:290 (1986).
71. H.E. Elsayed-Ali and G.A. Mourou, Appl.Phys.Lett., 52:103 (1988).
72. P.B. Sewell and M. Cohen, Appl.Phys.Lett., 11:298 (1967).
73. D.F. Mitchell, P.B. Sewell and M. Cohen, Surface Sci., 61:355 (1976); ibid, 69:310 (1977).
74. S. Ino, T. Ichikawa and S. Okada, Japanese J. Appl.Phys., 19:1451 (1980).
75. S. Hasegawa, S. Ino, Y. Yamamoto and H. Daimon, Japanese J.Appl.Phys., 24:L387 (1985).

LOW ENERGY ELECTRON MICROSCOPY (LEEM) AND PHOTOEMISSION MICROSCOPY (PEEM)

OF SEMICONDUCTOR SURFACES

E. Bauer, M. Mundschau, W. Święch* and W. Telieps[†]

Physikalisches Institut
der Technischen Universität Clausthal
and SFB 126 Göttingen-Clausthal
D-3392 Clausthal-Zellerfeld, Fed. Rep. Germany

INTRODUCTION

With a number of complementary surface imaging techniques such as conventional scanning electron microscopy (SEM), scanning tunneling microscopy (STM) and high energy reflection electron microscopy (REM) available for the study of semiconductor surfaces, what can be expected from still another technique (LEEM) and the revival of an old technique (PEEM)? This is the question which will be addressed in this paper and answered by first discussing the imaging features specific to LEEM and PEEM and then by illustrating them with some applications to Si(111) and Si(100) surfaces.

THE LEEM AND PEEM IMAGING PROCESS

Unlike SEM with secondary electrons or with unfiltered backscattered electrons LEEM uses elastically backscattered electrons. Unlike REM, which is done with forward-diffracted fast electrons at grazing incidence, LEEM makes use of back-diffracted slow electrons at normal incidence. Similar to REM, LEEM can either be done in the scanning or in the true imaging mode. Here only the true imaging mode will be considered. True imaging LEEM thus differs from the other surface imaging methods in the following major characteristics: (i) parallel instead of sequential image acquisition (compared to scanning imaging modes), (ii) normal incidence instead of grazing incidence (compared to REM) which eliminates foreshortening and depth of focus problems and (iii) imaging with diffracted instead of secondary or backscattered electrons (compared to SEM) which produces a completely different contrast. From these differences it is immediately evident that (nonscanning) LEEM will produce images much faster, without foreshortening and with good contrast also in specimens which do not produce contrast without diffraction. PEEM shares the advantage of no foreshortening with LEEM but suffers from lower intensity and produces a quite different contrast.

There are two other aspects of imaging which are important for practical applications: resolution and field of view. While STM is unbeatable with its atomic resolution it suffers from a limited field of view. SEM can now be done with nm resolution but image acquisition times for a large field of view are prohibitive. In REM a comparable resolution has been achieved but only in a region which is very narrow in the direction of the beam. On the other hand, LEEM has a limited resolution but a large field of view with constant resolution. Finally, the resolution of PEEM is even more limited but the field of view even larger.

Advantages and disadvantages of LEEM and PEEM compared to other techniques thus depend critically upon the problem to be studied, that is whether image acquisition time, foreshortening, type of contrast, resolution or field of view are the most important factors. Some of these factors depend upon the experimental set-up, others on the physics of the electron-solid and photon-solid interactions. These two aspects will be discussed next.

THE LEEM-PEEM INSTRUMENT

There are many ways in which such instruments can be built – and are being built now – but only one will be used here for illustration. It is the first and still the only one which actually produced acceptable LEEM images.[1] Fig. 1a shows its schematic, Fig. 1b its appearance. The heart of the instrument is the immersion objective lens 1 with the specimen 2 as cathode ("cathode lens") which in Fig. 1 is an electrostatic lens. The specimen is at a high negative potential U (typically −20 kV) so that slow electrons leaving the surface are accelerated in the lens to 20 keV energy with which they pass through the magnetic deflection field 3 and enter the imaging column whose major lenses are the intermediate lens 4 and the projector lens 5. The main purpose of the lens 4 is to image the diffraction pattern in the back focal plane 6 of lens 1 into the object plane of lens 5, but lens 4 serves also as a transfer lens of the specimen image in the center of the deflection field 3 to the object plane of the projective lens 5. Thus, by changing the excitation of lens 4 and inserting or removing the objective aperture 6, the LEEM image or the low energy electron diffraction (LEED) pattern can be observed alternately on the fluorescent screen 7 after image intensification with the channel plates 8. Image acquisition is either via still camera 9 or via video camera 9 and video recorder.

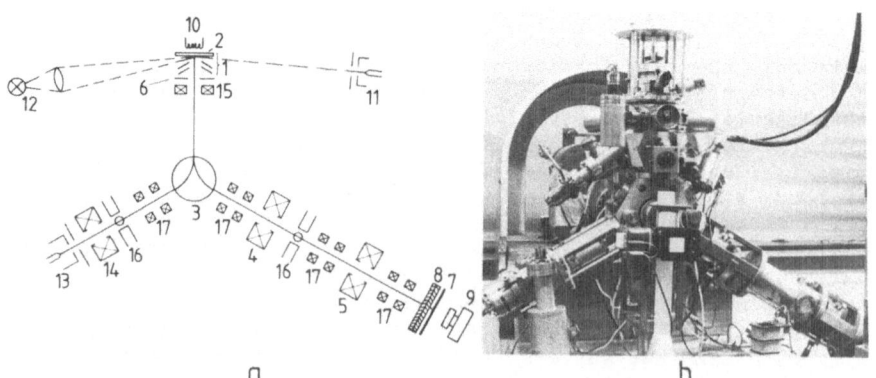

Fig. 1. (a) Schematic of a LEEM-PEEM microscope. For explanation see text. (b) LEEM-PEEM microscope at Clausthal. The hexagon is the beam deflector, the electron gun for LEEM is to the left, the specimen chamber and specimen manipulator on top of it.

The slow electrons can be created by heating (10) the specimen (thermionic electron emission), by bombardment with fast electrons from an auxiliary gun 11 (secondary electron emission), by illumination with UV light from a Hg lamp 12 or - and this is the main subject of this paper - by bombardment with slow electrons. These electrons come from a high coherence electron source 13 whose potential is $V = 0 - 500$ V more negative than that (U) of the specimen. The field-emitted electrons are accelerated to $e(U + V)$ eV and imaged with lens 14 onto the back focal plane 6 of the objective lens. The beam divergence in 6 determines the illuminated area on the specimen, the beam diameter in 6 the beam divergence on the specimen and the potential difference V determines the beam energy eV at the specimen. The astigmatism of the objective is corrected with the stigmator 15, while the quadrupoles 16 correct the residual astigmatism of the deflection field which is nearly nonfocussing. Finally, sets of deflection coils 17 serve for beam alignment. Several ports on the specimen chamber in addition to those for components 11 and 12 point towards the specimen so that surface processes which require accessories such as ion gun, evaporators or gas beams can be observed in situ. After bake-out the system reaches a base pressure in the specimen chamber in the low 10^{-10} to high 10^{-11} Torr range. As it is not magnetically shielded, DC and AC fields are compensated by large rectangular Helmholtz coils which are fed with a DC current and a phase-shifted AC current proportional to AC-$\vec{B}$-field in the specimen region. Mechanical vibrations are reduced by pressurized air springs which support a granite block on which the instrument is mounted.

Without AC field and vibrations the resolution of the instrument is limited by the objective lens. The homogeneous acceleration field in front of the specimen would allow in principle a resolution (in the Gaussian image plane) ranging from 2 nm with 200 eV electrons to 6 nm with 2 eV electrons for 20 kV acceleration potential,[2] but the aberrations of the electrostatic lens used in the present system increase these numbers by about a factor of 2^2. Replacement of this lens by a well-designed magnetic lens should, however, allow one to approach the limiting resolution of the homogeneous field. In PEEM the resolution is in general worse - and this is even more true in secondary electron emission - because in these cases electron energy E and energy width ΔE are in general comparable while in LEEM $\Delta E \ll E$, causing a larger chromatic aberration. Only when the highest energy $h\nu$ of the photons is just above the work function of the specimen is $\Delta E \approx E$ small enough for good resolution. The latter condition is usually fulfilled in thermionic emission but this imaging mode has rather restricted application.

THE ELECTRON-SOLID AND PHOTON-SOLID INTERACTION

Low energy electrons interact strongly with matter, both elastically and inelastically. Mean free paths for elastic scattering λ_e are usually only a few monolayers and those for inelastic scattering λ_i may be as low as 0.3 nm. As a consequence LEEM is dominated in general by the topmost atomic layers although in cases, in which λ_i is large, phenomena ("quantum size effects") are observed which require sampling depths of as many as 10 monolayers. As the scattering processes have been discussed elsewhere in more detail only the most important aspects from the practical applications point of view will be briefly discussed. First of all, below the threshold for volume plasmon creation ($\approx 10 - 20$ eV) inelastic scattering is usually weak compared to elastic scattering. Therefore, no energy filtering is required in this low energy range. Secondly, elastic backscattering is very strong at these energies and decreases in general strongly with energy. These two facts can be clearly seen in Figs. 2a[6,7] and 2b.[7] Fig. 2a shows the elastic reflectivity $R(E) = I/I_o$ of a W(110) surface at (near) normal incidence into the backward direction. Below 15 eV 25% - 60% of the

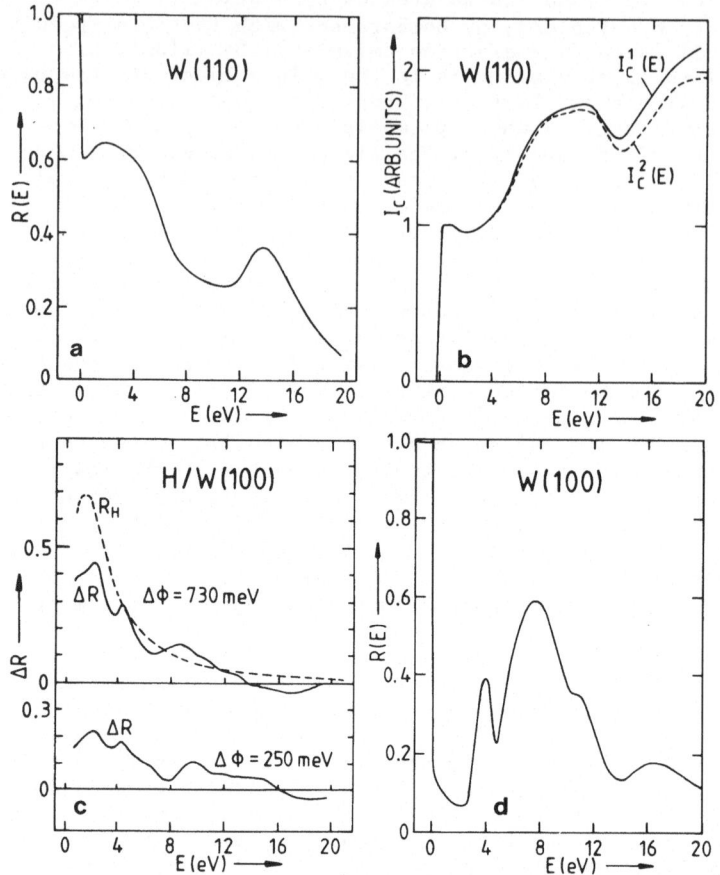

Fig. 2. (a) Fraction $R(E) = I/I_O$ of electrons which are elastically backreflected from a W(110) surface at near
normal incidence and reflection as a function of energy E. (b) Current $I_C(E) = I_O(1+R(E))$ collected by a
W(110) surface at near normal incidence without (I_C^1)
and with (I_C^2) inelastically scattered electrons.
(c) Reflectivity change $\Delta R(E)$ due to adsorption of approximately 1/4 (lower curve) and 3/4 (upper curve)
H monolayer on W(100). The dashed curve is a theoretical curve for a full monolayer. (d) $R(E)$ as in (a)
but for a W(100) surface.

incident electrons are reflected elastically. The complementary current
$I_C(E) = I_O(1 - R(E))$ into the crystal is plotted in Fig. 2b for two cases.
In one only elastically scattered electrons are collected (I_C^1), in the other
(I_C^2) also the inelastically scattered electrons. The difference $I_C^1 - I_C^2$
which represents inelastic scattering is seen to be less than 10% up to
12 eV and less than 20% up to 20 eV. Thirdly, light atoms whose 180° scattering cross-section is negligible at energies in the 10 - 100 eV range,
have large cross-sections at very low energies so that they become "visible". This is illustrated in Fig. 2c by the change $\Delta R(E)$ of $R(E)$ due to
hydrogen adsorption on a W(100) surface for about 1/4 and 3/4 monolayers.[8]

The reflectivity at 2 eV increases from the 7% of the clean surface (Fig. 2d)[6,7] to about 30% and 50%, respectively. As a consequence of these three facts it is in general advantageous to work at energies below 10 - 20 eV, at the cost of resolution.

Besides intensity and resolution, contrast is of fundamental importance in imaging. The main contrast mechanism in LEEM is diffraction contrast due to local differences in the backscattered intensity. Such differences arise in polycrystalline specimens from differences in grain orientation. This is well demonstrated by the comparison of Figs. 2a and 2d which show the reflectivity of two W surfaces with different orientations. At 2 eV the R values differ by a factor of 9! Strong diffraction contrast is also possible even on a single crystal surface provided that it has regions with different surface structure. A good example is the contrast between regions with (1x1) structure and regions with (7x7) structure on the Si(111) surface which will be discussed later. If there is no contrast between different regions because they are crystallographically equivalent at normal incidence as in the case of (1x2) and (2x1) domains on Si(100) surfaces, diffraction contrast can be achieved by tilting the incident beam so that the two domain orientations become inequivalent (see below). The beam tilt is achieved by displacing incident beam and objective aperture somewhat off the axis of the objective.[9] A beam displacement in the focal plane is equivalent to a change of angle of incidence in the specimen. Two kinds of contrast are possible in this case: (i) the specularly reflected beam ((00)-LEED beam) still passes through the aperture but has different intensity for the various domains ("bright-field imaging") or (ii) the (00) beam is intercepted by the aperture but a diffracted (hk)-LEED beam passes it ("dark-field imaging"). This second type of diffraction contrast is advantageous if there are (hk) beams with high intensity close to the (00) beam. An example for this situation is the (5x1) superstructure at low Au coverages on Si(111) (see below) or on the reconstructed Au(100) surface.[3,9]

Diffraction contrast always dominates when regions with different reflectivity exist and the surface is not so rough that strong field distortions on the specimen produce topography contrast. However, on homogeneous flat surfaces for which these contrast mechanisms fail, there is still another one which is typical for LEEM: the geometric phase contrast. Even the best prepared equilibrium single crystal surface has a large number of atomic steps. Electrons reflected from the two terraces next to a step have different optical path differences Δ with respect to each other and to the incident beam and, therefore, a phase difference $\mathcal{P} = 2\pi\Delta/\lambda$. By slight defocussing this phase difference can be converted into an amplitude difference resulting in a Fresnel diffraction image of the step. By changing the wave-length λ, i.e. the energy $E = 1.5/\lambda^2$ (λ in nm, E in eV), $\mathcal{P}$ can be made either $2n\pi$ or $(2n+1)\pi$ (n integer).[1] Thus, from the energies of maximum and minimum contrast, the step height $\Delta/2$ may be determined with the same accuracy as in LEED, but with the advantage that a single step is analyzed in LEEM while LEED determines the average step height within the coherence region. Pure geometric phase contrast at steps occurs only if there are no changes in interatomic distances close to the step. Otherwise the changes in the diffraction conditions in the distorted region around the step will produce strain contrast which, in principle can enhance or reduce the geometric phase contrast. The latter seems to be the case for Si. However, in contrast to REM in which the step contrast has been attributed to strains, geometric phase contrast is dominating in LEEM because of the small sampling depth of slow electrons.

In addition to diffraction contrast, topography contrast and geometric phase contrast there are also other contrast mechanisms such as atomic scattering factor contrast and inelastic scattering ("absorption") contrast which are due to differences in atomic backscattering and inelastic scattering, respectively. Both mechanisms are unimportant compared to the first three. There is, however, still another mechanism which is important in very thin films with parallel top and bottom faces: the "quantum size contrast".[10] Such films may be considered as one-dimensional potential wells normal to the surface capable of sustaining standing waves. For those wave-lengths for which $\lambda/4 = (2n+1)d$ the layer acts as an antiflection coating, for $\lambda/2 = nd$ it enhances the reflectivity of the surface, d being the film thickness. This contrast mechanism is different from diffraction contrast which is determined by the periodicity of the crystal. It can occur only within a limited thickness and energy range. The thickness must be small enough so that the elastic wave still "feels" the wall on the backside of the well. This means that d may only be a few times larger than λ_i and λ_e. As λ_i decreases rapidly from large values at E = 0 to 0.3 − 0.5 nm at 50 − 100 eV and λ_e usually increases rapidly with E, the suitable energy range is from several eV to several 10 eV in which d may be as large as 2 − 3 nm. By measuring the intensity oscillations as a function of energy not only d can be determined but also the mean inner potential in the film which together with E determines the wave-length.

Summarizing this section it can be stated that contrast in LEEM is similar but not identical to that in REM but completely different from that in SEM. Consequently, information can be obtained with LEEM which is not available from either SEM or REM. PEEM supplements LEEM: The oblique illumination produces strong topography contrast and the sensitivity of the photoemission yield causes strong work function contrast which is also of importance in secondary electron imaging in SEM. Many surfaces have work functions close to or above the cut-off of the best conventional UV radiation sources and windows. A small change of the work function due to adsorption can change, therefore, the PEEM intensity considerably. The details depend upon the density of state distribution below the Fermi energy. Very strong contrast can be achieved by proper choice of the adsorbate. A good example is the adsorption of Cu on Mo(110). Cu diffuses at elevated temperature to the steps at which it forms narrow bands with monolayer coverage and low work function while the remaining high work function surface stays clean.[11] Adsorption of electropositive atoms allows to vary the work function by a few eV and to make use of density of state differences between different regions of the specimen. Thus PEEM is in many aspects a valuable complementary technique to LEEM. In the following some examples of the application of LEEM and PEEM in semiconductor surface physics will be discussed.

THE SILICON (111) SURFACE

According to LEED and RHEED a thermally cleaned Si(111) surface can have either a (7x7) or (1x1) structure. The (1x1) structure is stable only above 1100 K but can be retained down to room temperature by laser quenching or trace impurity contamination. STM reveals that this "(1x1)" structure is by no means a true (1x1) structure but rather consists of a random distribution of small regions with a variety of superstructures. While LEEM cannot resolve this it nevertheless confirms that there are different states of the "(1x1)" structure which influence surface microstructure and surface processes in different manners.

This is best seen by the evolution of the (7x7) structure upon cooling by a few K below the transition temperature T_t. This causes steps decoration by preferred nucleation of the (7x7) structure at the steps. If

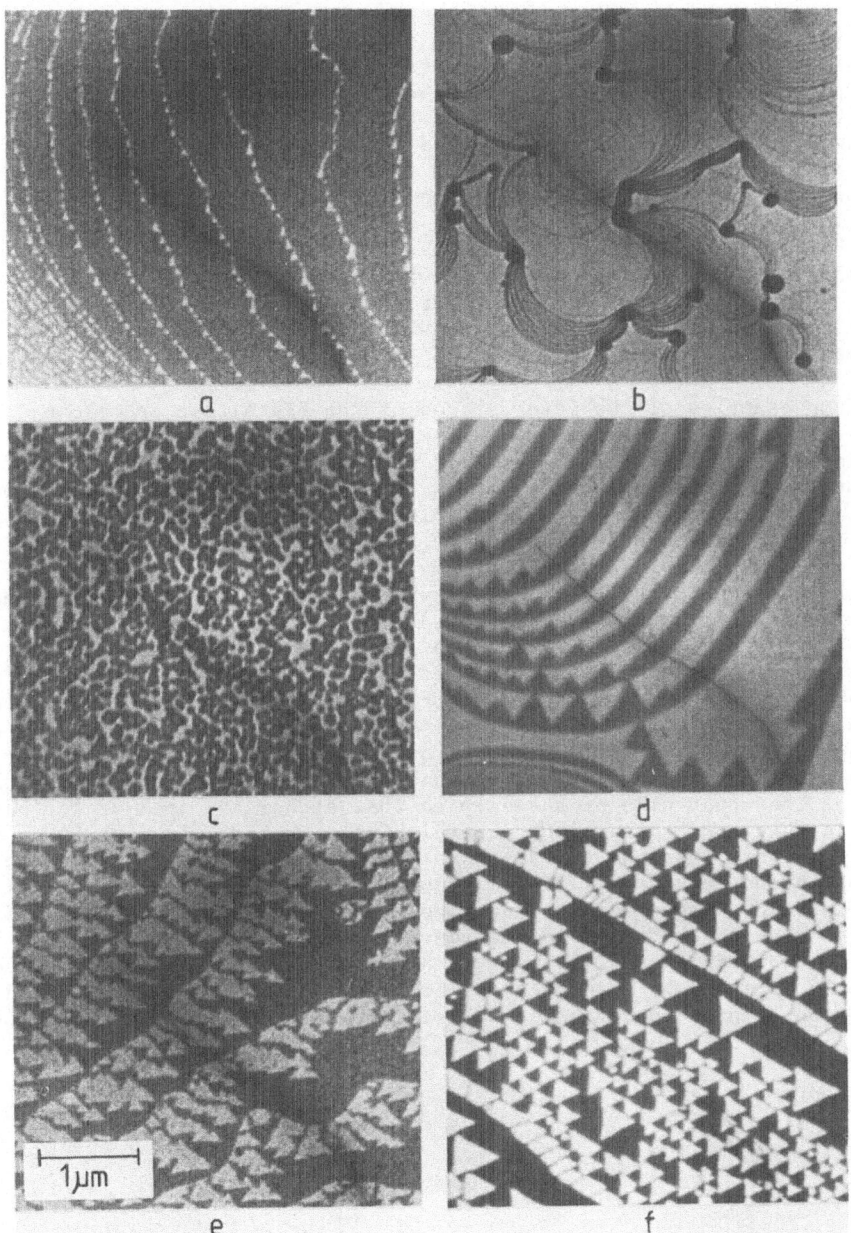

Fig. 3. LEEM images of various states of the Si(111) surface.
(a) Good step and terrace structure; (b) impurity-
generated step bunching with flat terraces; (c) irregular surface; (d) large (7x7) domains; (e) primary
and secondary (7x7) nucleation at steps; (f) (7x7) nucleation on terraces. The dark line in all figures is
caused by a crack in a channel plate. Energies 10.5,
10, 11, 10, 10.5 and 3 eV, respectively.

the surface-near region of the crystal is cleaned by heating to high temperatures, e.g. 1450 K, at which rapid evaporation and dissolution of impurities in the bulk occurs, a terrace-step structure with monatomic ter-

races is formed (Fig. 3a). If the crystal is heated at lower temperatures, e.g. 1100 - 1200 K, then many different surface configurations can develop, depending upon annealing time, impurity content, residual gas pressure and other parameters such as strains. Two such configurations are shown in Figs. 3b and 3c. In Fig. 3b step movement was impeded by impurity-induced pinning so that the steps have bunched into groups leaving large clean terraces in between them on which the (7x7) structure can grow unimpeded. The worst surface condition is seen in Fig. 3c. The random distribution of irregular features is seen both above and below T_t though with more contrast below T_t because the bright areas convert with decreasing temperature slowly into the (7x7) structure while the dark areas remain "(1x1)". Thus there is no unique (1x1) structure and the phase transition depends strongly on the state of the surface which is determined by the heat treatment and the impurity content.

Some examples of the later stages of the transition are shown in Figs. 3d - 3f. On a surface with a low density of defects only a few large two-dimensional (2D) (7x7)-"crystals" nucleate at the steps and grow when the surface had been exposed for many hours to the residual gas in the low 10^{-10} Torr range after the last cleaning (flashing to about 1450 K) (Fig. 3d).[3,12] Continued growth in this case requires increasing supersaturation, i.e. cooling. Apparently impurity adsorption impedes nucleation and growth. In contrast to this observation, strong primary and secondary nucleation occurs on a freshly cleaned surface with low defect density, even at low supersaturation (Fig. 3e). If the density of defects or impurities in the crystal is large, then (7x7) islands nucleate and grow not only at the steps but also in the terraces (Fig. 3f). Screw dislocations also are preferred nucleation sites. As long as the individual (7x7) crystals do not impede each other they grow in triangular shape with the apices pointing in the <112> directions. Nucleation at steps always takes place at the upper side of the step so that either the apex or the base point in the growth direction, depending upon whether the step is up or down (Fig. 4a). When the (7x7) crystals interfere with each other secondary nucleation occurs until finally domain walls visible as weak dark lines form when the crystals grow together. The kinetics of the processes involved have been studied in considerable detail.[13-15] It leaves no doubt that the transition is first order. The transition can, however, be considerably affected by imperfections so that in situations as depicted in Fig. 3c the impression of a second order phase transition arises in LEED.

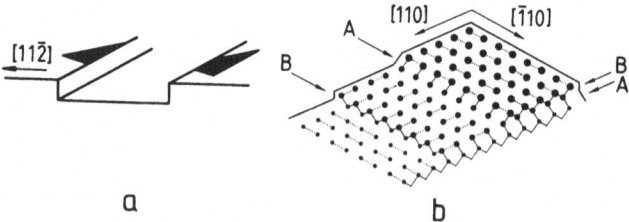

a   b

Fig. 4. (a) Schematic of (7x7) nucleation at steps on a Si(111) surface. (b) Schematic of step structure of a Si(001) surface.

This clearly demonstrates the importance of surface studies with good lateral resolution.

LEEM is also very well-suited for the study of the growth of metals and of their reaction with the substrate. They can be easily deposited in situ during observation at elevated temperature and their growth, disordering or dissolution in the bulk as well as their segregation upon cooling can be easily followed by LEEM. Examples studied briefly up to now include Au, Cu and Co. After annealing, Au forms several ordered structures as a function of coverage, the (5x1) being that with the lowest coverage. It disorders 80 K below the (7x7) structure of the clean surface and depresses the T_t of the clean surface by 10 K. Fig. 5a shows a LEEM image of triangular (5x1) islands in a sea of (7x7) structure at very low coverage. The ordered structure at the high coverage end, the (6x6) structure, on the other hand forms elongated islands with three equivalent orientations in a sea with (5x1) structure.

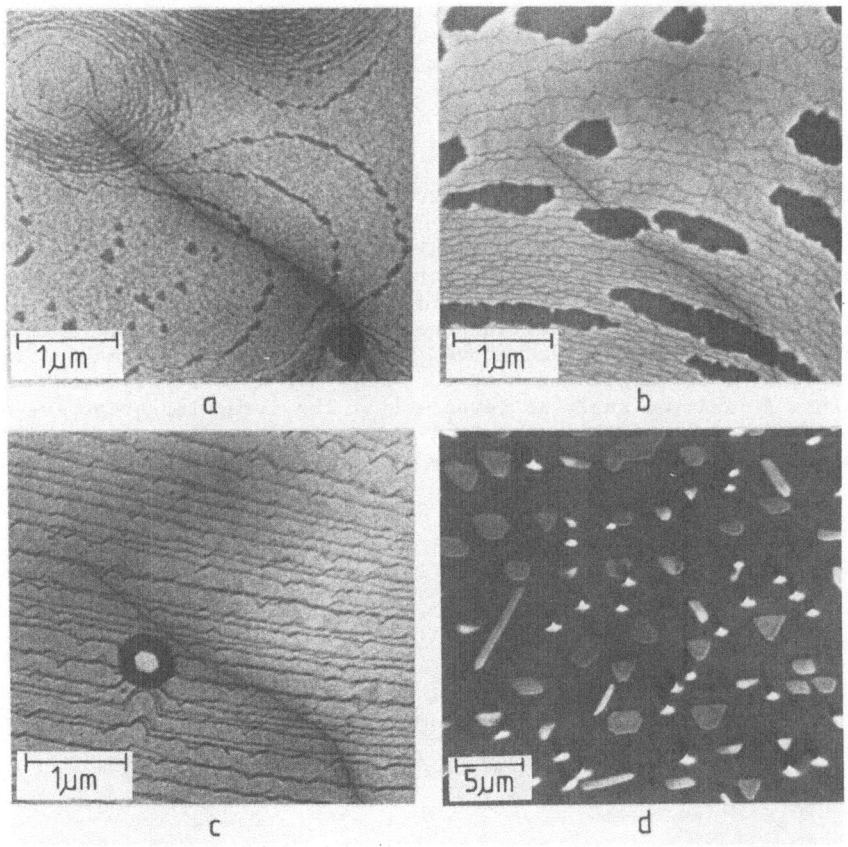

Fig. 5. (a) – (c) LEEM images of metal deposits on a Si(111) surface. (a) Islands with (5x1) structure at a very low Au coverage on a Si(111) surface. 4 eV. (b) Segregated "(5x5)" islands of Cu silicide. 10 eV. (c) A 3D Cu silicide crystal surrounded by 2D "(5x5)" structure, 4 eV. (d) PEEM image of a Si(111) surface covered with 2D Cu silicide with "(5x5)" structure and 3D silicide and SiC crystals.

In contrast to Au, which does not form a silicide in the monolayer range and only a metastable one at higher coverages, Cu reacts at elevated temperatures, e.g. at 850 K, already at low coverages with Si and forms an approximate, incommensurate "(5x5)" structure either during deposition or upon segregation from the bulk upon cooling. Simultaneously the step structure of the (7x7) regions surrounding the irregular "(5x5)" structure is considerably modified (Fig. 5b). This is even more the case at higher coverages when 3D Cu silicide islands have formed in the "(5x5)" sea. The steps are now facetted and bunched into groups of three monatomic steps along the $\langle 1\bar{1}0 \rangle$ directions (Fig. 5c).[16] Fig. 5d gives a PEEM overview of the layer from which Fig. 5c was taken by LEEM. A variety of crystal shapes and orientations is seen which can be selected for closer study by LEEM. For PEEM studies at magnifications comparable to LEEM neither resolution nor intensity are sufficient without work function reduction by electropositive adsorbates. Co reacts with Si already in the monolayer range and at room temperature. At higher temperatures flat crystals with well-developed hexagonal and triangular shape and (1x1) structure develop which are frequently twinned.[15] Growth at room temperature at which the nucleation density is very high and the island size is below the resolution limit of 10 - 20 nm is presently not accessible to LEEM.

THE SILICON (100) SURFACE

This surface has a (2x1) superstructure caused by the dimerization of the dangling bonds. Because these are rotated by 90° in successive layers two domain orientations result as indicated in Fig. 4b. The dimer bonds in the topmost layer are indicated by dotted lines, the bonds of the step atoms to the next lower layer by solid lines. At normal incidence the two domains are equivalent but tilting the beam, e.g. in the [001] azimuth, produces contrast as discussed above. Fig. 6a shows a LEEM image obtained in this manner. It is evident that the steps are alternately smooth and irregular. A detailed analysis reveals that the irregular steps are of type A, the smooth steps of type B.[12] The bonding configuration seen in Fig. 4b makes the different stability of the two step types understand-

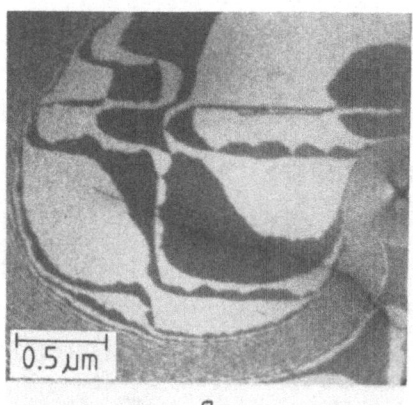
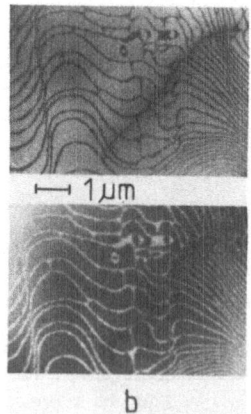

a   b

Fig. 6. LEEM images of Si(100) surfaces. (a) Typical large flat region with both (2x1) domains of comparable size, 6 eV. (b) Atypical flat region with one terrace dominating; beam tilt in [011] and [01$\bar{1}$] direction, 6 eV.

able. Si(100) surfaces tilted by $2^\circ - 3^\circ$ about one of the $\langle 011 \rangle$ directions have been reported to form terraces separated by double steps. The widths of these terraces (7.8 − 5.2 nm) is below the present resolution limit. However the tendency to double step formation can also be seen occasionally on less misoriented surfaces due to surface undulations produced by impurity-induced preferred and hindered evaporation. The closest approach to double steps is that shown in Fig. 6b which at the same time illustrates the contrast obtained by beam tilt in the two orthogonal $\langle 011 \rangle$ directions.

At high temperatures the sublimation can be observed via video camera until thermionic emission sets in which results in loss of contrast. Before this happens a transition from rapid orderly migration of steps to a chaotic generation of new steps and terraces is seen, which is believed to be the pre-roughening transition.[15] Cooling to lower temperatures, however, restores the large scale terrace and step structure. Film growth on this surface has not been studied up to now with LEEM. Such studies may be limited by the tendency of this surface to facet. An indication of this has been seen on a surface which was tilted 1° about a $\langle 011 \rangle$ axis and slightly Cu-contaminated. The tendency of Cu to induce facetting was already noted above where it produced facetting and agglomeration of steps on the (111) surface.

SUMMARY

The last two sections have shown that there is a wide range of phenomena on semiconductor surfaces which can be studied in situ by LEEM and PEEM. Phase transitions, sublimation, facetting, film growth, silicide formation and segregation were illustrated, but there are many other processes such as surface diffusion, ion beam and chemical etching, oxidation and nitridation, to name only a few. Up to what thickness the growth of insulating layers can be studied is not known at present. There are two possible limitations for such studies: charging and loss of contrast and intensity due to the disappearance of diffracted beams with increasing thickness of the amorphous layer. In the study of surfaces with thick insulating layers LEEM may well turn out to be inferior to SEM because it is not superior in contrast but lower in resolution. For all studies in which one of the LEEM-specific contrast mechanisms − diffraction contrast, geometric phase contrast or quantum size contrast − is available and which do not require the utmost in resolution but rather a large field of view, no distortion and/or the combination with LEED or PEEM, LEEM is superior to the other surface imaging techniques. LEEM is still in its infancy. Its full potential can only be judged once it has reached the level of sophistication which SEM, REM and STM have at present. One important advantage is evident already now: the short image acquisition time in LEEM which allows the study and monitoring of surface processes in real time.

ACKNOWLEDGEMENTS

One of the authors (M.M.) thanks the Alexander von Humboldt-Foundation for a research fellowship. Partial support by the Stiftung Volkswagenwerk is also gratefully acknowledged.

*On leave from Institute of Experimental Physics, University of Wrocław, PL-50-205 Wrocław, Poland.
†Deceased 31 May 1987

REFERENCES

1. W. Telieps and E. Bauer, An analytical reflection and emission UHV surface electron microscope, Ultramicroscopy 17:57 (1985).
2. E. Bauer, The resolution of the low energy electron reflection microscope, Ultramicroscopy 17:51 (1985).
3. E. Bauer and W. Telieps, Low energy electron microscopy, Scanning Microscopy Suppl. 1:99 (1987).
4. E. Bauer and W. Telieps, Emission and low energy reflection electron microscopy, in: "Study of Surfaces and Interfaces by Electron Optical Techniques", A. Howie and U. Valdré, ed., Plenum Press, New York, to be published.
5. E. Bauer, Low energy electron microscopy and normal incidence VLEED, in: "Elseviers Studies in Surface Science and Catalysis", J. Koukal, ed., Elsevier, Amsterdam, to be published (and references therein).
6. H.-J. Herlt, Elastische Rückstreuung sehr langsamer Elektronen an reinen und an gasbedeckten Wolfram-Einkristalloberflächen, Dissertation, Clausthal 1982.
7. H.-J. Herlt, R. Feder, G. Meister, and E. Bauer, Experiment and theory of the elastic electron reflection coefficient from tungsten, Solid State Commun. 38:973 (1981).
8. H.-J. Herlt and E. Bauer, A very low energy electron reflection study of hydrogen adsorption on W(100) and W(110) surfaces, Surface Sci. 175:336 (1986).
9. W. Telieps, M. Mundschau, and E. Bauer, Dark field imaging with LEEM, Optik 77:93 (1987).
10. M. Mundschau, E. Bauer, and W. Święch, Initial epitaxial growth of Cu on Mo{011} by low energy electron microscopy and photoemission electron microscopy, to be published.
11. M. Mundschau, E. Bauer, and W. Święch, Photoemission microscopy and atomic steps on Mo{011}, Surface Sci., 203:412 (1988).
12. W. Telieps, Surface imaging with LEEM, Appl. Phys. A44:55 (1987).
13. W. Telieps and E. Bauer, The (7x7)⟷(1x1) phase transition on Si(111), Surface Sci. 162:163 (1985).
14. W. Telieps and E. Bauer, Kinetics of the (7x7)⟷(1x1) transition on Si(111), Ber. Bunsenges. Phys. Chem. 90:197 (1986).
15. M. Mundschau, unpublished.
16. M. Mundschau, E. Bauer, W. Telieps, and W. Święch, In situ studies of epitaxial growth in the low energy microscope, Surface Sci., to be published.

TRANSMISSION ELECTRON MICROSCOPY OF IN-SITU DEPOSITED

FILMS ON SILICON

J.M. Gibson *, J.L. Batstone ** and M.Y. Lanzerotti ***

*AT&T Bell Laboratories, 600 Mountain Avenue, Murray Hill, NJ 07974
**Dept. of Materials Science and Engineering, The University
Liverpool, England
***Dunster House, Harvard University, Cambridge, MA 02138

ABSTRACT

We discuss applications of an ultra-high vacuum TEM to the study of clean Si surfaces and in-situ deposited films. For the NiSi$_2$ on Si system, we show the importance of metastable phases during growth. For native oxidation of Si, the behavior of individual atomic steps is viewed. In summary, moderate resolution TEM and diffraction is shown to have a great deal to contribute to semiconductor surface science primarily because of the kinematical diffraction by monolayers and the penetration to view sub-surface phenomena.

INTRODUCTION

The transmission electron microscope (TEM) is most commonly used to study specimens in a destructive manner. That is, the prepared specimen is examined and then discarded as useless for other experiments. As a result, although TEM is tremendously powerful, it is not viewed as one of the in-situ characterization techniques which the crystal grower employs to perfect his art. Since TEM is in principle compatible with ultra-high vacuum technology (UHV), in recent years interest has arisen in developing in-situ characterization of crystal growth and surfaces. Cherns and Stowell[1] demonstrated the in-situ growth of Pd on Au with a high-vacuum instrument. Yagi et. al.[2] modified a JEOL 100B TEM to obtain UHV necessary for most semiconductor studies, concentrating initially on reflection electron microscopy, although some studies were done with TEM.[3] Takayanagi demonstrated one extremely useful feature of TEM in surface science in this instrument: he solved the structure of the Si(111) 7 × 7 reconstruction.[4] This feat proved possible, despite the onslaught of every surface science characterization technique over 20 years, because of the simple kinematical nature of diffraction of electrons by monolayers at high accelerating voltage. Fig. 3(a) shows an example of the diffraction from a Si(111) 7 × 7 reconstruction of the type seen by Takayanagi. An additional important advantage of TEM over other surface science techniques is its penetration enabling study of deep surface layers. This, of course, is critically important in the study of epitaxial growth. In this paper we describe the application of our own modified UHV TEM to the study of Si surfaces and in-situ grown films. At this time several groups around the world are developing such instruments and examples of in-situ studies in the semiconductor field will undoubtedly become more common.

The instrument used in this study is a modified JEOL 200CX top-entry 200kV TEM. A differentially pumped specimen chamber has a base pressure of ~1×10^{-9}τ, obtained with an ion pump, a Ti sublimation pump and liquid He cryo-paneling. The specimen is held in a top-entry loaded non-tilting cartridge made from Ta, in which it can be directly heated resistively to the melting point of Si. In-situ evaporation of up to ~50Å of material onto the top-side of the specimen is achieved by pulse-heating a Ta filament coated in a separate evaporator. Gas exposure can also be achieved through a controlled leak valve and partial pressures are measured with a quadrapole mass spectrometer. Details of the design are given by M. McDonald et. al.[5]

Clean Si surfaces are obtained with mechanically-dimpled and chemically-thinned specimens by heating *in-situ* to ~1200°C. Initially thin specimen areas are lost in this process but are regenerated by surface diffusion and evaporation at high temperatures. Such areas are often atomically flat over ~1μm and are ~2000Å thick. These regions are suitable for plan-view imaging and diffraction. Even in these relatively thick specimens, monolayer diffraction is readily seen (if periodic). Some examples of clean surface studies are given elsewhere.[6,7]

NICKEL SILICIDE FORMATION

Tung et. al.[8] showed that extremely high quality crystalline thin films of $NiSi_2$ can be grown on Si(111). This metallic silicide has a cubic structure (CaF_2) with a lattice constant only 0.5% less than silicon. However, it had proven previously impossible to grow perfect single crystal films of the material by vacuum evaporation of Ni and furnace annealing.[9,10] These films contained both double-positioned orientations: type-A (in which the silicide and silicon substrate are mutually aligned) and type-B (in which there is a 180° mutual rotation about the (111) growth direction). Tung et al.[8] were able to grow single crystal films of either type-A or type-B orientations by employing extremely clean growth conditions: deposition of Ni in-situ in a Molecular Beam Epitaxy (MBE) chamber on clean reconstructed Si(111) surfaces. After mild annealing at 450°C (in comparison to ~750°C required for less clean vacuum evaporated films),[9,10] $NiSi_2$ forms. In an unusual but highly reproducible observation, Tung et. al.[8] reported that the final orientation of the $NiSi_2$ layer is a function only of the initial room temperature deposited Ni film thickness before annealing. Nickel deposits of thickness ~8-10Å result on annealing in exclusively type-B films whereas those 16-20Å result in the type-A orientation (others yield A+B). These layers were dubbed "templates" by Tung et al.[8] since after formation thicker films of the same orientation could be readily overgrown. A consequence of this "black magic" is that physical properties of the type-A and type-B interfaces could be measured independently: specifically an anomalous variation in Schottky Barrier height was observed.[11] The origin of the type-A/type-B template phenomenon remained a mystery until recently when it was elucidated by in-situ TEM studies.[12,13] The template phenomenon provides ideal fodder for the in-situ TEM technique since it involves the structure of highly reactive layers deposited in UHV conditions but of thickness $\geq$ 10 monolayers and thus not readily accessible to many conventional surface science techniques.

The detailed results of our in-situ study and those of other complementary techniques is listed in detail elsewhere.[13] Briefly, the key new result which emerged was observed on annealing in-situ Ni films of thicknesses at which some type-A $NiSi_2$ resulted. Fig. 1 shows a series of diffraction patterns of such a film with nominal thickness (of deposited Ni) 10Å. On annealing at ~350°C a strong diffraction spot occurs at the 1/3 422 position which we have identified as the 100 diffraction spot from the hexagonal phase $\Theta-Ni_2Si$. On further annealing the spot weakens in intensity as the $\Theta-Ni_2Si$ phase is replaced by $NiSi_2$ at ~450°C. If such a sample is removed from the microscope below 400°C, then the $\Theta-Ni_2Si$ phase is stable and can be observed in a TEM with tilting facilities. This permitted confirmation of the 3-D diffraction expected from $\Theta-Ni_2Si$. Dark-field images taken with the $\Theta-Ni_2Si$ 100 reflection during in-situ annealing reveal that it transforms exclusively into type-A $NiSi_2$ on further annealing (Fig. 2). Type-B $NiSi_2$ appears to form immediately on

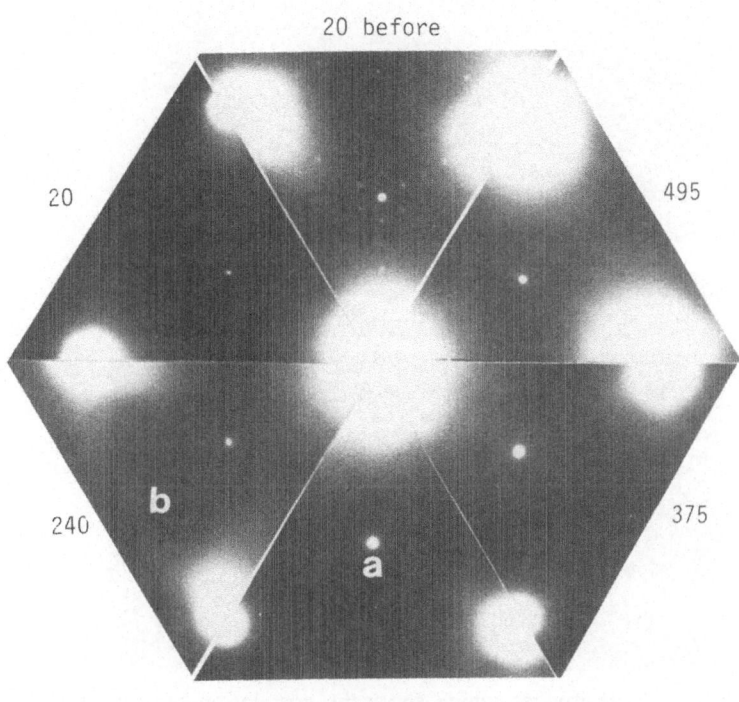

Fig. 1   A series of diffraction patterns as a function of temperature (in °C) from a 10 Å Ni film deposited and annealed on Si (111) in-situ. "Before" refers to the surface prior to deposition.

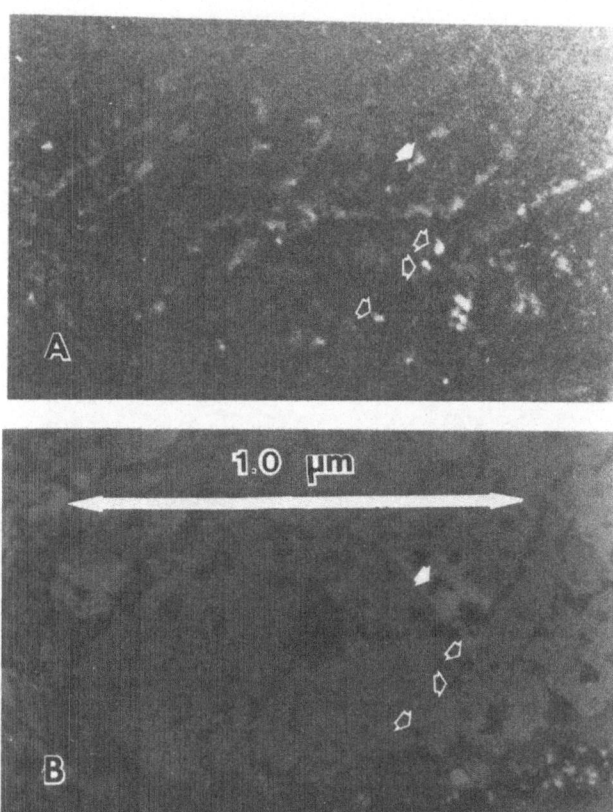

Fig. 2 Two dark-field TEM images which show the correlation between the growth of the
Θ–Ni_2Si phase during in-situ annealing and the subsequent growth of the type-A
$NiSi_2$ phase. (a) is a 1/3 422 (equivalent to 100 Θ–Ni_2Si) dark-field image at
400°C, where Θ–Ni_2Si regions are bright. (b) is a 111 dark-field image, taken near
the type-B 112 pole in a Phillips 420 TEM from the same area, after growth. The
latter reveals the type-B regions as bright and the type-A regions (including a small
number of holes in the silicide) are dark. The correlation is actually quite exact, at
any given temperature the Θ–Ni_2Si phase does not exactly match because some has
either not yet transferred or already converted to type-A $NiSi_2$.

deposition and is covered with unreacted Ni for coverages in excess of 10Å. If there is sufficient unreacted Ni, annealing causes complete transformation to Θ–Ni_2Si to take place, yielding a single-crystal type-A $NiSi_2$ film on further annealing. A key further piece of the template puzzle is that for Ni coverages in excess of ~20Å the Θ–Ni_2Si phase does not occur on annealing but the orthorhombic δ–Ni_2Si phase appears. This is because the Θ–Ni_2Si phase is metastable: it occurs on the bulk phase diagram only above 900°C. The δ–Ni_2Si phase is however stable in bulk at room temperature and has previously been observed in annealed vacuum deposited Ni films.[10]

The occurrence of the metastable Θ–Ni_2Si phase can be related to the lowering of energy for metastable phases by epitaxy. This has been observed by several workers in other systems, starting with Schulz[14] for CsCl on NaCl and more recently with α–Sn on In Sb.[15] In binary silicide systems we expect epitaxial metastability to be very common due to the large number of available phases and our studies show these phenomena to account for many of the template observations. In general a critical thickness is expected for metastable phases resulting in unusual thickness dependent microstructure such as the type-A/type-B $NiSi_2$ enigma. Metastable phases may interfere with the sequence of chemical phase formation.

The importance of metastability extends to $NiSi_2$ growth on (100)Si. Tung et. al. had shown that templates were again useful in growing good quality (100) films with flat interfaces.[8] At high thicknesses (~15Å Ni) poor quality films result. Our in-situ studies first confirmed the total absence of the Θ–Ni_2Si phase, presumably due to the fourfold substrate symmetry on (100) Si which raises its interface energy from poor epitaxial match. At low thicknesses, direct transformation to $NiSi_2$ is seen for Ni deposited in-situ on (100)Si, without intermediate phases. However, for high coverages transformation to the δ–Ni_2Si phase is seen, which subsequently produces poorer quality $NiSi_2$ films. Related phenomena have also been studied for Co on (100)Si in detail.[16]

OXIDATION OF SILICON

There have been many studies of the interface structure of SiO_2 on Si, because of its technological importance. We have recently begun an in-situ study of the oxidation process in the UHV TEM in the hope of directly observing the behavior of surface steps as the surface transforms into a buried interface. To do so in plan-view surface/interface imaging we take advantage of an effect first noted experimentally by Cherns[17] and theoretically by Lynch.[18] Certain Bragg reflections, for example 1/3 422 in the f.c.c. system, whilst forbidden in the bulk can occur from single monolayers or thin foils with a non-integral number of unit cells. Images taken with such reflections can exhibit a change in intensity on crossing a monatomic step on either surface of a thin foil, so that monatomic steps can be seen in plan-view. Cherns showed this effect experimentally for Au(111) foils.[17] An alternate view of the forbidden surface sensitive reflections is as reciprocal lattice rods extending from higher order Laue zones.[17,18] For example, the 1/3 422 is associated with a 111 reflection in the first order Laue zone. The intensity oscillates with period $\frac{1}{s} = \sqrt{3}\, a_o$. In general these reflections have been difficult to observe experimentally in non-noble metals: we shall come back to this later. Using very clean and flat in-situ prepared thin foils of Si the $\frac{1}{3}$ 422 reflections are readily observed from (111) surfaces.[4] Fig. 3 shows an example from the Si(111) 7×7 surface. In Fig. 3a) we show a dark-field image taken with this reflection with an objective aperture of radius 0.1 Å^{-1}. Image contrast is consistent with that expected and each change from light to dark can be related to a monatomic step on either foil surface. The step spacing on one surface is ~1000Å. Fig. 3(b) shows the effect of exposure of this surface to ~ 1000 ML O_2 at $10^{-6}\tau$ and re-evacuation to ~$10^{-9}\tau$. Steps

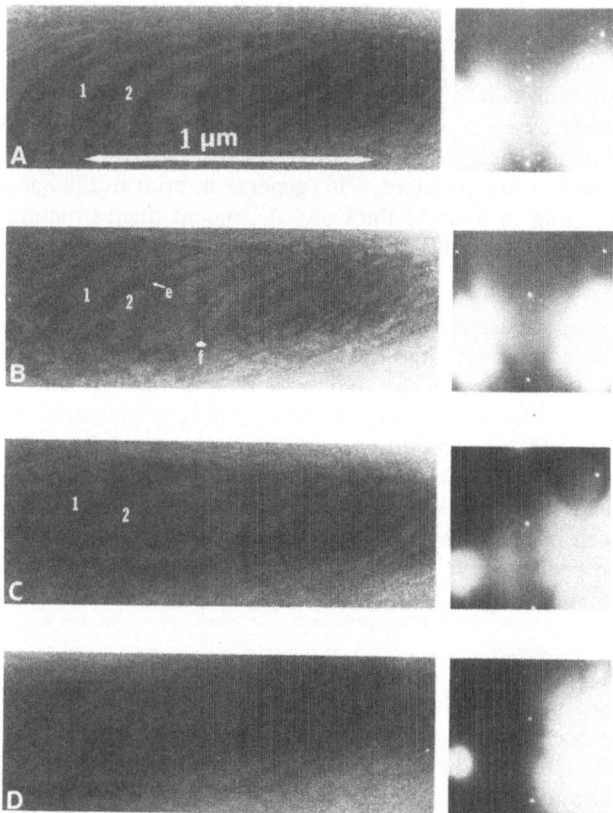

Fig. 3   Images taken with 1/3 422 reflections and revealing atomic terraces on a thin (~1000 Å thickness) Si specimen in a UHV transmission electron microscope at 100kV.   Diffraction patterns are inset showing (a) the clean Si (111) 7×7 superstructure (with the 1/3 422 diffraction spot arrowed); (b) partial transformation to a 1×1 surface after 600 ML O_2 exposure; (c) the 1×1 unreconstructed nature of the native oxide/Si interfaces and (d) the effect of stripping the oxide in an aqueous HF solution.   The images reveal the behavior of atomic steps and are discussed in the text.

have been moved by the interaction of O_2 and the 7×7 has transformed partially to a 1×1 structure.

The oxidation process can be studied even after the formation of a native oxide, in Fig. 3(c), by exposure to air for 12 hours. The native oxide, about 20Å thick,[19] does not obscure the contrast from terraces and steps at the buried Si/SiO$_2$ interface. The step density at this interface is unchanged by oxidation and the buried Si/SiO$_2$ interface is as flat as the original surface. More surprisingly, the step arrangement at the buried interface is almost identical to that on the original surface. This implies that the oxidation process occurs by attack on terraces and not by step propagation, for the latter would lead to randomization of the step distribution after growth of 1 monolayer of oxide. Another interesting result is the effect of 5% HF:H$_2$0 etching on the same sample: after stripping for 10 minutes, which removes the native oxide, the sample is rapidly dried and transferred into the microscope. Image (d) shows that the surface step distribution does not represent that at the buried interface. This may have a bearing on the detailed study of Si/SiO$_2$ interfacial roughness by Henzler et. al.[20] using LEED to study the HF stripped surface. Clearly the ability to study steps at the buried interface without removal of the oxide is a great advantage of the TEM technique. Also, the technique posesses advantages over the high resolution cross-section method since it does not suffer from projection limitations.[21]

To image steps requires very flat interfaces on both sides of the sample, as occurs in the in-situ experiments. Also, the presence of diffuse scattering from the substrate typically limits the resolution of steps to ~30Å. However, it appears that statistical information on step spacing is available more readily from diffraction patterns, even when one surface is quite rough. It can be shown[22] that a gaussian randomly rough surface with average step spacing L and height a gives a diffraction spot due to a termination reflection with profile

$$I(s_x, s_z) \sim \frac{\pi s_2 a}{\sin(\pi s_2 a)} \left\{ \frac{(s_z a)^2/L}{\left[\frac{\pi(s_z a)^2}{L}\right]^2 + s_x{}^2} \right\} \tag{1}$$

For the 1/3 422 spot in (111) $s_z = \frac{1}{\sqrt{3}a}$. The Lorentzian line shape of the 1/3 422 due to broadening allows readily determination of the step spacing L. For very rough surfaces the spot may become invisible in the background, since the peak intensity drops as L increases. This accounts for the difficulty of observing the 1/3 422 spot (or 110 spot on (100)) from reactive materials such as Si, Al and Cu. Only for "exceptionally thin and flat specimens"[23] has the 1/3 422 been observed previously in Si, without UHV annealing.[24] However, we find that well-annealed SiO$_2$/Si interfaces prepared by conventional thermal oxidation are sufficiently flat for sharp 1/3 422 and 110 spots to be visible. We have developed a digital quantification system for accurately measuring integrated intensity and peak shape from several such diffraction patterns and can use this in conjunction with equation (1) to estimate the step spacing on (111) and (100) surfaces. Fig 4 shows an example of a digitized background subtracted peak with a Lorentzian fit. Table 1 shows the effect of some processing parameters on the Si/SiO$_2$ interfacial roughness. Note the tremendous effect of post-oxidation annealing, noted by Henzler et. al.[20] but here observed to be much more dramatic for both (111) and (100) interfaces.

Measurements of such images show that intensities are close to those expected from well-terminated Si surfaces, with no evidence for additional diffraction from epitaxial phases under the conditions used here for in-situ and ex-situ oxidation. Finally, a study is under way to solve the structural damage of O$_2$ attack on the 7×7 by Takayanagi's method.[4]

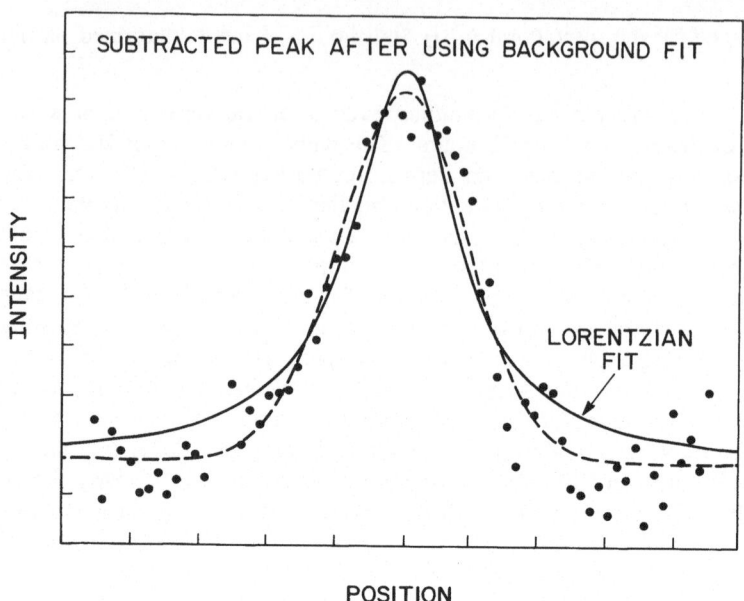

POSITION

Fig. 4 Digitized intensity data from a 1050°C dry oxidation on Si(111) given a one hour post-oxidation anneal, showing the Lorentzian fit after background subtraction.

Table 1

EX-SITU OXIDES

Interfacial roughness on (111) probed by 1/3 422 spot in plan-view TEM

OXIDATION CONDITIONS	THICKNESS	HWHM ($\mathring{A}^{-1}$)	L=Step Spacing ($\mathring{A}$)
Dry 1050°C	670$\mathring{A}$	$1.7 \pm .7 \times 10^{-2}$	62 ± 24
Dry 1050° + 1 Hr Post Oxidation Anneal in N_2	640$\mathring{A}$	$2.9 \pm .2 \times 10^{-3}$ (resolution $\sim 1 \times 10^{-3}$)	361 ± 26
Wet 1050°C	1000$\mathring{A}$	$> 2 \times 10^{-2}$	<40

CONCLUSION

The in-situ experiments described here were designed to take advantage of the unique features of transmission electron microscopy and diffraction in the study of surfaces: kinematical diffraction and penetration. The study of Ni on Si surfaces required a technique with ability to give simple diffraction information from ~10 monolayer thick films to allow the understanding of the importance of metastable phases in the growth of silicide films. For studies of the step distribution at buried interfaces, during and after oxidation, the use of "termination" Bragg reflections is of great advantage and allowed both reliable quantitative information of interface roughness from plan-view samples and step propagation studies during in-situ oxidation.

The author is grateful for collaborations with V. Elser, R. T. Tung, D. Loretto and M. L. McDonald.

REFERENCES

[1] D. Cherns and M. Stowell, Scripa. Met. **7** 489 (1973).

[2] N. Osakabe, Y. Tanishiro, K. Yagi and G. Honjo, Surf. Sci. **97**, 393 (1980).

[3] K. Takayanagi, Proc. of 34th Annual EMSA Meeting, p. 205, (1981), edited by Bailey, Claitor, Baton Rouge, LA.

[4] K. Takayanagi, K. Yagi, K. Kobayashi and G. Honjo, J. Phys. E **11**, 441 (1978).

[5] M. L. McDonald, J. M. Gibson and F. C. Unterwald, J. Sci. Inst., to appear.

[6] J. M. Gibson, M. L. McDonald and F. C. Unterwald, Phys. Rev. Lett. **55**, 1765 (1985).

[7] J. M. Gibson, M. L. McDonald, J. L. Batstone and J. M. Phillips, Ultramic. **22**, 35 (1987).

[8] R. T. Tung, J. M. Gibson and J. M. Poate, Phys. Rev. Lett. **50**, 429, (1983).

[9] K. C. R. Chiu, J. M. Poate, J. E. Rowe, T. T. Sheng and A. G. Cullis, Appl. Phys. Lett. **38**, 988 (1981).

[10] H. Foll, P. S. Ho and K. N. Tu, J. Appl. Phys. **52**, 250 (1981).

[11] R. T. Tung, Phys. Rev. Lett. **52**, 461, (1984).

[12] J. M. Gibson, J. L. Batstone, R. T. Tung and F. C. Unterwald, Phys. Rev. Lett. **60**, 1158 (1988).

[13] J. M. Gibson and J. L. Batstone, Surface Science, to appear.

[14] L. G. Schulz, Acta. Cryst., **4**, 487 (1951).

[15] R. F. C. Farrow, D. S. Robertson, G. M. Williams, A. G. Cullis, G. R. Jones, I. M. Young and P. N. J. Dennis, J. Cryst. Growth **54**, 507 (1981).

[16] D. Loretto, J. M. Gibson, S. M. Yalisove, R. T. Tung, Proc. of the 46th Annual Meeting of the Electron Microscopy Society of America, **84**, edited by G. W. Bailey (San Francico Press) 1988.

[17] D. Cherns, Phil. Mag. **30**, 549 (1974).

[18] D. Lynch, Acta Cryst., **A27**, 399 (1971).

[19] J. H. Mazur and J. Washburn, AIP Conf. Ser. **122**, 52 (1984).

[20] P. O. Hahn and M. Henzler, J. Vac. Sci. Tech. A **2**, 574, (1984).

[21] S. M. Goodnick, D. K. Ferry, C. W. Wilmsen, Z. Liliental, D. Fathy and O. L. Krivanek, Phys. Rev. B **32**, 8171 (1985).

[22] J. M. Gibson, M. Y. Lanzerotti and V. Elser, to be published.

[23] A. Ourmazd, G. R. Anstis and P. B. Hirsch, Phil. Mag. A **48**, 139 (1983).

[24] S. Iijima, Ultramic. **6**, 41, (1981).

SURFACE STUDIES BY SEM AND STEM

J.A. Venables[*†] and P.A. Bennett[†]

*School of Mathematical & Physical Sciences
University of Sussex, Brighton BN1 9QH, U.K.
†Department of Physics, Arizona State University
Tempe, AZ 85287, USA

INTRODUCTION

Scanning electron (SEM) and scanning transmission (STEM) electron microscopy are versatile, well established, techniques for characterisation of materials. Other papers in this volume attest to their widespread use for understanding semiconductors, and devices based on these various material combinations. This paper concentrates on studies performed in ultra-high vacuum (UHV), so that clean surfaces can be produced and maintained during the experiments. Under such conditions, several SEM and STEM signals have sensitivity at the monolayer (ML) level, so that true surface studies can be carried out.

Several reviews are available which chart the course of these developments over the last ten years [1-3]. Over the same period we have seen the rapid emergence of scanning tunnelling microscopy (STM) [4], and also of Low energy (LEEM)[5], Transmission (TEM) and Reflection (REM) electron microscopy, as techniques which can be applied to similar problems [6]. The particular strengths of SEM- and STEM-based techniques arise primarily from their analytical capability. This means that compositional, structural, microstructural, and in some cases electrical and optical, information can be correlated on the same area of the sample. In the context of surface studies, SEM and STEM have the ability to examine rough (highly 3-dimensional) samples, and to correlate surface and sub-surface information.

The geometry of SEM and STEM signals is illustrated schematically in Fig. 1. Both techniques use a fine-focussed electron probe on the sample, with serial recording of the collected signal to form the image as a function of the probe position (x,y). The distinction between the two is that SEM is traditionally done on bulk samples situated beyond the final lens, as seen in Fig. 1(a). This gives excellent sample access, with lateral resolution easily reaching 20 nm and extending in some machines with field emission guns (FEG's) to below 5 nm. The higher resolution STEM configuration is achieved by immersing the thin foil sample into a highly excited condenser-objective lens, illustrated in Fig. 1(b). Lattice resolution below 0.2 nm and point resolution less than 0.5 nm can be achieved in a dedicated STEM equipped with a high brightness FEG [7].

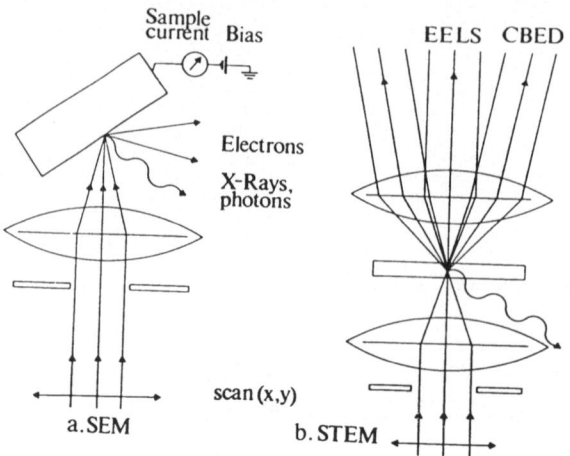

Fig. 1. Signals in a) SEM and b) STEM configurations

There are several surface-analytical signals which can be obtained in these SEM and STEM configurations. Best known is perhaps Auger electron spectroscopy (AES), which provides surface chemical analysis via energy analysis of the electrons emitted in SEM. The SEM-AES combination, or scanning Auger microscopy (SAM), is widely available commercially. The Auger electrons have strong surface sensitivity via their short inelastic mean free path, which is typically λ less than 1nm at energies E below 500 eV, rising to λ greater than 2 nm at E above 1500eV.

Reflection high energy electron diffraction (RHEED) can be obtained easily in SEM, by turning the sample to glancing angle and simply observing a fluorescent screen [2]. The combination SEM-AES-RHEED is particularly powerful and has been installed in several laboratories. We have also found that a very simple extension of SEM, called biassed secondary electron imaging or b-SEI [7], is particularly valuable in a surface context. Some examples of these developments are described in the next section.

Although sample access is severely restricted in the STEM geometry, there are some fortunate aspects of signal collection. The post-specimen lens (Fig. 1(b)) compresses the angular range of the transmitted electrons. Hence it is possible to collect a relatively wide angle, up to 20° off-axis, convergent beam electron diffraction (CBED) patterns, and to do detailed crystallographic studies. The inelastic electrons used in electron energy loss spectroscopy (EELS) go through the lens at very small angles; and x-ray emission can be collected in an energy dispersive (EDX) detector [8]. None of these signals is specifically surface sensitive. However, in films less than a few 10 nm thick, surface signals can be detected via the high surface to volume ratio.

The development of specific surface sensitive techniques in conjunction with UHV-STEM is a current development project, and progress is described in the third section. Emphasis is given to secondary and Auger electrons; these electrons with energies up to E ~ 2 keV, spiral in the strong magnetic field and emerge along the axis of the objective lens. Preliminary experiments indicate that such developments will be successful, and will enable surface topographic, chemical and electronic information to be correlated with the other analytical signals available in a modern FEG-STEM.

SEM STUDIES OF SURFACES

The SEM-AES-RHEED combination

An ultrahigh vacuum SEM, with AES and RHEED facilities, has been installed in several laboratories [2,9-12]. This combination is extremely versatile. The examples described below concentrate on developments at Sussex and Arizona State Universities. Other developments are mentioned briefly in the last sub-section.

Surface diffusion and crystal growth studies using b-SEIs

The present arrangement at Sussex is shown schematically in Fig. 2; the system, based on a cold FEG operating typically at 30kV, has been used to study the growth of metal on metal (e.g. Ag/W(110) [13]) and on semiconductor (e.g. Ag/Si(100) and (111) [14]) surfaces.

For recent studies on these systems, the development of biassed secondary electron imaging (b-SEI) has been most useful [15]. In such experiments, the metal is deposited through a mask of holes, shown in Fig. 2, and the sample is biassed negatively to a few hundred volts. Under these simple conditions the secondary electron signal has a sensitivity better than 0.1 ML in the cases studied. More recently, the collected specimen current has been shown to give a (reversed) signal of comparable (5-10%) contrast [16]. A comparison of the two images for a 1 ML Ag deposit on Si(111) is shown in Fig. 3. The effects are caused by changes in the work-function and band-bending [15]. In the case of metals on metals, only the work function change is important, as evidenced by our work on Cs and Ag deposited on tungsten. However, for semiconductor surfaces, the effects of band-bending can also be significant, as seen in the case of Ag/Si(111). Further work is in progress on this point.

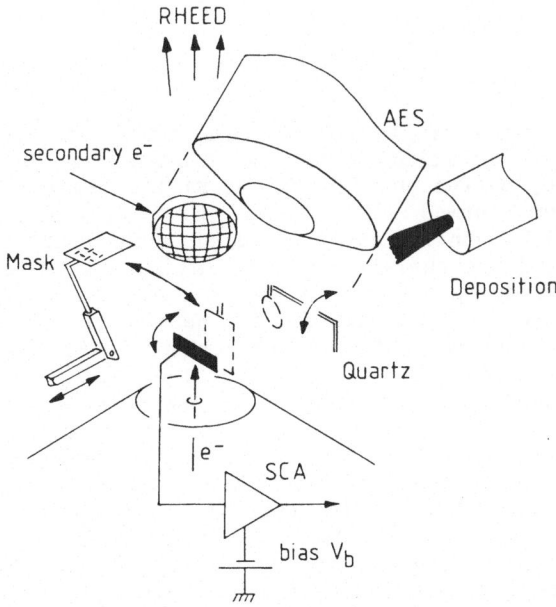

Fig. 2. SEM-AES-RHEED geometry in the VG HB50 [16].

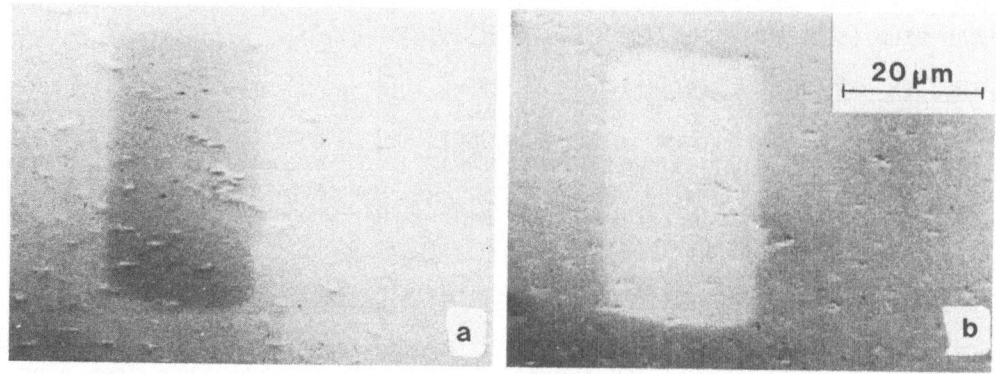

Fig. 3.   Comparison of (a) biassed specimen current image with (b) biassed
secondary electron image for 1 ML Ag/Si(111), at V_b = -200 V [16].

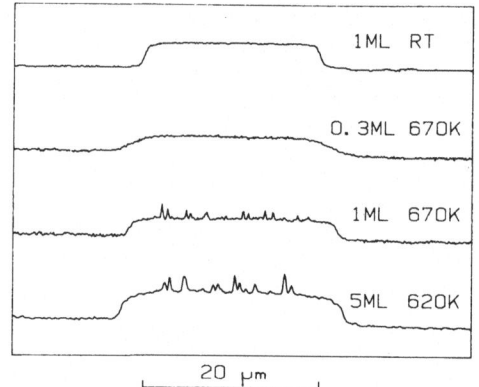

Fig. 4.   Typical b-SEI line scans showing a range of contrast for different
doses, as well as the presence of islands at 1 and 5 ML [18].

Quantitative measurements of surface diffusion have been made for
Ag/W(110) [17] and Ag/Si(111) [18].   At elevated sample temperatures, the
patches broaden by diffusion.   In the Ag/Si(111) system, the image of the
intermediate layer formed (the so-called √3 layer) gets wider.   This
broadening can be quantitatively studied with b-SEI line scans [18].
Examples, including the nucleation of Ag islands on top of the √3 layer at
moderate temperatures, are shown in Fig. 4.   The width observed, after a 5
ML dose of Ag atoms has been delivered from the silver source, exhibits a
strong peak as a function of temperature, shown in Fig. 5.

At high temperature, diffusion is in competition with re-evaporation,
allowing us to deduce a value of E_a-E_d, where E_a and E_d are the
activation energies for adsorption and diffusion respectively.   At moderate
temperatures, diffusion and nucleation both occur, leading to the formation
of Ag islands in the centre of the deposit; this competition is determined
by Ag-adatom binding (E_b) and E_d .   Detailed kinetic models have been
developed and used to deduce atomic parameters (E_a, E_d, E_b) with high
precision.   Our best values for this system are E_a = 2.35 ± 0.1, E_d = 0.35
± 0.05 and E_b = 0.10 ± 0.03 eV [18].

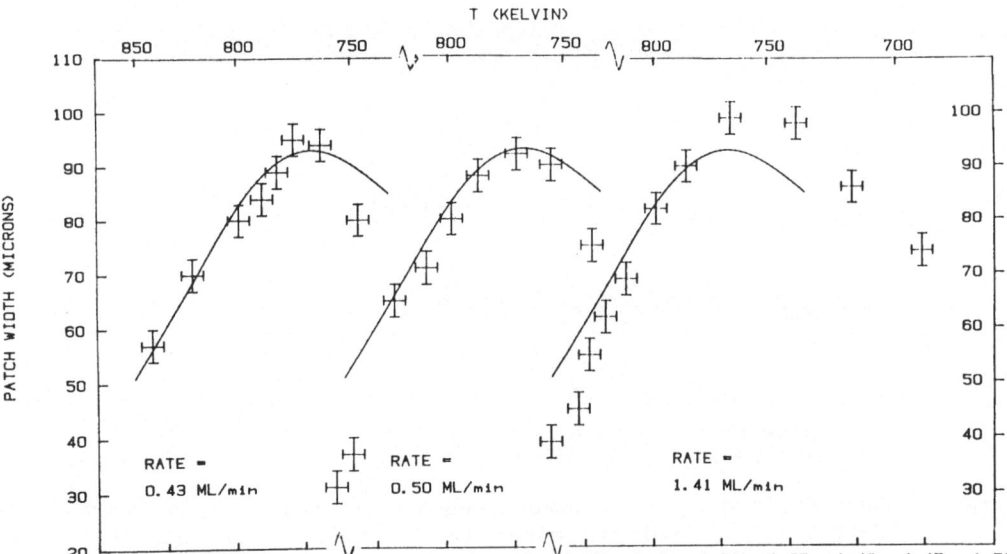

Fig. 5. Patch width as a function of deposition temperature T(K) for a 5
ML dose, deposited at the indicated rates. Calculation for R = 1
ML/min, E_a = 2.3, E_d = 0.42 and E_b = 0.13 eV [18].

Silicide formation studied by scanning RHEED

In the above examples, the main focus has been on SEM, with AES and
RHEED used as ancillary techniques to monitor surface composition and
crystallography. In other studies, similar instrumentation has been used
with different priorities. At Arizona State, a compact SEM-AES-RHEED
machine has been built using a 'bolt-on' FEG. The system is typically used
at 15kV and the FEG is operated in the thermal field emission mode, which
is very stable at high emission currents [9].

The initial growth of nickel silicides has been extensively studied.
Nickel is deposited through a similar mask to that illustrated in Fig. 2,
but with the mask placed further away from the sample, so that a known
thickness gradient is established. Thus a single deposition can be used to
take RHEED patterns from several coverages (of Ni) which are spatially well
separated.

Fig. 6 is a scanning RHEED dark field image using a large diffraction
aperture centered on the (400) Kikuchi band of Si(111). It shows three
patches of nickel about 4 nm thick at their centers and tapering down to
zero coverage at their edges, after annealing at 600°C. At this annealing
temperature, an epitaxial $NiSi_2$ layer is formed with three different
configurations: B-type $NiSi_2$ is essentially twinned (at the substrate
interface) compared to A-type $NiSi_2$ which is a lattice continuation of the
substrate. These form at coverages of < 1 nm and 2 nm, respectively, while
both A and B-type form at coverages above 3 nm. This thickness dependence
is clearly visible in the dark field image, with contrast arising from the
Kikuchi band intensity, which is strong for Si(111) and A-type $NiSi_2$, and
weak for B-type and mixed A + B-type $NiSi_2$. By annealing to well defined
temperatures and repeating the patterns, kinetic 'phase-formation diagrams'
showing the evolution of the various silicide phases and their epitaxial
orientations can be rapidly established. The resulting diagram is shown in
Fig. 7 [9].

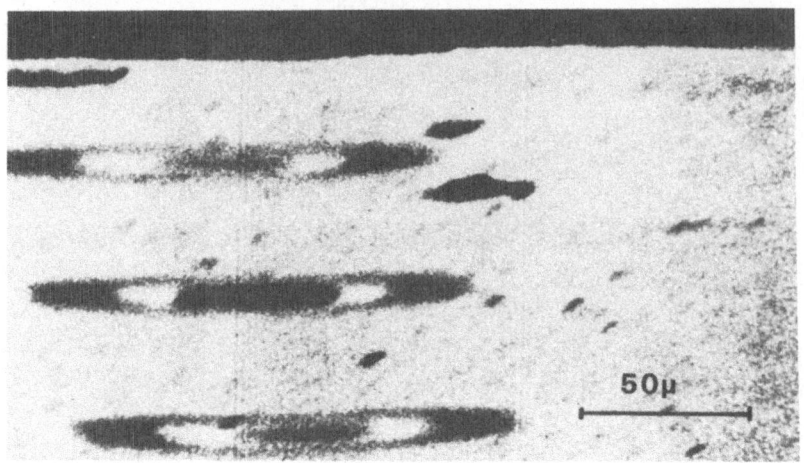

Fig. 6. Dark-field image of three annealed patches showing A-type and B-type NiSi$_2$, and the mixed (A+B) types in the centre of the patches [9].

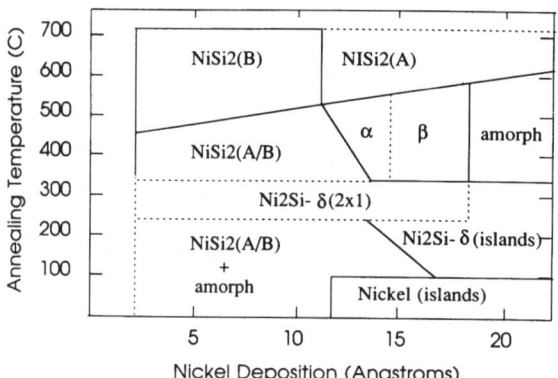

Fig. 7. Phase-formation diagram representation of coverages and annealing temperatures at which the various silicide structures are formed in the Ni-Si system. Solid lines show distinct boundaries, dotted lines show coexistence [9].

It should be noted that RHEED is a surface sensitive probe, and that the diffraction patterns may not correctly represent the state of the entire film thickness. However, when the film is a single phase, such as an epitaxial single crystal, or when it is a homogeneous multi-phase with correct surface stoichiometries, which often occurs for three-dimensional island structures, it commonly does. Of course the entire thin film reaction may be dominated by stoichiometries and reactions at the surface [19], so the information provided by RHEED and Auger is crucial to understanding these systems. In this sense, the surface sensitive probes are complementary to the penetrating probes such as UHV-TEM and STEM which provide information about the entire film thickness, and are uniquely suited for probing structures and reactions at buried interfaces [20].

Other studies based on the SEM-AES-RHEED combination

It is well known that the intensity of RHEED spots varies during crystal growth of semiconductors by molecular beam epitaxy (MBE), with a period of 1 ML, as the surface alternates between atomically rough and smooth [21]. By stopping the deposition when the layers were partially complete and using the specular RHEED spot intensity as the signal in a scanning REM mode, Ichikawa et al [10] have succeeded in visualizing the nucleation pattern of Si deposited onto Si(111), when the steps are relatively widely separated. These pictures are valuable confirmatory evidence of the models of nucleation in competition with step growth in semiconductor MBE.

Other workers in Japan and Germany [11] have concentrated on lower energy electron diffraction, in the LEED-MEED range, where the angle of incidence θ_0 is larger, and the foreshortening less severe than in REM. At lower probe energies, $E_0 < 1$ keV, there is also substantially increased backscattered signal intensity and contrast. The spatial resolution, however, deteriorates unless electrostatic immersion lens techniques are used, as in Bauer's LEEM [5]. It is possible that a scanning version of this instrument can also be developed to work at very high spatial resolution, but the constraints on source brightness are extremely severe.

The relatively recent practice of collecting Auger electrons using undifferentiated spectra, in $N(E)$ or $E.N(E)$ form, is helpful in the quest for quantification, since information is also contained in the background intensity and its energy dependence. Depending on the probe energy E_0, the angle of incidence θ_0 and the analysed energy E, the background can have largely backscattered or secondary electron character. Prutton and coworkers [12] have studied this background quantitatively and found that it often can be well represented by a power law AE^{-m} [21], similar to EELS, but with $m < 1$ [22]. These studies, and also those of Batchelor et al [23, are important in establishing how well AES can be quantified in the context of scanning Auger instruments.

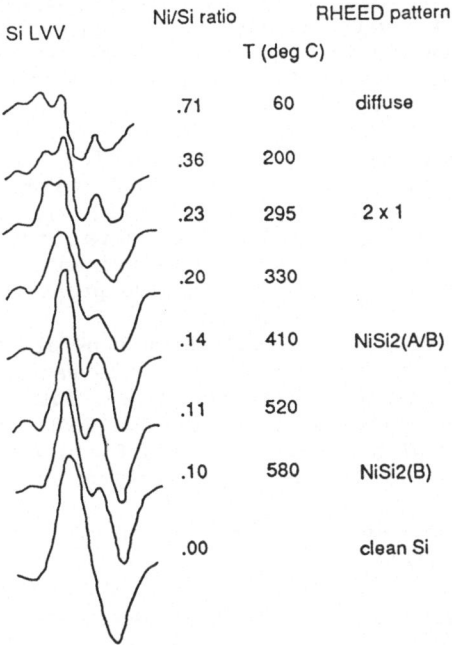

Fig. 8. Auger lineshape (d^2N/dE^2) spectra for Si LMM (92 eV), as modified by bonding to Ni, under various annealing conditions [24].

An alternative use of AES is as a 'fingerprint' of the bonding state of atoms in the surface region. The transitions which are most affected are those involving valence electrons. An example is shown in Fig. 8 for Si LVV (92 eV), as modified by bonding to Ni in the nickel silicides [24]. In this case second differential (d^2N/dE^2) spectra are shown, and the way in which the spectral shape changes with varying Ni content in the deposition and annealing sequence is clear. In the coexistence regions, seen in the phase diagram of Fig. 6, the spectra can be synthesised by linear combinations of the adjacent phases [25]. In the case of Fig. 8, an auxiliary wide electron beam was used to take Auger spectra with good signal to noise ratio from the general area probed by the micro-RHEED beam.

In most applications of AES on a microscopic scale, and especially in SAM, the low signal to noise ratio is a problem, particularly for quantitative analysis. Hence it is useful to be able to correlate AES with other signals, which, while not chemically specific, are much stronger. The b-SEI and RHEED signals described here are cases in point. The energy loss (EELS) signal, which can also be obtained in a scanning instrument, may also be useful in certain cases [26].

INSTRUMENTAL DEVELOPMENTS FOR STEM AND SEM

Development of an UHV-STEM for surface studies

The successful development of the FEG-STEM has depended crucially on rigorous application of UHV techniques (< 10^{-10} Torr) in the gun region for the effective use of cold field emission. It is in a sense surprising that, given this technology, a UHV-STEM for surface studies has taken a long time to be developed. However, other features are also needed, including in-situ sample preparation facilities, which are easier to organise with a side entry stage, and welding, and sealing to, soft magnetic materials. A major step has been the demonstration that double viton 'O'-ring seals, with a pumped interspace, can reach true UHV specification after baking to temperatures approaching 200°C. This allows the necessarily complex system to be demounted much more straightforwardly for repairs and other changes.

A system of this type has been developed for the NSF HREM facility at Arizona State University. The system, codenamed MIDAS (a Microscope for Imaging, Diffraction and Analysis of Surfaces), is based on the VG HB501 100kV FEG-STEM, but incorporates several novel design features. These include improved column optics and post-specimen lenses, and a versatile eucentric stage which is coupled to extensive preparation chambers [27].

All the signals (EELS, CBED, EDX) shown schematically in Fig. 1(b) are available in this machine. In early tests, the vacuum was <2.10^{-10} Torr in the sample chamber itself, measured in an intentionally unfavourable position; the lattice planes of both Au(200) 0.204 nm, and MgO(220) 0.148 nm have been resolved with the Angular Dark Field (ADF) detector; and high quality CBED patterns of Si, and EELS spectra of Al have been obtained [28]. Many applications will result from these features alone. But in addition provision has been made for low energy electron spectroscopy and imaging as described below.

Electron spectroscopy and microscopy using magnetic parallelizers

The key to low energy electron spectroscopy in a STEM is that the high magnetic field of the objective lens acts as a highly efficient electron collector and collimator. Low energy electrons form tight spirals in the magnetic field, the outer diameter, d (mm), being given by

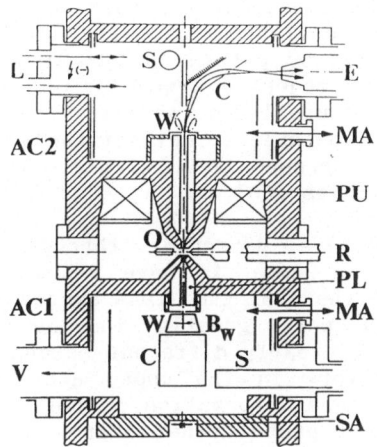

Fig. 9. Arrangement for analysis of low energy electrons in 'MIDAS' [27].

$d = 0.135 \ E_i^{\frac{1}{2}} . \sin\theta_i / B_i$.

For an initial energy E_i = 100 eV and magnetic field B_i = 1 Tesla, all the electrons are confined within d = 0.135 mm. As the magnetic field is reduced away from the centre of the objective lens to a value B_f, the angle θ_f scales [29], as

$\sin\theta_f / \sin\theta_i = (B_f / B_i)^{\frac{1}{2}} . (E_i / E_f)^{\frac{1}{2}}$.

Thus, if B_f = 0.01T, all the electrons are confined within $\sin\theta_f$ = 0.1 if $E_f = E_i$; i.e. within a cone θ_f = 5.74°, or even less if the electrons are accelerated so that $E_f > E_i$. Thus all the electrons emitted are collimated, or 'parallelized' into this cone, whose angle is within the acceptance angle of a (commercial) Concentric Hemispherical Analyser (CHA).

The MIDAS system has been 'stretched' beyond a standard STEM to allow us to detect these electrons, as illustrated in Fig. 9 [27,29]. There are two analysis chambers (AC1 and AC2), and the back bores of the objective lens (O) contain lower and upper 'parallelizer' coils (PL and PU) terminated by magnetic apertures (MA). As explained in more detail elsewhere [29], these apertures reduce the field B_f abruptly to zero, causing the electrons to stop spiralling and to proceed in straight lines away from the axis, within the cone defined by θ_f.

The next problem is how to deflect the low energy electrons off the axis. We have chosen to do this with a small Wien ($E \wedge B$) filter followed by a sector of a gridless Cylindrical Mirror Analyser (CMA). The Wien filter (W) and CMA (C), plus secondary electron detectors (S) are shown in two projections in the analyser chambers on Fig. 9. In this way the cone of low energy electrons is transferred from the exit of the parallelizer to an intermediate focus (F) and then into an energy analyser (E), while the Wien filter keeps the 100 keV beam on-axis. Secondary electron detection (without analysis) is achieved simply by reversing the sign of the fields in the Wien filter.

These ideas have been tested by building deflectors and simulating the performance of the parallelizer with a scanned low energy electron gun. The position and size of the focus have been found for the prototype [30] and this has provided sufficient information to construct a final design. Essentially all the electrons go through a line focus around 4 x 10 mm. Various options are then available to form spectra and energy selected images. About 3% energy resolution is available directly at F, and higher resolution can be achieved by putting a CHA at E so that the dispersion plane is vertical. The projected transmission and energy resolution of such a scheme are highly competitive; assuming that selected energy imaging is the main goal, we will be able to collect the vast majority of electrons emitted at energies up to around 1keV, with a slow fall-off in collection efficiency at higher energies [29].

Secondary electrons are detected 'through the lens' in several instruments and have been shown to have resolution in the 1 nm range [31,32]. In the initial tests of the MIDAS system [28], secondary electron signals received at S were greatly increased by the use of the parallelizers. Moreover, clearly different secondary electron images were obtained with the detectors in the upper and lower analyser chambers, showing that genuine surface information is being obtained. This example is shown in Fig. 10; we expect further improvements to be possible as a result of optimising the collection geometry further. The correlation of secondary electrons showing surface structure, with the ADF signal showing heavy atoms in the bulk has been demonstrated previously [3,31,32], and will be an extremely useful feature of the new machine.

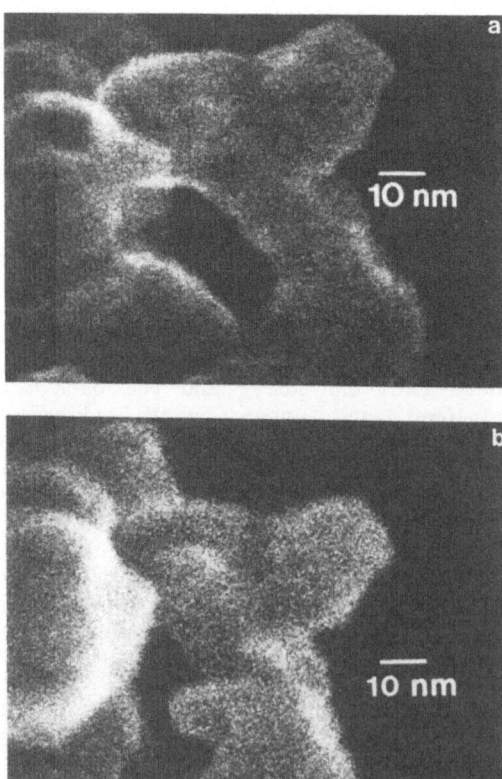

Fig. 10. Secondary electron images from a) upper and b) lower side of a carbon black sample in MIDAS [28].

In a SEM configuration, with the sample outside the lens, two choices
have traditionally been made to collect and analyse electrons emitted from
the sample. These are to use a CHA, usually with input electrostatic
lenses, or to use a CMA. The CHA has the advantage that it can be a
'bolt-on' accessory, and that it does not take up too much solid angle.
However, this means that the collecter signal is correspondingly low. The
CMA has a larger collection efficiency; but as a 'bolt-on' addition it
suffers from being very bulky and typically has to be positioned with its
axis at a large angle (90° or more) to the probing electron beam. The
concentric geometry, with the probing beam along the axis of the CMA, has
various advantages, but has to be considered integrally with the whole
instrument. The major development of this geometry has been done in
connection with commercial Auger microprobes, but there is also scope for
special purpose instruments [33].

At Sussex, we have developed an experimental microscope based on this
coaxial configuration, as shown in Fig. 11. The CMA has been designed with
a large collection angle, $\Omega > 1$ sterad, and a modest-energy resolution $\Delta E/E$
~ 2% [34]. By settling on this resolution from the start, a factor of two
improvement in collection efficiency has been designed in. The detector
slits can also be adjusted to change the resolution and detected signal by

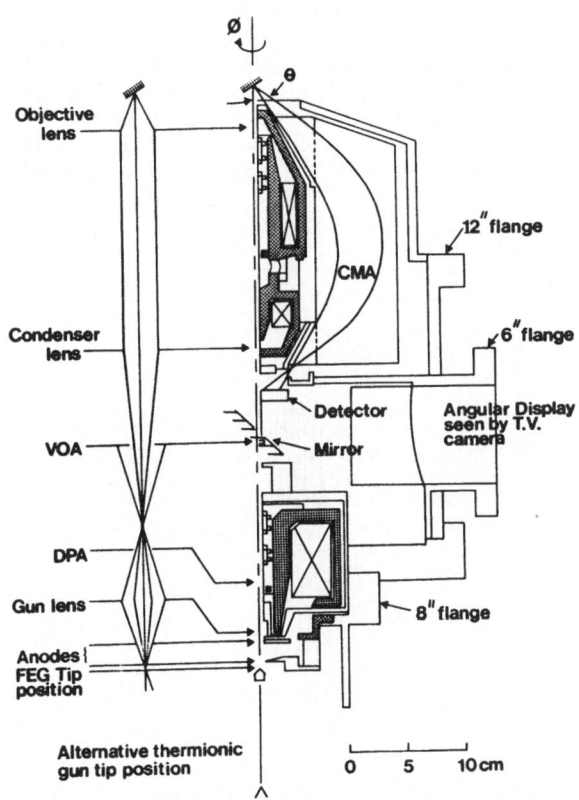

Fig. 11. The Sussex experimental SEM-SAM configuration. The column is
based around a large CMA with a ring detector, which has high
collection efficiency, and allows us to explore angular resolved
spectroscopy [34].

a factor of order three; initial tests have achieved the design energy resolution and collection efficiency [35].

The design is based on a rather large diameter CMA, which means that high voltages up to around 10 kV can be applied to the outer cylinder, so as to analyse the whole of the electron energy spectrum. There is a lot of information in the overall form of the spectrum, including the back-scattered and secondary electron regions [22,23] as well as the Auger peaks, which can be used for qualitative and quantitative analysis. A further advantage of the larger analysis is the increased volume of space in which the sample is in focus, and the less restrictive mechanical tolerances required. However, the resolution is sensitive to stray magnetic fields from the concentric magnetic optics, which have to be compensated for low energy electrons. Although the magnetic parallelizer configuration has the highest collection efficiency at low energies, the CMA solid angle for a given energy resolution ($\Delta E/E$ or ΔE depending on retardation and operating mode) is constant, and so eventually wins at high energies, $\geqslant$ 2 keV. A numerical comparison of these analyser systems is given in more detail elsewhere [36].

The off-axis ring detector, indicated in Fig. 11, will enable us to experiment with angular resolved spectroscopy, as the ϕ information, and some θ information is preserved. Calculations have been made of the expected angular resolution, taking into account the refraction effect of the input grid structure, which in this case are thin wires parallel to the axis. This effect is shown in Fig. 12, for the extremal trajectories, θ = 28.5° and 53.5° [34]. The refraction effect is stronger for the lower θ, but these trajectories hit the detector at larger radius r than the higher θ trajectories. The effective resolution $\Delta\theta$, $\Delta\phi$ is $\approx \pm$ 5° which should be useful for angular resolved Auger and backscattering spectroscopy up to several keV energy. The important point is that these (θ,ϕ) images can be collected in parallel, thus opening the way for the use of such signals as 'fingerprints' of surface crystallography and adsorbate geometry from microscopic areas.

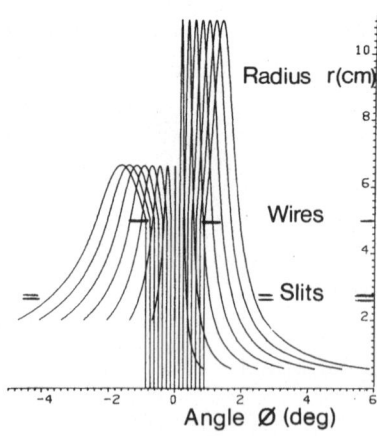

Fig. 12. Calculated r(ϕ) trajectories for the CMA with input wires, for the two extremal values of θ_0 (28.5°, left, and 53.5°, right). The trajectories terminate at the detector position [34].

ACKNOWLEDGEMENTS

Our research has been supported by the SERC (Sussex) and in Arizona by NSF (DMR-84-12232, and -85-00659), ONR (N-00014-84-G-0203) and AFOSR (87-0367), as well as Arizona State University. We also thank several coworkers at both universities who have contributed centrally to the projects described.

REFERENCES

1. J.A. Venables, Ultramicroscopy 7, 81 (1981); in: Chemistry and Physics of Solid Surfaces IV, Eds. R. Vanselow and R. Howe (Springer, Berlin, 1982) Ch. 6.

2. J.A. Venables, D.R. Batchelor, M. Hanbücken, C.J. Harland, G.W. Jones, Phil. Trans. Roy. Soc. A318, 243 (1986).

3. J.A. Venables, D.J. Smith and J.M. Cowley, Surface Sci. 181, 235 (1987), and refs. quoted.

4. For recent STM conferences proceedings, see Surface Sci. 181 (1987); J. Vac. Sci. Tech. (1988, in press); J. Microscopy (1988, in press).

5. W. Telieps and E. Bauer, Ultramicroscopy 17, 57 (1987); Scanning Microscopy Suppl. 1, 99 (1987) W. Telieps, Appl. Phys. A44, 55 (1987); E. Bauer, this volume, and refs. quoted.

6. K. Yagi, J. Appl. Cryst. 20, 147 (1987).

7. J.A. Venables and G. Cox, Ultramicroscopy 21, 33 (1987) and refs. quoted; C. Mory, C. Colliex and J.M. Cowley, Ultramicroscopy 21, 171 (1987).

8. The techniques CBED, EELS and EDX are extensively covered in other papers in this volume.

9. P.A. Bennett, B.N. Halawith and A.P. Johnson, J. Vac. Sci. Tech. A5, 2121 (1987); Phys. Rev. B37, 4268 (1988).

10. M. Ichikawa, T. Doi, M. Ichihashi and K. Hayakawa, Jap. J. Appl. Phys. 23, 913 (1984); Appl. Phys. Lett. 50, 1141 (1987).

11. T. Ichinokawa and Y. Ishikawa, Ultramicroscopy 15, 193 (1984); T. Ichinokawa, Y. Ishikawa, M. Kemmochi, N. Ikeda, Y. Hosokawa and J. Kirschner, Scanning Microscopy Suppl. 1, 93 (1987).

12. M. Prutton, R. Browning, M.M. El Gomati and D.C. Peacock, Vacuum 32, 351 (1982); M. Prutton and M.M. El Gomati, Inst. Phys. Conf. Ser. 93, 255 (1988).

13. G.D.T. Spiller, P. Akhter and J.A. Venables, Surface Sci. 131, 517 (1983).

14. M. Hanbücken, M. Futamoto and J.A. Venables, Surface Sci. 147, 433 (1984).

15. M. Futamoto, M. Hanbücken, C.J. Harland, G.W. Jones and J.A. Venables, Surface Sci. 150, 430 (1985); C.J. Harland and J.A. Venables, Ultramicroscoy 17, 9 (1985); J.A. Venables, Proc. Int. Cong. on Electron Microscopy, Kyoto 1, 75 (1986).

16. C.J. Harland, G.W. Jones, T. Doust and J.A. Venables, Scanning Microscopy Suppl. 1, 109 (1987).

17. G.W. Jones and J.A. Venables, Ultramicroscopy 18, 439 (1985).

18. J.A. Venables, T. Doust and R. Kariotis, Materials Research Symp. 94, 3 (1987); to be published.

19. E.J. van Loenen, J.F. van der Veen and F.K. LeGoues, Surface Sci. 157, 1 (1985).

20. J.M. Gibson, J.L. Batstone, R.T. Tung and F.C. Unterwald, Phys. Rev. Lett. 60, 1158 (1988).

21. See e.g., P.J. Dobson, these proceedings, and refs. quoted.

22. J.A.D. Matthew, M. Prutton, M.M. El Gomati and D.C. Peacock, Surf. Interface Analysis 11, 173 (1988).

23. D.R. Batchelor, P. Rez, D.J. Fathers and J.A. Venables, Surf. Interface Analysis in press; D.R. Batchelor, H.E. Bishop and J.A. Venables, ibid, submitted.

24. P.A. Bennett, X. Tong and J.R. Butler, J. Vac. Sci. Tech. B6, 1336 (1988).

25. P.A. Bennett, J.R. Butler and X. Tong, J. Vac. Sci. Tech. in press.

26. M.M. El Gomati and J.A.D. Matthew, J. Microscopy 147, 137 (1987); Appl. Surface Sci. 32, 320 (1988).

27. J.A. Venables, J.M. Cowley and H.S. von Harrach, Institute of Physics Conf. Ser. 90, 85 (1987).

28. The tests were performed by S. von Harrach, R.J. Keyse, G.G. Hembree and J.M. Cowley.

29. P. Kruit and J.A. Venables, Ultramicroscopy 25, 183 (1988).

30. G.G. Hembree, Luo Chuan-Hong, P.A. Bennett and J.A. Venables, Proc. 46th EMSA meeting (1988) 666.

31. J. Liu and J.M. Cowley, Scanning Microscopy 2, 65 (1988); Ultramicroscopy 23, 463 (1987).

32. D. Imeson, R.H. Milne, S.D. Berger and D. McMullan, Ultramicroscopy 17, 243 (1985).

33. R.L. Gerlach and N.C. McDonald, Scanning Electron Microscopy 1, 199 (1976); ibid 1, 213 (1979). G. Todd, H. Poppa and L.H. Veneklasen ibid 1, 207 (1979); Thin Solid Films 57, 213 (1979).

34. C.J. Harland, G. Cox, D.J. Fathers, P.S. Flora, M. Hardiman, G. Raynerd, M. Whitehouse-Yeo and J.A. Venables, Inst. Phys. Conf. Ser. 90, 9 (1987).

35. J.A. Venables, D.R. Batchelor, P.S. Flora, C.J. Harland, G.G. Hembree and Luo Chuan-Hong, J. Micr. et Spectr. Electronique, in press.

36. P. Kruit and J.A. Venables, Scanning Microscopy Suppl. 1, 115 (1987).

TRANSMISSION AND REFLECTION ELECTRON MICROSCOPY ON

CLEAVED EDGES OF III-V MULTILAYERED STRUCTURES

Philippe-André Buffat+, Jean-Daniel Ganière* and Pierre Stadelmann+

*Inst. Micro- et Opto-électronique
+Inst. Interdépartemental Microscopie Electronique
 Ecole Polytechnique Fédérale, CH-1015 Lausanne, Switzerland

INTRODUCTION

The growth by molecular beam epitaxy of III-V layers with reduced thickness permits the synthesis of new materials. The optical and electrical properties of these structures are strongly related to the roughness of the hetero-interfaces, the chemical composition and the accurate thickness of the layers. Electron microscopy is a direct way to get local information. Despite its rather limited resolution power, SEM is quite commonly used. Routine TEM applications are limited due to the time consuming nature of the thin foils preparation process and the artefacts associated. Our observations on cleaved samples demonstrate that Wedge Transmission Electron Microscopy (WTEM) and Reflection Electron Microscopy (REM) offer some unique advantages on the previous methods in terms of specimen preparation, layer thickness determination, estimation of interface abruptness, chemical composition information and parallelism of the epilayers.

LIMITS OF SEM AND TEM

The main advantage for the use of the SEM is the possibility to study clean bulk samples simultaneously with different contrast modes (secondary electrons, EBIC, VC, CL,...) over quite large areas. Nevertheless, in most cases of multilayered epitaxial structures, information on the nanometer scale is required and the resolving power of the SEM becomes a critical parameter. The secondary electron contrast mode is then the only one possible. Most of the layers cannot be distinguished directly from the change in secondary electron yield due to a chemical or an electrical contrast, even if layers of different doping can sometimes produce different secondary electrons yields, or collection efficiency, due to electric effects. The sample then needs to be chemically etched with a convenient mixture to produce some topographic contrast or a stain which can be associated with the layers or the hetero-interfaces. Figure 1 was taken on a SEM with LaB6 gun (3.5nm nominal resolution at 40 kV) and illustrates the power and the limitations of that technique. Another limit concerning the geometric parameters estimation arises from the distortions of the scanned raster in the electron column and in the cathode ray tube. This causes the local magnification to vary significantly over the micrograph area and to curve straight lines. If the former contribution decreases with magnification and is really important only at low magnification, the latter one is constant on the micrograph irrespective of the magnification.

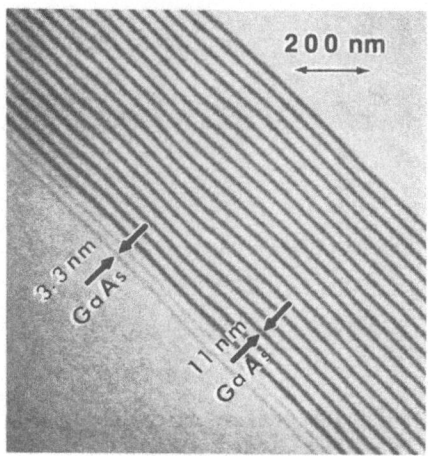

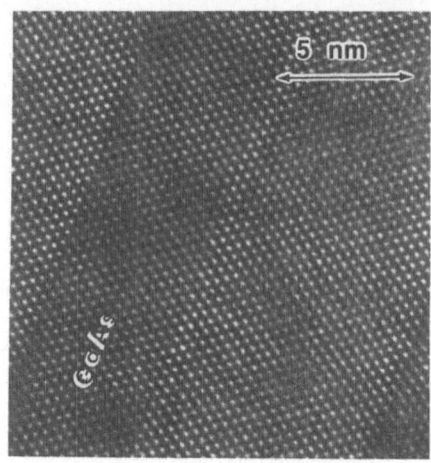

Fig. 1. SEM picture of a MQW structure made of AlGaAs/GaAs, x=0.2. The layer apparent dimensions are obviously wrong.

Fig. 2. Cross-section of an AlAs/GaAs MQW. The irradiation damage reduces the information content.

Diffraction contrast and higher resolving power in TEM allows us to overcome these limitations and a resolution of a few tenths of a nanometer can be attained. The main drawback of the TEM is the time consuming procedure used to prepare the thin foils, especially when cross-sections are required for edge-on studies. In this case, bonding pieces face to face with glue, mechanical prepolishing and ion bombardment or chemical etching for thinning to perforation has to be carried out[1]. This can rarely be done in less than one day. In addition, these processes induce more or less severe artifacts depending on the materials. Such effects are, in particular, buckling of the foil in the thin areas due to strain relaxation and ion implantation, uncontrolled thickness variation[2] due to uneven sputtering or preferential etch and ion irradiation damage[3] (fig. 2) or amorphous surface films. Image contrast interpretation is strongly limited by these effects.

WEDGE TRANSMISSION ELECTRON MICROSCOPY (WTEM)

Cleavage has been extensively used to produce thin flakes at the early stage of TEM (see for example references in Hirsch[4]). Most of the III-V compounds used in the semiconductor industry crystallize in the zincblende structure and can be easily cleaved on the {110} planes. Usually, the wafer orientation is [001] and cleavage along the [±110] planes produces a perfect 90⁰ wedge. This is transparent to electrons over a distance of a few hundred nanometers from the edge. Observation is often done along, or close to, the [100] zone axis, i.e. with the epilayers parallel to the incident electron beam (fig. 3a). A simple method to mount the sample is to stick it on a home-made copper grid as shown in figure 3b.

Wedge microscopy is interesting in several aspects:
- The method of specimen preparation is quite fast, it avoids artefacts due to the conventional thinning process and needs only a few square millimeters of material.
- The contrast interpretation is made easier due to the precise knowledge of the observed area thickness.
- The proximity of the thicker part of the sample reduces significantly buckling and strain relaxation effects.
- The steep variation of thickness across the sample allows new possibilities to gain chemical composition information.

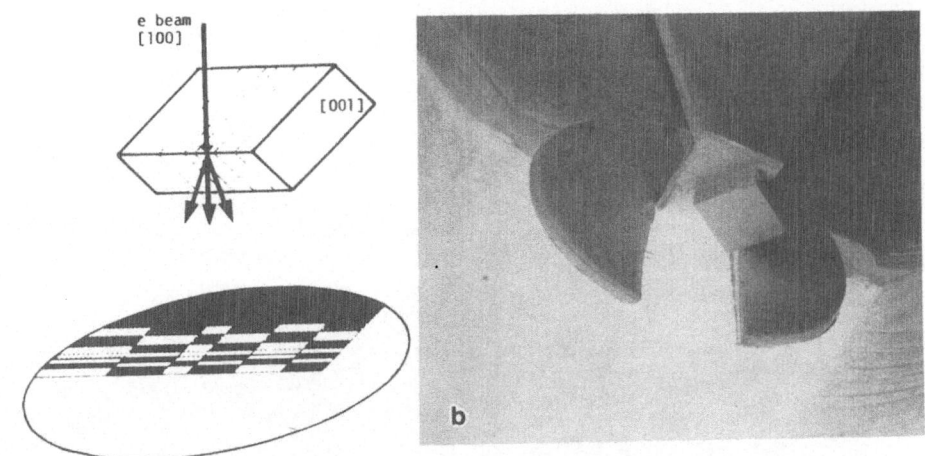

Fig. 3. Sketch of Wedge Transmission Electron Microscopy: a) orientation of the specimen under the beam, b) specimen setting on the special grid.

In contrast to conventional TEM on thin foils, WTEM takes advantage of the change in thickness over the observed area. The wedge shape of the specimen governs directly the observed contrast. In bright field and in dark field, the equal thickness fringes are always present. Their profile depends on the chemical composition of the material and discontinuities are observed[5,6,7,8] at the hetero-interfaces. For instance in AlGaAs based material, as long as the difference in Al content between adjacent layers exceeds a few percent, it is possible, just by visual inspection, to estimate the layer thickness (fig. 4) with an accuracy only limited by the interface abruptness and the microscope resolution as in usual TEM on thin foils. In addition to the latter, if the interfaces are not abrupt, or if there is a gradient of Al concentration - for instance a graded index of refraction structure (GRINSCH) (fig. 5) - WTEM gives unique information of the spatial extent of these chemical heterogeneities. This information is essential for the interpretation of photoluminescence spectra.

Figure 6 illustrates the usefulness of the WTEM technique applied to a surface laser structure grown by MBE. The structure of the $(AlAs)_2$-$(GaAs)_9$ superlattice is easily resolved and composition instabilities are seen in the buffer. The large shift and the curvature of the thickness fringes in the AlAs layers indicates a topographical effect. It is due to a chemical etch prior to observation as a consequence of the strong reactivity of that material with air. The interfaces bounding the AlAs layers are flatter on the substrate side than on the free surface side, highlighting the difficulties to grow thick high quality AlAs epilayers.

HREM observations can be carried out on wedges. Each micrograph is then a "thickness series". Artefacts like irradiation damage during ion beam thinning, amorphous surface layers or preferential etching are avoided. Figure 7 was taken on one of the $(AlAs)_2$-$(GaAs)_9$ superlattice of the sample above. Its periodicity (10.1±0.3 (200) planes) can be easily and more precisely deduced than on the corresponding diffraction pattern by counting a sufficient number of (200) planes along the edge (at constant thickness). Moreover, local fluctuations also can be deduced. The precise partition between AlAs and GaAs would require an optimal choice of defocus to highlight the contrast difference in the thinnest area and fast operation of the microscope to limit the contamination to a minimum. In this respect, preliminary results show that with InP/InGaAs material, which has more favorable structure factors, it is easiest to get a good delineation between the two phases, despite its strong sensitivity to be damaged by electron irradiation. Comparison with simulated images of wedges (fig. 8) is in progress. It should be noted that both experimental and simulated pictures give the impression that the layer

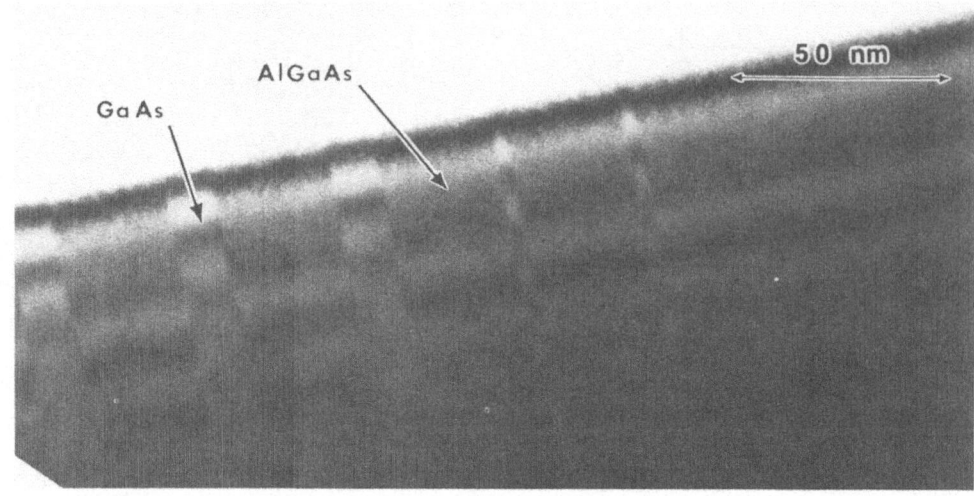

Fig. 4. WTEM micrograph of the same AlGaAs/GaAs (x=0.2) MQW sample as for figure 1. The changes in the thickness fringes profile correspond precisely to the hetero-interfaces and the layer thickness can be accurately measured. [100] bright field, 300 kV

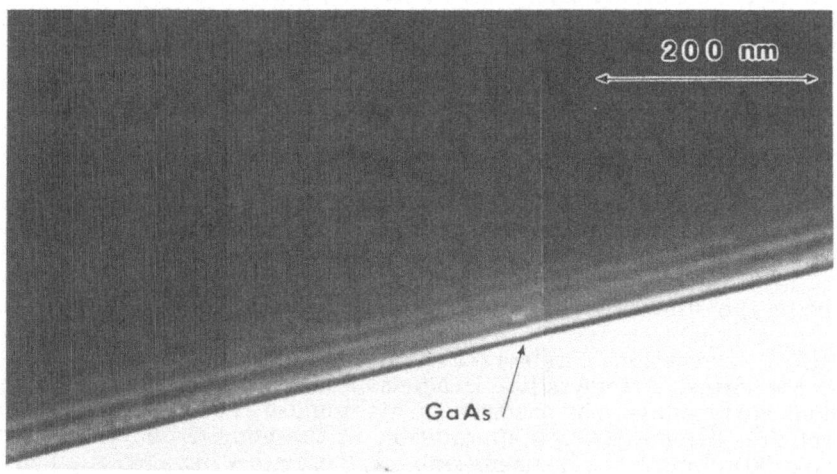

Fig. 5. Graded index AlGaAs (GRINSCH) material around a single GaAs well. The gradient in composition can be followed by the continuous change in the profile of the thickness fringes. On the substrate side (on left on the picture), the fringes appear fuzzy in a portion of the layer. That effect corresponds to an uncontrolled chemical composition produced by temperature oscillations of the MBE sources.

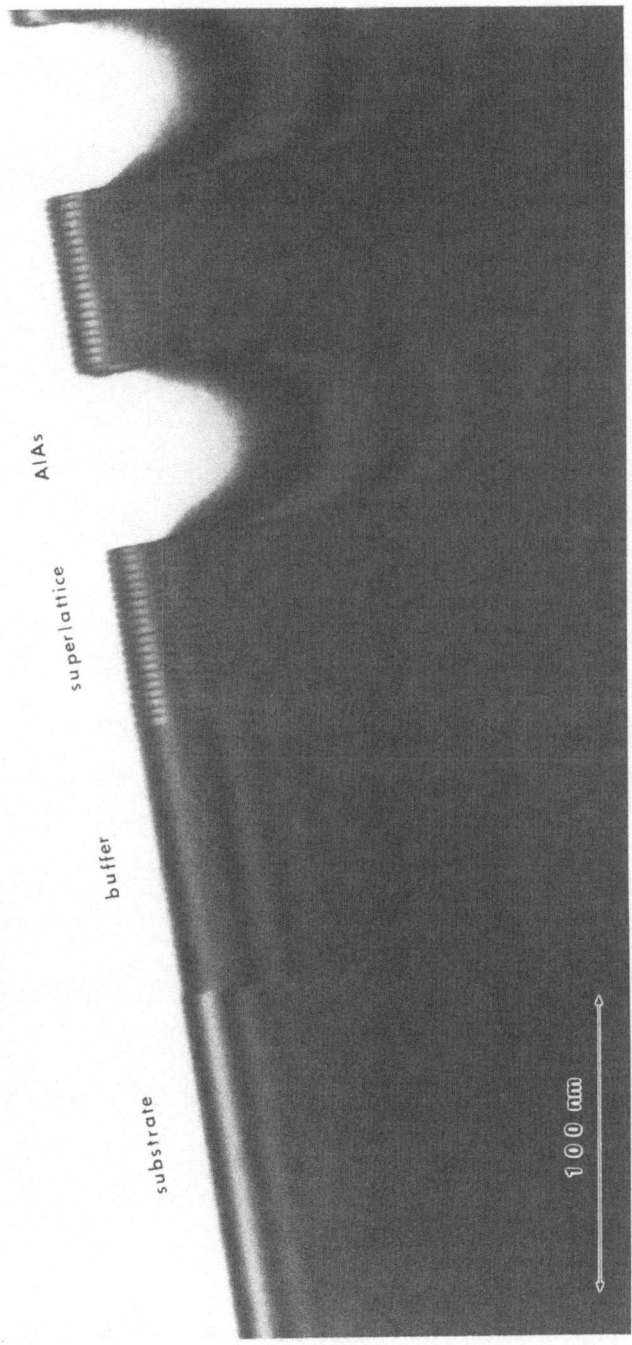

Fig. 6. Surface laser structure grown by MBE. From left to right: n doped GaAs substrate, AlGaAs buffer, first layers of the Bragg reflector made of $(AlAs)_2(GaAs)_9$ superlattices and 58 nm AlAs layers. The fluctuations of composition into the buffer result of an insufficient substrate rotation speed. The bending of the thickness fringes in the AlAs layers correspond to a topographical effect and is due to a decomposition of AlAs under contact with air prior the observation. Referred to the growth direction, the AlAs/superlattice interfaces exhibit a noticeable roughness at contrary of the superlattice/AlAs ones. WTEM picture: accelerating voltage 300 KV, [100] zone axis bright field.

323

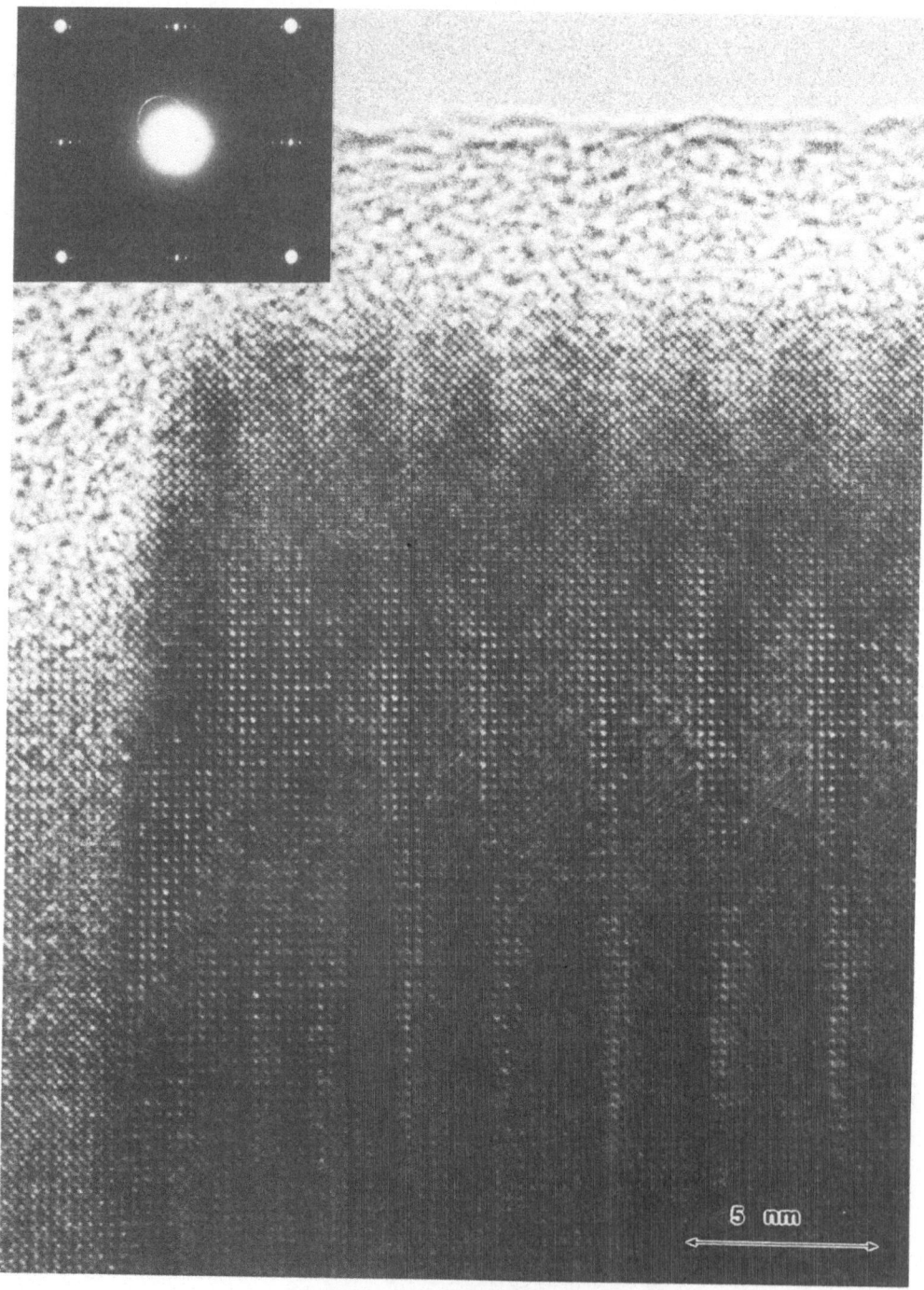

Fig. 7.   HREM on a cleaved wedge (slightly out of [100]). First layers of a (AlAs)$_2$-(GaAs)$_8$ superlattice. The images width of the layers seems to vary with the wedge thickness because of the contrast reversal. In that area, the growth of the layers has been disturbed by the surface roughness of the underlying AlAs layer. The [100] diffraction pattern exhibits a superstructure corresponding to the superlattice.

thickness varies with the sample thickness. This effect, due to the reversal of contrast with thickness, confirms that naïve interpretation associating the position of the atoms with the observed black or white contrasts may most often lead to erroneous conclusions.

The profile of the thickness fringes of a (hkl) beam is a function of the composition, of absorption and Debye-Waller coefficients of the sample, of the precise direction of observation and, of course of the thickness change across the specimen. At least in ternaries, i.e. when the proportion can only vary between two elements, WTEM thickness fringes can be used to derive quantitative information about the local chemical composition[5,6,8] with a spatial resolution of about 2 nm.

The accuracy assessment of that method to measure the Al content in AlGaAs material is under investigation. Bright field along the [001] zone axis has been chosen. This orientation was found to be easy to align and gave reasonable extinction distances in comparison with the transparency of the sample. Observations in Reflection Electron Microscopy (REM) show that the cleaved surfaces are flat and do not contain large steps. Steps of atomic height are scarce and do not introduce a large uncertainty on the thickness. More important is the question of the precise shape of the edge. The first comparison between HREM pictures and simulation suggest that some rounding may happen. However, the angle between the [110] and [-110] faces bounding the wedge is 90^0. Then, on the image, the thickness difference between two points in a (200) plane is twice their distance. The profile of the thickness fringes have been calculated in a Bloch wave approach with the EMS programs of P. Stadelmann[9]. Calculations of the profile of the [100] bright field thickness fringes at 300 kV were carried out using

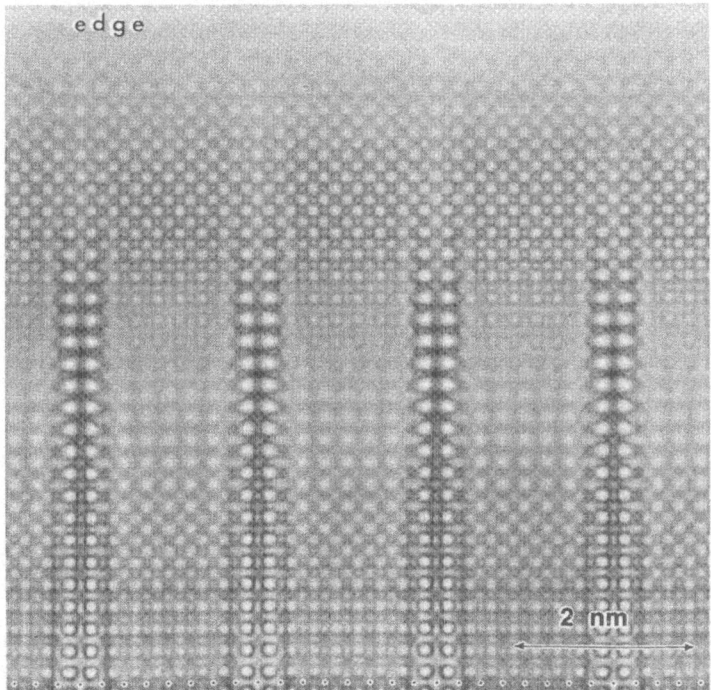

Fig. 8.   HREM image simulation of a wedge shaped (AlAs$_2$)-(GaAs$_6$) using Bloch-wave approach and a supercell containing 8192 atoms and a sampling of 128x512 pixels. E=300 kV, defocus 60nm, Cs=1.2mm, beam divergence=0.8mrad, defocus spread 12nm

81, 121 or 161 beams (fig. 9a) and show that beams in addition to 121 do not greatly change the profile. Experimentally, the alignment of the specimen on the [100] zone axis is ascertained from the quality of the match between the (200) and (220) Kikuchi lines with the corresponding spots. It is estimated to be better than a tenth of g_{220} under visual observation of the microscope screen. The effect of such a slight misalignment was estimated by moving the center of the Laue circle - defined by the intersection of the Ewald sphere and the zero order Laue zone - out of (000). It is found to be of very little importance (fig. 9b). If comparison of experimental micrographs with computed profile is required, the Debye-Waller correction has to be taken in account. Figure 9c shows the profiles obtained using three diffrent Debye-Waller factor. Again, the overall effect is quite low, but results in a slight shift of the thickness fringes, the larger Debye-Waller temperature factor the shorter the extinction distance.

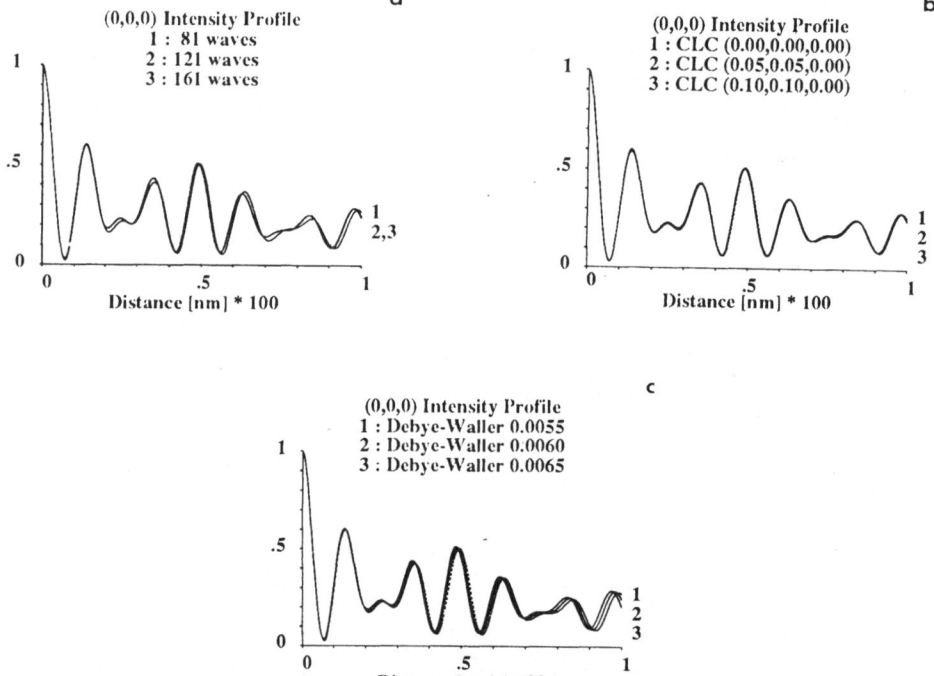

Fig. 9.   Bloch wave calculation of the thickness fringes profiles in $Al_{0.2}Ga_{0.8}As$; [100] bright field, 300 kV: a) Effect of the number of beams considered along the zone axis. Calculations for 81 beams (curve 1), 121 beams (curve 2) and 161 beams (curve 3). The differences are less than a few percents and there is no need for a higher accuracy. b) Comparison between profiles for perfect alignment on the zone axis and slight misalignment: center of the Laue circle at (000), (0.05 0.05 0.05) and (0.10 0.10 0.10) for curves 1,2,and 3 respectively. The experimental inaccuracy in setting the orientation of the sample is certainly smaller and is seen to induce a negligible effect on the intensities. c) Effect of the value chosen for the Debye-Waller factor. Curves 1,2,3 correspond respectively to 0.0055, 0.0060 and 0.0065 nm^2. If the overall shape of the profile remains unchanged, the larger Debye-Waller factor the shorter the extinction distance.

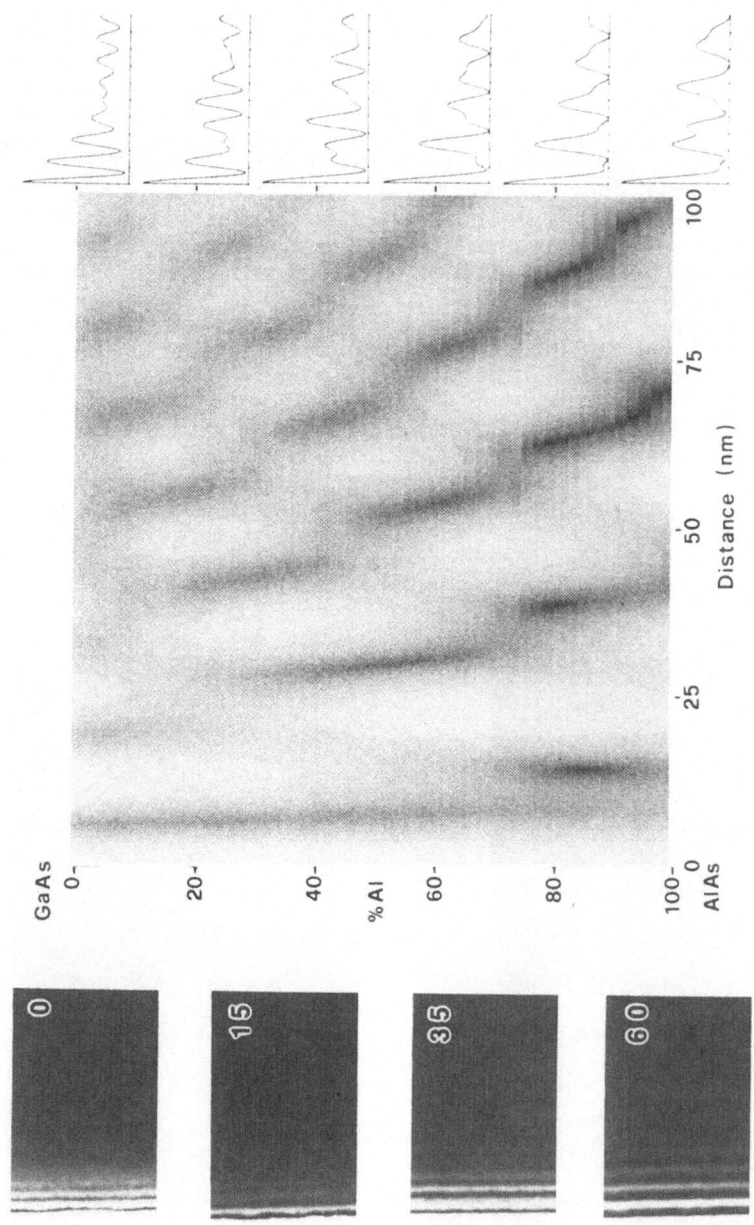

Fig. 10. Map of the calculated intensities of the thickness fringes in 2% steps of the Al composition for AlGaAs material (300 KV, [100] bright field). It is clearly seen that, even if the shift of the maxima with composition is quite low, the general outlook over 4 to 5 fringes gives already a good indication on the Al content.

327

In conclusion, a reasonable estimation of the Al content in AlGaAs can be deduced from the overall shape of the thickness fringes profile and the distances between major lines. A map of the thickness fringes has been simulated for each Al content in steps of 2% (fig. 10) for 300 keV electrons (BF [100], 121 beams, Debye-Waller factor[10] of 0.006 nm^2. Using that map, Al concentration across the GRINSCH shown in figure 5 was estimated to vary from 18% to 40%.

A higher accuracy would require a quantitative comparison of the experimental profile shape with references or at least the ratio of the fringe intensities. Possible ways could use an atlas made of experimental profiles of well known composition samples with interpolation routines or use computed profiles. In the latter case, a better knowledge of the absorption coefficients is still required[8]. But a more difficult question arises from the need for quantitative measurements of intensities. This has to be solved in both cases. The large intensity variation across the profile does not allow to record them on a photographic media without escaping from the "linear" part of the film response. To overcome this difficulty, the characteristic curve of the emulsion would have to be exactly known and the development conditions perfectly controlled. Direct recording of the intensities, possibly including an EELS filter, should also be considered too. Different electronic sensors can be used, for example slits and photomultipliers, STEM line intensity recording (with parallel illumination) or television cameras (if a noise reduction procedure allows a sufficient number of grey levels to be recorded).

Topographical information on surfaces can be gained with the WTEM technique too. For example, the etch rate of mixture of H_2O_2 and NH_4O (pH=7.05) which should only attack GaAs can be calibrated. The wedge shown on Figure 11a was etched on one face prior the cleavage of the second one. The depth of attack can be deduced from the height of the steps along the edge. In addition, at the border of the GaAs layer, the thickness fringes reveal a transition zone where AlGaAs (x=0.28) is slightly attacked.

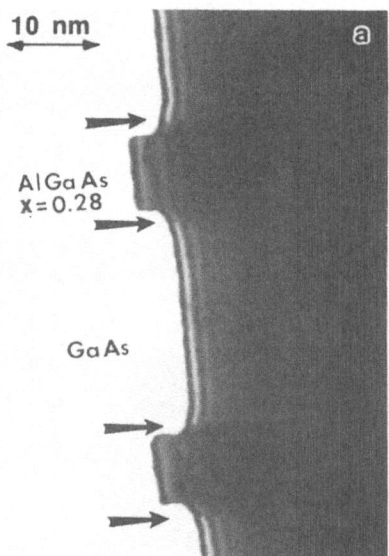 

Fig. 11. Examples of topographical information gained using WTEM. a) One face of that wedge was chemically etched prior to the cleavage of the second face. Bright field WTEM along [100] reveals the profile of the etched groove magnified by $2^{1/2}$. In addition, the thickness fringes show that the AlGaAs has been slightly attacked. b) The high definition profiling of the grooves on this holographic grating has been made by WTEM. The sample has to be precisely oriented for the electron beam running in a plane normal to the cleaved surface and parallel to the grooves .

The performance of holographic gratings with small periods are directly in relation to the shape profile. This profile can be accurately observed (fig 11b) on (single) cleaved edge if the grating is nearly parallel to the incident electron beam (shadow image).

REFLECTION HIGH ENERGY ELECTRON MICROSCOPY (RHEEM)

Reflection of High Energy Electron Diffraction (RHEED) is performed by letting the incident electron beam fall under grazing incidence on the surface of a bulk sample (fig. 12a). Reflection High Energy Electron Microscopy (RHEEM, or more simply, REM) is obtained in a TEM when a RHEED diffracted beam is selected by the objective lens aperture to form a dark field image[11]. A possible mount, inspired from Hsu design[11,12], is shown on figure 12b. A distinction should be made between true surface studies and sub-surface analysis. In the former case, the scattering has to occur on the topmost atomic layers and the reciprocal lattice points degenerate into rods[13] when very shallow incidence is used. It is then a true surface probe able to monitor surface structure, surface films or surface cleanliness[14,15]. These observations require a well controlled environment, often including UHV and in-situ surface preparation[16]. In the latter case, the incidence angle can be larger, the beam penetration deeper and diffraction occurs mainly under the surface. TEM microscopes of recent design have proved to have a sufficient vacuum quality for that application. Most of the picture of that study were taken in a Philips EM 430ST microscope, some in a Philips EM300. The information gained is then a volume information on the sub-surface structures. Here, the advantage of RHEED and REM is mainly the absence of thinning procedure. The only requirement being to have flat or convex[17] surfaces, free of dust or particles in order to avoid uncontrolled absorption or scattering of the incident and diffracted beams (shadow effects). In REM, the sample is viewed under the direction of the selected reflection. As Bragg angles are small, that particular perspective introduces a strong foreshortening in the direction of the microscope column while retaining the nominal magnification in a plane normal to it.

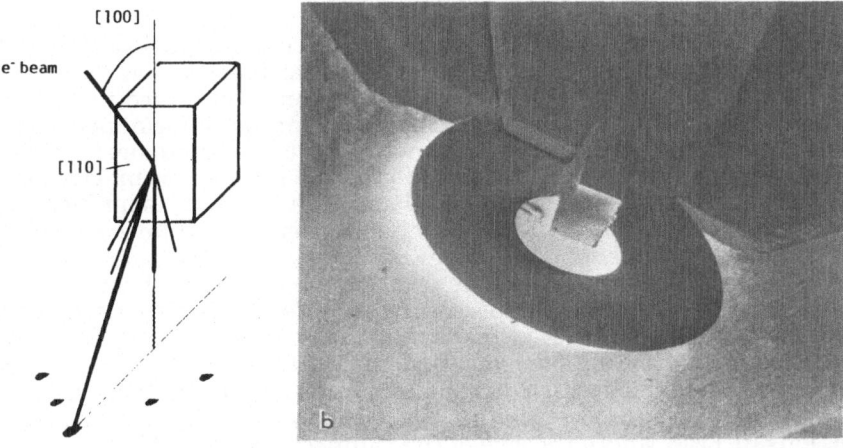

Fig. 12. Sketch of Reflection Electron Microscopy (REM): a) Geometric relationship between sample and electron beams for diffraction. One scattered beam is chosen with the objective aperture (not drawn) to produce a dark field image. b) Specimen setting on the special grid. If a large tilt sample holder is available, WTEM and REM can be carried out on the same sample.

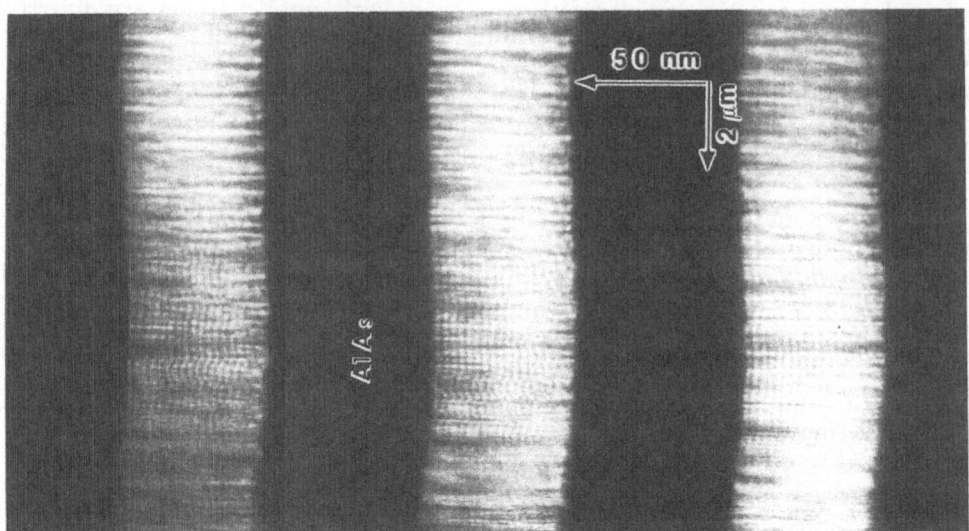

Fig. 13. High magnification of a REM micrograph of a surface laser. Despite the reduced resolving power of this imaging technique compared to TEM or WTEM and surface contamination, likely due to the presence of reactive AlAs layers, the $(AlAs)_2$-$(GaAs)_8$ superlattice is resolved.

The resolution is degraded by the contribution of the numerous inelastic electrons and the low brightness of the dark field images which limits the quality of the astigmatism correction. However, resolutions of 1 nm or better are routinely attained[17,18] as observed on the surface laser sample of figure 13. The studied surface extends nearly almost one millimeter in a plane parallel to the electron beam and it can not be observed on a single micrograph. A first limitation arises from the finite depth of focus of the microscope. A second limitation, the lack of parallelism of the illumination beam when strongly excited objectives are used[19], is more stringent than the first one and limits the field of view in all directions.

In III-V multilayered material characterization, REM is performed on [110] cleaved surfaces to observe the stacking of the layers[12,18,20]. It is a unique method to observe the interface parallelism or bending over a few micrometers. In effect, roughness at the nanometer scale can be observed in TEM on cross sections or in WTEM on cleaved wedges. Long range information can be obtained from optical or mechanical flatness well above the micrometer. When the layers are observed in REM with the direction of the incident beam close to [100] (ie the incident beam lying in the layers plane), the nominal magnification is, in first approximation, retained in the direction normal to the layers while the magnification in the plane of the layers is foreshorten by some 50 to 100 times. Decooman[20] gave a detailed description of the magnification calculation. As shown on figure 14, this perspective highlights the deviations of the layer planes and the bumps observed correspond to hills in the growth direction viewed in cross-section extending over microns with a total height of some nanometers to some tens of nanometers. Such shallow hills can not be seen in SEM due to the distortions and limited resolving power inherent in that technique, nor on cross-sections in TEM where the size of the thinned area would be too small.

It has been suggested that the observed bumps could result from a topographical effect induced by the cleavage, like hills or grooves in the cleaved surface itself. The three pictures of the figure 15 were taken at the same location on a cleaved surface of the laser already shown on figure 6, but with different diffraction conditions close from (880),(882) and (88-2). It is clearly seen that, whatever

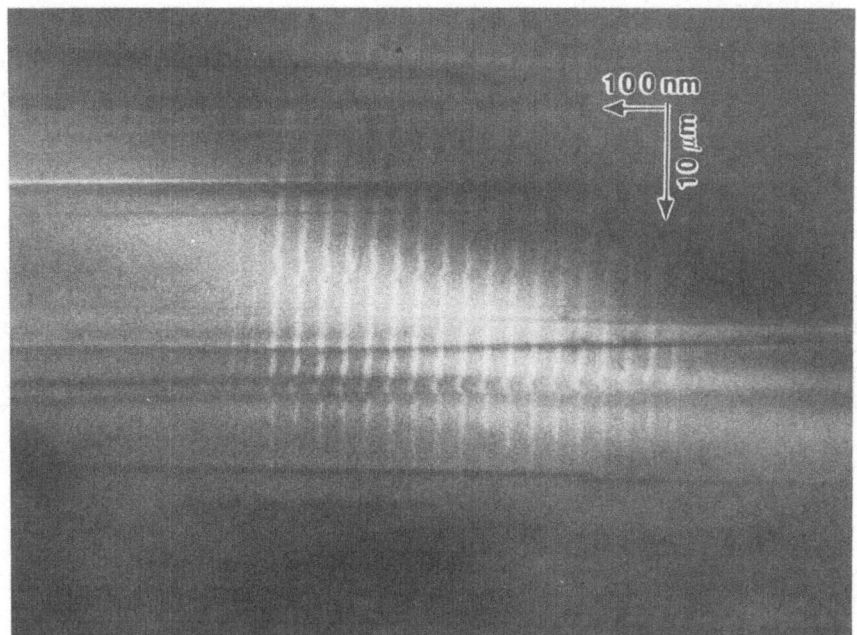

Fig. 14. REM micrograph of the same MQW structure shown in figure 1 (SEM) and 4 (WTEM). The surface was freshly cleaved (in air) and free of contamination. The quality of the cleaving process is assessed by the presence of only a few steps on the surface. The 3.3nm thick GaAs layers are accurately resolved. The bumps observed along the layers are cross-sections of hills of some tens nanometer high extending over a few micrometers.

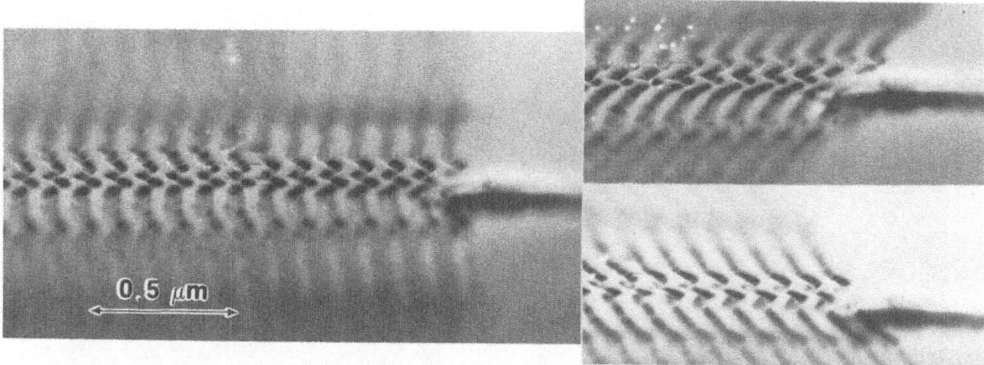

Fig. 15. Bumps or kinks observed on a single REM micrograph can be interpreted either as steps on the cleaved surface or as cross-sections of layer hills. These three pictures taken under different orientations prove unambiguously the hill nature of the contrast.

the observation direction is - along the layers, on left or on right of them - the bumps direction is not reversed and hence a topographical effect induced by the cleavage itself can be excluded.

Figure 16 illustrates the use of REM and WTEM for multilayered material characterization in surface lasers structures made by MBE. It compares the structure of the AlAs layers in the mirrors with and without stabilizing the growth of AlAs layers by inserting thin GaAs layers during the growth.

CONCLUSIONS

The use of TEM is often considered as a cumbersome, time consuming and costly technique. It is certainly true when all the resources of this technique must be employed. Nevertheless, in numerous applications, only quite simple morphological or chemical composition information are required. In that respect, Wedge Transmission Electron Microscopy (WTEM) and Reflection Electron Microscopy (REM) have been proven to be greatly helpful and to offer fast answers.

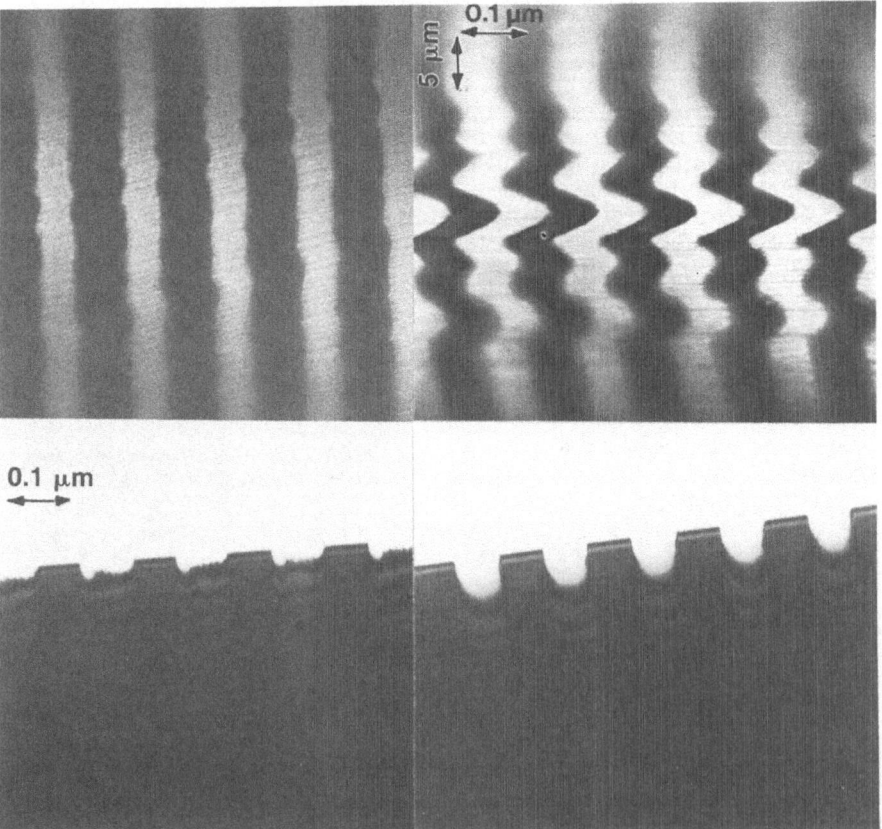

Fig. 16. The association of REM (top) and WTEM (bottom) allows a unique characterization of multilayered structures. Compared to the structure on the right-hand side, the introduction of GaAs wells into the AlAs layers of the structure on the left-hand side has reduced the roughness of the layers and improved the optical performances of this surface laser.

Typically, results can be obtained in about 2 hours including specimen preparation. Thickness measurement of the layers is found to be more accurate and more reliable than in SEM. In addition, unique observations can be performed as the control of the chemical composition stability within each layers, the existence of gradients at the hetero-interfaces, and the roughness of the interfaces in the micron range or below. Eventually, it should be possible to derive quantitative assessment of chemical composition within a few percents if the intensities of the thickness fringes are recorded and compared to computed ones.

REFERENCES

1   J.C. Bravman and R. Sinclair, The Preparation of Cross-section Specimens for Transmission Electron Microscopy, **J. Electron Microsc. Tech.**, 1:53 (1984)

2   C.W.T. Bulle-Lieuwma and P. C. Zalm, Suppression of Surface Topography Development in Ion-Milling of Semiconductors, **in** "Surface and Interface Analysis", ECASIA (1986)

3   N.G. Chew and A. G. Cullis, The Preparation of Transmission Electron Microscope Specimens from Compound Semiconductors by Ion Milling, **Ultramicroscopy**, 23:175 (1987)

4   P.B. Hirsch, A. Howie, R. B. Nicholson, D. W. Pashley and M. J. Whelan, "Electron Microscopy of Thin Crystals", Butterworths, London (1965)

5   H. Kakibayashi and F. Nagata, Simulation Studies of a Composition Analysis by Thickness-Fringe (CAT) in an Electron Microscope Image of $GaAs/Al_xGa_{1-x}As$ Superstructure, **Jpn. J. Appl. Phys.**, 25:1644 (1986)

6   H. Kakibayashi and F. Nagata, Composition Dependence of Equal Thickness Fringes in an Electron Microscope Image of $GaAs/Al_xGa_{1-x}As$ Multi-layer Structure, **Jpn. J. Appl. Phys.**, 24:L905 (1985)

7   C. B. Boothroyd, E. G. Britton, F. M. Ross, C. S. Baxter, K. B. Alexander and W. M. Stobbs, Methods for the Assessment of Layer Orientation, Interface Step Structure and Chemical Composition in GaAs/(Al,Ga)As Multilayers, **in** "Microscopy of Semiconducting Materials, 1987", A. G. Cullis and P. D. Augustus, ed., Institute of Physics, Bristol and Philadelphia (1987)

8   C. J. D. Hetherington, D. J. Eaglesham, C. J. Humphreys and G. J. Tatlock, TEM Compositional Microanalysis in III-V Alloys, **in** "Microscopy of Semiconducting Materials, 1987", A. G. Cullis and P. D. Augustus, ed., Institute of Physics, Bristol and Philadelphia (1987)

9   P. Stadelmann, EMS-a Software Package for Electron Diffraction Analysis and HREM Image Simulation in Material Science, **Ultramicroscopy**, 21:131 (1987)

10 K. Lonsdale, Temperature and other Modifying Factors, **in** "International Tables for X-Ray Crystallography III", The Int. Union of Cryst., Kynoch Press (1968)

11 T. Hsu, A Laboratory Guide for Reflection Electron Microscopy (REM), **Philips Electron Optics Bull**, 120:1 (1984)

12 T. Hsu, S. Iijima and J. M. Cowley, Atomic and other Structures of Cleaved GaAs(110) Surfaces, **Surf. Sci.**, 137:551 (1984)

13 L. Reimer, "Transmission Electron Microscopy", Springer-Verlag, Berlin Heidelberg New York Tokyo (1984)

14 T. Hsu and L.-M. Peng, Experimental Studies of Atomic Step Contrast in Reflection Electron Microscopy (REM), **Ultramicroscopy**, 22:217 (1987)

15 K. Takayanagi, Surface Atomic Structure Study by UHV-Electron Microscopy and Diffraction, **in** "Proc. Int. Congress Electron Microscopy Kyoto 1986", **J. Electron Microsc.**, 35(Suppl):133 (1986)

16 N. Shimizu, Y Tanishiro, K. Kobayashi, K. Takayanagi and K. Yagi, Reflection Electron Microscope Study of the Initial Stage of Oxidation of Si(111)-7x7 Surfaces, **Ultramicroscopy**, 18:453 (1985)

17 T. Hsu, Reflection Electron Microscopy (REM) of Vicinal Surfaces of Fcc Metals, **Ultramicroscopy**, 11:167 (1983)

18 B. C. De Cooman, K.-H. Kuesters, C. B. Carter, Cross-sectional Reflection Electron Microscopy of III-V Compound Epilayers, **J. Electron Microsc. Tech.**, 2:533 (1985)
19 K. K. Christenson and J. A. Eades, On "Parallel" Illumination in the Transmission Electron Microscope, **Ultramicroscopy**, 19:191 (1986)
20 B. C. De Cooman, K.-H. Kuesters, C. B. Carter, T. Hsu and G. Wicks, Reflection Electron Microscopy of Epilayers Grown by Molecular Beam Epitaxy, **Phil. Mag.** A, 50:849 (1984)

DISLOCATION GENERATION AND ELIMINATION IN GaAs ON Si

P.D. Augustus, P. Kightley, R.R. Bradley and R.J.M. Griffiths

Plessey Research Caswell Ltd
Caswell, Towcester, Northants, NN12 8EQ

ABSTRACT

Transmission Electron Microscopy is shown to be the key analytical
technique in assessing the crystalline quality of thin epitaxial layers
of GaAs on Si. Its use is demonstrated in assessing initial nucleation
conditions, dislocation introduction and elimination and to show the
benefit of strained layer superlattices in dislocation reduction.

INTRODUCTION

Many new electronic devices are possible if mismatched epitaxial layers
can be fabricated with a minimum number of threading dislocations in the
upper layers which will contain active device areas. For minority
carrier devices this minimum is around 10^4 dislocations per cm^2. One
such mismatch system which has commanded a great deal of attention is
the growth of GaAs on Si the device possibilities of which have been
described by Kroemer[1].

Recent developments have shown substantial improvement in the quality of
epitaxial layers of GaAs on Si. Many of the crystallographic defects
reported earlier have been eliminated and the indications are that the
remaining impediments may be overcome. Gross three dimensional growth,
stacking faults, microtwins and anti phase domains reported earlier[2]
can all be eliminated by careful control of growth conditions. Research
into the epitaxial growth has centred around; choice of suitable
substrate orientations, substrate cleaning procedures and control of the
initial nucleation and island coalescence. With careful control of
these features a suitable growth template exists, the next major
problems are the mismatch in lattice parameters (4%) and the difference
in thermal expansion coefficients between GaAs and Si. The coefficient
for GaAs is about three times that of Si. As the structure is cooled
from the growth temperature the GaAs tries to contract more than the Si.
The stress produced in the GaAs may lead to warpage of the wafer and

cracking of the GaAs when the overlayer is greater than about 4 microns thick.

Dislocations must be introduced to take up the misfit and threading portions of the dislocation networks controlled by suitable application of strained buffer layers. Experiments in using strained-layer -superlattice (SLS) buffers[3] suggest that this is the way forward to reducing the density of threading dislocations whilst keeping the overall thickness of epitaxial layer to a minimum in order to reduce stress, warpage and cracking. Pearton et al[4] have demonstrated that in straightforward growth of GaAs on Si, without SLS's, the quality of the near-surface GaAs increases significantly with increasing film thickness and decreasing lattice defects to an extent where at 4 microns thick, layers have a deep level density, backscattering yield, minority-carrier lifetime and implant activation efficiency comparable to the same parameters in bulk and homoepitaxial GaAs. It is the aim of this work to obtain the same quality of material in thinner GaAs layers whilst having a density of threading dislocations suitable for the fabrication of minority carrier devices. We have found that Transmission Electron Microscopy (TEM) is an essential tool for monitoring the crystalline quality of the epitaxial growth and for the study of the performance of buffer layers. Substantial progress has been achieved by using plan view TEM on a run to run basis and by using cross-section TEM for specific defect studies.

EXPERIMENTAL

TEM studies were performed on plan view, bevel section and cross section samples. Of major benefit to this programme was the discovery that jet etching the silicon from the back of the wafer using a standard etch for silicon, i.e. 4 parts HNO_3 to 1 part HF, produced a polished taper section on the GaAs with a large area of electron transparent material. One would not normally attempt to jet etch GaAs with HNO_3:HF because it would not produce a smooth polished surface but in this case, with a thin epitaxial layer, the resulting GaAs surface finish was as good as that achieved by the more usual Br or Cl in methanol etch and had the advantage of being a one step process taking only a few minutes.

Where it was necessary to examine portions of the structure further than 0.5 microns from the top surface, layers were etched away from the surface prior to jet thinning or bevel sections were made. Extensive use of stereo pairs enabled us to determine dislocation directions. This gave a wider view than that achieved with cross-section TEM. Cross sections do have a place as they give an immediate visual impact but their use for dislocation counting is severely limited, only being of use for densities greater than $10^7 cm^{-2}$. In the course of this work all dislocation counts were made from plan view samples.

TEM cross sections were made by lapping and polishing samples to 50 microns thickness followed by ion, or atom, beam thinning. The TEM studies were performed on (001) plan view and (011) cross section samples using a Jeol 120CX at 120KV.

MOCVD growth was made on nominally (001) silicon wafers tilted up to 4[o] for some experiments. The standard RCA clean[5] was used. Growth was in two stages, the first 20nm at 400°C followed by a thermal anneal at 750°C for 20 mins and the main GaAs growth was at around 720°C. Strained layers were incorporated by the introduction of GaInAs of composition ranging from 10% In 90% Ga to 30% In 70% Ga.

Initial Growth Morphology

Early growth is strongly dependant upon the condition of the silicon surface when the GaAs is nucleated. Lessons can be learnt from the epitaxy of silicon on silicon to show what crystallographic defects will result from poor surface cleaning. Of most importance is to remove the surface oxide without creating SiC nuclei, both oxide and carbide are responsible for stacking fault generation. The dryness of the MOCVD reactor, its pipework and gasses are also important in preventing the formation of silicon oxides.

Early attempts made by growing GaAs at 720°C directly onto a poorly cleaned silicon surface gave large 3 dimensional islands which coalesced without completely wetting the silicon surface; small voids were seen at the interface and there were many microtwins and stacking faults. Improvements to the initial growth conditions eliminated these defects.

Apart from better surface cleaning and reactor housekeeping the main improvements came from the incorporation of the 2 stage growth process and by making the first stage an AlGaAs layer. AlGaAs was shown to completely cover a Si surface where GaAs would not. This is probably due to Al having a greater affinity for a lightly oxidised surface but there is still the question of whether the growth is initiated by a single AlGaAs layer or by discrete growth islands. Where large oxide islands were present a thin AlGaAs layer did not appear to cover it, at least not with epitaxial material.

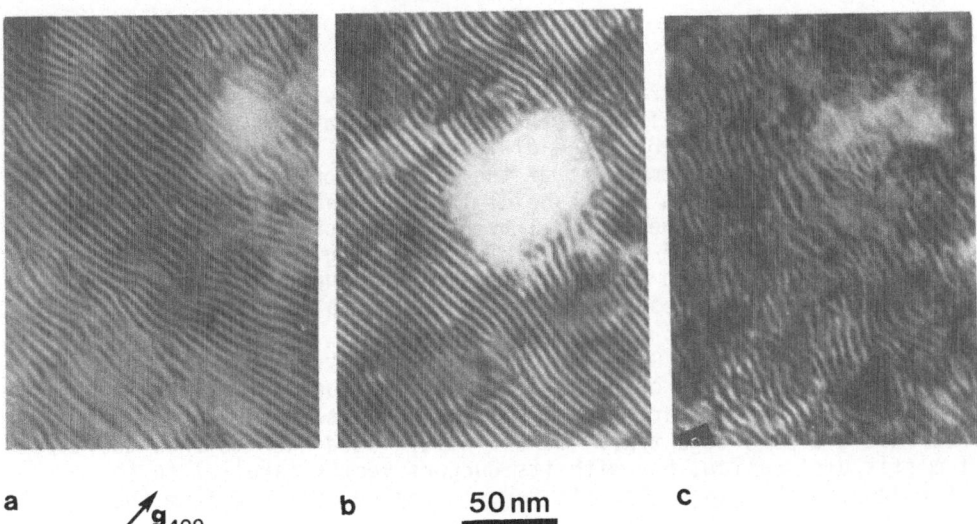

a g_{400} b   **50 nm**   c

Fig.1. Thin AlGaAs films on Si showing moiré patterns perpendicular to the [200] diffraction vector, (a) HF clean and anneal (b) anneal but no HF clean (c) HF clean but no anneal.

Fig.1. shows examples of early growth phenomena. In each case a layer of AlGaAs has been deposited on silicon and examined in plan view. Moiré fringes from the Si/AlGaAs bicrystal show how the AlGaAs layer is oriented with respect to the substrate. In Fig.1a a good epitaxial relationship is shown by the predominantly parallel moiré fringes. This sample had an HF clean to remove surface oxide and post deposition anneal at 740^0C for 20 mins. Sample b had the anneal but the HF clean had been omitted, a 50nm amorphous patch can be seen in the micrograph although the rest of the layer is shown by the fringes to be crystalline. This patch was one of many and because the HF dip was omitted it is assumed that they are oxide islands. The sample shown in Fig.1c has had the HF clean but no anneal, it can be seen from the moiré fringes that the 400^0C growth is crystalline rather than amorphous but there is a wide spread of disorientation. Comparing Fig.1a with 1c it can be seen that the anneal produces a solid phase epitaxial regrowth and the resulting improved crystalline state gives a good template for subsequent layers. The HF dip, low temperature AlGaAs and anneal combination was responsible for a reduction in stacking fault density from 4×10^6cm^{-2} to less than 10^5cm^{-2}.

Returning to Fig.1 the initial growth islands are seen to be disorientated with respect to the substrate and each other. In each case the GaAs to Si misfit could be responsible for the rotation, however, the orientation is improved during the annealing stage. For this ordering to occur it must be facilitated by the glide of grain boundary dislocations formed during the coalescence of disorientated grains.

An aspect of GaAs on Si growth that might appear to be an intractable problem is "antiphase" domains (APD's) where Ga/Ga and As/As bonds would be formed along domain boundaries. Although these APD's were seen in early layers using a convergent beam technique[2] they do not occur in more recent material grown using the preparation techniques outlined above[6].

Misfit Dislocations

The textbook image of strained heteroepitaxial systems shows a planar array of misfit dislocations at the exact substrate to epitaxial layer interface. The spacing of these dislocations will depend upon the magnitude of the edge component of the dislocation Burgers vector. The length of dislocation in the plane of the interface is always expected to be substantial and the possibility of very short lengths is not considered. Evidence of inplane dislocation length cannot be obtained by cross-section TEM and this is not a feature that, to our knowledge, has previously been investigated in this epitaxial system.

The 4% mismatch between GaAs and Si requires 10^{12} $\frac{1}{2}$[110] type edge dislocations running in orthoganal [110] directions to take up this difference in lattice parameter. Not all the dislocations in the interface are pure edge type, Otsuka et al[7] used HREM to show two types of misfit dislocation, one with its Burgers vector parallel to the interface and the other with its Burgers vector inclined from the interface by 45^0. Eaglesham et al[2] pointed out that HREM will correctly identify the dislocations provided (i) the dislocation structure projects along the beam direction (ii) The Burgers vector is always $\frac{1}{2}$[110] and (iii) the images are not unduly affected by strain.

However, strain effects are always visible at the interface and the first two assumptions are not necessarily correct. Eaglesham et al[2] attempt to avoid any confusion produced by the HREM by supplementing these results with weak beam images from cross section samples tilted out from $\lceil 011 \rceil$ to $\lceil 111 \rceil$. The problem that we have experienced in attempting this type of analysis is that the tilt produces overlapping GaAs and Si in the beam direction and the main features observed are moiré fringes which have similar spacings to the expected misfit dislocations. We have established that these are moiré fringes by observing their change of direction as the diffraction vector is altered.

We have adopted a different approach to the examination of interfacial dislocations. The GaAs was etched back to leave approximately 50nm remaining on the Si. Plan view samples were then made which enabled extensive areas of the interface region to be observed. Of course moiré fringes again filled the field of view but dislocations could also be observed. Fig. 2. is a weak beam g(2g) 400 image from one of these samples. Note that no misfit grid of dislocations running in $\lceil 110 \rceil$ directions can be seen at the interface. Some dislocations can be seen but few lie along the orthagonal $\lceil 110 \rceil$ directions. Analysis showed that these were predominantly mixed 60^0 dislocations but in general the length lying in the plane of the interface was short and not necessarily running in a $\lceil 110 \rceil$ direction.

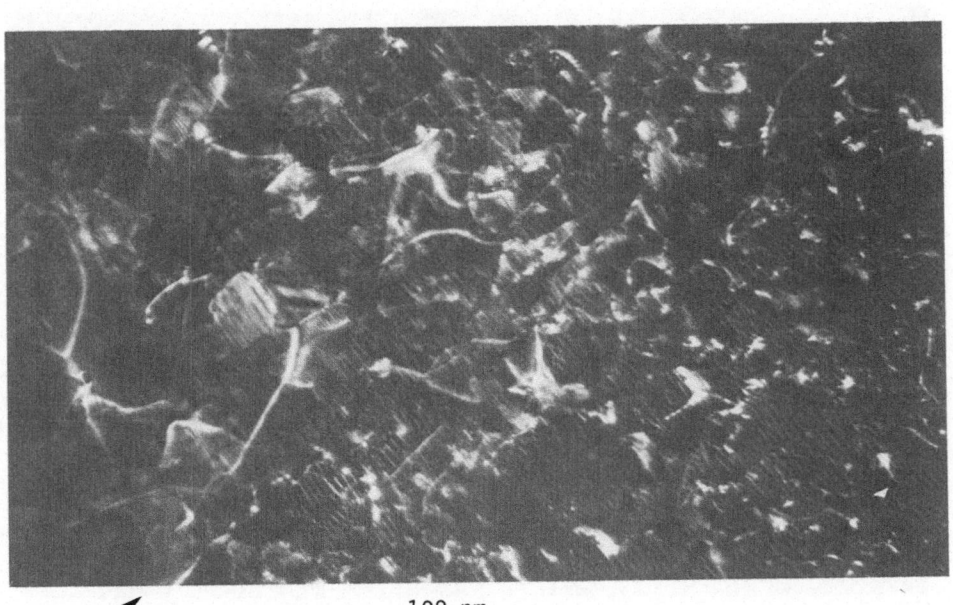

$\mathbf{g}_{400}$

100 nm

Fig.2.   Thin AlGaAs film on Si imaged in a dark field weak beam g (2g) 400 reflection. Dislocations appear but not as orthogonal $\lceil 110 \rceil$ arrays of misfit dislocations. Etched back sample.

Consideration should be given to the mechanism of dislocation introduction. If perfect layer by layer growth were to take place by the propagation of growth steps the first GaAs or AlGaAs layers will be constrained to fit the Si lattice and tetragonal distortion will occur in the direction normal to the growth surface. This is known as pseudomorphic growth. The large misfit should provide sufficient energy for dislocation generation and subsequent motion during growth of the layer. The relaxation of this layer will take place with the introduction of misfit dislocations which must originate from within the GaAs or at its surface. Fresh dislocations must be introduced because there is an insufficient number of threading dislocations emerging from the silicon substrate to turn over in the plane of the interface and take up the misfit. The nature of the dislocations introduced will depend on whether the critical epilayer thickness for their formation is exceeded before the initial growth islands coalesce. We have shown how the three dimensional aspect ratio of islands depends upon the cleanliness of the Si surface and the "wetting" ability of AlGaAs compared with GaAs. If dislocations are introduced before coalescence they cannot have a length lying in the plane of the interface greater than the length of the initial islands, unless they meet exactly with the dislocations in adjacent islands.

We should also consider the dislocations that may be introduced due to the mutual disorientation between islands. The moiré fringes of Fig. 1. show the degree of disorientation that exists before annealing and dislocations will be formed at the intersection of islands. These dislocations may well take up a configuration relieving misfit between adjacent islands and will not be dispersed by the anneal.

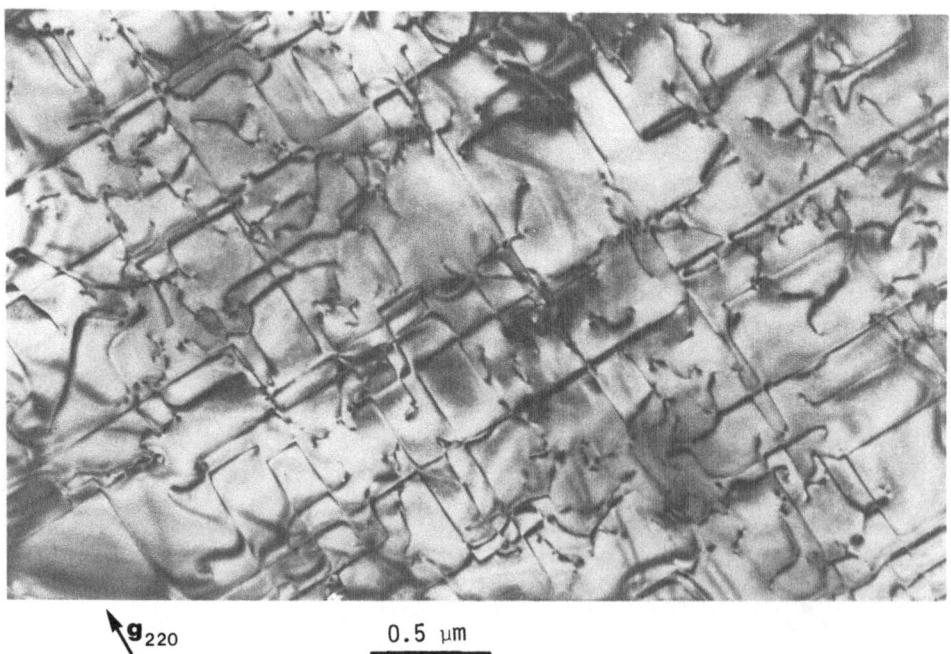

g_{220}　　　　　0.5 μm

Fig.3.　Bright field g220 image of a thin GaAs layer etched back to within 50nm of the Si interface. Stereographic analysis shows predominantly threading dislocations.

If we compare the GaAs on Si results with those from another epitaxial system having more favourable growth conditions we see a different effect. The MBE growth of Si with Si/Ge layers starts with a Si buffer layer. Growth here will be by step propagation and discrete islands will not form even when Ge is introduced. Dislocation introduction will be into a uniform layer which has reached the critical thickness and the evidence of Eaglesham and co-workers[8] shows up to $10\mu m$ lengths of edge dislocations lying in orthogonal $\lceil 110 \rceil$ arrays at the Si to SiGe interface. The nucleation source for these dislocation has not been shown. Dodson[9] discusses several possible mechanisms and concludes that the most likely mechanism, when growth takes place on a perfect substrate, would be heterogeneous loop formation at areas of high local stress. As our GaAs on Si growth does not have a similar dislocation array and has only short lengths of dislocation in the plane of the interface we conclude that the dislocations are introduced before or at island coalescence.

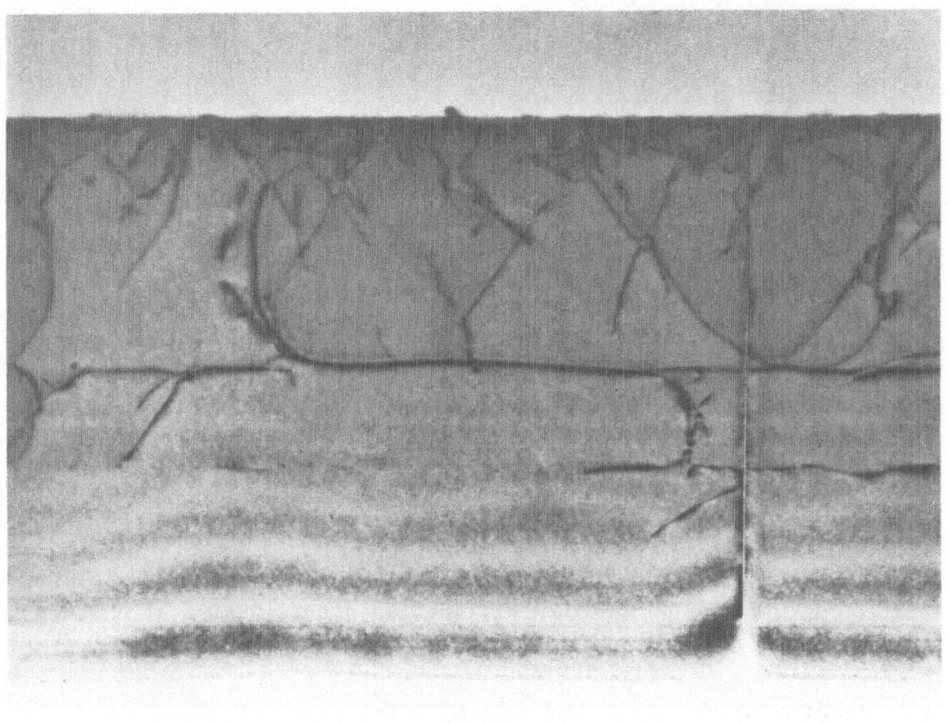

← g_{220} 200 nm

Fig.4. Cross-section of a GaAs on Si epitaxial layer. B=$\lceil 110 \rceil$.

By studying bevel section samples in plan view TEM and applying stereographic analysis we have observed that dislocations from close to the interface thread upwards through the foil. Because of the high density of dislocations, interaction and annihilation readily occurs within the first half micron from the interface. Fig.3. shows such an area with the GaAs etched back close to the Si interface. Although there is a tendency to take up $\lceil 110 \rceil$ orientations the dislocations are predominantly threading from bottom to top of the foil. This view is

341

reinforced by the cross section of Fig. 4. which shows a marked reduction in dislocation density in the first quarter micron of growth. The position where dislocations turn over and run parallel with the substrate interface is at the introduction of a strained layer superlattice, not visible in Fig. 4. imaged with a ⌈220⌉ diffraction vector. Considerable dislocation annihilation occurs in the first quarter micron of growth where the dislocation density is high. To continue this process at the maximum rate it is necessary to turn over the threading dislocations into a horizontal direction, increasing their path lengths. Dislocations are forced to bow under the elastic stresses of the strained layer until they form a misfit length in the plane of the superlattice interface.

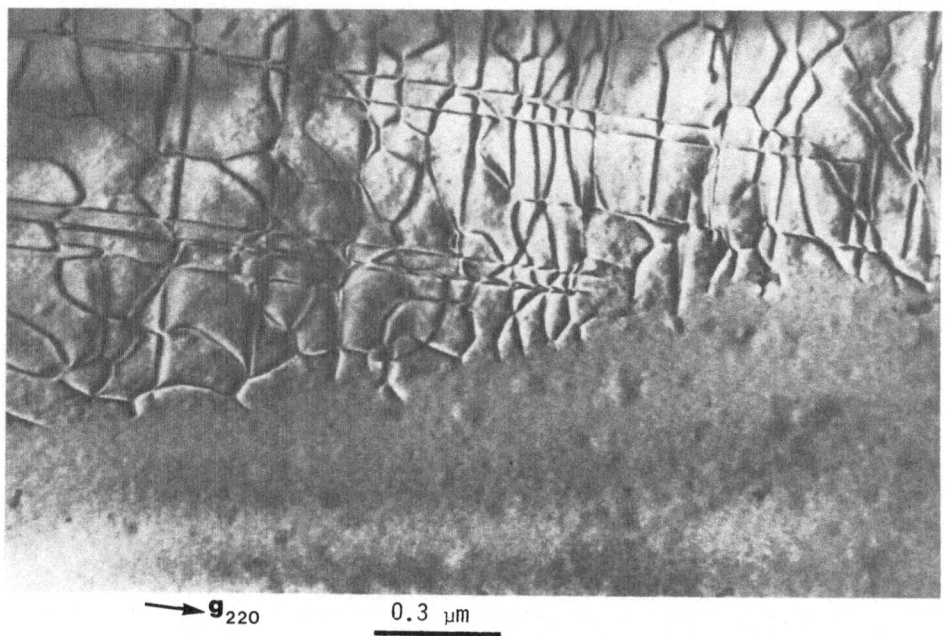

$\rightarrow$ **g**$_{220}$ 0.3 μm

Fig.5. Bevel section TEM of a dislocation array located at a SLS and the dislocation free GaAs above the SLS. Bright field g 220.

Fig. 5. shows a bevel section through material containing a strained layer superlattice at approx. 1 μm from the epitaxial layer to substrate interface. The dislocation array is clearly visible and is in the plane of the superlattice. The dislocations in this array are predominantly 60^0 type, some pure edge dislocations were found but no screw dislocations. Close examination of these arrays shows that individual dislocations only travel a few microns in the plane of the network before reverting to a threading direction. The bevel section was made in such a way that the lower portion of the micrograph is a transmission image through GaAs above the GaInAs superlattice. Although this area appears to be devoid of dislocations, examination of the same region at a lower magnification shows 10^7 dislocations per cm^2 threading upwards. To obtain further reductions in dislocation density further strained layer superlattices must be introduced to turn over these threading dislocations once again. With each array in the plane of the interface more of the mismatch is accommodated and there is further opportunity for dislocations to interact and annihilate one another. However, as the density of dislocations is reduced the misfit accommodation is reduced and the chances of dislocation annihilation is reduced.

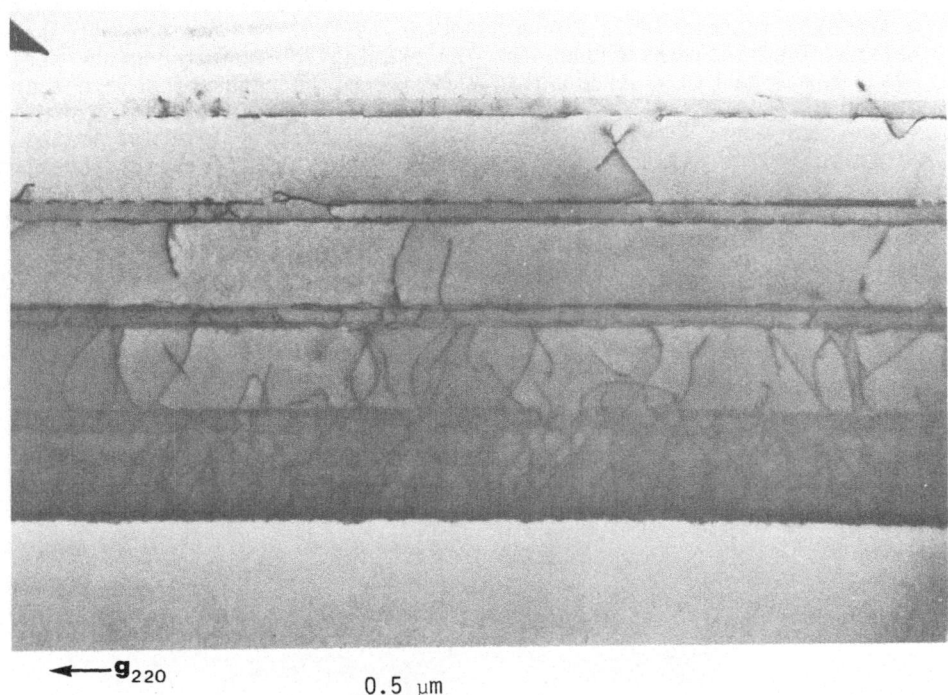

g_{220}

0.5 μm

Fig. 6. Cross-section of a GaAs on Si epitaxial layer with horizontal bands of dislocations at the 4 SLS's. B = [110].

Fig. 6. is a cross section TEM micrograph of GaAs on Si growth with 4 strained layer superlattices each having 10 layers of $Ga_{0.9}In_{0.1}As$ with thickness 5nm and spacing 5nm. The total layer thickness is 2μm and the topmost GaAs layer was shown to have a dislocation density of $10^7 cm^{-1}$. Without the superlattices it was necessary to grow 4μm of plain GaAs to achieve the same dislocation reduction[4]. With closer spacing of the sets of superlattices it should be possible to achieve this quality of material in layers less than 1μm thick.

Growth on Patterned Substrates

The patterning of mesa structures on epitaxial wafers is an accepted part of optical device technology. If the patterning is taken back to the stage before epitaxial growth and patterns made on the silicon substrate raised islands or stripes of epitaxial material may be created. Growth in this way has two potential advantages over planar epitaxial growth; if the width of the stripes is less than the minimum crack spacing it is expected that no cracks will form on the top of the mesas and the mesa edges will provide an escape route or sink for threading dislocations that have been turned over by the superlattices. This idea of reducing the area of substrate that is grown on was suggested by Lee and co-workers[10] and demonstrated by Hodson et al[11]. Specimens for this TEM examination were prepared in the manner described by Hodson. The effectiveness of small islands in reducing dislocation density is expected to increase as the island diameter is reduced but the smallest islands could not be assessed for dislocations due to the difficulty in thinning a 200μm diameter island from the back of the wafer. The specimens chosen for TEM examination were therefore stripe mesas 8μm wide Fig. 7. shows plan view TEM micrographs of adjacent areas on and off the mesa (a) and (b) respectively. The dislocation densities in the two areas were 10^8 and 5×10^8. Of further interest is the distribution of dislocations across the mesa, most of the dislocations reaching the top surface were at the centre of the mesa and the edges were denuded showing the effects of either epitaxial layer relaxation at the edges or the sinking of dislocations on the side walls.

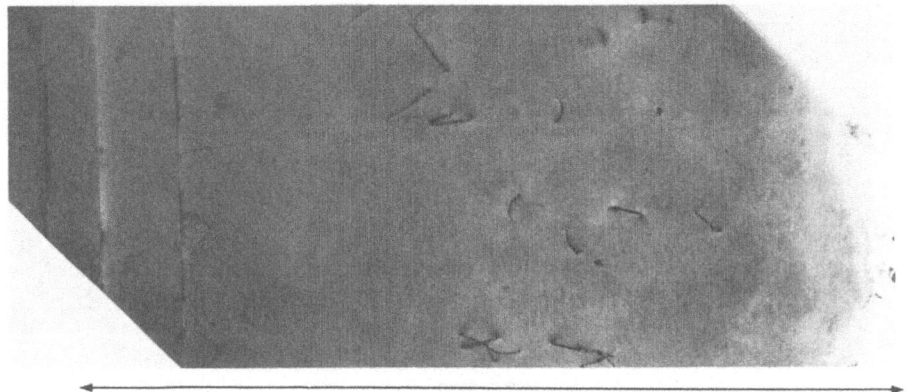

mesa width 8 μm

a

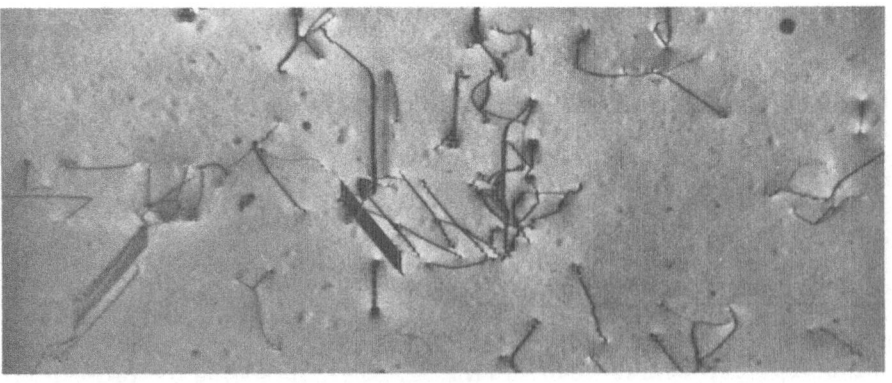

g_{220}

b

Fig. 7. Plan view TEM of selective area growth of GaAs on Si.
(a) on the mesa. (b) in the land between mesas.

Cross-section TEM of the mesas shows the way in which growth around the edges has occurred. Fig. 8. is a dark field 400 image of a typical mesa edge. A reduced GaAs and GaInAs growth rate at the sidewall is indicated by the narrower superlattice band and the dark field micrograph shows how non-epitaxial grains can occur in this region. The actual dislocation densities in this sample are not impressive but nevertheless there is a substantial difference on and off the mesa. If we apply the same reduction factor to the best planar GaAs on Si growth then a figure of $10^5 \mathrm{cm}^{-2}$ near the edges of a large mesa or in the middle of a small mesa would be possible. The reason for the high dislocation density for growth on the patterned substrate was the problem of Si surface cleaning after patterning experienced in this experiment.

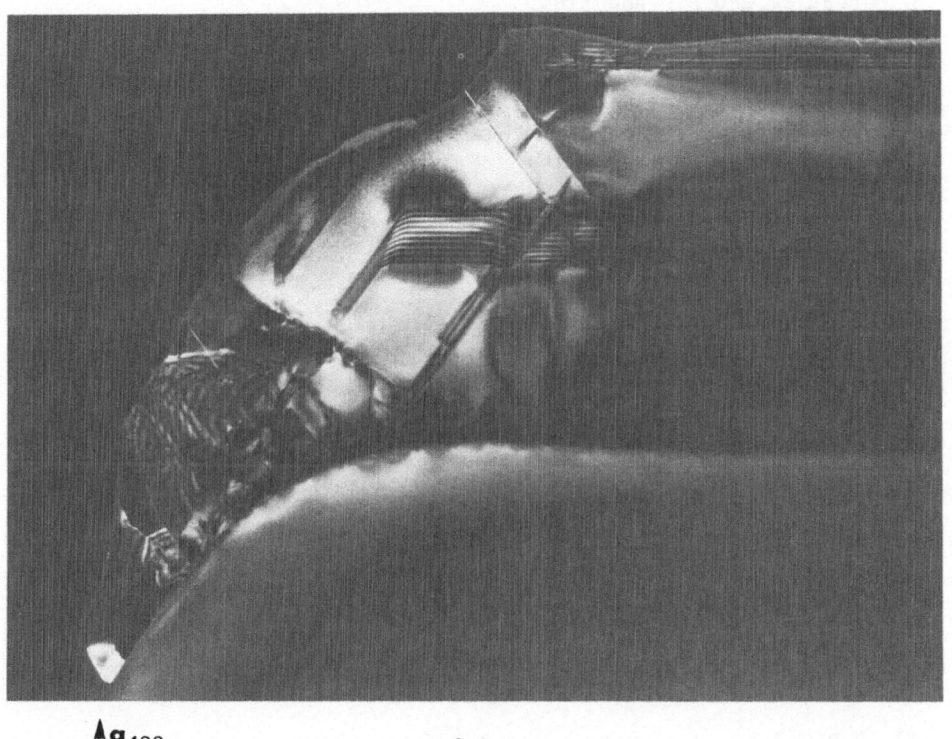

↑g_{400} 0.3 μm

Fig. 8.   Cross-section TEM of the edge of a mesa. Dark field g 400 reflection. Note, part of the layer was lost during thinning.

It has been shown that the silicon surface preparation and control of the initial nucleation conditions are important factors in the growth of good quality GaAs on silicon. Dislocation Engineering combined with selective area growth show the possibility of producing optoelectronic quality material on a silicon substrate.

ACKNOWLEDGEMENTS

The authors wish to thank T B. Joyce and J. A. Beswick for support with MOCVD growth and G B. Davies for help with TEM specimen preparation. Part of the work described here was carried out under a US Department of Defence contract.

(Contract number N00014-86-R-WC05).

REFERENCES

[1]   H B Kroemer. Proc. Mater Res Soc 67 (1986) 3.

[2]   D J Eaglesham, R Devenish, R T Fan, C J Humphreys, H Morkoc, R R Bradley and P D Augustus.
Inst Phys Conf Ser 87 (1987) 105.

[3]   T Soga, S Hattori, S Sakai, M Takeyasu, M Umeno.
J Appl Phys 57 (1985) 4578.

[4]   S J Pearton, C R Abernathy, R Caruso, S M Vernon, K Short, J M Brown, S N G Ohu, M Stavola and V E Haven.
J Appl Phys 63 (1988) 775

[5]   W Kern and D A Puotinen, RCA Review June (1970) 187.

[6]   D J Eaglesham, private communication.

[7]   N Otsuko, C Choi, Y Nakamura, S Nagakura, R Fischer, C K Peng and H Morkoc.
Appl Phys Lett 49 (1986) 277.

[8]   D J Eaglesham, E P Kvam, D M Maher, C J Humphreys, G S Green, B K Tanner, J C Bean.
Appl Phys Lett 53 (1988) 2083.

[9]   B W Dodson, C J Humphreys, G S Green, B K Tanner and J C Bean.
App Phys Lett 53 (1988) 2083.

[10]   H P Lee, S Wang, Y-H Huang and P Yu.
App Phys Lett 52 (1988) 215.

[11]   P D Hodson, P Kightley, R C Goodfellow, T B Joyce, J R Riffat, R R Bradley and R J M Griffiths.
Semicond Sci Technol 3 (1988) 715.

THE MICROSTRUCTURE OF GaAs/Si FILMS STUDIES

AS A FUNCTION OF HEAT TREATMENT

A. Rocher, H. Heral[1], M.N. Charasse, A. Georgakilas,
J. Chazelas, J.P. Hirtz[2], H. Blanck[3], and J. Siejka[4]

[1]Laboratoire d'Optique Electronique du CNRS-29
rue Jeanne Marvig, F-31400 Toulouse, France
[2]Thomson-CSF/LCR - Domaine de Corbeville
F-91401 Orsay, France
[3]Thomson-SC/DAG - Domaine de Corbeville
F-91401 Orsay, France
[4]G.P.S./E.N.S., Université Paris VII Tour 23
F-75005 Paris, France

ABSTRACT

     The effect of heat treatments applied to a 400 nm GaAs
layer grown by MBE on a (001) silicon substrate is discussed.
These heat treatments have been applied during or after the
growth of the GaAs, in order to improve the quality of the
layer. A substantial improvement of the crystalline quality,
measured by RBS, is observed. The density of threading
dislocations decreases after heat treatments. Specimens have
been also studied by TEM. X-TEM observations show an
interface roughness of about 1.5 nm and both 60° and Lomer
interfacial dislocations are seen. Misfit dislocation
networks attain a limited size. Threading dislocations are
often located at the limit of these dislocation networks.

INTRODUCTION

     The heterostructure of GaAs thin films on silicon
substrates (GaAs/Si) has attracted considerable interest in
recent years, mainly for two reasons: 1) the possibility of
fabricating existing GaAs-based devices on large and solid Si
substrates, and 2) the exciting potential of monolithic
integration of GaAs-based electronic and optoelectronic
devices with Si integrated circuits. However, the density of
structural defects such as dislocations, stacking faults and
microtwins in GaAs on Si heteroepitaxy is still too high for

the different lattice constants and thermal expansion coefficients of the substrate and the epilayer. As a result of these mismatches, defects in the epilayer are formed initially during the growth process or during postgrowth cooling by propagation into the epilayer. Even for GaAs grown on Si(100), where a large fraction of the dislocations formed at the interface have Burgers vectors in the interfacial plane, dislocation densities in the range of 10+6 to 10+7 cm-2 are usually found. This is over three orders of magnitude greater than the dislocation density for GaAs films grown directly on GaAs substrates. The main problem is to know how this density can be reduced. One can prevent many threading dislocations from reaching the surface by using a strained-layer super-lattice (SLS). The strain of the SLS will bend the threading dislocations and reduce the dislocation density near the free surface /2/.

Recent publications have shown that rapid thermal annealing (RTA) /3/ or long thermal annealing (LTA) /4,5/ lead to a reduction of the dislocation density in the GaAs epilayer /6/. The goal of this work is to study the evolution of the crystalline quality in relation with these two thermal processes on a 400 nm GaAs. Rutherford Backscattering Spectroscopy (RBS) allows us to obtain an estimation of the quality of the layer. Transmission Electron Microscopy (TEM) gives information about the nature of defects in the epilayer.

EXPERIMENT

The samples are grown by Molecular Beam Epitaxy in a Varian Gen II MBE system. The (001) silicon substrates are misoriented by 4° toward <110>. The substrate preparation consists of a degreasing followed by 10 mn in (HF/H$_2$O) (1/10) and then 10 mn in hot (HNO$_3$/H$_2$O) (1/1). Under UHV the sample is heated for 30 mn at 800°C and 1 mn at 1000°C. The temperature is then lowered to 300-400°C and a prelayer of As is deposited before the growth. The samples consist of a 400 nm GaAs layer grown at 0.4 μm/h with a temperature ramp from 350°C to 450°C. The epilayer is then encapsulated in a 150 nm AlAs layer, deposited at 630°C, to prevent the GaAs from evaporating during the annealing process at high temperature.

Long thermal annealing is made in situ at 720°C under As4 overpressure during one hour. Rapid Thermal Annealing is performed ex situ on half of the specimen. RTA is made with a quartz chamber heated by twelve 2.5 kW halogen lamps. The sample is placed between two silicon wafers, the temperature of which is measured with a thermocouple. The temperature flash is started at 300°C and a temperature of 870°C is reached in 7 seconds. The lamps are then extinguished.

Thus three samples are studied and compared : # 37 as grown, # 37 with ex situ RTA and # 119 with in situ long thermal annealing just after growth.

The samples are studied only from a structural point of view by Rutherford Backscattering Spectroscopy (RBS) and by Transmission Electron Microscopy (TEM).

The evolution of crystalline quality has been studied by RBS. This technique gives significant information about the depth profile of point and extended defects. This information is obtained by comparison of aligned spectra on a reference bulk GaAs target and on the sample analysed, and of aligned and random spectra obtained on the sample analysed.

Crystalline defects are characterized by TEM in the conventional mode and the High Resolution mode in both cross-section and plan-view. The <110> cross-sections are obtained by mechanical grinding and argon ion milling. The plan-views are prepared by chemical etching of the rear side of the silicon substrate. The TEM observations are performed in a JEOL 200CX, with a point-to-point resolution of about 0.27nm at 200 kV.

RESULTS AND DISCUSSION

GaAs crystalline quality

The crystalline quality of the three GaAs epilayers is evaluated from the RBS spectra shown on the fig. 1, 2 and 3.

The spectra shown in Fig. 1 correspond to the as grown specimen. The spectrum of Fig. 1b indicates a crystallographic quality much poorer than the bulk GaAs. The aligned spectrum, shown in Fig. 1a, tends to approach to the random one, which confirms this low quality. The count ratio between random and channelling spectra measured just after surface peaks, Xmin, is about 35%.

The RBS spectra of Fig. 2 show an improvement of the quality of the specimen # 119. The backscattering signal obtained for the aligned geometry comes close to the reference bulk GaAs one, and it is relatively much smaller than the random signal compared to the as grown specimen # 37. The measured Xmin is about 8%.

RTA improves the crystalline quality as shown through the the RBS spectra of Fig. 3. At the surface of the GaAs layer, the signal is not very far from the bulk GaAs signal. The measured Xmin is now only 3.3%.

Fig. 4 shows two micrographs of the specimen # 37, as grown and after RTA. The TEM specimens are cross-sections of the 4° misoriented interface. In accordance with RBS observations, it is evident from these pictures that the dislocation density is largely reduced by RTA. Sample # 119 has a density of defects equivalent to that of # 37 after RTA. Such results are in good agreement with those given by CHOI et al /4/.

Roughness

Fig. 5 shows the HREM images of the interfaces GaAs/Si of the as grown and RTA processed specimens. In both cases the interfaces are not perfectly planar, but present a roughness of about 6 or more atomic layers. Similar observations are discussed by HULL et al. /7/. There are two

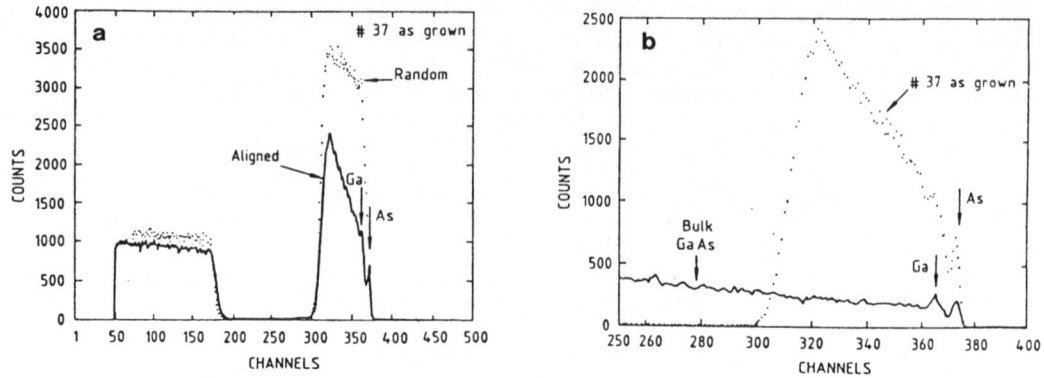

Fig. 1. 2.3 MeV ion channeling of #37 as grown
(4.2 keV/channel), a) aligned and random spectra, b) aligned
spectra of #37 as grown and a bulk GaAs.

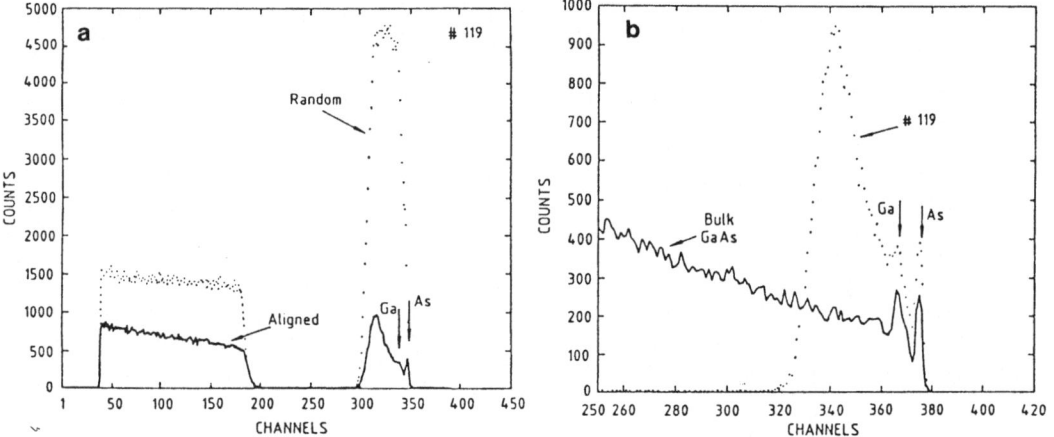

Fig. 2. 2.3 MeV ion channeling of #119 (3.8 keV/channel),
a) aligned and random spectra, b) aligned spectra of #119
and a bulk GaAs.

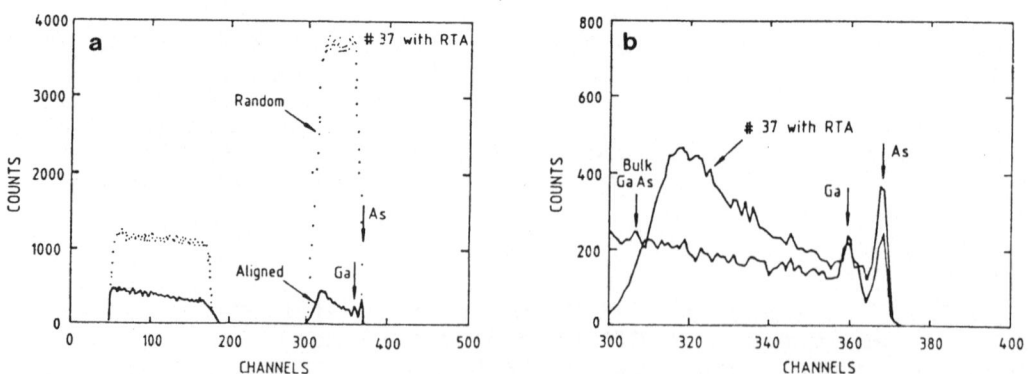

Fig. 3. 2.3 MeV ion channeling of #37 with RTA
(3.7 keV/channel), a) aligned and random spectra,
b) aligned spectra of #37 with RTA and a bulk GaAs.

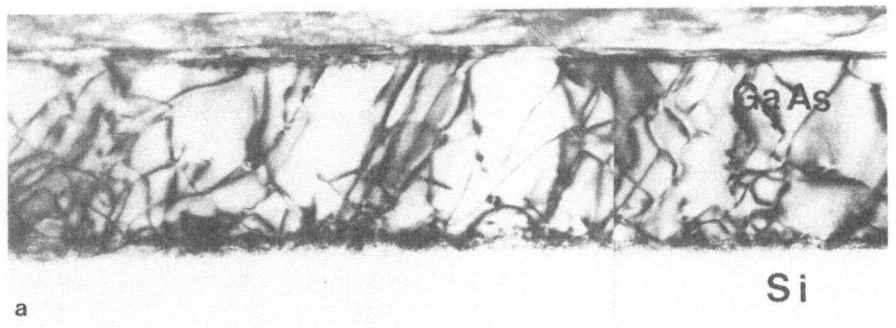

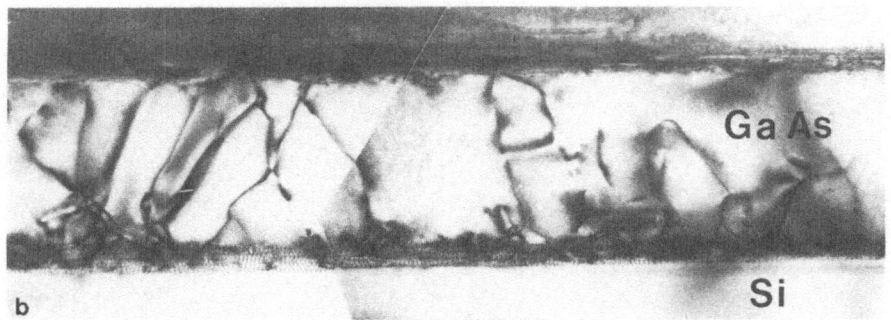

Fig. 4. bright field image of a cross-section, a) as grown sample, b) sample after RTA process.

possible reasons for roughness. The first is related to the roughness of the surface of the silicon substrate itself. The second is a surface reaction between Ga, As and Si occuring at the beginning of the growth. This point might be related to the RHEED observations performed during the GaAs growth: the RHEED pattern becomes very spotty just at the opening of the Gallium shutter.

Interfacial dislocations

Like OTSUKA et al. /8/, we found a high concentration of Lomer dislocations at the misoriented interface as shown on fig. 5. For this interface, the proportion of the Lomer to the total number of dislocations is 60% in the RTA processed sample and about 90% in the as grown GaAs/Si. This result seems to be different from that given by TSAI and LEE /9/, but the 60° dislocations, as shown on Fig. 5b, are paired and only about 1.5 nm apart. 60° dislocations and Lomer dislocations probably have different mechanism of creation as described by NARAYAN et al. /10/.

Fig. 6 shows a plan-view of the GaAs/Si interface of # 37 after RTA. The typical result is shown in Fig. 6a and 6b. Note the moiré fringes observed on the bright field image of Fig. 6a. The calculated moiré fringe spacing assuming bulk GaAs and Si lattice constants is 5 nm for the 220 reflection; this agrees well with the observed value /11/. Fig. 6b is a

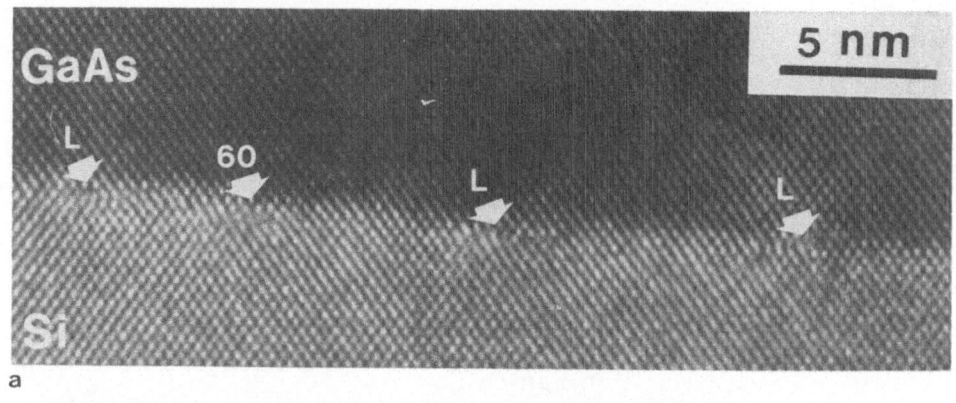

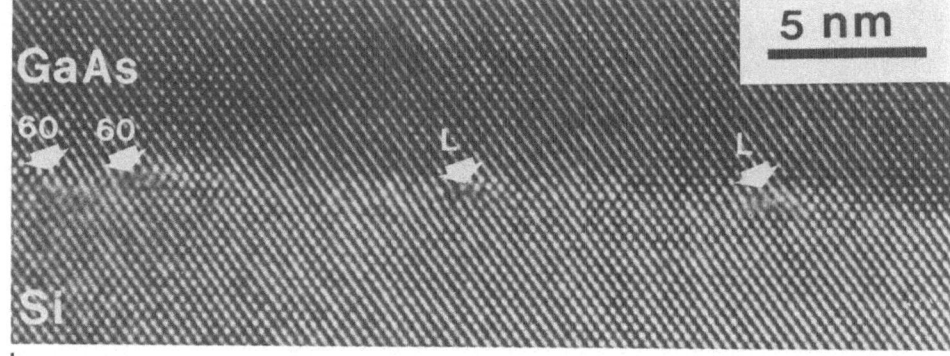

Fig. 5. HREM images of misoriented GaAs/Si
interface. a) as grown sample, b) sample with RTA.
Dislocations are characterized as 60° or Lomer
dislocations.

220 weak beam image of the GaAs/Si interface of the same area
as the bright field image. With this observation condition,
only one family of dislocations is seen. The spacing between
dislocations is equal to 10 nm. The comparison between these
two values is an indication that the misfit dislocations are
mainly Lomer type with a Burgers vector 1/2(110). In
addition, we can also observe on Fig. 6b some areas where the
dislocations are spaced by 5 nm. Such dislocations are in
this case characterized as 60° dislocations. Similar results
are obtained for the other family of misfit dislocation. The
moiré fringes are not so straight and disappear locally. Such
observations are related to partially relaxed stresses and
threading dislocations. The moiré fringe defects, like S on
fig. 6a, are often localized at a discontinuity of the network
of dislocations as observed by the C-arrows on the weak beam
image of fig. 6b. These discontinuities seem to be organized
to limited areas of the misfit dislocation network.

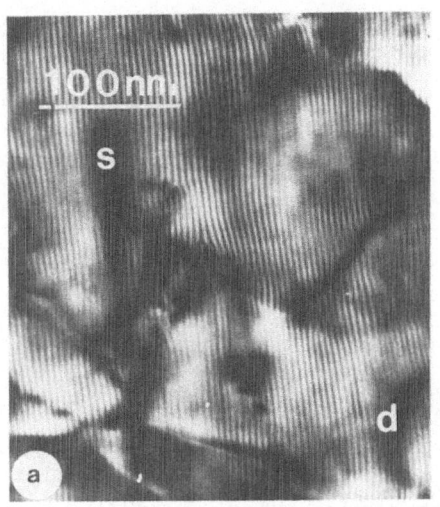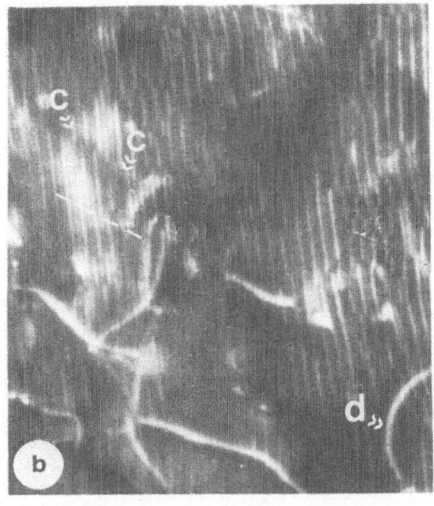

Fig. 6.   Plan-view of the RTA processed sample = 37.
a) the bright field image shows a moiré pattern. b)
weak beam image shows a dislocation array mainly
characterized as Lomer dislocations and locally 60°
dislocations.

Threading dislocations

Most of threading dislocations are created mainly during
the cooling process. The misfit parameter varies by 5% when
the temperature decreases from 500°C to room temperature.
There are 5% of the misfit dislocations in excess. There are
two possible behaviours : the first is that the residual
stresses are not relaxed and a curvature of the wafer can be
induced by the epilayer; a concavity could then be directly
associated with the differential thermal expansion effect.
The second is the relaxation of the stresses by emission of
the dislocations in excess in the interface. These
dislocations can reach the free surface. The threading
dislocations are in this case two segments of the dislocation
merging from the interface. The density of threading
dislocations is then probably related to the size of misfit
array network. This size is probably limited by the
nucleation process in relation with the nature and the quality
of the surface.

CONCLUSION

In conclusion, we have proved that both annealing
techniques are very effective in reducing the defect density
of thin GaAs/Si epilayers. According to CHOI et al /4/, these
techniques are very effective for improving the

microstructures of epilayers having a high density of defects due to nonideal growth conditions. Despite the progress made to date, the reproducible optimization of the growth condition of GaAs on Si has not been achieved as yet. Finally, we think that the reduction of dislocation density in the GaAs layer grown on silicon needs a better understanding of the role of the three dimensional growth on the mechanism of creation of defects.

References

/1/ H.KROEMER, Mat. Res. Soc. Symp., 67 , 3, 1986.
/2/ Z.LILIENTAL-WEBER, E.R.WEBER, J.WASHBURN, T.Y.LIU and H.KROEMER, NATO Advenced Research Workshop Heterostructure on Si. Cargese, France (1988).
/3/ N.CHAND, R.PEOPLE, F.A.BAIOCCHI, K.W.WECHT and A.Y.CHO, Appl. Phys. Lett. 49 , 815, (1986).
/4/ C.CHOI, N.OTSUKA, G.MUNNS, R.HOUDRE, H.MORKOC, S.L.ZHANG, D.LEVI and M.V. KLEIN, Appl. Phys. Lett. 60 , 992, (1987).
/5/ R.M.LUM, J.K.KLINGERT, B.A.DAVIDSON and M.G.LAMONT, Apll. Phys. Lett. 51 , 36, (1987).
/6/ H.HERAL, A.ROCHER, M.N.CHARASSE, A.GEORGALIKAS, J.CHAZELAS, J.P.HIRTZ, H.BLANK and J.SIEJKA, Mat. Res. Soc. Symp., 102 , 51, (1987).
/7/ R.HULL, S.J.ROSNER, S.M.KOCH and J.S.HARRIS, Jr., Appl. Phys. Lett. 49 , 1714, (1986).
/8/ N.OTSUKA, C.CHOI, Y.NAKAMURA, S.NAGAKURA, R.FISCHER, C.K.PENG and H.MORKOC, Appl. Phys. Lett. 49 , 277, (1986).
/9/ H.L.TSAI and J.W.LEE, Appl. Phys. lett. 51 , 130, (1987).
/10/J.NARAYAN, S.SHARAN, A.R.SRIVATSA and A.S.NANDEDKAR, Mat. Sci. and Eng., B1 , 105, (1988).
/11/ K.ISHIDA, M.AKIYAMA and S.NISHI, Jap. J. Appl. Phys. 25, L288, (1986).

ELECTRON MICROSCOPY OF Ge$_x$ Si$_{1-x}$ / Si STRAINED LAYER SUPERLATTICES

D.D. Perovic *, G.C. Weatherly * and D.C. Houghton[+]

* Department of Metallurgy and Materials Science
  University of Toronto, Toronto, Canada M5S 1A4
+ Division of Physics, National Research Council of Canada
  Ottawa, Canada K1A 0R6

ABSTRACT

Problems associated with the interpretation of conventional electron diffraction images from Ge$_x$ Si$_{1-x}$ / Si strained layer superlattice structures (SLS) and relaxation of the strain field of a SLS by dislocation generation and dislocation filtering mechanisms are reviewed. Surface relaxation in cross-sectional TEM samples is modelled using a Fourier series solution and good agreement is found between experimental and computed diffraction contrast images for a single layer structure. Methods to handle the extension to a multiperiod SLS structure are suggested. In a 40-period SLS of relatively low Ge fraction (x= 0.17), loss of coherency is typically observed on annealing at the first Ge$_x$Si$_{1-x}$ /Si interface. For higher Ge concentrations (x= 0.25) loss of coherency occurs at several Ge$_x$Si$_{1-x}$ /Si interfaces in the superlattice. The use of SLS as dislocation "filters" is briefly reviewed and the limitations of this approach to obtaining low dislocation density epitaxial films are considered.

INTRODUCTION

The lattice deformation associated with the coherent growth of Ge$_x$Si$_{1-x}$ /Si strained layer superlattices (SLS) and heterostructures can have a dramatic effect on their electrical and opto-electronic properties[1,2]. This has led to the development of IR photodetectors[3], modulation-doped field effect transistors[4] and resonant tunneling diodes[5]. In order to produce device quality material, close control must be exercised over the growth conditions so that a perfect crystal which is compositionally uniform and has atomically sharp interfaces is produced. The strain distribution in the heterostructures is important not only in modification of the band structure within a multiple quantum well region, but also in dictating the critical dimensions at which a structure loses coherency either during growth or post-growth annealing treatments.

In this paper, a number of topics are considered which bear directly or indirectly on the nature of the strain field in Ge$_x$Si$_{1-x}$ /Si heterostructures: the relaxation of strains in thin film samples prepared for TEM studies; mechanisms of the loss of coherency in multi-layer structures; the use of strained layer superlattices for dislocation filtering, and the role that substrate cleaning procedures exercises in determining the perfection of the strained layer superlattice. Before discussing the experimental results, the strain distribution expected in a SLS as grown (ie.bulk) and after thinning for TEM examination is briefly reviewed.

Stresses in Multilayered Thin Films

The coherent growth of a SLS involves the deposition of a discrete number of alloy layers, usually followed by a capping layer, onto a substrate whose thickness is very much greater than the combined thicknesses of the deposited layers. Under these conditions the analysis given by Suhir[6,7] appears to be the most complete as it considers both the biaxial strain associated with coherency and thermal mismatch in addition to the strains due to wafer bending which must accompany this deposition procedure. If a discrete number of alloy layers (n_i) are deposited, the biaxial stress in the i th layer is given by

$$\sigma_i = E_i' \, \varepsilon_i \, [1-\exp{(-k(r-y))}] \tag{1}$$

In eqn.(1), E_i', the "biaxial modulus" is $2\mu(1+\nu) / (1-\nu)$ for elastically isotropic materials, where μ represents the shear modulus and ν is Poisson's ratio. For the anisotropic case $E_i' = c_{11} + c_{12} - 2 \, (c_{12}^2 / c_{11})$, where c_{ij} are the elastic constants referred to the cubic system. If the thermal strain contribution is ignored, $\varepsilon_i \approx \Delta a/a$, where Δa is the difference in the lattice parameters (a) of the substrate and deposit. r is the radius of the substrate (assumed to be a thin circular wafer); y is a measure of the radial distance from the centre of the wafer and k is a constant $>>1$, whose exact value depends on the thickness and elastic constants of the substrate and film[6]. Except at the wafer edges, eqn.(1) demonstrates the well-known result that the strains (and stresses) associated with the growth processes are constant and are accommodated in the alloy layers. The biaxial stresses approach zero at the end of the layers (ie. as $y \to r$).

Bending introduces a number of other stresses into the problem. These are usually ignored but could be important in analyzing loss of coherency or film fracture. A small biaxial stress is introduced into the substrate, whose magnitude* at the interface with the SLS is of the order

$$\sigma_{substrate} \approx - (t_f \, / \, t_s) \, \sigma_i \tag{2}$$

where t_f is the thickness of the deposited film and t_s is the thickness of the substrate. In addition, an interfacial stress develops at the ends of the wafer $(y \to r)$ whose maximum value at the substrate interface is

$$\tau = - k \sum_{i=1}^{n} E_i' \, t_i \, \varepsilon_i \tag{3}$$

The summation is carried out for n layers, each of thickness t_i and misfit strain ε_i .

Surface Relaxation of Stresses

The simplest case to consider is a single alloy layer grown on a substrate with a fairly substantial capping layer. On thinning a sample removed from the central portion of the wafer for cross-sectional TEM, the stresses, which for this geometry are wholly contained in the alloy layer are relaxed near the top and bottom surfaces of the foil. The geometry which we have adopted to solve this problem is shown in Fig. 1. The top and bottom surfaces are rendered stress-free by imposing surface tractions equal in magnitude but opposite in sign to the stresses given by eqn. (1) (when $\exp(-k \, (r-y)) \to 0$). The exact solution to this problem has been given by Timoshenko and Goodier [8]. The strain in the y-direction is given by

$$\varepsilon_{yy} = \frac{1}{E} \frac{qa}{1}(1+\nu) + \frac{4q}{\pi} \sum_{m=1}^{\infty} \left[\frac{\sin(\alpha a)\cos(\alpha y)}{m \, (\sinh(2\alpha c)+(2\alpha c))} \right] \left[\begin{array}{l} (1+\nu)\alpha c \, \cosh(\alpha c)\cosh(\alpha x) \\ -(1-\nu-2\nu^2)\sinh(\alpha c)\cosh(\alpha x) \\ -(1+\nu)\alpha x \, \sinh(\alpha x)\sinh(\alpha c) \end{array} \right] \tag{4}$$

where $\alpha = (m\pi / l)$.

---

* The exact value would depend upon the composition and temperature of deposition of the alloy and capping layers.

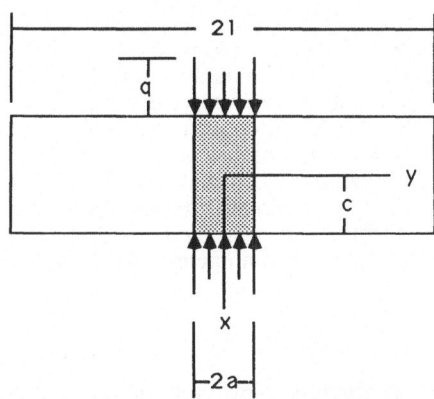

Fig. 1 Diagram illustrating the coordinate system used in the Fourier series solution; q represents the symmetrical load required to balance the internal stress due to misfit in the strained layer.

The dimensions l, a and c are defined in Fig. 1; q is the symmetrical load required to balance the internal stresses, and $\alpha = (m\pi / l)$. An identical expression was given by Gibson and Treacy[9]; these authors suggested that the solution could account for stress relaxation in a multiple layer structure with the strains (and stresses) partitioned between the alloy and silicon phases. We believe that this is incorrect. The correct form for ε_{yy} with strain partitioning is

$$\varepsilon_{yy} = \frac{1}{E}\frac{q_1-q_2}{2l} a (1+\nu)$$
$$+ \frac{2(q_1+q_2)}{\pi}\sum_{m=1}^{\infty}\left[\frac{(1-\cos(\alpha a))\cos(\alpha y)}{m\,(\sinh(2\alpha c)+(2\alpha c))}\right]\left[\begin{array}{l}(1+\nu)\alpha c\,\cosh(\alpha c)\cosh(\alpha x)\\ -(1-\nu-2\nu^2)\sinh(\alpha c)\cosh(\alpha x)\\ -(1+\nu)\alpha x\,\sinh(\alpha x)\sinh(\alpha c)\end{array}\right] \quad (5).$$

In this equation, q_1 and q_2 are the loads required to balance the internal tensile and compressive stresses in the two layers (ie. Si and Ge_xSi_{1-x} respectively) that form the repeating structure and l now corresponds to one superlattice period. Accordingly, the relative value of q_1 and q_2 will depend on the degree of strain partitioning between the layers.

In the analysis described in this section, we have used eqn.(4) to describe the strain relaxation effect in a single layer. For solving the contrast expected from surface relaxation effects, the local rotation of the lattice planes (dR_y /dx) with respect to the unrelaxed crystal is required[10]. This is given by

$$\frac{dR_y}{dx} = \frac{4\varepsilon_0}{\pi}\frac{(1+\nu)}{(1-\nu)}\sum_{m=1}^{\infty}\left[\frac{\sin(\alpha a)\sin(\alpha x)}{m(\sinh(2\alpha c)+(2\alpha c))}\right]\left[\begin{array}{l}(\alpha c)\cosh(\alpha c)\sinh(\alpha y)\\ -2(1-\nu)\sinh(\alpha c)\sinh(\alpha y)\\ -\alpha y\cosh(\alpha y)\sinh(\alpha c)\end{array}\right] \quad (6).$$

EXPERIMENTAL PROCEDURE

MBE Growth Conditions
The growth of $Ge_x Si_{1-x}$ /Si strained layer superlattices were carried out using a Vacuum Generators V80 MBE system. A base pressure of $\approx 5 \times 10^{-11}$ torr was obtained using a combination of liquid nitrogen-trapped oil diffusion and Ti sublimation and ion pumps. The

epitaxial layers were grown on 100 mm diameter, <100> oriented Czochralski-grown Si substrates. The initial *ex-situ* substrate preparation involved UV ozone exposure in a reactor for ≈ 45 min to remove hydrocarbon contamination immediately before introduction into the vacuum system. Subsequently, oxide removal was carried out *in-situ* by heating the wafer to ≈ 900 °C in a Si flux ≈ 0.1 Å/sec for 15 min prior to cooling to the growth temperature in the range 500-550 °C. During growth, the combined Si and Ge deposition rate was typically 5 Å/sec and fluxes were controlled using Sentinel III optical sensors. The vacuum pressure during growth was ≈ 5 x 10^{-10} torr during growth. Reflection high energy electron diffraction indicated clean surfaces are obtained under proper preparation conditions. Improper *in-situ* cleaning results in the entrainment of small particles at the substrate/epilayer interface.

Annealing Treatment

The post-growth annealing treatments were carried out in high vacuum (≈10^{-7} Pa) for durations varying from 30 min to 4 hrs in the temperature range 600-900 °C. Rapid thermal annealing treatments were also carried out for 30 sec in the range 700-850 °C in a nitrogen environment.

TEM Sample Preparation

Samples were prepared for cross-sectional transmission electron microscopy using standard methods. The surface normal for all samples was <011>. The samples were thinned in an Ion Tech FAB 306 atom mill using 4-5 keV Ar atoms incident at shallow angles to minimize the depth of the amorphous surface layers. The samples were examined on an Hitachi H-800 operating at 200 kV and a Philips EM 430T electron microscope at 250 and 300 kV.

SURFACE RELAXATION EFFECTS

A qualitative interpretation of relaxation images at single layer interfaces has been given by Weatherly et al.[11] based on the solution of a line force acting on an elastic half-space. The solution can be applied in relatively thick foils wherein the strain fields at the two surfaces are separated far enough so that they can be considered independently as bounding semi-infinite solids. However, in the case of relatively thin foils, one must employ a solution which accounts for the interaction effects between the strain fields at the two surfaces. This can be done using a Fourier series expression for vertical loading along the upper and lower edges of a beam[8] as given in eqn. (4).

In this paper, we will consider the agreement between computed and experimental images for a single strained layer using both solutions. Fig. 2 compares the experimental and computed images for a single Ge$_{0.3}$Si$_{0.7}$ strained layer, thickness 10 nm, and capped with a Si layer of 500 nm.

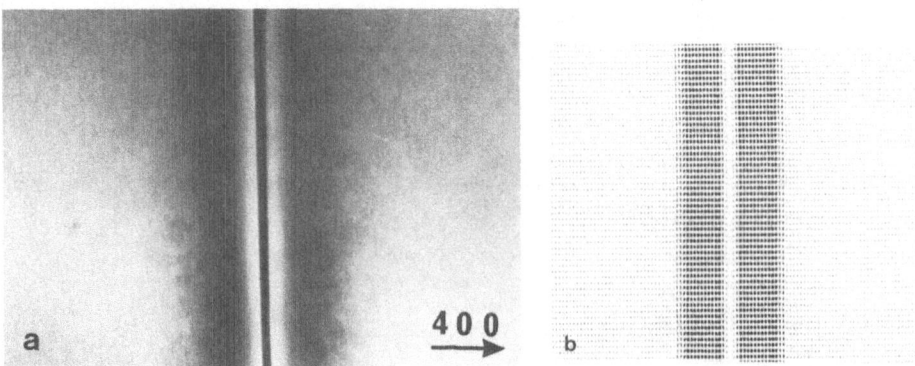

Fig. 2 Experimental (a) and computed (b) bright field diffraction contrast images taken with the **g**= 400 (w=0) reflection for a single Ge$_{0.25}$Si$_{0.75}$ strained layer. The images are from areas 1 ξ_g thick.

The foil thickness is $\approx 1\xi_g$ for the $\mathbf{g}= 400$ reflection and is oriented at the exact Bragg diffracting condition (w=0). The computed images were generated from the Howie-Whelan two-beam dynamical diffraction equations and the column approximation[10] using a modification of the method of Head et al.[12] to integrate the differential equations[13]. In order to simplify the analysis, both the alloy layer and substrate were assumed to be elastically isotropic, with $\nu = 0.3$. The normal and anomalous absorption coefficients required in the Howie-Whelan equations were assumed to be 0.1 both in the alloy layer and the substrate (This assumption ignores the contribution of "structure factor" to the image contrast.) In moderately thick foils, the alloy layer is always darker than the surrounding matrix with $\mathbf{g}= 400$ (see Fig. 2); this effect has not been included in the simulated images. The values for the lattice plane bending were calculated from eqn. (6) by setting $(a/l)<<1$. The comparison in Fig. 2 comes from a relatively thin region of the sample, $\approx 1\xi_g$ thick. In thicker regions anomalous absorption effects become important, particularly in interpreting the dark field image which shows asymmetric dark-light contrast with $\mathbf{g}= 400$. Computed and experimental dark field images are compared in Fig. 3 for a sample that is $8\xi_g$ thick. Good agreement is found at all foil thicknesses using the Fourier series solution for the relaxation displacement field, both for the image width and the details in the image - see, for example the small changes in the dark contrast band about 80 nm from the alloy layer in the dark field image shown in Fig. 3.

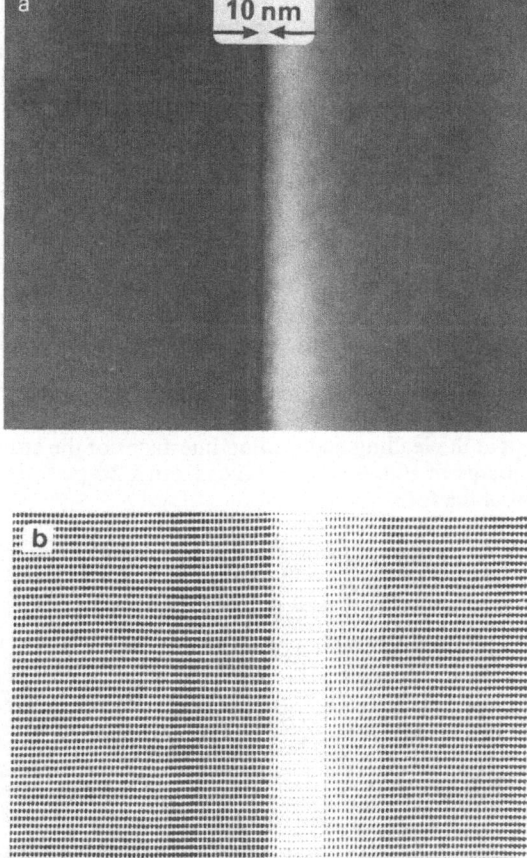

Fig. 3 Experimental (a) and computed (b) dark field images of the single period $Ge_{0.25}Si_{0.75}$ strained layer taken from a thick region in the foil $\approx 8\xi_g$ using a $\mathbf{g}= 400$ reflection; anomalous absorption effects result in an asymmetry of the relaxation strain field about the layer.

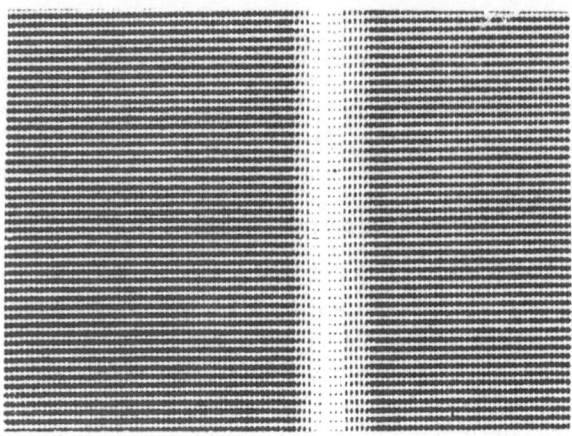

Fig. 3 cont. (c) Computed diffraction contrast image using the line force solution[11].

Image simulations using the line force solution[11] agreed fairly well in predicting the strain field width for thicker foils (Fig. 3c). However, the details of the computed image do not match the experiment as well as the Fourier series solution. The advantage of the line force solution is that one is not required to sum large numbers of Fourier coefficients in calculating the displacement field. This results in a reduction in the computing time by about two orders of magnitude for the computation of single layer images. It should be mentioned that the width of the anomalous strain field associated with elastic relaxation remains constant with varying foil thickness under fixed diffraction conditions. This has been observed in both experimental and computed diffraction contrast images.

The extension of this approach to a multiple alloy layer situation is complicated. We have already noted that eqn's (4) and (6) only apply to a single alloy layer and the multiple alloy layer <u>cannot</u> be handled by selecting varying values of (a / l). The correct method for a discrete number of alloy layers (with again a substantial capping layer) would be to superimpose the displacements associated with each alloy layer, treating each one separately as though it were embedded in a thin plate with (a / l) <<1. Qualitatively, it is obvious that in a multiple SLS structure, the displacements associated with lattice plane bending will tend to cancel one another except at the leading and trailing interfaces of the structure. This is clearly shown in the dark field image of Fig. 4 which comes from a 20-period superlattice (x=0.25) in a relatively thin region of the foil.

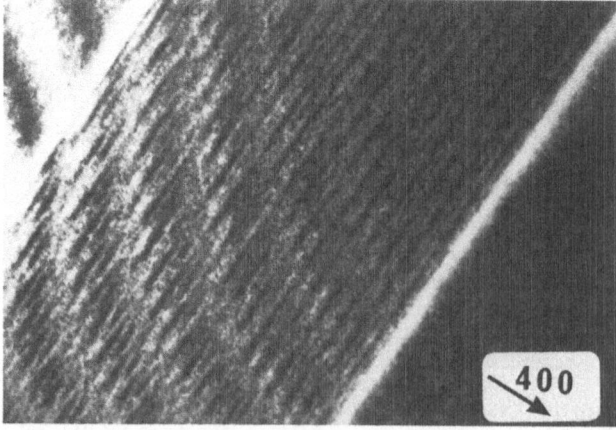

Fig. 4 **g**= 400 dark field image of a 20-period superlattice (x=0.25) tilted away from the exact Bragg diffracting condition (w=0.5).

The bright band of contrast at the substrate and capping layer interfaces is associated with lattice plane bending, while the contrast within the SLS arises principally from structure factor effects due to the different extinction distances between the Ge_xSi_{1-x} and Si layers. This conclusion is further supported by the bright field image shown in Fig. 5, taken from the same 20-period superlattice structure of Fig. 4. Pronounced lattice plane bending contrast is confined to the region of the first two alloy layers.

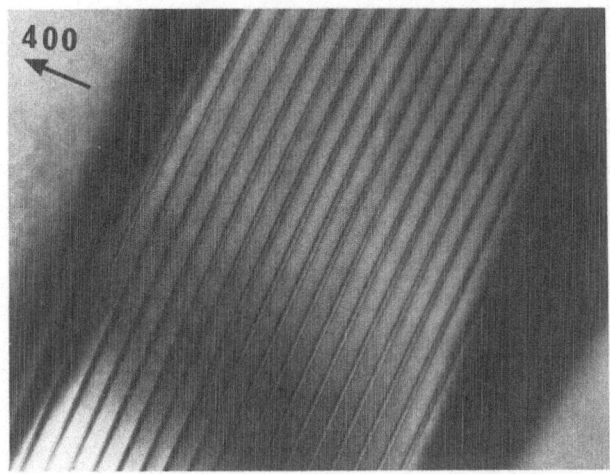

400

Fig. 5 $g = 400$ (w=0) diffraction contrast image of a 20-period $Ge_{0.25}Si_{0.75}$ SLS; note the broad dark strain field contrast at the outer layers of the SLS. Structure factor contrast is also evident within the superlattice structure.

EPITAXIAL GROWTH DEFECTS

During the course of our studies on Si-Ge heterostructures, we have frequently encountered a curious defect which is visible by strain field contrast in cross-sectional TEM samples. Two examples of these defects are shown in Fig. 6. For obvious reasons we have chosen to name these defects "pagodas". Similar observations have been reported by Hull et al.[14] and ascribed to "buckling" of the thin foil samples, but we have found a low density of "pagoda-defects" in otherwise perfect samples (Fig. 6a). A higher density of "pagodas" is often observed in samples which are partially incommensurate (Fig. 6b). Although our analysis of these defects is as yet incomplete, their occurrence in multilayer structures correlates well with the nature of particles formed at the original substrate due to imperfect cleaning procedures prior to film growth. Direct lattice resolution and strain field contrast of these particles demonstrate that they are often fully coherent with the surrounding matrix, in agreement with the findings of Chrenko et al.[15]. The composition of the particles has not been determined, but SIMS analysis suggests that they are either SiO_2 or SiC. Cubic SiC particles have been observed at Si/SiO_2 interfaces, epitaxially related to the Si substrate[16], and SiC can be epitaxially deposited onto (001) Si substrates despite the 20% lattice misfit between the two crystal structures[17].

If the particles are fully coherent, the SLS film is perfect, free of "pagoda-defects". On the other hand if the particles have lost coherency, pagodas are commonly observed in the first few layers of a SLS structure lying immediately above or at an angle corresponding to the trace of {111} planes to the incoherent particle (cf. Fig. 7). The strength of the strain field for the "pagoda-defect" decays progressively into the layers of the film and the strain field itself has a characteristic asymmetry, always pointing towards the original substrate. The strain contrast from the "pagodas" is complicated by the interaction with the lattice plane bending contrast discussed previously. One possible mechanism which could explain the occurrence of these defects is the propagation of atomic step structures from the particle-epilayer interface during growth which persists into the SLS itself, disrupting the atomic abruptness and perfection of the epilayer interfaces. In this model the defect might be characterized by a circular step (one or two atom planes in height) whose radius decreases as growth proceeds. Alternatively the pagoda defects might be caused by relaxation of the strain

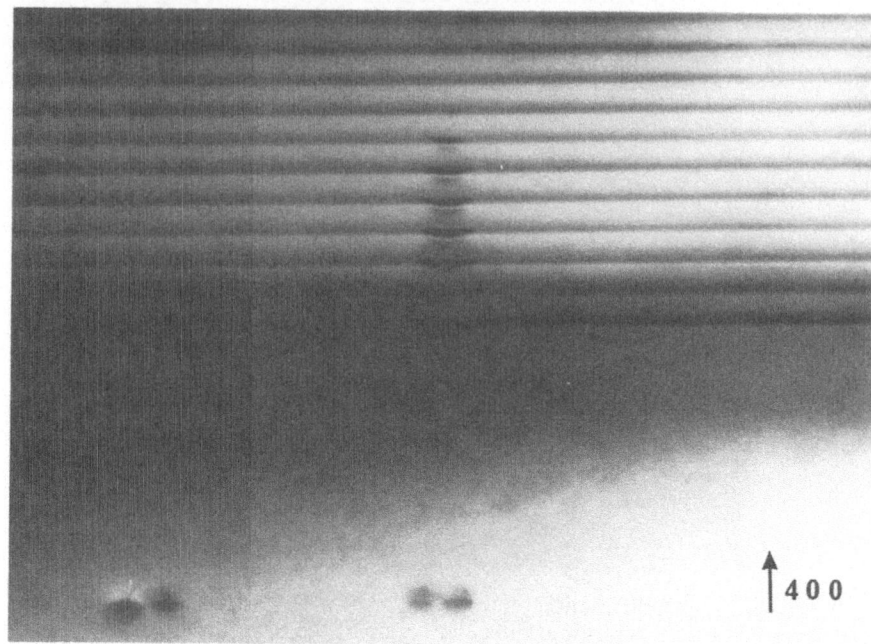

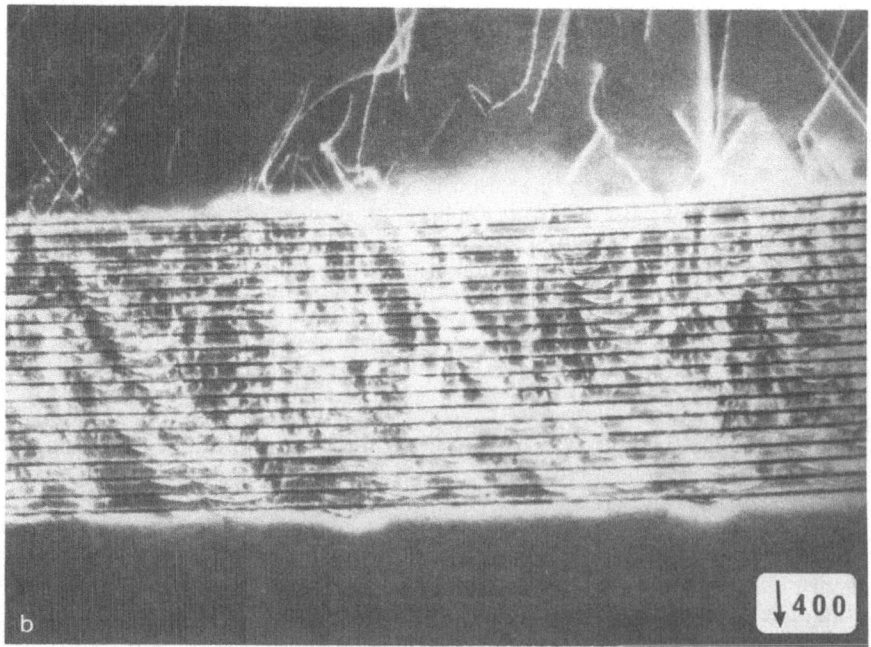

Fig. 6 Diffraction contrast images showing "pagoda defects" in 20-period superlattices with (a) x=0.25 and (b) x=0.45. The higher Ge concentration in (b) has resulted in incommensurate growth at an early stage. In both cases "pagodas defects" are seen to propagate through the superlattice structure.

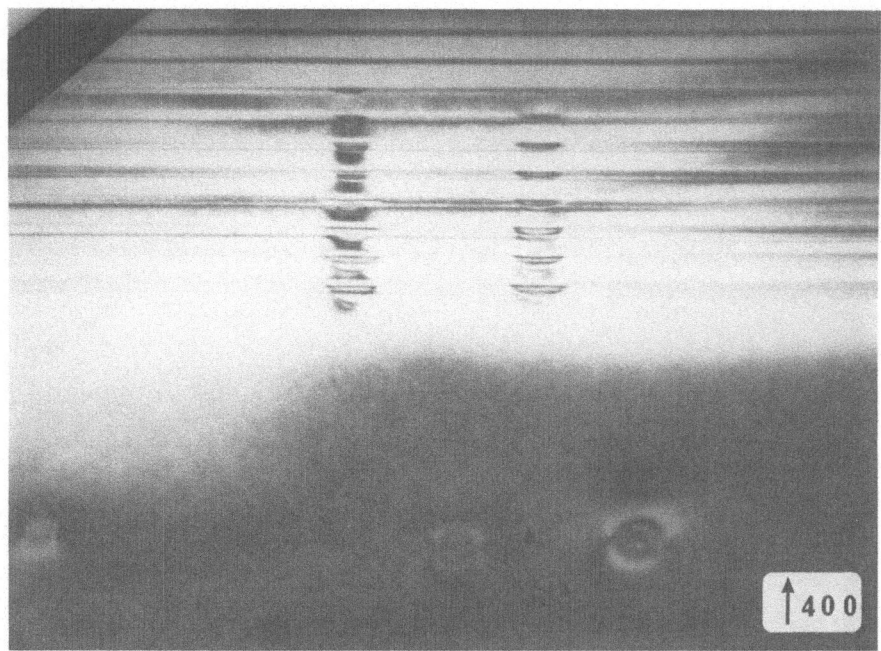

Fig. 7 Diffraction contrast image (g=400) showing several small particles at the original substrate-buffer interface. The "pagoda" defects may be correlated with particles which are not fully coherent with Si.

field of the particles by glide and climb of dislocation loops punched out by the SiC particles through the SLS on {111} planes.

DISLOCATION INTERACTIONS

Loss of Coherency Studies

The mechanisms of coherency loss on SLS structures have been extensively studied in Si-Ge alloys because of the critical role played by the strain field in the alloy layers in producing high quality devices. Several different theories have been developed to account for the loss of coherency, which fall into two broad categories. The first, due to van der Merwe and Ball[18], and Matthews[19], assumes that relaxation of the coherency of the SLS occurs by the glide and climb of pre-existing threading dislocations when a critical thickness is reached in the alloy layer. These theories (or modifications of them) are useful in discussing the application of SLS's as dislocation "filters" to minimize the threading of dislocations through a strained heterostructure- see below. The second set of theories recognizes that in semiconductor films (having the diamond or zinc-blende structure) grown on nearly perfect substrates (dislocation densities $\approx 10^3$ /cm^2), a barrier to dislocation nucleation allows the growth of fully coherent metastable films to much greater thicknesses than are predicted by the equilibrium models[18,19]. The first attempt at predicting the critical film thickness for loss of coherency under these conditions was made by People and Bean[20]. A number of modifications of the People and Bean theory have been suggested; a recent review by Maree et al.[21] summarizes these. The favoured site for dislocation nucleation is thought to be at a free surface in a strained layer where a half loop can form on an inclined (111) plane and glide down to the interface to relieve the misfit.

In our work we are addressing the problem of how coherency is lost on annealing a fully coherent 40-period SLS. The annealing temperatures in these experiments was significantly greater than the growth temperature and depending on the temperature and Ge content of the alloy layers, progressive relaxation of the stresses was found on annealing[22,23]. Two examples of different stages in this process are illustrated in Fig. 8.

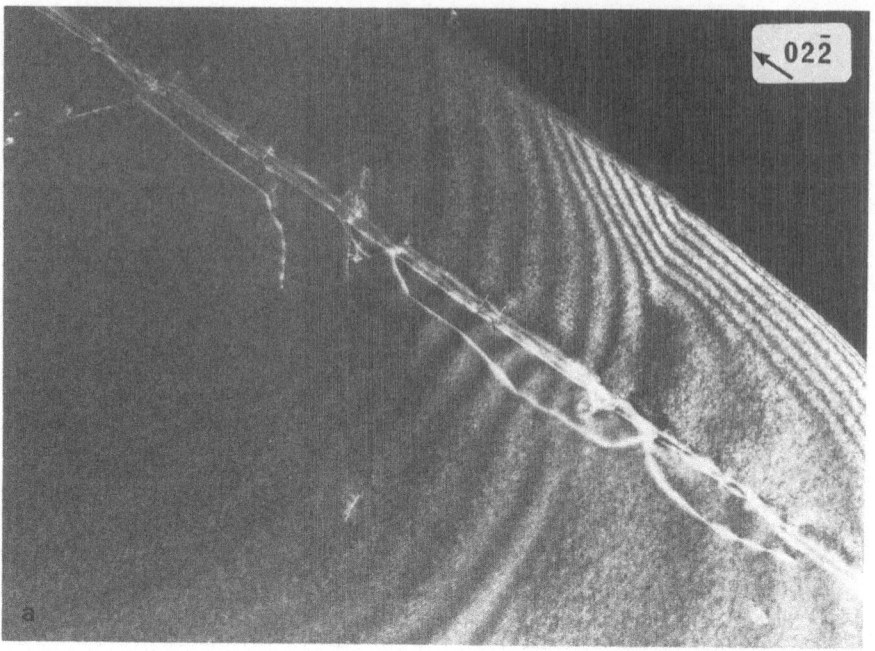

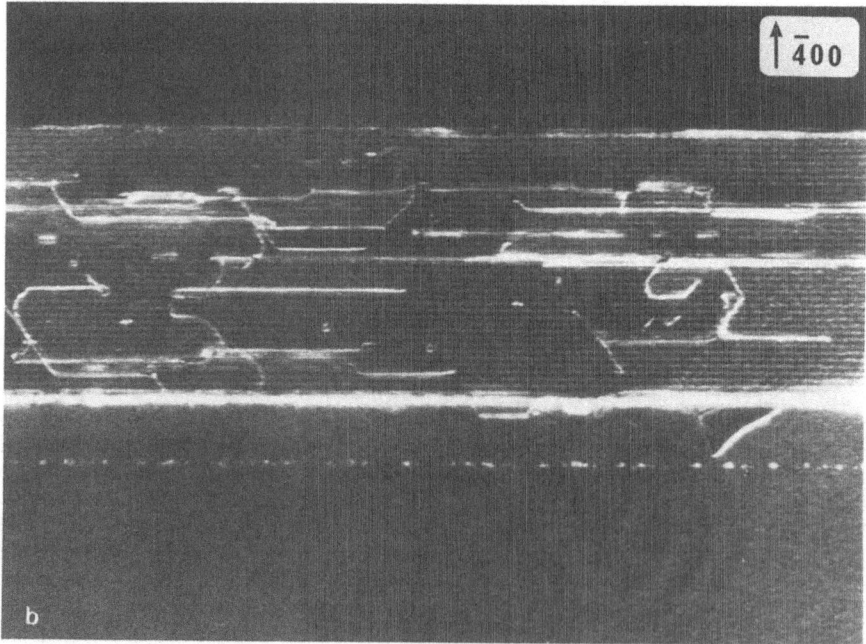

Fig. 8   Weak beam images (g-3g) showing strain relaxation in annealed (2000 sec at 800°C) superlattice structures for a: (a) 40-period $Ge_{0.17}Si_{0.83}$ SLS; (b) 40-period $Ge_{0.25}Si_{0.75}$.

The dislocations in Fig. 8a were characterized by a standard **g•b** analysis. The segments lying in the (100) interfacial plane have **b**= ± a/2[101]; these are 60° mixed dislocations which are less efficient in relieving the misfit strain than dislocations of pure edge character (ie. a/2[011] or a/2[01$\bar{1}$]). It can be seen in Fig. 8a that the strained layer interfaces are fully coherent. This is due to the relatively low Ge concentration in the alloy layers (x= 0.17) such that each strained layer is below the critical thickness for dislocation generation. In fact, loss of coherency is observed at the first Ge_xSi_{1-x}/Si interface. In this way the whole 40-period SLS acts as a unit which is decoupled from the substrate by the generation of dislocations at the first layer. As a result the misfit strain of the alloy layers are no longer accommodated solely within the Ge_xSi_{1-x} layers but are reduced by a factor of ≈2 as the adjacent Si spacer layers expand in tension, ie. the misfit strains are now partitioned between the Ge_xSi_{1-x} and Si layers of the SLS.

At higher Ge fractions the misfit strain of each Ge_xSi_{1-x} layer will exceed some critical value such that dislocations will generate at any Ge_xSi_{1-x}/Si interface of the SLS. This is seen in Fig. 8b where both threading and interfacial misfit dislocations are observed. The dislocations have the same Burgers vector as before (ie. **b**= a/2[101]). There are several examples in Fig. 8b which illustrate how threading dislocations form interfacial misfit dislocation segments due to the strain field of the SLS as first described by Matthews and Blakeslee[24]. The preliminary results shown here indicate that a surface nucleation mechanism[20,21] for dislocation generation cannot be invoked.

We do not yet understand how dislocations are introduced at the first alloy layer. The largest stresses and strains are in the alloy layers (the biaxial stresses discussed in §2), and to a first approximation these are independent of position in the SLS array. The observations might be explained by the role played by the interfacial shear stresses introduced by wafer bending, but further studies are required of the first stages of relaxation to substantiate this.

Dislocation Filtering

Several studies have shown that strained layer superlattices can act as effective dislocation filters[25,26], and this method has been used in an attempt to produce high quality Ge films on (100) Si substrates through compositional grading of a SLS structure[27]. In practise there are a number of problems associated with this technique and the quality of the Ge films proved to be inferior to those produced by growing Ge films directly onto Si substrates, followed by a post-growth annealing treatment [27]. In addition to the difficulties of maintaining good two-dimensional growth conditions in alloy layers at high Ge contents[27], a detailed study of the dislocation-SLS interactions reveals two dislocation-specific problems. These are illustrated in Fig. 9 which comes from a $Ge_{0.7}Si_{0.3}$ strained layer superlattice of fixed strained layer thickness and varying spacer layer thickness grown on Si (100) with a 500 nm Ge buffer.

The first SLS which has a spacer thickness of 30 nm are clearly effective in reducing the dislocation density by causing many of the threading dislocations to be deflected so that they relieve the misfit at the interface plane, as first described by Matthews and Blakeslee[24]. However the **g•b** analysis shown in Fig. 9 demonstrates that some dislocations are observed to pass through the SLS; these are nearly pure edge in character with **b**= ±a/2[011] or ±a/2[01$\bar{1}$] and lie predominantly along the [100] growth direction. According to Matthews and Blakeslee[24], the force (F_ε) on a threading dislocation penetrating a strained interface is a function of both the misfit strain (ε) and thickness (t) of the layer. This is given by

$$F_\varepsilon = 2\mu \frac{(1+\nu)}{(1-\nu)} b\, t\, \varepsilon\, \cos\lambda \qquad (7)$$

where μ is the shear modulus, ν is Poisson's ratio, b is the magnitude of the Burgers vector of the threading dislocation and λ is the angle between **b** and the direction in the interface perpendicular to the intersection of the slip plane and the interface. For the dislocations observed in our studies, if they lie on {111}, the angle λ is 90° such that there is no force exerted on the threading dislocations by the stress field of the strained layers. Accordingly,

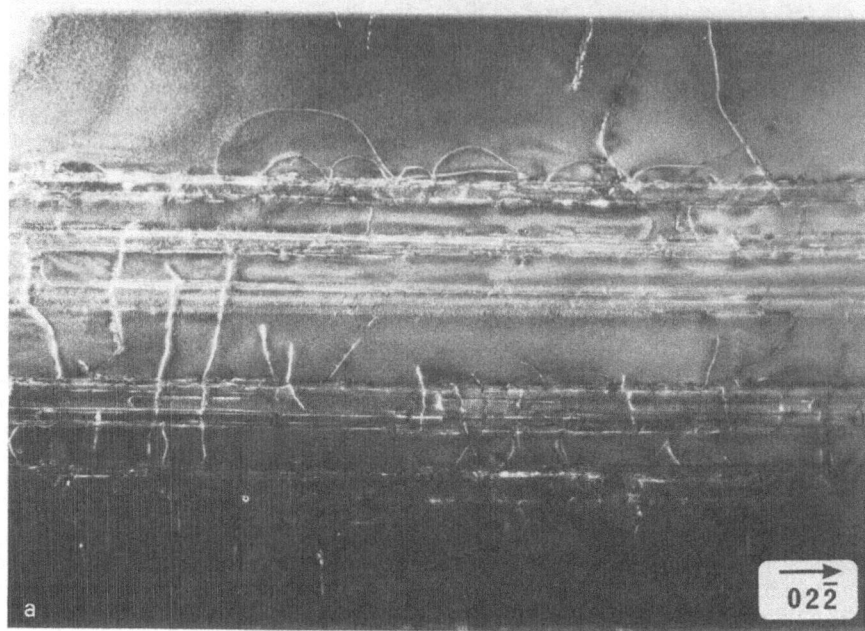

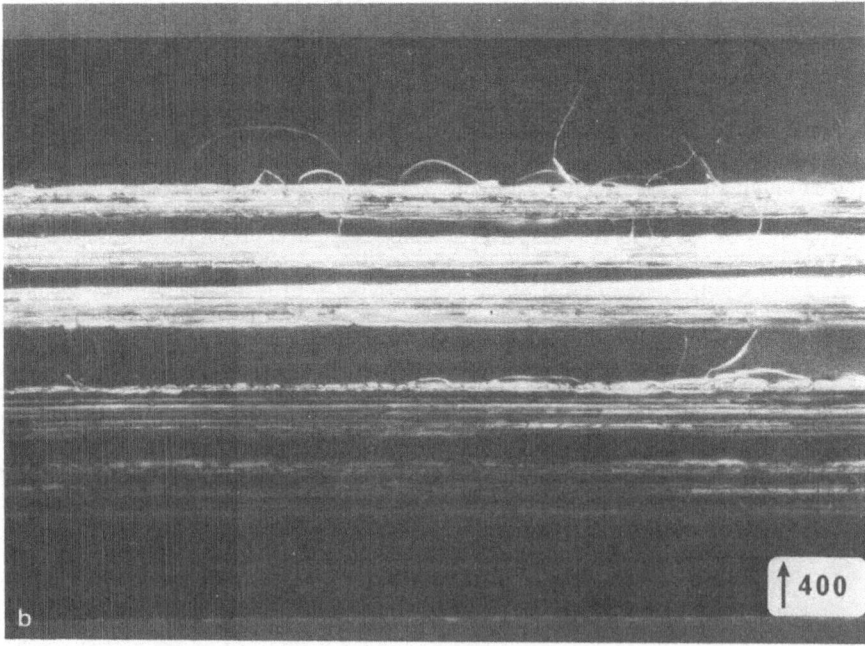

Fig. 9 Weak-beam images (g-3g) for a $Ge_{0.7}Si_{0.3}$ SLS grown on Si with varying spacer layer widths: (a) g= 022; the interaction of threading dislocations with the SLS is evident; (b) g= 400; the threading dislocations are effectively invisible under this diffracting condition.

the dislocations will propagate through the superlattice layers unperturbed by the misfit strain of the SLS. However the dislocations seen to penetrate the SLS in Fig. 9 appear to have **u**, the dislocation line direction parallel to [100] and may not lie on a slip plane. In this case they could only relieve misfit by substantial climb so that **u** lies in (100). However, at the low growth temperatures employed in MBE growth, appreciable dislocation climb is unlikely.

These effects plus the possibility of the SLS itself generating dislocations (as described in the previous section) limits the efficiency of a SLS as a threading dislocation filter.

REFERENCES

1. R. People, *IEEE J. Quant. Electron.*, **QE22**, 1696 (1986).
2. J.C. Bean, L.C. Feldman, A.T. Fiory, S. Nakahara and I.K. Robinson, *J. Vac. Sci. Technol.*, **A2**, 436 (1984).
3. S. Luryi, A. Katalsky and J.C. Bean, *IEEE Trans. Electron Devices*, **ED31**, 1135 (1984).
4. H. Daemokes, H.J. Herzog, H. Jorke, H. Kibbel and E. Kasper, *IEEE Trans Electron Devices*, **ED33**, 633 (1986).
5. H.C. Liu, D. Landheer, M. Buchanan and D.C. Houghton, *Appl. Phys. Lett.*, 52, 1809 (1988).
6. E. Suhir, *Mat. Res. Soc. Symp. Proc.*, **91,** 73 (1987).
7. S. Luryi and E. Suhir, *Appl. Phys. Lett.*, **49**, 3 (1986).
8. S.P. Timoshenko and J.N. Goodier, *Theory of Elasticity*, 3rd ed., New York, McGraw-Hill (1970).
9. J.M. Gibson and M.M.J. Treacy, *Ultramicroscopy,* **14**, 345 (1984); J.M. Gibson, R. Hull, J.C. Bean and M.M.J. Treacy, *Appl. Phys. Lett.*, **46**, 649 (1985).
10. P.B. Hirsch, A. Howie, R.B. Nicholson, D.W. Pashley and M.J. Whelan, *Electron Microscopy of Thin Crystals,* Florida, R.E. Kreiger (1977).
11. G.C. Weatherly, D.D. Perovic and D.C. Houghton, *Inst. Phys. Conf. Ser.*,**87**, 237, (Proceedings of Microsc. Semicond. Mater. Conf., Oxford, 6-8 April, 1987).
12. A.K. Head, P. Humble, L.M. Clareborough, A.J. Morton and C.T. Forwood, *Computed Electron Micrographs and Defect Identification*, Amsterdam, North Holland (1973).
13. D.D. Perovic, *Transmission Electron Microscopy of Elastic Relaxation Effects in Ge_xSi_{1-x} Strained Layer Superlattices,* M.A.Sc.Thesis, University of Toronto (1988).
14. R. Hull, J.C. Bean, F. Cerdeira, A.T. Fiory and J.M. Gibson, *Appl. Phys. Lett.*, **48**, 56 (1986).
15. R.M. Chrenko, L.J. Schowalter, E.L. Hall and N. Lewis, *Mat. Res. Soc. Symp. Proc.*, **56**, 27 (1986).
16. A. De Veirman, K. Yallup, J.Van Landuyt, H.E. Maes and S. Amelinckx, *Inst. Phys. Conf. Ser.*, **87**, 403, (Proceedings of Microsc. Semicond. Mater. Conf., Oxford, 6-8 April, 1987).
17. P. Pirouz, C.M. Chorey, T.T. Chang and J.A. Powell, *Inst. Phys. Conf. Ser.*, **87**, 175, (Proceedings of Microsc. Semicond. Mater. Conf., Oxford, 6-8 April, 1987).
18. J.H. van der Merwe and C.A.B. Ball, in *Epitaxial Growth*, edited by J.W. Matthews, Academic Press, New York, Part B, Chap. 6 (1975).
19. J.W. Matthews, *ibid*, Part B, Chap.8 (1975).
20. R. People and J.C. Bean, *Appl. Phys. Lett.*, **47,** 32 (1985); Erratum, *ibid*, **49,** 229 (1986).
21. P.M.J. Maree, J.C. Barbour, J.F. van der Veen, K.L. Kavanagh, C.W.T. Bielle-Lieuwna and M.P.A. Vegrs, *J. Appl. Phys.*, **62**, 4413 (1987).
22. D.J. Lockwood and J.-M. Baribeau, *Can. J. Phys.*, in press (1988).
23. J.-M. Baribeau, S. Kechang and K. Munro, submitted to *Appl Phys. Lett.* (1988).
24. J.W. Matthews and A.E. Blakeslee, *J. Cryst. Growth*, **27**, 118 (1974).
25. J.W. Matthews, A.E. Blakeslee and S. Mader, *Thin Solid Films*, **33**, 253 (1976).
26. J.W. Matthews and A.E. Blakeslee, *J. Cryst. Growth*, **32**, 235 (1976).
27. J.-M. Baribeau, T.E Jackman, D.C. Houghton, P. Maigne and M.W. Denhoff, *J. Appl. Phys.*, **63**, 5738 (1988).

DEFECT STRUCTURE IN LOW AND HIGH MISFIT SYSTEMS

Horst P. Strunk

Technical University Hamburg–Harburg
D-2100 Hamburg 90, FRG

INTRODUCTION

One of the most important concerns in semiconductor heteroepitaxy is the formation of dislocations and similar defects as a result of misfit stresses. In general these defects are harmful to the electronic/optonic properties of the material and the primary interest is to avoid the defects; where not possible, as an alternative, mechanisms are to be found that reduce the defect density or the presence of defects should be restricted to areas, where they may be tolerated. Unfortunately, the mechanisms that operate to nucleate, multiply and propagate dislocations depend in many cases on the heteroepitaxial system under consideration; especially the degree of misfit, growth temperature and growth mechanism may influence the motion of dislocations and thus the defect structure that develops in the system.

Generally, a discussion of misfit dislocation formation considers a critical thickness (see e.g. /1/) of the heteroepitaxial layer beyond which the defect-free but strongly strained misfitting epilayer state is replaced by a then more favorable state that is elastically relaxed due to the introduction of misfit dislocations (or more generally of defects that may compensate the strain, such as twins, stacking faults). One fact, however, was sometimes not properly considered in discussing misfitting systems in terms of critical thickness: for the considered defects to form, a defect process must be available to the crystal. Thus, only in cases where the nucleation and/or multiplication of defects is 'easy' (e.g. practically not rate determining) a correspondence of experimental and theoretical critical thicknesses can be expected.

All other cases have to deal with the details of defect formation and multiplication, and, thus, with the condition set by the considered system and the experimental parameters. A whole variety of such defect processes are possible therefore and a thorough treatment requires first an experimental analysis of each considered misfit system. In the following we shall discuss two extreme cases as is critical thickness concerned: the cases of low and high misfits.

Low misfit, i.e. large critical thickness, has the advantage of permitting the defect process to be described in "classical" terms of plasticity and diffusion, such as glide or climb of individual dislocations and their interactions. High misfit, i.e. small critical thickness, may be described the same way using the elements detected in low misfit systems. We will summarize results on initial dislocation processes that were obtained during an extended research effort on the system Ge on GaAs /2/. At an ('effective') critical thickness in the order of a few atomic layers, however, this approach may become invalid since growth mechanism and misfit defect formation will be coupled. Description in terms of "molecular processes", such as surface diffusion or local attachment of atoms (say, in form of surface agglomeration) might be more appropriate. These processes, which are very difficult to access experimentally, are presently in the center of research activities (e.g. corresponding papers in /3/). We will consider the system Ge on Si; in order to put emphasis on the

369

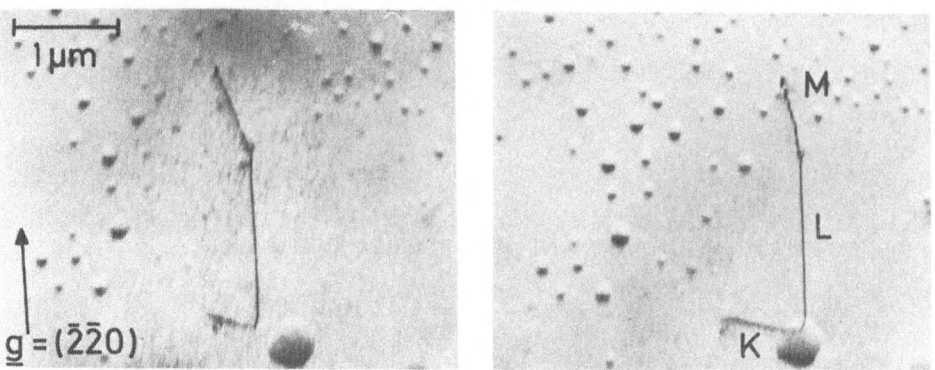

Fig. 1.   Threading dislocation that extended a segment of misfit dislocation L. K: Segment that is contained in the GaAs substrate, M: dislocation segment capable of glide in the Ge epitaxial layer. Stereo micrograph.

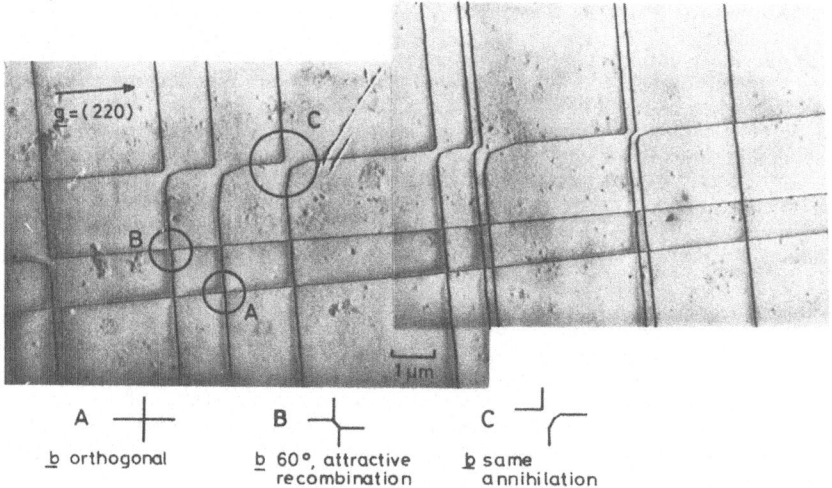

Fig. 2.   Misfit dislocation network at a Ge/GaAs epitaxial interface. Different types of dislocation crossing are marked by circles A,B, and C and are sketched at the bottom of the figure. For details see text.

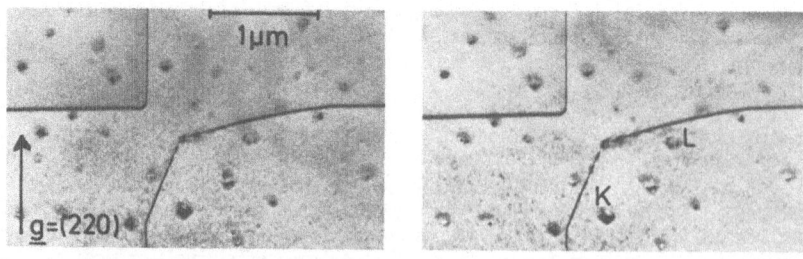

Fig. 3.   Misfit dislocation configuration of the type marked C in Fig.2. The segmented angular dislocation line (K and L) leaves the interface plane towards the surface of the Ge epitaxial layer. Stereo micrograph.

molecular type of the processes we will discuss essentially the case of defect-free seeded lateral overgrowth of Ge over SiO_2 and propose a novel type of misfit compensation on a molecular scale at the amorphous-crystalline interface. As a last topic, the problem of creating the first dislocation in an otherwise dislocation-free misfitting substrate-epilayer system will briefly be addressed.

EXPERIMENTAL PROCEDURES

Low misfit: Ge on GaAs

The Ge layers were grown by chemical vapor deposition from GeH_4 at 870K to thicknesses between 0,5 and 2μm. The orientation of the GaAs substrates is {001} with a deviation amongst the different substrates between 0^0 and 3^0 towards a <110> direction. The etch pit density of the substrates was in the order of $10^7\,m^{-2}$.

High misfit: Ge on Si

The Ge(Si) and nearly pure Ge layers were grown by liquid phase epitaxy from In and Bi solution, respectively. The dislocation-free Si substrates were oriented {111} to within one degree. For seeded lateral overgrowth the substrates were covered with thermal oxide 0.5 to 1μm thick into which stripes serving as seeding areas, with widths up to 100um, were etched. The growth temperature was around 1100 K with a growth temperature interval between 30 and 1 K and a cooling rate between 30 and 2K/h.

Transmission electron microscopy

Because of the low defect density the Ge on GaAs layers were prepared for TEM analysis in plan view. Information about the defect distribution was obtained by stereo micrographs. The samples were mechanically thinned from the GaAs substrate side to approximately 30μm; subsequently the GaAs was chemically etched using solution H_2SO_4 : H_2O_2 : H_2O (3:1:1) until a final thickness of up to 5μm depending on the thickness of the Ge layer was obtained. These specimens were mounted on a brass ring for the TEM investigation. Careful surface-parallel grinding provided for a specimen that was homogeneously thick over large areas (diameter typ. 1mm). These specimen thus contained the whole Ge layer and the top part of the GaAs substrate and were transparent in a high-voltage TEM (HVEM) operated at 1 MV. This experimental procedure permitted a detailed and statistically sound analysis of the defect structure even if there was a very low defect density.

The high misfit Ge(Si) on Si epilayers were investigated by using cross-sectional specimens. These were prepared by following the conventional scheme /4/ by gluing a stack of material together surface to surface and cutting these stacks into disks approximately 0.5mm thick. The disks were then ground to approx. 40 μm thickness and further thinned using an ion miller until a hole appeared.

INITIAL DISLOCATION MECHANISMS IN Ge EPILAYERS ON GaAs

Observations and evaluation

As may be expected from the {001} substrate orientation, the misfit dislocations are distributed at right angles near the interface. In-situ x-ray topography performed during growth of the Ge layers indicate the elongation of contrast lines along the surface which can be interpreted as extension of misfit dislocation segments /5/. In fact HVEM corroborates this view. Fig. 1 shows a stereo micrograph of what is obviously a threading dislocation (segment K) the segment M of which is contained in the Ge layer and has moved by glide some distance and extended a misfit dislocation L.

In accordance with these observations, the misfit dislocation structure in slightly thicker Ge layers consists of an orthogonal pattern of 60^0 dislocations lying at about the interface (Fig. 2). A first result to be mentioned is that the dislocations are bunched together contrary to an equidistant distribution which one could expect on grounds of arguments of optimal stress relaxation. The reason for bunching can be seen in a dislocation source intrinsic to this misfit dislocation arrangement. For this discussion the crossing points

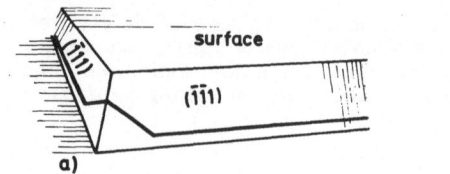
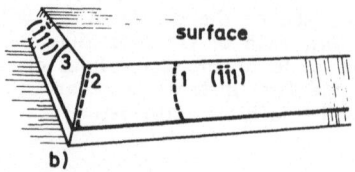

Fig. 4.   (a) Spatial shape of the segmented angular dislocation.
(b) Formation of a segmented angular dislocation by cross-slip of a dislocation segment that extends a misfit dislocation by glide.

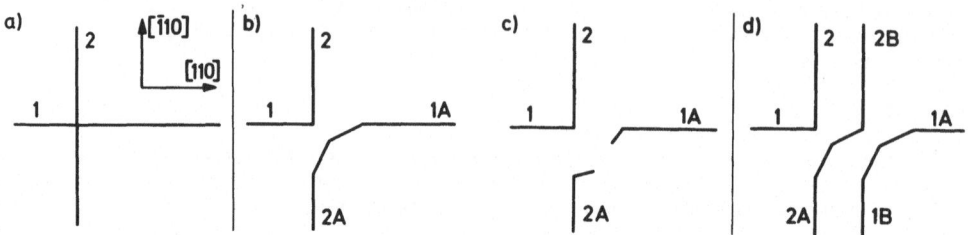

Fig. 5.   Schematic of the segmented angular dislocations and misfit dislocation source, seen along the surface normal.
a,b: Reaction leading to the segmented angular dislocation,
c: this dislocation, on intersection with the layer surface, forms two independent dislocation segments.
d: Glide of these segments, with corresponding cross-slip to form further misfit dislocations.

of the dislocations have to be considered. Three types differing in the angles between the two Burgers vectors of the crossing dislocations exist (circled in Fig. 2): (i) 60⁰ leading to a recombined dislocation segment, (ii) 90⁰ without noticeable interaction, and (iii) 0⁰, in which case a reformation of the crossing point into two angularly shaped dislocations occurs.

This last configuration deserves further discussion, as it is asymmetrical in shape. Fig. 3 shows such a configuration in more detail in a stereo micrograph; inspection indicates, that the rectangular dislocation is confined to one plane (which corresponds roughly to the interface), whereas the segmented angular dislocation line leaves this plane towards the surface of the epilayer. In Fig. 4a, this configuration is depicted in perspective view; it can be seen, that formation of this particular shape occurs due to dislocation line length reduction aided obviously by the attractive image force exerted by the epilayer surface. This process of local rearrangement cannot occur, as discussed earlier /2/, at the other angular dislocation, since length reduction would require glide into the substrate, thus against the exerted image force. This particular crossing point type can occur in four different configurations according to the four-fold symmetry of the substrate normal. Moreover, each of these configurations is, by origination, uniquely linked to one of the four possible 60⁰ misfit dislocation types; pure inspection of the configuration type thus gives the Burgers vector of the respective dislocations. This consequence holds also for analogous crossings occurring with other substrate orientations, especially {111} (see /6/). Of course, the segmented angular dislocations can also result from a respective cross-slip process of a gliding screw (or threading) dislocation segment as indicated in Fig. 4b.

Figures 5a and b show sketches of the formation of the segmented arrangement just described as projected along the surface normal of the epilayer. An important consequence is added to this sketch (Figs. 5c and d): In a certain thickness range of the epilayer (essentially up to around the "height" of the segments), the dislocation corner of the segmented arrangement may reach the surface to form two independent dislocation segments. A stereo micrograph of this configuration is shown in Fig. 6. These dislocation segments are capable of glide and may extend further misfit dislocations as sketched in Fig. 5d (see /7/). This "secondary misfit dislocation source" (as opposed to the primary source creating the first independent misfit dislocation) leads to bunching, i.e. non-equidistant distribution of misfit dislocations /2/; such elements may be recognized in Fig. 2.

372

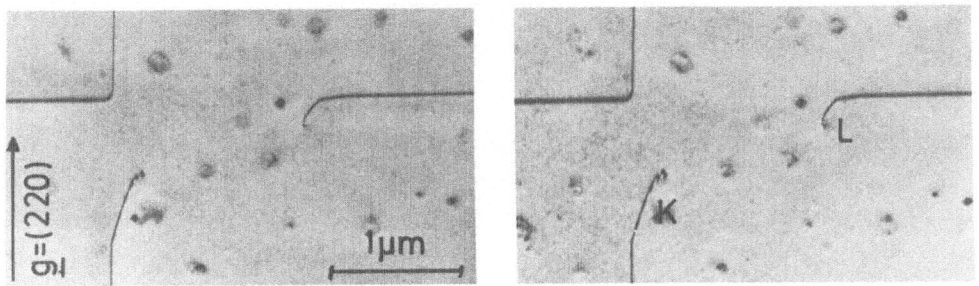

Fig. 6.   Segmented angular dislocation that happens to intersect the layer
           surface. Stereo micrograph. Two independent glissile dislocations (K
           and L) are formed.

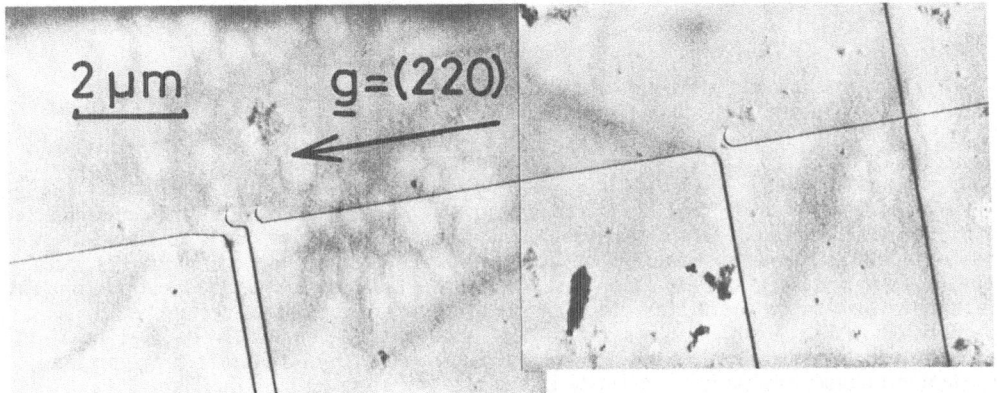

Fig.7.   Misfit dislocation arrangement that occurred due to glide-induced
           activation of threading dislocations by gliding dislocation segments.

Another type of secondary misfit dislocation source encountered in the low misfit
system is shown in Fig. 7. Stereo micrographs indicated that the segments attached to each
of the three misfit dislocations extend into the substrate /8/. The explanation points to a
glide-induced misfit dislocation source: a gliding dislocation segment (coming from the left
in this example and extending a misfit dislocation) encounters a grown-in threading
dislocation; at the same time the original gliding segment cross-slips (e.g. Fig. 4b) and
develops the shape of the segmented angular dislocation. In Fig. 7 this glide-induced
activation occurred three times, which is not typical, of course, since generally threading
dislocations are statistically distributed and are not arranged in <110> directions as indicated
in Fig. 7. The activation process, of course, is most efficient when dislocations with the
same Burgers vector and same sign are involved which happened to be the case in Fig. 7
also. Opposite sign of the Burgers vectors would lead to partial recombination and to
formation of extended misfit dislocations with substrate segments at both ends, which in
fact were occasionally observed.

Secondary sources and misfit dislocation distribution

The present misfit structure is produced by glide only. In this case two secondary
misfit dislocation sources were identified to produce additional misfit dislocations once the
first misfit dislocations have formed:
a. glide activation of grown-in dislocations and
b. creation of new dislocations segments capable of glide at crossing points of dislocations
with same Burgers vector ("Hagen-Strunk-source", see recent literature /9,10,11/).

373

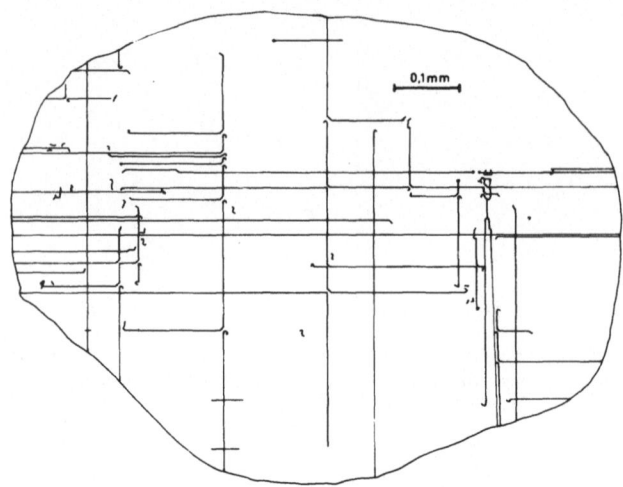

Fig. 8.   Schematic drawing of a misfit dislocation array at the Ge/GaAs interface, evaluated by HVEM.

Whereas activation of the first source is generally purely statistical, as it depends on the distribution of activated grown-in dislocations, the second source leads to bunching and thus an inhomogeneous distribution of dislocations. Moreover, depending on the Burgers vector of the dislocations of the first crossings, the profuse multiplication by this mechanism may cause the preference of a specific Burgers vector in certain areas. This is exemplified in Fig. 8 which shows a record of an evaluated comparatively large misfitting region. Inspection corroborates this conclusion, since in fact two different configurations of segmented angular dislocations dominate in the left and right half of the figure. As a result of the screw components of the mixed misfit dislocations, a twist around the surface normal is created which is opposite in the two halves of the sample. Thus the operation of this source enhances the effect of the screw components and leads to an energetically rather unfavorable misfit array; a dislocation array, in which the Burgers vectors alternate, would effectively reduce the influence of the screw components (a similar arrangement was discussed regarding dislocations at oxide-nitride-mask edges /12/).

Some remarks concerning the limited activity of the secondary source at segmented angular misfit dislocation should be added. It is to be expected from the model that the source can be active in a limited thickness range of the epilayer only. The lower limit d_{min} may be seen in the critical thickness d_{crit}, as misfit dislocations have to be available already.

$$d_{min} \sim d_{crit} \qquad (1)$$

d_{crit} is, for a given misfit dislocation system, essentially dependent only on the inverse of the misfit parameter f /1, 13/:

$$d_{crit} \sim k/f \qquad (2)$$

The quantity k depends on the elastic constants. The upper limit d_{max} may be obtained from the notion that above this thickness the image stress T_i acting on the dislocation is smaller than the stress T_0 to move the dislocation:

$$T_0 \geq T_i = \frac{Gb}{2cd} \qquad (3)$$

Hence

$$d_{max} = \frac{Gb}{2cT_0} \qquad (4)$$

Here c denotes a constant which accounts for the details of stress fields and geometry, G and b are shear modulus and Burgers vector, resp.; the factor of 2 is kept because the distance between dislocation and its mirror image is roughly double the epilayer thickness d. The stress T_0 can be regarded as sort of critical stress at which the dislocation starts to glide with reasonable velocity to undergo the annihilation at the surface. Although crude, this estimate shows that the thickness range increases (Eq. 4) with increasing shear modulus G of the epilayer and with decreasing stress T_0. The latter conclusion indicates that the maximum thickness for source operation increases with increasing growth temperature (because T_0 then generally decreases) and, more importantly, may strongly depend on the doping level. It is known from measurements of dislocation velocities (e.g. /14,15,16/) that the ease of glide, as symbolized by T_0 here, is strongly influenced by type and concentration of doping (i.e. by the Fermi level). This topic shall not be detailed here.

It is interesting to note that, within the present estimate, a critical misfit can exist below which the source cannot operate. This occurs when the minimum thickness equals or exceeds the maximum thickness, i.e.

$$d_{min} \geq d_{max} \qquad (5)$$

Thus, with eqs. 2 and 4:

$$f \leq 2ckT_0/G \qquad (6)$$

A very rough estimate (2ck: 0,1...1, T_0: 1MPa, G: 10...50GPa) yields $f \leq 10^{-4}... 2 \times 10^{-6}$, which corresponds to very low misfit systems. This result, however, should only be taken as indication for the existence of such a region of inactivity; quantification of the model requires a much more detailed consideration of stress fields and geometry.

Thus far "intrinsic" properties of the source have been considered; there can also be thought of external influences on its operation. The surface which has to be cut by the segmented angular dislocation, is crucial in this respect. The cutting process may be prevented by a surface coating or other type of additional layer, such as an amorphous layer which exists after ion milling for TEM in-situ observations. In any case, such a barrier to the source operation may be useful in situations in which misfitting systems are used under conditions of possible dislocation glide.

Climb misfit dislocations

The 60^0 dislocations considered thus far are ineffective in relieving misfit stresses as compared to 90^0 dislocations, i.e. dislocations whose Burgers vectors lie in the interface. Although 90^0 dislocations may form by recombination of "glide misfit dislocations" (e.g. /2/), this process is very unlikely to provide a regular misfit dislocation array in low misfit systems. Rather, climb is required and such a mechanism occurs frequently during diffusion where point defects are involved. As an example the diffusion of phosphorus into silicon to form an emitter contact shall briefly be considered. Fig. 9 shows a very early and a more developed stage of such climb misfit dislocations. This case is especially interesting: The undersized phosphorus atoms lead to tensional stress in the diffused volume; this tension can

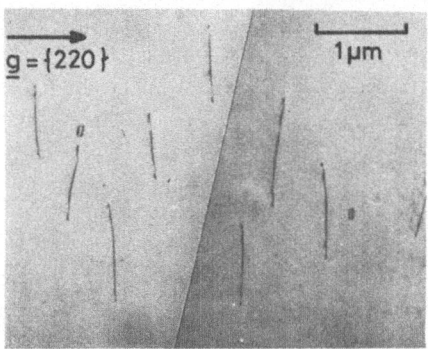 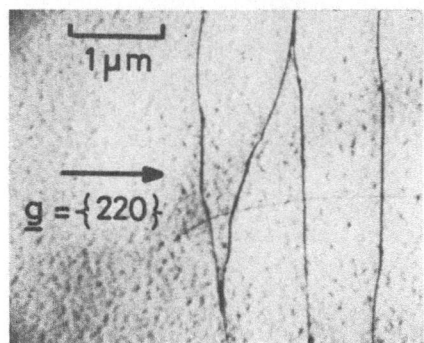

Fig. 9.   Formation of misfit dislocations by climb from the surface due to phosphorus diffusion into silicon
(a) Early stage of diffusion, (b) Later stage of diffusion

be relieved by 90° dislocations that introduce additional half planes into the diffused volume. Thus climb from the surface requires either emission of vacancies from the cores or attachment of interstitials to the cores of the dislocations. The latter occurs in the present case, since phosphorus diffusion causes a supersaturation of silicon self-interstitials /17/. The interesting aspect now is, that the chemical force due to these interstitials (whose supersaturation is independently determined by the diffusion conditions) supports the elastic force acting on the dislocations due to the misfit in the system.

HIGH MISFIT, REDUCTION OF DISLOCATION DENSITY IN Ge EPILAYERS ON Si

Defect structure in epitaxial layers

Figure 10 shows the interface structure between a Si substrate and an SiGe overgrowth as seen in a cross-sectional sample tilted obliquely to the electron beam of the microscope. Thus the high dislocation density at the interface is visible as a band of fine contrasts. A few other dislocation lines are also visible near this interface. These dislocations in all cases grew into the SiGe layer (Fig. 11) and form a dense network there. In addition to these features planar defects were detected in this layer to lie approximately parallel to the interface, but within the epilayer. These defects are visible in Fig. 10 at the top and in Fig. 11, there are two at the bottom. Origin and nature of these planar defects is not yet clear; judging from the complicated fringe contrast they do not represent simple stacking faults. It was observed that these defects effectively may capture dislocations that emanate from the interface (e.g. /18/); some of these dislocations are visible in Fig. 10. It appears possible to utilize these defects for reducing the dislocation density in the grown Ge or GeSi-layers; however, very probably, these are not capable of a reduction to almost zero density. Such a goal may be reached by seeded lateral overgrowth.

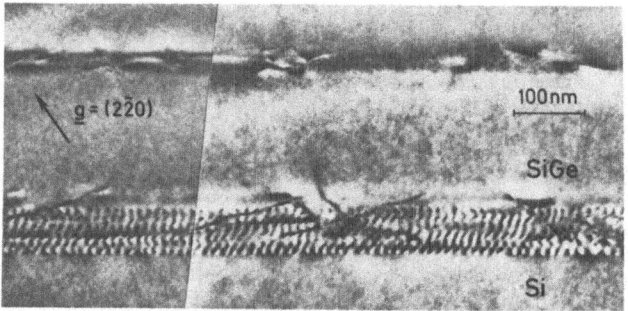

Fig. 10.   Defect structure at interface between SiGe and Si substrate; epitaxial growth from In-solution. XTEM, specimen tilted obliquely to the electron beam to display the interface as a band (at bottom).

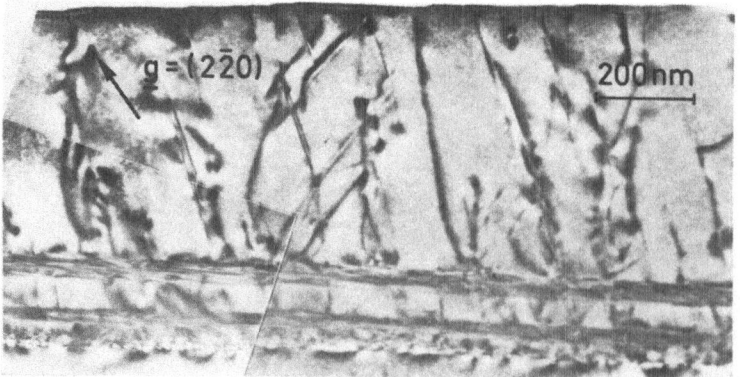

Fig. 11.   Defect structure in SiGe on Si. XTEM, interface can be seen as a fine band at the very bottom of the micrograph.

Seeded lateral overgrowth of Ge on SiO₂/Si

Figure 12 shows a cross-sectional TEM micrograph of the edge of a window in a SiO₂ mask on silicon; in the window a Ge layer was grown epitaxially from Bi solution. Contrary to what is generally obtained in CVD experiments of this type, (e.g. /19/), no defects are created in this case at the interface SiO₂/Ge. In fact, this result is even more noteworthy as this interface is very rough (the window was produced by etching); contrast experiments in addition revealed, that there are even no stress concentrations at this interface as recognizable by corresponding stress contours (e.g. those visible in Fig. 11 at the interface at the very bottom). The same result, "no defect generation", is obtained after lateral overgrowth as observed far from the window edge (Fig. 13, cf. /20/ also).

It was already pointed out very early /21/, that "steps" in the surface of amorphous layers may lead to dislocations, stacking faults, twins and related lattice defects in a crystalline overgrowth because of accommodation reasons. This does clearly not occur in the present system Ge on SiO₂ (seeded on Si substrate) as confirmed by other techniques like etching and EBIC.

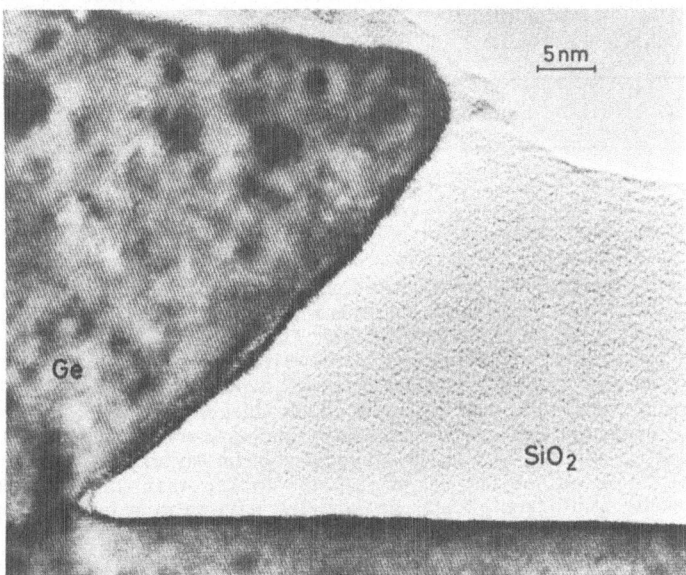

Fig. 12.   High resolution electron micrograph of a Ge layer grown from Bi-solution in a window of a SiO₂ mask. XTEM, structure imaging. No defects have nucleated at the Ge/SiO₂ interface.

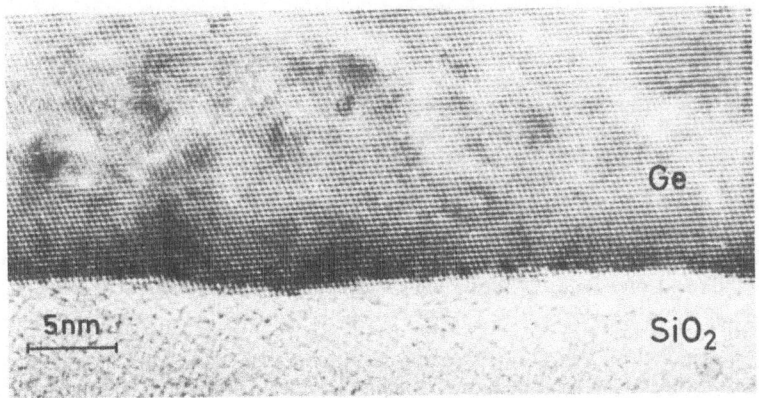

Fig. 13.   High resolution electron micrograph of the Ge/SiO₂ interface in the region of overgrowth; no defects have nucleated at the comparatively rough interface.

A tentative explanation, still to be confirmed experimentally, results from the fact that the four elements present near the SiO_2-Ge(Bi) interface may form a number of Bi-compounds. These compounds offer a number of lattice parameters that range around the Ge-{111}-interplane distance (Table 1) stress-driven formation of the appropriate compound, possibly accompanied with some degree of non-stoichiometry, may effectively compensate the local corrugations of the SiO_2 surface. More generally spoken, the present growth experiment uses a system which is capable of locally selecting at the SiO_2/Ge interface a chemical composition such as to accommodate misfit on a molecular scale /22/.

Table 1. Some Bi-compounds and selected lattice plane distances

Compound	Structure	Set of planes	Distance [A]
α-Bi_2O_3	hexagonal	121	3.254
$Bi_{12}GeO_{20}$	cubic	310	3.208
$Bi_{12}SiO_{20}$	cubic	111	3.210
$Bi_{12}(SiO_4)_3$	cubic	310	3.257
Ge	diamond	111	3.266

THE FIRST MISFIT DISLOCATION

As indicated by the previous considerations, a number of multiplication mechanisms to form misfit dislocations at the interface are available to a misfitting system, once a first dislocation capable of glide or climb is available. The necessary but certainly not sufficient condition is that the strained epilayer exceeds the critical thickness as defined by Matthews /1/. In fact, very careful growth of epilayers, which avoids grown-in dislocations and other types of dislocation formation, may result in much thicker dislocation-free epilayers than predicted by this criterion. Bean et al. /23/ have impressively corroborated this possibility by growing Ge_xSi_{1-x} - alloys onto Si by molecular beam epitaxy. These authors obtained thicknesses more than one order of magnitude thicker than predicted by Matthews' criterion. The results could theoretically be modeled with success by equating the specific energy in the dislocation-free overgrowth against the self-energy of an isolated first dislocation /24/. This self-energy is essentially represented by the core energy of the dislocation, whereas the energy component stored in the long range strain field of the dislocation is essentially the entity that enters Matthews' criterion. A similar approach that considers the self-energy also was discussed already very early by Queisser /25/ in treating misfit dislocations in boron doped silicon.

Two consequences have to be considered. Firstly, the epilayers with thickness beyond the Matthews critical thickness are inherently unstable against misfit network formation. Once a first dislocation is formed in these layers by whatever mechanism, this dislocation may multiply in the volume of the epilayer by one of the discussed mechanisms to form dislocations at the interface and, certainly enough, in the epilayer volume also. Such a sudden transition of a highly strained heteroepitaxial layer into the dislocated state may occur during processing steps, such as ion implantation, diffusion, etc., following layer growth.

Secondly the theoretical model of People and Bean /24/ does not detail the mechanism by which the first dislocation forms. In fact, not much is known about such mechanisms from experiment and one possible evidence discussed earlier /26/ will briefly be considered. The possible mechanism bases on a study by high resolution electron microscopy of phosphorus diffusion in silicon /27/ and replaces the athermal formation of the first dislocation, as assumed in People and Bean's treatment /24/ (and in Queisser's as well /25/) by a sequence of thermally activated steps, at the end of which a dislocation is formed. The electron microscope observations /27/ revealed that after predeposition of a phosphorus-doped glass, a high density of small silicon phosphide precipitates (size typ. 10 nm) exist at the silicon surface. These precipitates were partly associated with tiny stacking faults or dislocation loops. For the discussion here the following steps are interesting: In the course of drive-in, which is performed after removal of the glass, the dislocation loops may grow, essentially due to the Si self- interstitial supersaturation, that is associated with phosphorus-diffusion /17/. Because of the decreasing concentration level of phosphorus at the surface during the diffusion treatment the precipitates may dissolve eventually. The nucleated defects, however, will remain generally and form sources of misfit dislocations.

This nucleation mechanism is very likely of general importance for all misfitting layers caused by diffusion of under- or over-sized dopants into semiconductors. It also bears relevance for heteroepitaxial misfitting layers; formation of precipitates or inclusions at the surface of a growing layer is very likely due to the presence of inadvertently introduced impurities. Corroboration of this nucleation mechanism is seen in the recent observation of 'diamond-like' defects /28/ that acted as misfit dislocation sources. Unfortunately, only the dislocation reactions could be modeled and nothing is known presently about the formation and nature of the defect.

CONCLUSIONS

The discussion showed that the formation of misfit dislocations in low misfit systems can be described and understood in terms of 'classical' dislocation behavior. A misfit dislocation source formed at crossings of misfit dislocations with same Burgers vectors is shown to lead to energetically less favorable bunching of misfit dislocations. The dislocation mechanism discussed may also occur in systems with high misfit, where it is difficult to detect. In any case, these misfit dislocation mechanisms occur in the volume of the epilayer and consequently cause a certain dislocation density within the epilayer, be it low or high misfit.

The experiments performed suggest that the density of these dislocations may be reduced by several experimental provisions. Especially the case of lateral overgrowth of Ge over SiO_2, seeded on Si, is discussed, in which no defects nucleate at the Ge/SiO_2 interface. The reason for the growth of this highly perfect Ge-layers is seen in the accommodation of the molecular height fluctuations in the SiO_2-surface by local variation of the chemical composition and, thus, lattice parameter of the growing Ge layer.

In highly misfitting systems formation of dislocations, i.e. more precisely the formation of the first dislocation being capable of glide, can be suppressed as shown for example by R. Hull /28/ even if the obtained thickness of the epilayers largely exceeds the critical thickness as defined by the mechanical equilibrium criterion. However, it has to be born in mind that such layers are inherently unstable against introduction of misfit dislocations during subsequent processing steps.

ACKNOWLEDGMENT

The author is grateful for continuous cooperation with Dr. E. Bauser, Dr. H. Cerva, and Dr. J.H. Werner. Thanks are due to Mrs. A. Kessler and Mr. N. Strunk for help during preparation of the manuscript. Furthermore, the author acknowledges a discussion with Prof. H.J. Queisser on aspects of misfit dislocations.

REFERENCES

1. J. W. Matthews, Coherent interfaces and misfit dislocations, in: "Epitaxial Growth", J.W. Matthews, ed., Academic Press, New York, London, (1975)

2. H. Strunk, W. Hagen, and E. Bauser, Low density dislocation arrays at heteroepitaxial Ge/GaAs interfaces investigated by high voltage electron microscopy, Appl. Phys. 18: 67 (1979)

3. R. Hull, J.M. Gibson, and D.A. Smith, eds., "Initial Stages of Epitaxial Growth", (Mat. Res. Symp. Proc. Vol. 94), Materials Research Soc., Pittsburgh, PA, USA (1987)

4. M. S. Abrahams and C.J. Buiocchi, Cross-sectional specimens for transmission electron microscopy, J. Appl. Phys. 45: 3315 (1974)

5. W. Hagen and H.J. Queisser, In-situ x-ray topography of epitaxial Ge layers during growth, Appl. Phys. Lett. 32: 269 (1978)

6. H. Strunk, W.Hagen, and B.O. Kolbesen, Observation of individual misfit dislocations by high-voltage electron microscopy, J. Physique, Colloque C6, 40: C6-213 (1979)

7. W. Hagen and H. Strunk, A new type of source generating misfit dislocations, Appl. Phys. 17: 85 (1978)

8. W. Hagen and H. Strunk, Glide activation of grown-in dislocations in epitaxial films having almost critical thickness, in: "Electron Microscopy 1980", Vol.4, P. Brederoo and J. van Landuyt, eds., 7.European Congr. on Electron Microscopy Foundation, Leiden, Belgium (1980), p. 372

9. Yu. A. Tkhorik and L.S. Khazan, "Plastic Deformation and Misfit Dislocations in Heteroepitaxial Systems", Naukova dumka, Kiev, USSR (1983) (in russian)

10. V. J. Vdovin, L.A. Matveeva, G.N. Semenova, M. Ya. Skorohod, Yu. A. Tkhorik, and L.S. Khazan, Mechanism of misfit dislocation network formation in the heteroepitaxial system Ge-GaAs {001}, phys. stat. sol. a 92: 379 (1985)

11. K. Rajan and M. Denhoff, Misfit dislocation structure at Si/Si_xGe_{1-x} strained-layer interface, J. Appl. Phys. 62: 1710 (1987)

12. H. P. Strunk and B.O. Kolbesen, Dislocations in silicon devices, in: "Defects in Crystals", E. Mizera, ed., World Scientific, Singapore (1987), p. 208

13. C. A. Ball and H.J. van der Merwe, The growth of dislocation-free layers, in: "Dislocations in Solids", Vol. 6, F.R.N. Nabarro, ed., North Holland Publ. Co., Amsterdam, New York, Oxford (1983)

14. P. B. Hirsch, Dislocations in Semiconductors, in: 'Dislocations and Properties of Real Materials', The Institute of Metals, London (1985), p. 333

15. K. Sumino, Dislocations in GaAs crystals, in: "Defects and Properties of Semiconductors: Defect Engineering", J. Chikawa, K. Sumino, and K. Wada, eds., KTK Scientific Publ., Tokyo (1987), p. 3

16. K. Sumino, Interaction of dislocations with impurities in silicon, ibid., p. 227

17. H. Strunk, U. Goesele and B.O. Kolbesen, Interstitial superstration near phosphorus-diffused emitter zones in silicon, Appl. Phys. Lett. 34: 530 (1979)

18. M. I. Alonso, H.P. Trah, H. Cerva, H.P. Strunk, and E. Bauser, Heteroepitaxy and seeded lateral overgrowth on silicon substrates by liquid phase epitaxy, in: "Silicon Molecular Beam Epitaxy", J.C. Bean and L.J. Schowalter, eds., The Electrochemical Soc. Inc., Pennington, N.J., USA (1988), p. 313

19. J. T. McGinn, L. Jastrzebski, and J.F. Corby, Defect characterization in monocrystalline silicon grown over SiO_2, J. Electrochem. Soc. 131: 398 (1984)

20. H. P. Trah, M.I. Alonso, M. Konuma, E. Bauser, and H.P. Strunk, Liquid phase epitaxy of $Si_{1-x}Ge_x$ (0<x<1) on partially masked Si-substrates, in: "Heteroepitaxy on Silicon II", J.C.C. Fan, J.M. Phillips, and B.-Y. Tsaur, eds., (Mat. Res. Soc. Symp. Proc. Vol. 91), Materials Research Soc., Pittsburgh PA, USA (1987), p. 393

21. R. H. Finch, H.J. Queisser, G. Thomas, and J. Washburn, Structure and origin of stacking faults in epitaxial silicon, J. Appl. Phys. 34: 406 (1963)

22. H. Cerva and H.P. Strunk, to be published

23. J. C. Bean, L.C. Feldman, A.T Fiory, S. Nakahara and J.K. Robinson, Ge_xSi_{1-x}/Si strained layer superlattice grown by molecular beam epitaxy, J. Vac. Sci. Technol. A2: 436 (1984)

24. R. People and C.J. Bean, Calculation of critical layer thickness versus lattice mismatch for Ge_xSi_{1-x}/Si strained-layer heterostructures, Appl. Phys. Lett. 47: 322 (1985)

25. H. J. Queisser, Slip patterns on boron doped silicon surfaces, J. Appl. Phys. 32: 1776 (1960)

26. H. P. Strunk and B.O. Kolbesen, Microscopy of process-related defects in silicon devices, in: " Gettering and Defect Engineering in the Semiconductor Technology", H. Richter, ed., Institute for Physics of Semiconductors, Frankfurt/Oder, GDR (1985), p. 347

27. A. Bourret and W. Schröter, HREM of SiP precipitates at the (111) silicon surface during phosphorus predeposition, Ultramicroscopy 14: 97 (1984)

28. C. J. Humphreys and R. Hull, this workshop

IN-SITU ELECTRON MICROSCOPE STUDIES OF MISFIT DISLOCATION

INTRODUCTION INTO Ge_xSi_{1-x}/Si HETEROSTRUCTURES

R. Hull, J.C. Bean, D. Bahnck, J.M. Bonar and C. Buescher

AT&T Bell Laboratories
600 Mountain Avenue
Murray Hill, NJ 07974, USA

ABSTRACT

An outstanding question in semiconductor strained layer epitaxy is the details of lattice mismatch relaxation via the introduction, propagation and interaction of misfit dislocations. In this paper, we review present understanding of the strained layer relaxation process and describe recent in-situ relaxation experiments in a transmission electron microscope which, to our knowledge, have enabled us for the first time to directly observe misfit dislocation phenomena in strained layer semiconductors in real-time. These experiments have provided detailed understanding of defect nucleation, propagation and interaction events during elastic strain relaxation in Ge_xSi_{1-x}/Si(100) epitaxy and have allowed quantitative measurement of physical parameters such as activation energies which describe these processes.

1. INTRODUCTION

Constant development and refinement of advanced crystal growth techniques such as Molecular Beam Epitaxy (MBE) and Organometallic Vapor Phase Epitaxy (OMVPE) in recent years have enabled synthesis of highly perfect epitaxial semiconductor structures when the constituent layers are closely lattice-matched. Examples of such systems are $Al_xGa_{1-x}As$/GaAs and $In_{0.53}Ga_{0.47}As$/InP structures which have provided new insights into basic physics and enabled new high speed electronic and optoelectronic device structures. Extension of such epitaxial structures to systems containing materials with significantly different lattice parameters has lead to the concept of "strained layer epitaxy" (1,2). As illustrated in Figure 1, it is generally found that it is possible for low coverages to grow the epitaxial layer such that its atoms are in registry with the substrate, adopting the lattice parameter of the substrate in the interfacial plane. This causes an in-plane stress which produces a corresponding distortion of the unit cell along the growth direction, the sense of the normal relaxation being opposite to the sense of the in-plane strain. Such a configuration contains considerable elastic strain energy, and at a characteristic epilayer thickness known as the "critical thickness", h_c, it becomes energetically favorable for interfacial dislocations to relax this strain energy by allowing the epitaxial layer to relax towards its bulk lattice parameter (3,4). The magnitude of h_c will clearly depend upon the magnitude of the lattice mismatch between substrate and deposit (3,4) and, more subtly, upon growth temperature and growth rate (5,6). Many theoretical models (e.g. 3,4,5,7) have been developed to describe the transition between the strained and dislocated states and to predict the magnitude of h_c. Most of these theories recognize that the transition from totally strained epitaxy to the equilibrium relaxed structure is not totally abrupt, and thus as has been pointed out by Fritz (8), the exact magnitude of h_c will depend upon the sensitivity of the experimental technique used to detect lattice relaxation misfit dislocations. Nevertheless, the concept of a characteristic thickness at which dislocation introduction at least dramatically accelerates is widely accepted.

Despite the plethora of theoretical models describing this transition, experimental understanding of the strain relaxation process is still very limited. Critical thickness values as a function of lattice strain have been experimentally determined for a number of systems (e.g. 2,9), but little is known about the detailed processes involved in the strain relaxation. In this paper we describe in-situ strain relaxation experiments in a transmission electron microscope (TEM) which allow the processes of misfit dislocation propagation and interaction to be directly studied in detail, providing a unified understanding of critical relaxation phenomena in strained layer epitaxy.

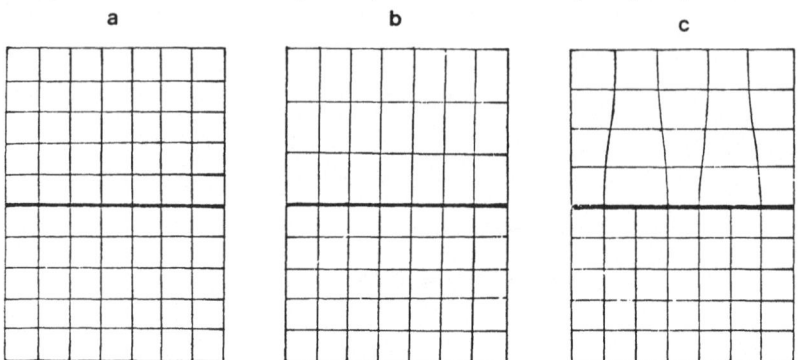

Figure 1. Schematic diagram of (a) lattice-matched epitaxy (b) coherently strained lattice-mismatched epitaxy (c) relaxed lattice-mismatched epitaxy.

2. EXPERIMENTAL

Shown in Figure 2 is an experimental plot (as obtained from plan-view TEM, X-ray diffraction and ion channelling measurements (2), with an experimental sensitivity ~ 1 part in 10^3 in strain relaxation) of critical thickness vs. composition in the $Ge_xSi_{1-x}/Si(100)$ system, for an MBE growth temperature of 550°C. Also shown are equilibrium predictions of the critical thickness in this system, based upon the analysis of Matthews and Blakeslee (4), who derived an expression for critical thickness by balancing the forces on a dislocation threading from the substrate in a direction approximately perpendicular to the interface. The magnitude of h_c was obtained by balancing the force due to misfit stress in the epitaxial layer with the restoring force exerted by the line tension of the dislocation. This latter force is configuration dependent, thus we have modified it for the configuration appropriate to the present system. The original Matthews/Blakeslee formulation was derived for consideration of III-V heteroepitaxy at a time when typical substrate dislocation densities were of the order $10^6 cm^{-2}$, which is a sufficient density to act as the source for the numbers of misfit dislocations required for strain relaxation (in the Matthews and Blakeslee model the threading dislocations are deflected into the interfacial plane, where they propagate during growth to produce misfit dislocation segments). In contemporary Si substrates, threading dislocation densities are $< 100 cm^{-2}$ (although defect densities in the homoepitaxial Si buffer layer typically deposited before Ge_xSi_{1-x} heteroepitaxy may be higher), thus as will be argued later in this paper, dislocation loop nucleation and growth will be necessary at some point in the epilayer to act as the misfit defect source. We have therefore in our calculations used the line tension appropriate to a half-hexagonal dislocation loop, with one side in the interfacial plane, and the other two threading to the surface. The dislocation Burgers vector is assumed to be of the 60-degree, $\frac{1}{2}<011>$ type, which may move solely by glide on the appropriate $\{111\}$ slip plane (these are the dislocations observed in this system for $x < \sim 0.25$, as will be discussed later). Elastic constants appropriate to the $Ge_xSi_{1-x}/Si(100)$ system are used.

It can be seen that the experimentally determined values of h_c are significantly larger than equilibrium predictions, especially for lower values of x in Ge_xSi_{1-x} (note that this trend is also qualitatively true if the original Matthews/Blakeslee term for dislocation line tension is used). This suggests that the as-grown structures at 550°C are metastable, and that activation barriers with respect to dislocation nucleation and/or growth are prohibiting strain relaxation at this relatively low temperature. This model is supported by the substantially lower critical thicknesses measured for $Ge_xSi_{1-x}/Si(100)$ grown at 750°C (10), by subsequent theoretical modelling incorporating dislocation propagation activation energies (5) and by direct observations of strain relaxation upon thermal annealing for structures grown at 550°C (6,11,12).

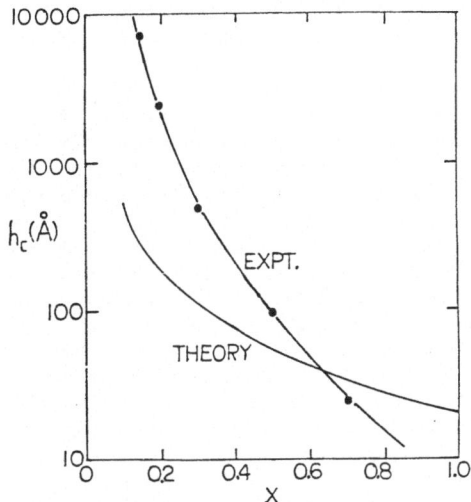

Figure 2. Experimental (MBE (2) substrate temperature = 550°C) and theoretical equilibrium (following Matthews and Blakeslee (4), for 60° dislocations) critical thickness curves for the $Ge_xSi_{1-x}/Si(100)$ system.

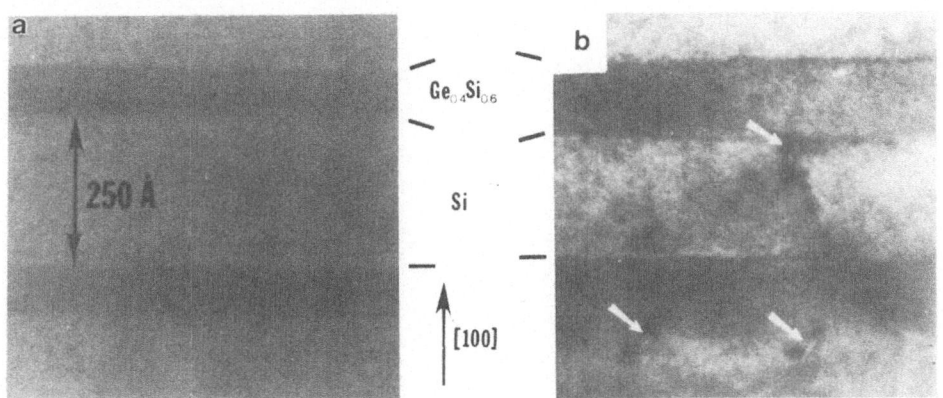

Figure 3. Cross-sectional <011> TEM images of a 20-period 75Å $Ge_{0.4}Si_{0.6}$/225Å Si superlattice structure on Si(100) (a) as-grown at 530°C (b) following bulk ex-situ annealing at 775°C for 30 minutes.

As an example, shown in Figure 3 are TEM cross-sectional images of part of a 20 period 75Å $Ge_{0.4}Si_{0.6}$/225Å Si superlattice grown on Si(100) at 530°C. The as-grown structure, 3(a), exhibits no misfit dislocations to the sensitivity detectable by cross-sectional TEM ($\sim 10^7 cm^{-2}$ at low magnification). The structure shown in 3(b) has been annealed ex-situ in a furnace to 775°C, and exhibits an extremely high dislocation density, indicating activation barriers have been overcome. Note also that strain relaxation has proceeded partially by interdiffusion of the layers (11).

In the experiments which will subsequently be described here, the annealing of metastable $Ge_xSi_{1-x}/Si(100)$ structures is done in-situ in a TEM, such that we may dynamically observe in real-time the strain relaxation processes induced by misfit dislocation nucleation, propagation and interaction. Structures are grown by MBE at 550°C such that they are in the metastable regime between the experimental and equilibrium h_c curves of Figure 2. Thin-foil TEM samples are then made of the material. These samples are always prepared in the plan-view geometry; in the cross-sectional geometry the Ge_xSi_{1-x}/Si interface will be exposed to the top and bottom thin foil surfaces, and thus surface diffusion across the interface might be expected to dominate the experiment. In the plan view geometry, the interface is always buried away from free surfaces.

Sample dimensions are crucial in ensuring that thin foil effects do not invalidate quantitative measurements from the experiments. As shown in Figure 4, the primary consideration is that the rigid substrate approximation still be reasonably valid in the thinned TEM samples. For 200 kV electrons, the maximum penetration depth is ~ 1 micron. Thus, if we require that the thinned substrate thickness is > one order of magnitude larger than the epilayer thickness, then it is required that the epilayer thickness be of the order of hundreds of Å. By reference to Figure 2, this will require that x in Ge_xSi_{1-x} be relatively high. Unfortunately, the tendency towards surface roughness also increases at higher x (2), thus at too high a value of Ge concentration, the surface modulation amplitude may become a significant fraction of the epilayer thickness. We thus determined that values of x ~ 0.25 − 0.30 were optimum for these experiments, as h_c ~ 500Å and the measured surface roughness from cross-sectional TEM was < 20 Å. As indicated in Figure 4, sample regions substantially removed (> ~ 5 micron) from the foil edge were imaged, again to minimize thin foil relaxation effects. Note that the effects of differential thermal expansion between Ge_xSi_{1-x} and Si are of secondary importance in these experiments: the difference in thermal expansion coefficients, K, between Ge and Si are such that in the temperature range we explore here, the stresses induced by the differences in K_{Ge} and K_{Si} are ~ an order of magnitude lower than stresses due to lattice mismatch. In principle, structures which are largely relaxed at the highest annealing temperature may further deform during cooldown due to differential thermal expansion, although we have rarely observed this in thin Ge_xSi_{1-x} films.

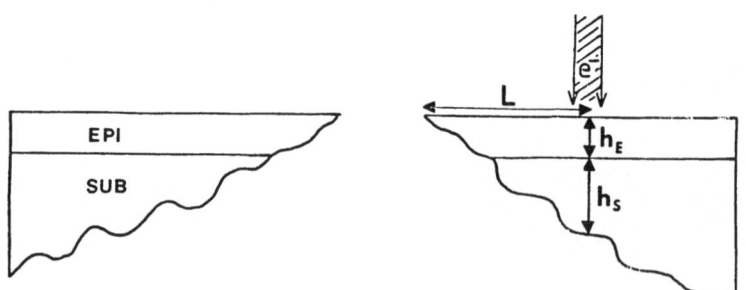

Figure 4. Schematic illustration of sample geometry for in-situ TEM Ge_xSi_{1-x}/Si relaxation experiments.

Plan view TEM samples were prepared by backside etching in an acetic:nitric:hydrofloric acidic etch. The samples were imaged in a JEOL 2000FX transmission electron microscope operated at 200 kV. Diffraction contrast experiments were performed either in a double tilt (±30, ±45 degree) holder at room temperature, or in a Gatan single tilt (±45 degree) heating holder operated between room temperature and ~ 900°C. Images were recorded either statically using conventional photographic negatives, or dynamically using a Gatan video camera and image intensifier coupled to a conventional video cassette recorder operating at conventional TV rates. Note that use of a single tilt heating holder made accurate diffraction contrast conditions difficult to establish during dynamical heating experiments, both in terms of obtaining strong 2-beam conditions, and in accurately controlling the deviation parameter as the thin strained films tended to bend at the thin foil edges. Thus, detailed deduction of dislocation Burgers vectors was established at different temperatures by transferring the specimen from the single tilt heating to double tilt ambient holders.

Ge_xSi_{1-x} heterostructures were deposited onto Si(100) surfaces by MBE (2, and references contained therein). Substrate surfaces were cleaned by Ar^+ ion sputtering prior to deposition of a 2000Å Si buffer layer. Ge_xSi_{1-x} heteroepitaxy was then commenced at a growth temperature of 550°C, unless stated otherwise in the text.

To accurately confirm MBE growth calibrations, selected Ge_xSi_{1-x}/Si heterostructures were independently analysed for composition and layer thickness using a combination of Rutherford Backscattering and cross-sectional TEM.

3. RESULTS

The plan view images of Figure 5 show typical misfit dislocation microstructures as functions of in-situ annealing temperature of a 350 Å $Ge_{0.25}Si_{0.75}$/Si(100) heterostructure. As can be seen from the images, the initially relatively low dislocation density (average spacing of the order of microns) at the growth temperature significantly relaxes at higher annealing temperatures, confirming the metastability of the as-grown structures. The slightly "mottled" contrast visible in the Ge_xSi_{1-x} material in these images is, we believe, strain contrast arising from slight variations in epilayer thickness. The intensity of the mottled contrast is generally observed to reduce as strain is relaxed during annealing, consistent with this hypothesis. It is also less visible in structures of lower Ge concentration, which we expect to be more planar. The exact intensity distribution of the mottling is extremely sensitive to deviation parameter (accounting for much of the variation in Figure 5 (a) - (c)). In Figure 6, the relaxation process is quantitatively displayed by plotting the average distance between dislocations, p, vs. annealing temperature for 300 and 350Å thick $Ge_{0.25}Si_{0.75}$/Si(100) structures. It can be observed that the relaxation process (which is slower in the thinner film, due to the lower initial stress state in this structure) is relatively gradual over the entire temperature range. Even at the highest annealing temperature of $\sim$900°C (where we might expect layer interdiffusion to become significant), only $\sim$30% of the strain expected in the equilibrium state is relaxed in the thicker structure. Thus the strain relaxation process in the Ge_xSi_{1-x} /Si(100) system, at least for these particular combinations of film thickness and composition is relatively sluggish. This is partially compounded by the fact that a significant proportion of the misfit dislocations observed of these films are of pure edge (90° type, with the Burgers vector lying in the interfacial plane), which must either move by slower (as opposed to dislocation glide of 60° dislocations) mass transport processes involved in dislocation climb, or possibly by a cooperative motion of two 60-degree components. The proportion of 90° dislocations increases with annealing temperature; in the as-grown films the defects are predominantly 60° at this composition.

By analysis of dynamic video images, it has been possible to directly measure the velocity of misfit dislocations, as shown in Figure 7 which plots observed velocity of 60° defects vs. annealing temperature in $Ge_{0.25}Si_{0.75}$ films. These velocities are measured using frame-by-frame (i.e. time resolution of 1/25 sec) analysis of the video recording. The upper limit to dislocation velocity we measure is set by the time taken for a defect to move across the field of view at the lowest usable magnification; with the objective lens excited this produces a minimum magnification of $\sim$75000x onto the TV monitor allowing measurement of velocities up to $\sim$100micron.sec^{-1}. The finite number of frames required for the defect to traverse the field of view at these higher velocities causes the relatively large error bars in this regime in Figure 7.

It can immediately be seen that dislocation velocities are relatively low at the MBE growth temperature of 550°C, being less than $\sim$5micron.sec^{-1}. With v=3 micron sec^{-1} and a growth time of 200 seconds for a 350Å $Ge_{0.25}Si_{0.75}$ film, this would produce a maximum dislocation length in the growth process of 0.6 mm. In practice, observed dislocation lengths are very much less then this because: (i) dislocation growth probably

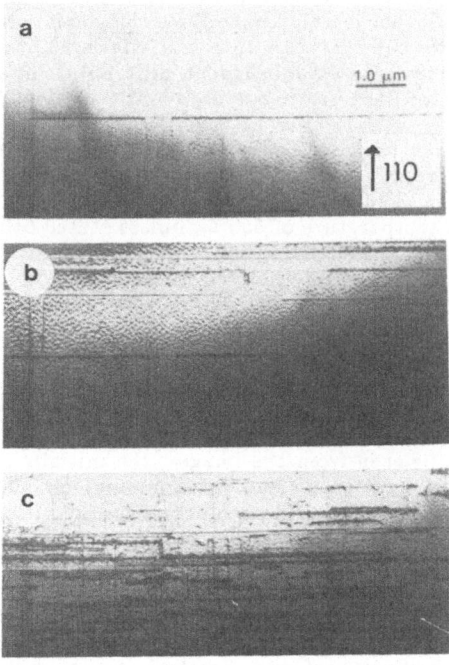

Figure 5. Plan view TEM <022> bright field images of a 350Å $Ge_{0.25}Si_{0.75}/Si(100)$ structure grown at 550°C (a) as-grown and annealed in-situ in the TEM to (b) 700°C (c) 900°C.

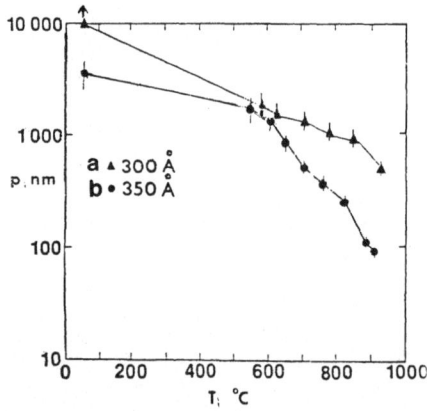

Figure 6. Variation of average distance between misfit dislocations, p, vs. annealing temperature for $Ge_{0.25}Si_{0.75}/Si$ structures (a) 300Å thick and (b) 350Å thick. The samples were successively annealed for ∼ 4 minutes at each temperature.

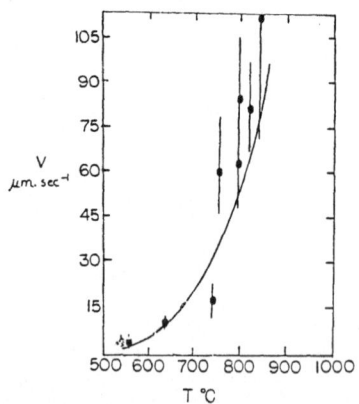

Figure 7. Variation of 60° misfit dislocation velocity vs. temperature during relaxation of $Ge_{0.25}Si_{0.75}/Si(100)$ films.

only occurs towards the end of the film growth time, when the film stress is sufficient to encourage defect motion and (ii) as will be shown later, defect interactions discourage dislocation growth. The above figure immediately shows, however, why there are high threading defect densities in the material (defects which traverse the thickness of the epitaxial layer, as opposed to being constrained to the interfacial plane). As illustrated in Figure 8, for a given amount of strain relaxation (defined by the total dislocation line length and the individual dislocation Burgers vectors), the ideal case would correspond to effectively infinite dislocation lengths, terminated only by the boundary conditions at the edge of the wafer. In the case, such as observed experimentally in this system, where average line lengths are $<<$ wafer diameter, individual misfit dislocation segments have to terminate on the nearest free surface, which in general will be the growth surface. Thus each misfit defect segment will have two threading ends associated with it (this condition will only be abrogated if the misfit segment terminates at the wafer edge, forms a node with another dislocation, or forms a complete loop upon itself) and for a given amount of relaxation, the shorter the average dislocation length the higher the threading defect density. A simple geometrical relationship (13) may be derived between the areal density of misfit dislocation ends, n, the average spacing between misfit dislocations, p, and the average dislocation line length, l, yielding:

$$l = \frac{16}{\pi^2 pn}$$

The average dislocation line lengths, l, deduced from the above formula and the measured values of p and n for annealing of a 350Å $Ge_{0.25}Si_{0.75}$ film are shown in Figure 9. It can be seen that as the relaxation process proceeds (p decreases), more and more defects are generated (n increases), but the average dislocation line length l remains relatively constant (and even drops slightly at higher temperatures) at a few microns. This shows that generation of extra dislocation line length does not occur solely by growth of original defect sources (as would be the case for the Matthews and Blakeslee threading defect source), but occurs at least partially by generation of large numbers of new defects. The observation that l does not increase during the relaxation process strongly suggests that defect interactions, as will be discussed further below, strongly limit growth of individual misfit dislocation segments.

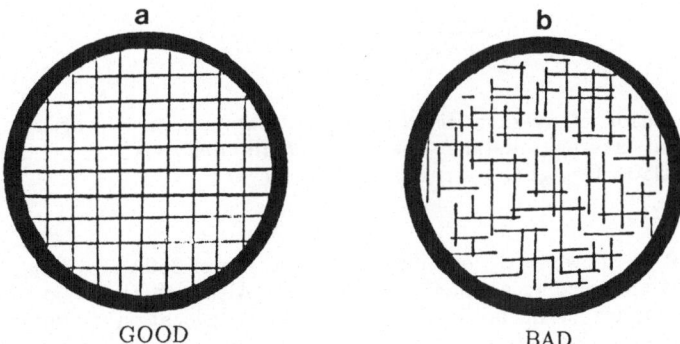

Figure 8. Schematic illustration of the relationship between average dislocation line length and threading dislocation density. For a given amount of lattice relaxation (i.e. a given amount of total dislocation line length) (a) shows the ideal case of infinitely long misfit dislocations terminating at the wafer edges and (b) shows the more realistic case of finite misfit dislocation segments terminating by threading to the epilayer free surface.

In the $Ge_{0.25}Si_{0.75}$ structures discussed so far, where the TEM sample dimensions and geometry are such that quantitative analysis of relaxation is possible, we have obtained quantitative measurements of the activation energies for dislocation nucleation and propagation (13). In the temperature range appropriate for MBE growth of these structures, say 550°C—750°C, the measured activation energies are 0.3±0.2 eV for nucleation and 1.1±0.2 eV for propagation. These figures show that at moderate temperatures, nucleation of defects is achieved more easily than propagation of defects. It thus appears that the "critical thickness" of the heterostructure for this growth temperature and composition is a function more of the stress required to enable significant defect growth than a function of the defect nucleation process. During thermal relaxation of the as-grown heterostructure, increasing temperature favours defect growth over nucleation, but as shown by Figure 9, defect interactions prevent growth becoming the strongly dominant relaxation mechanism.

It is found that the defect microstructure and relaxation mechanisms are strongly dependent upon the Ge concentration x, and hence also upon the epilayer thickness. Increasing x favors greater proportions of 90° dislocations with respect to 60° dislocations and causes more sluggish layer relaxation. This latter observation may partially be explained by the slower nature of climb as compared to glide motion, but is also strongly dependent upon dislocation interaction forces as functions of Ge concentration and epilayer thickness, as will now be discussed.

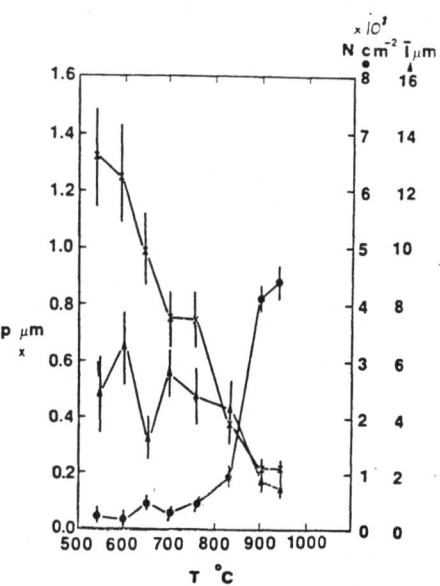

Figure 9. Variation of average dislocation line length, $\bar{l}$, areal threading dislocation density, n, and average distance between misfit dislocations, p, during thermal relaxation of a 350Å $Ge_{0.25}Si_{0.75}$ structure.

In Figure 10, we show the dislocation microstructure of 350Å $Ge_{0.25}Si_{0.75}$ and 3000Å $Ge_{0.15}Si_{0.85}$ films annealed to similar temperatures. Although the magnitude of strain relaxation is comparable in both films, the misfit dislocation structures are very different. In the $Ge_{0.15}Si_{0.85}$ film, the defects are almost exclusively of the 60° type, are relatively long (> 50 micron) in average length and cross orthogonal defects relatively easily. Thus in the field of view of Figure 10(a), only one threading dislocation end (arrowed) is visible. In contrast, the $Ge_{0.25}Si_{0.75}$ film, contains a significant proportion of 90° defects, has an average dislocation length ∼5 micron, and it is observed that intersection of orthogonal misfit dislocation segments is ∼ two orders of magnitude more likely to produce a defect pinning event than in the lower Ge composition film. Although Figure 10(b) has a similar field of view to that of 10(a), many dislocation ends are visible in the higher x film. (Note that for the $Ge_{0.15}Si_{0.85}$ films, the epilayer thicknesses are sufficiently great to abrogate the rigid substrate approximation discussed earlier for TEM films. We are thus not confident about extracting quantitative activation energies from these lower x films. Qualitative deductions, such as those discussed immediately above, however, should still be valid: we are simply observing these processes at a slightly lower stress than that appropriate to a rigid substrate). These different probabilities for defect interactions arresting dislocation growth allow the lower mismatch films to relax much more abruptly with temperature. Shown in Figure 11 is the variation of p with annealing temperature for structures very similar to the two films imaged in Figure 10. It can be seen that the $Ge_{0.15}Si_{0.85}$ film relaxes relatively rapidly in the temperature range 650—750°C. This significantly more abrupt relaxation in the more dilute Ge film is a general result we have observed on several occasions and has important consequences with respect to thermal stability of these mismatched structures: although higher mismatched layers will relax more rapidly with respect to layer thickness, their stability with respect to thermal relaxation is greater than the lower mismatch structures, i.e. they are less metastable. This is also consistent with the critical thickness data of Figure 2.

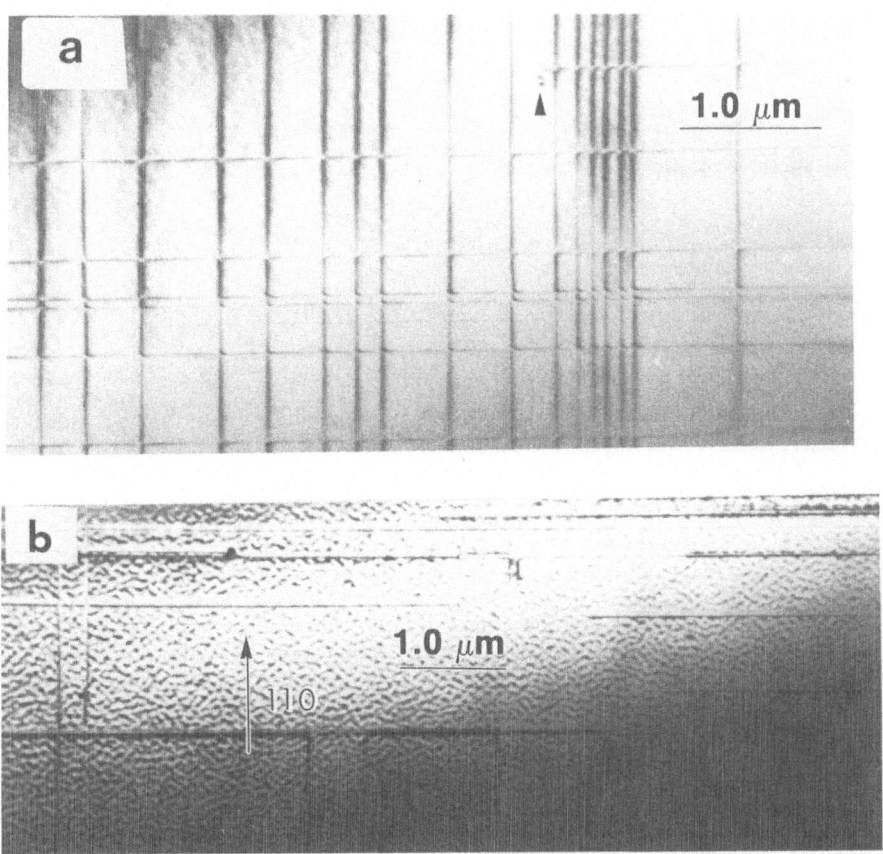

Figure 10. Plan view TEM images of (a) ~2500Å $Ge_{0.15}Si_{0.85}$/Si(100) annealed to ~700°C (single threading dislocation arrowed) (b) ~350Å $Ge_{0.25}Si_{0.75}$/Si(100) annealed to ~700°C.

By considering the forces acting on a propagating dislocation (14), we have been able to model and predict this composition-dependence of the defect interaction probability. In ref. (14), it is shown that this dependence arises naturally if the image, misfit stress, line tension and inter-dislocation forces are considered.

The final primary defect process to be discussed is perhaps the least understood, the nucleation stage. As has been discussed earlier, the conventional substrate threading defect source generally assumed for III-V heteroepitaxy does not appear appropriate to low defect Si substrates. In this case, we require a source which generates misfit dislocation loops or half-loops either at the epilayer surface, the interface or within the bulk of the epilayer, as illustrated in Figure 12. These loops then grow under the influence of the misfit stress until they consist of a misfit segment in the interfacial plane coupled to threading segments terminating on the growth surface. As the loop sizes and populations increase, defect interactions become important, as previously discussed.

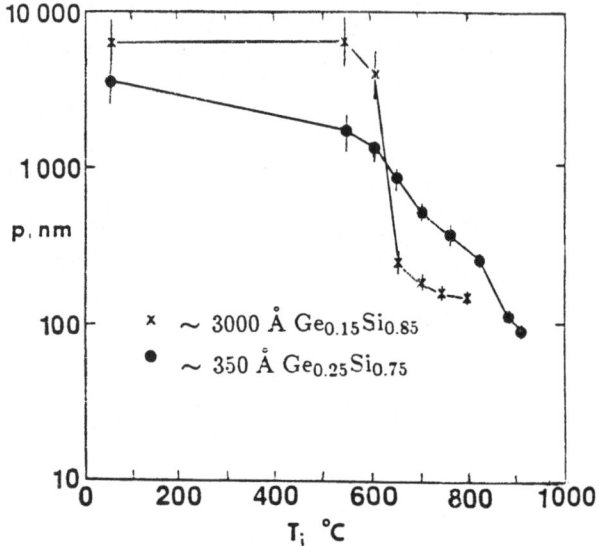

Figure 11. Variation of average misfit dislocation spacing during thermal relaxation of $Ge_{0.15}Si_{0.85}/Si$ and $Ge_{0.25}Si_{0.75}/Si$ structures.

Perhaps the classic mechanism to assume for homogeneous defect nucleation in this geometry would be generation of a half-loop at the growth surface. The energetics of this process may be calculated by balancing the self energy of the loop, the elastic strain energy relieved by the loop, and the energies associated with step creation/removal on the free surface and the stacking fault energies for dissociated dislocations, where appropriate. Such calculations have suggested that for moderate lattice mismatches $< \sim 2\%$, activation barriers for this process are tens of eV or greater for the materials parameters appropriate to the $Ge_xSi_{1-x}/Si(100)$ system (e.g. 15,16,17). Similar constraints would apply to generation of defects as complete loops within the epilayer or at the epilayer/substrate interface.

One is thus forced to consider, theoretically and experimentally, heterogeneous sources for nucleation. In our experimental observations we have encountered a large number of nucleation events over a wide range of epilayer thicknesses and compositions, and do not believe that a single ubiquitous defect source is operating. In agreement with other work (18), the characteristic defect distributions we observe are unevenly spaced groups of long (> 50 micron) $60°$ defects at lower mismatch (say $x < 0.2$) and a much higher density of short (a few micron) $90°$ defects at higher mismatch ($x \geq 0.25$). For these $90°$ defects, we are able to directly observe the nucleation event and are able to study the defect microstructure along the entire dislocation length: no obvious precursor stage to the defect nucleation is observed.

The geometry of these high mismatch defects is strongly suggestive of dislocation half-loops nucleating at the growth surface. To reconcile this geometry with the predicted high activation energies discussed above, several mechanisms for favoring defect nucleation can be envisioned such as multi-atomic layer steps (19), Ge clusters, impurities or particulates. In particular, we have previously argued that even random (Gaussian) statistical variations locally in composition can enhance the stress in small volumes sufficiently to enable defect nucleation at lower average film compositions than bulk elasticity theory would predict (17). Shown in Figure 13 are the Gaussian probabilities (using the binomial approximations for large N that $\sigma(N_{Ge})^2 = Nx(1-x)$ and $\bar{N}_{Ge} = Nx$) that a local volume containing N atoms, N_{Ge} Ge atoms and of average Ge content x in Ge_xSi_{1-x} is locally enhanced to a Ge content x+0.1. Also shown are the required probabilities per cluster to produce different numerical densities of nucleation sites, where the number of sites is calculated from the inverse cross-sectional area of a Ge-rich cluster around the nucleating dislocation loop, such that half the dislocation strain field is contained within the cluster. Detailed analysis (17) shows that the required number of atoms within each cluster is ~ 800, thus it can be seen from Figure 13 that significant densities of nucleation sites are produced with locally enhanced Ge concentration.

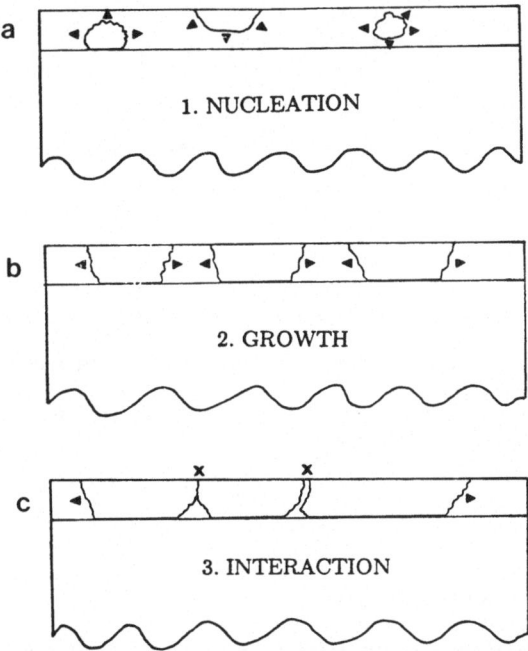

Figure 12. Schematic illustrations of the processes by which misfit dislocations relax elastic strain in lattice-mismatched Ge_xSi_{1-x} epitaxy: (a) dislocation nucleation (b) dislocation propagation (c) dislocation interaction. Dislocation segments in the interfacial plane are misfit relieving, those terminating to the growth surface are threading defects.

For low mismatches ($x < \sim 0.2$) in the Ge_xSi_{1-x}/Si system, activation barriers for misfit dislocation loop nucleation are very high ($> \sim 100$ eV), and the above arguments relating to random clustering cannot reconcile calculations with physically reasonable activation energies. In this case, an extrinsic source for dislocation nucleation may be required such as impurities or contamination, substrate or buffer layer defects, gross surface roughness, non-random clustering of Ge or thermally-induced stresses. At first sight, it appears unlikely that any of these potential sources are present in sufficient densities to produce the observed defect densities. Two other sources have been proposed and observed which may account for defect nucleation in this regime: (i) the Hagen-Strunk defect multiplication source (20,21) which generates new defects via intersection of orthogonal dislocations of equal Burgers vectors. We note, however, that to date we have not directly observed this source in the $x > \sim 0.15$ films we have studied. (ii) The "Eaglesham-Kvam" defect (16), observed as a source in Ge_xSi_{1-x} films for $x<\sim0.2$, consisting of a $\frac{1}{6}<411>$ planar fault lying within the epitaxial film: the origin and nature of this defect has not been ascertained, but has been shown to act as a regenerative nucleation source via dissociation into $\frac{1}{2}<011>$ misfit dislocations. Again, we note that we have not systematically observed this defect in the composition range we have studied. The detailed nature of dislocation generation in low-mismatch epitaxy thus remains unclear, and indeed may be a strong function of deposition conditions and cleanliness.

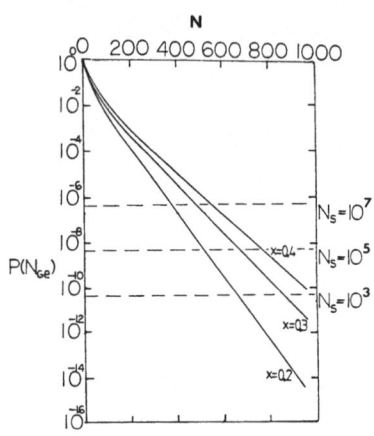

Figure 13. Gaussian probabilities of a local volume containing N atoms in a Ge_xSi_{1-x} alloy randomly having an enhanced Ge composition x+0.1. Also shown are the required probabilities per cluster to achieve given densities of nucleation sites (N_s, cm^{-2}), based upon nucleation in these Ge rich regions.

4. DISCUSSIONS AND CONCLUSIONS

The above results conclusively demonstrate that nucleation, propagation and interaction processes are all important in determining the rate at which misfit dislocations relieve elastic strain in lattice-mismatched epitaxy. The relative importance of these processes as a function of Ge concentration in Ge_xSi_x/Si heterostructures define different strain relaxation regimes. For $x < \sim 0.20$, energetic calculations of dislocation loop formation energies predict extremely high activation energies. In addition we note that homogeneous half-loop or loop formation is to first order independent of epitaxial layer thickness, depending upon the layer strain but not upon the total stress (15,16,17). Dislocation formation in this regime thus requires heterogeneous, probably growth technique-induced, nucleation sites. The relatively low density of these sites, and the stress which appears to be necessary to activate them, means that significant layer thicknesses are required before high defect populations are established. Once nucleated, defects can propagate relatively quickly by glide as they are generally of the 60° type. We also cannot rule out the possibility that once a sufficient total line length of dislocation has been established and intersection of orthogonal dislocations becomes frequent, dislocation multiplication sources such as the Hagen-Strunk source become significant (although we have not directly observed these sources for $x>0.15$). The balance of forces acting on propagating dislocations in these thicker epitaxial layers (of the order of thousands of Å in the critical thickness regime for this composition range) also enables orthogonal defects to move past each other relatively easily, producing long misfit dislocation segments and lower threading dislocation densities. The difficulty in nucleating defects in these structures, and thus in establishing a measurable dislocation line length, explains the large extent of the metastable regime at low mismatch in Figure 2, whilst the ease of defect propagation and lack of pinning interactions contribute to the strong metastability of these structures with respect to thermal annealing, as shown in Figure 11.

At higher mismatch (x > ~ 0.25), defect nucleation via loop formation starts to become energetically feasible so extra paths for nucleation exist. Significant defect populations are established at lower film stresses, and the extent of the metastable growth regime with respect to film thickness correspondingly decreases. The increasing preponderance of 90° defects with increasing lattice mismatch, however, appears to place increasing reliance on bulk transport processes involved in dislocation climb or on cooperative motion of 60-degree components, and defect interactions strongly limit dislocation growth. The metastability with respect to temperature of these higher mismatch structures is therefore less than for the lower mismatch structures.

In summary, many of these processes have been elucidated for the first time by relaxing the structures in-situ in the TEM, and directly recording dynamic dislocation processes. This combination of real-time observation with more detailed and quantitative analysis of statistically large numbers of defects recorded using conventional still photographic negatives has produced a far more detailed understanding of the strain relaxation process. In using this technique, considerable attention has to be paid to the experimental limitations imposed by the thin-foil TEM geometry, but as discussed in the experimental section of these papers, provided the structure is optimized the in-situ approach here can provide a significantly improved qualitative and quantitative understanding of misfit dislocation phenomena in strained layer epitaxy.

5. ACKNOWLEDGEMENTS

We would like to acknowledge important discussions with D.J. Eaglesham, J.M. Gibson, E.P. Kvam, D. Loretto and D.M. Maher; technical assistance from R.E. Leibenguth and D.J. Werder; and Rutherford Backscattering measurements by K.T. Short and A.E. White.

6. REFERENCES

(1) G.C. Osbourn, IEEE J. Quant. Electron. QE-22, 1677 (1986) (1985)
(2) See J.C. Bean in Proc. Mat. Res. Soc. 37, ed. J.M. Gibson and L.R. Dawson (Materials Research Society, Pittsburgh, PA, 1985), p.245.
(3) J.H. Van der Merwe and C.A.B. Ball in Epitaxial Growth, Part b, edited by J.W. Matthews (Academic, New York, 1975), pp. 494-530
(4) J.W. Matthews, J. Vac. Sci. Technol. 12, 126 (1975) and references contained therein
(5) B.W. Dodson and J.Y. Tsao, Appl. Phys. Lett. 51, 1325 (1987); J.Y. Tsao, B.W. Dodson, S.T. Picreaux and D.M. Cornelison, Phys. Rev. Lett. 59, 2455 (1987)
(6) R. Hull, A.T. Fiory, J.C. Bean, J.M. Gibson, L. Scott, J.L. Benton and S. Nakahara, Proc. 13th Int. Conf. on Defects in Semiconductors, Coronado, CA Aug. 1984, ed. L.C. Kimmerling and J.M. Parsey, Jr. (AIME, Warrendale, PA)
(7) R. People and J.C. Bean, Appl. Phys. Lett. 47, 322 (1985); 49, 229 (1986)
(8) I.J. Fritz, Appl. Phys. Lett. 51, 1080 (1987)
(9) I.J. Fritz, S.T. Picreaux, L.R. Dawson, T.J. Drummond, W.D. Laidig and N.G. Anderson, Appl. Phys. Lett. 46, 967 (1985)
(10) E. Kasper, H-J. Herzog and H. Kibbel, Appl. Phys. 8, 199 (1975)
(11) A.T. Fiory, J.C. Bean, R. Hull and S. Nakahara, Phys. Rev. B 31, 4063
(12) R. Hull, J.C. Bean, D.J. Werder and R.E. Leibenguth, Appl. Phys. Lett. 52, 1605 (1988)

(13) R.Hull, J.C. Bean, D.J. Werder and R.E. Leibenguth, submitted to Phys. Rev. Lett.

(14) R. Hull and J.C. Bean, accepted for publication in Appl. Phys. Lett.

(15) J.W. Matthews, A.E. Blakeslee and S. Mader, Thin Solid Films 33, 253 (1976)

(16) D.J. Eaglesham, E.P. Kvam, D.M. Maher, C.J. Humphreys and J.C. Bean, accepted for publication in Phil. Mag.

(17) R. Hull and J.C. Bean, to be published in Jul/Aug 1989 issue of J. Vac. Sci. Tech. A

(18) E.P. Kvam, D.J. Eaglesham, D.M. Maher, C.J. Humphreys, J.C. Bean, G.S. Green and B.K. Tanner, Proc. Mat. Res. Soc. 104, ed. R.T. Tung, L.R. Dawson and R.L. Gunshor, (Materials Research, Pittsburgh, PA), p. 623.

(19) B.W. Dodson, Appl. Phys. Lett. 53, 394 (1988)

(20) W. Hagen and H. Strunk, Appl. Phys. 17, 85 (1978)

(21) K. Rajan and M. Denhoff, J. Appl. Phys. 62, 1710 (1987)

MISFIT DISLOCATIONS IN $In_xGa_{1-x}As$/GaAs HETEROSTRUCTURES NEAR THE CRITICAL THICKNESS

D. Cockayne[*], P. Orders[+], A. Sikorski[*], B. Usher[+], and J. Zhou

[*]Electron Microscope Unit, University of Sydney, N.S.W. 2006 Australia and Beijing Laboratory of Electron Microscopy, Academia Sinica, China and [+]Telecom Research Laboratories, Victoria 3168 Australia

INTRODUCTION

High quality strained $In_xGa_{1-x}As$/GaAs (001) superlattices are of increasing interest because the effective band-gap (1.45 – 0.45eV (λ = 0.85 – 3.1μm)) is of considerable importance for optical fibre communication, and its value can be controlled by altering x. However, in growing the layered or graded heterostructures, misfit strain is often accommodated by misfit dislocations, which can degrade device properties. An understanding of the nature of these dislocations, and their distribution in the heterostructure or superlattice, is therefore of importance in optimising the performance of the materials in device applications. A number of studies have been made of the nature of the dislocations in this system, and several mechanisms for their introduction into the structure have been proposed. In particular, attempts have been made to characterise the thickness h_c of epilayer at which misfit dislocations induced by stress first occur, and to identify the nature and source of these dislocations.

Using X-ray topography, Ahearn, Laird and Ball[1] studied VPE-grown $Ga_{.95}In_{.05}As$/GaAs for an epilayer thickness t = 8μm > h_c. They observed an orthogonal cross-grid of dislocations lying close to the (001) interface plane, with dislocation line directions in or near to $[1\bar{1}0]$ and [110]. They postulated that the majority of dislocations were generated by interactions of gliding threading dislocations. Rajan, Devine, Moore and Maigne[2] investigated dislocation structures in a superlattice system grown by MBE with x ~ 0.3, in which the superlattice layers individually had t < h_c. They found an (001) network of 60' and edge dislocations lying along $[110]$ and $[1\bar{1}0]$, together with individual dislocations penetrating into the substrate. For single stepped layers with x = 0.13 and t ~ 1.1 μm (> h_c ~ 0.1μm), Fitzgerald, Ast, Kirchner, Pettit and Woodall[4] found an interfacial network of predominantly 60' dislocations, lying along [110] and [110], together with individual sessile edge dislocations lying in the buffer layer up to 400 nm below the interface. They deduced that the sessile dislocations were formed by the 60' dislocations from the interface network gliding into the buffer layer and interacting. Hockly, Al-Jassim, Booker and Nicklin[5] studied graded layers of InGaAs on GaAs substrates, and found a series of (100) networks of predominantly 60' dislocations, together with some sessile edge dislocations, and linked by dislocation segments lying on the four inclined {111} planes.

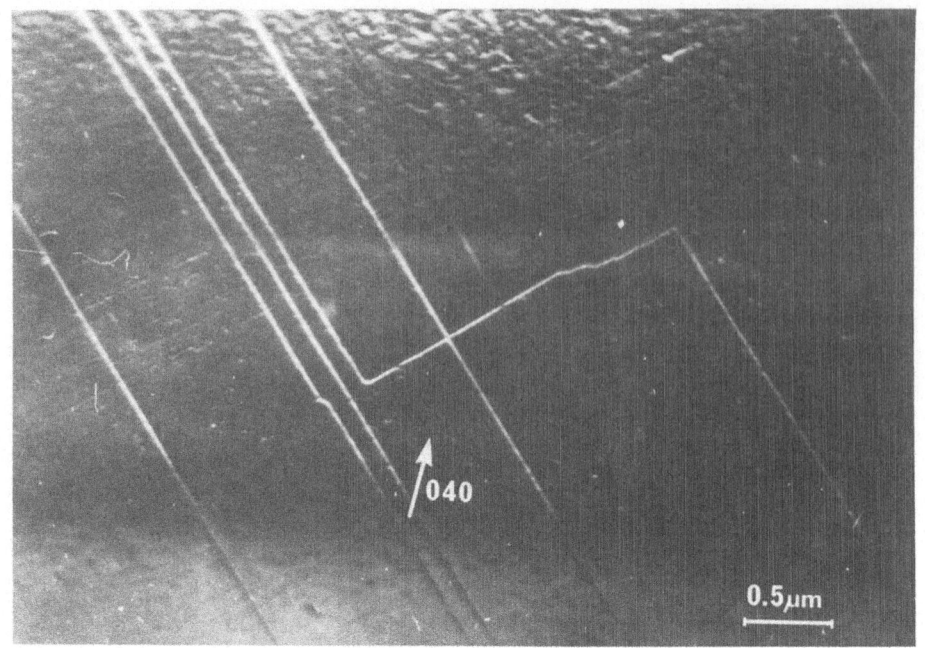

Fig. 1.   60' dislocations lying along ⟨110⟩ directions in the (001)
plane.   t= 20 nm, x= 0.3.

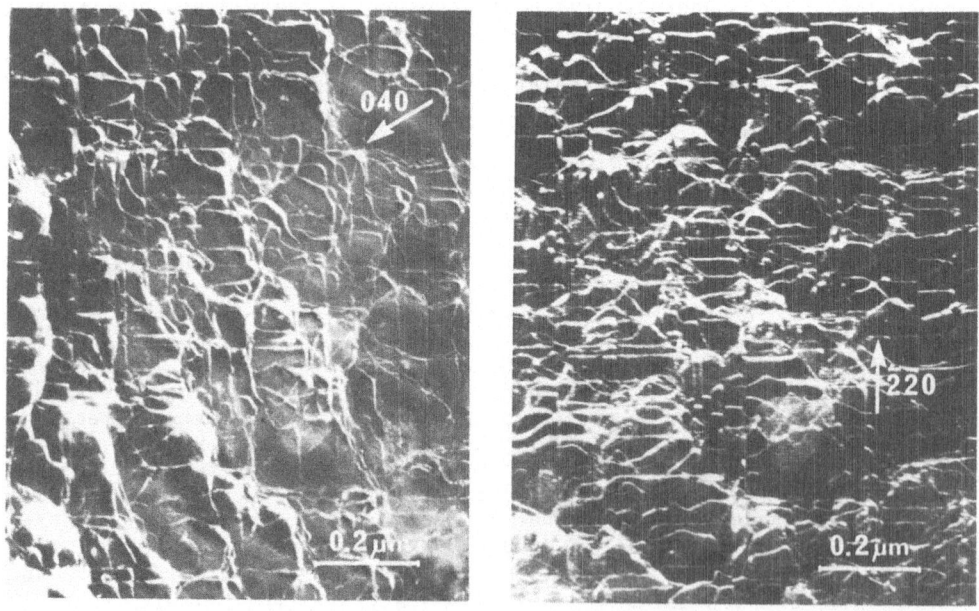

Fig. 2.   A typical dislocation network for t = 100nm, x = 0.3.   The
dislocations lie predominantly along ⟨110⟩ directions, but
deviations are clear.   Most dislocations are of 60' type, but
there are many edge segments.   The images are taken with the g
vectors indicated.

From these studies it can be concluded that in the InGaAs/GaAs stepped layer system, misfit is accommodated by both 60' and sessile edge dislocations, and that these dislocations are generally in an (001) planar network, with line directions along ⟨110⟩. Additionally dislocations are found both in the substrate and in the epitaxial layer, to an extent dependent upon t and x. However it is not evident from these earlier studies how the dislocation network develops near $t = h_c$, and for this reason a systematic study of this question has been made.

MATERIALS

Single-step strained layer heterostructures of $In_xGa_{1-x}As$/GaAs were grown by MBE using a Varian 360 system. A 0.3μm GaAs buffer layer was grown on an undoped (100) GaAs substrate at 590'C, followed by a layer of $In_xGa_{1-x}As$ grown at 530'C. An As stabilized surface was maintained during the growth, and the Ga flux was unchanged for the growth of the buffer and $In_xGa_{1-x}As$ layers. Further details are given in Orders and Usher[3]. A suite of samples was prepared, with x = 0.3 and t = 7,10,20,30,50,100,300 and 500 nm.

Approximately 2 mm thick slices were cut from the wafers using a wire saw, and thinned to approximately 0.1 mm by hand polishing. The specimens were etched to perforation using a solution of H_2SO_4, H_2O, H_2O_2 (8:1:1 by volume), washed in water and then in acetone and finally in methanol, and mounted on slotted grids for electron microscope examination. Cross-section samples were prepared by gluing two specimens together, epitaxial layers facing, and then by following the thinning procedure described above. Final thinning of these samples was carried out by ion-beam thinning.

The specimens were examined in a 300kV Philips EM430 transmission electron microscope. Techniques of dark-field and weak-beam imaging were used to identify dislocation Burgers vectors, geometries and densities. High resolution electron microscopy was also used to study the dislocation geometries in the cross-section samples.

DISLOCATION CHARACTERISATION

No dislocations were found in specimens with t = 7nm or 10nm. Dislocations were found in the specimen with t = 20nm, and an example is seen in Figure 1. The dislocations form a square grid of 60' dislocations, lying in the (001) plane (the interface plane) and with one direction of the grid predominating. They have the Burgers vectors b = a/2 ⟨110⟩ inclined to the (001) interface plane, their line directions being either [1̄10] or [110]. In the light of earlier observations, it is relevant to point out that these Burgers vector determinations were not straightforward, partly because the dislocations were dissociated (see later), and partly because the displacement field of misfit dislocations is not the same as for isolated dislocations in the bulk, being influenced by the displacement field of the strained lattice. Cross section samples showed that the network of dislocations was planar (to ~ 5 nm), and no dislocations were found outside the network.

For t > 20nm, the dislocation density increased, but the network retained its essentially planar form. As in Figure 2, deviations of the dislocation line direction from ⟨110⟩ were evident. Dislocation interactions by repulsion or attraction were observed, similar to those analysed by Strunk, Hagen and Bauser[6] in Ge/GaAs. Burgers vector analysis of the resulting interacting segments showed them to have edge

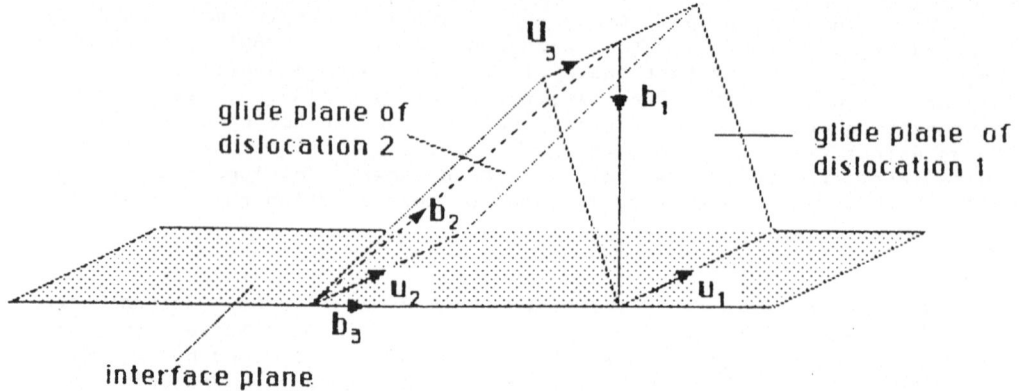

Fig. 3. Two 60' dislocations with line $\underline{u}_1$ and $\underline{u}_2$ and Burgers vector $\underline{b}_1$ and $\underline{b}_2$ interact to form the sessile edge dislocation with Burgers vector $\underline{b}_3$.

character. The proportion of segments with edge character increased with t, until for t ~ 500nm, most segments were of edge character.

These observations can be explained in terms of the model shown in Figure 3. Sixty degree dislocations relieve misfit strain through the edge component of $\underline{b}$ lying in (001). However they are inefficient in relieving the misfit stress, since other components of $\underline{b}$ cause bending of the epilayer about an axis in (001). In Figure 3, two of these dislocations with line directions $\underline{u}_1 = \underline{u}_2 = [110]$ in the (001) plane of the interface but with different {111} glide planes, with $\underline{b} = a/2[10\bar{1}]$ and $a/2[011]$ respectively, glide out of the network plane on {111}. (Whether the direction of glide is towards or away from the epilayer surface is not clear from the data, although from careful inspection of the cross-section samples it appears to be the former.) The dislocations interact in $\underline{u}_3$ to form sessile edge dislocations with $\underline{b} = a/2[110]$. This interaction removes the components of $\underline{b}$ causing the bending referred to above, and the consequent lowering of the total dislocation energy provides the driving force which causes the dislocations to glide away from the interface.

In considering dislocation mechanisms and sources, it is important to recall that, in general, 60' glide dislocations in GaAs are known to be dissociated into two Shockley partials[7,8]. Weak-beam images of the relatively isolated dislocations in specimens with t = 20 and 30 nm showed them to be dissociated on their {111} glide planes in the same way. This was established by putting each partial out of contrast in turn, and also by imaging the stacking fault using a reflection for which $\underline{g}.\underline{b}_{total} = 0$. Further evidence is shown in Figure 4 , where the dislocation dissociation is clearly seen in the high resolution image. The dissociation width is 5 nm, which is close to the equilibrium dissociation width of dissociated dislocations in GaAs[7]. We can deduce from this that the dislocation dissociation is close to the equilibrium value for isolated dislocations in bulk.

GENERATION OF MISFIT DISLOCATIONS

A number of mechanisms have been proposed for the introduction of stress-relieving misfit dislocations in strained layer systems. Matthews

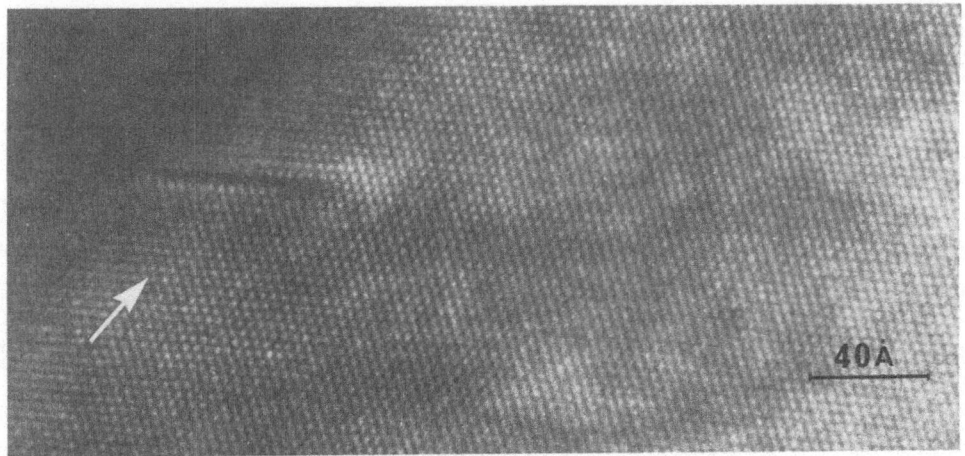

Fig. 4. High resolution image of misfit dislocation showing the
dissociation on the inclined {111} plane. The approximate
position of the interface is indicated.

and Blakeslee[9] considered the mechanical equilibrium of a grown-in
threading dislocation in the strained lattice. In their model, the
critical thickness is exceeded when it is energetically favourable for
the threading dislocation to bow out in the interface plane, under the
influence of the misfit stress, to form a misfit dislocation in or near
the interface plane. Hagen and Strunk[10] have identified a dislocation
source in the intersection of glide misfit dislocations. Matthews[11] and
Ball and Van der Merwe[12] investigated the conditions for the nucleation
and expansion of half loops. People and Bean[13] estimated the critical
thickness by determining the minimum areal energy density required to
form a dislocation of minimum energy, which they took to be a screw
dislocation. This model has been refined by Maree, Barbour, van der
Veen, Kavanagh, Bulle-Lieuwma and Viegers[14], who have taken the
dislocation of minimum energy to be a dissociated half loop forming at a
free surface.

These various mechanisms have recently come under scrutiny because
they predict widely differing values of h_c. Experimental values of h_c
determined from X-ray rocking curves (e.g. ref. 3) appear to be in good
agreement with the values predicted by People and Bean[13] and by Maree et
al[14]. However Gourley, Fritz and Dawson[15,16] found that measurement of
h_c determined using X-ray rocking curves gave significantly higher
values than those obtained using photoluminescence microscopy. Their
values of h_c agreed with those predicted by the model of Matthews and
Blakeslee[9], as have values determined in several other systems (see ref.
16).

The samples used in this study come from the same suite of
specimens as used by Orders and Usher[3], who have shown that their
experimental values of h_c, determined from X-ray rocking curves, agree
well with the energy balance model of People and Bean[13]. This model
gives h_c = 18 nm for the system considered here, which agrees well with
the observation of 10 < h_c <20 nm deduced from the observations reported
above.

In considering possible sources of misfit dislocations, the high
nucleation energies estimated for nucleation of surface half loops
suggests that such a source is energetically unlikely[17,18].

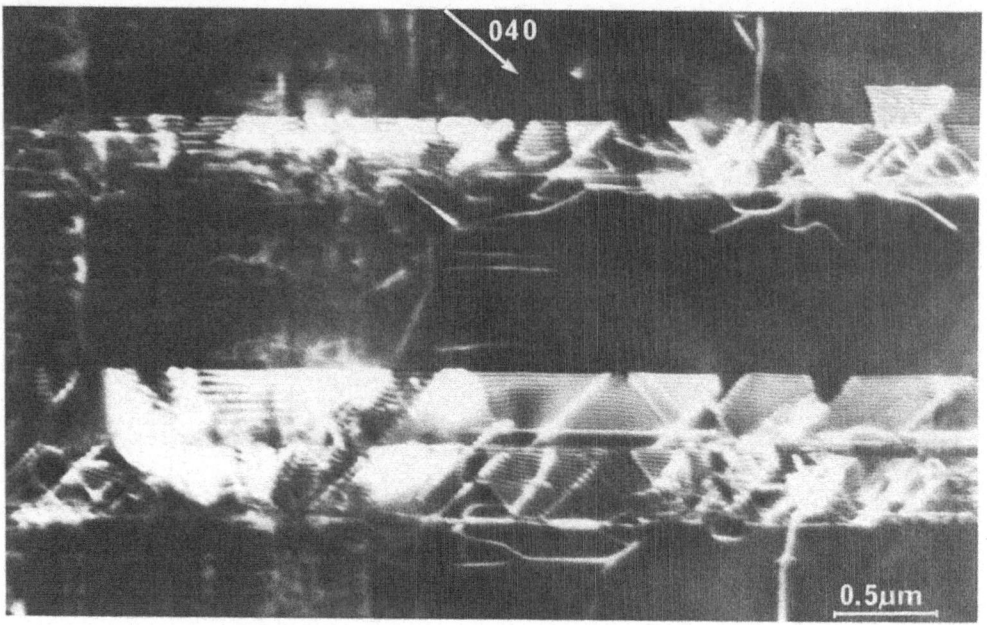

Fig. 5. A GaAs/InGaAs/GaAs heterostructure in plan view. The interfacial network is seen on the left, with dissociated dislocations on the inclined {111} planes in the GaAs layer which is in tension.

Nevertheless, there is a considerable amount of experimental evidence[18,9,19] that the surface does act as a source. This discrepancy may arise because of heterogeneous stresses causing surface nucleation of dislocations[18], which is not taken into account in the theoretical treatment.

From this summary, it is evident that the mechanisms of misfit dislocation generation are incompletely understood.

DISCUSSION

We consider the consequence to this study if the source is in the free surface. If we assume that nucleation of a 60' glide misfit dislocation occurs at the free surface, any proposed mechanism must take into account the dissociation of the dislocation into a 30' and a 90' Shockley partial. If the stacking fault of the dissociated dislocation is to be intrinsic in nature, the leading partial must be the 30' partial if the stress field is compressive, and the 90' partial if it is tensile. Since the resolved shear stress on the {111} glide plane is at 60' to the 30' partial but parallel to the 90' partial, the force on the 90' partial is greater than the force on the 30' partial by a factor of two. In a compressive field, the leading partial must be the 30' partial, if the contained stacking fault is to be intrinsic in nature. Consequently the 30' partial must be nucleated first, but, because of the greater force on the 90' partial, it will be followed rapidly by the 90' partial. The greater force on the 90' partial will ensure that the two glide together on {111}. On the other hand, in a tensile field, the leading partial is the 90' partial. In this case the smaller force on the 30' partial will cause it to lag behind, producing extended regions of fault on the {111} glide plane.

Evidence for this mechanism has been sought in a study of a three layer GaAs/In$_{0.14}$Ga$_{0.86}$As/GaAs heterostructure. For this system, GaAs is in tension while InGaAs is in compression. In the material studied, t > h$_c$ for both epilayers. In the GaAs epilayer, widely extended dislocations were found on the {111} glide planes, sometimes extending from the upper (GaAs/InGaAs) interface to the surface. Figure 5 shows an example. The foil has been thinned so that in the left side of the image the dislocation network in this interface is retained within the thin foil. In the right half of the image the foil contains the upper GaAs epitaxial layer only. Shockley partial dislocations are seen gliding on closely spaced {111} planes, and forming large ribbons of fault. Similar faulted regions were not observed in the InGaAs epilayers of either the two- or three-layer systems, where the dislocation dissociation was found to be close to the equilibrium value in bulk (see above). These observations are in agreement with the discussion above since InGaAs is in compression while GaAs as an epilayer on InGaAs is in tension[20].

It is of interest that in Figure 5, the partials, being on the same or closely spaced {111} planes, must originate from a common source. If this source is a surface step, acting as a strain concentrator, repeated operation of the source will increase its effectiveness.

A further consideration for the 60' dislocations in the compound semiconductors, AB, such as GaAs, is that they can be of two different types depending upon whether the terminating extra half-plane (in the undissociated form) terminates in group III or group V (II or VI) atoms. If the glide model of the dislocation is accepted rather than the shuffle model[21], then these two types of dislocation are referred to as A(g) and B(g). For misfit 60' dislocations, constraints upon the direction of b mean that in (001) epitaxial systems the 60' dislocations with line direction along [1$\bar{1}$0] will be of the opposite type to those with line direction along [110].

A number of authors[21,22,23] have shown that there are differences in the threshold stresses for producing dislocation movement for A(g) and B(g) dislocations, and in the mobilities of the two types. Consequently an asymmetry in the number of misfit dislocation lines along [110] and [1$\bar{1}$0] might be expected. Such effects have been observed previously in GaAlAsP/GaAs[19,24,25], in InGaAs/GaAs[26], and in InGaP/GaP[27], and are reported above in this study.

REFERENCES

1. J. S. Ahearn, Jr., C. Laird and C. A. Ball, The misfit dislocation structure of an InGaAs/GaAs heterojunction with low misfit. Thin Solid Films 42:117 (1977)
2. K. Rajan, R. Devine, W.T. Moore and P. Maigne, Dislocation structure in In$_x$Ga$_{1-x}$As/GaAs strained-layer superlattices, J. Appl. Phys 62:1713 (1987)
3. P. J. Orders and B. F. Usher, Determination of critical layer thickness in In$_x$Ga$_{1-x}$As/GaAs heterostructures by X-ray diffraction, Appl. Phys. Lett. 50:1604 (1987)
4. E. A. Fitzgerald, D. G. Ast, P. D. Kirchner, G. D. Pettit and J. M. Woodall, Structure and recombination in InGaAs/GaAs heterostructures, J. Appl. Phys. 63:693 (1988)
5. M. Hockly, M. Al-Jassim, G. R. Booker and R. Nicklin, Electron microscope studies of VPE GaInAs layer structures suitable for use as infrared LEDs, J. Microscopy 118:117 (1980)

6. H. Strunk, W. Hagen and E. Bauser, Low-density dislocation arrays at heteroepitaxial Ge/GaAs-interfaces investigated by high voltage electron microscopy, Appl. Phys. 18:67 (1978)

7. A. M. Gomez and P. B. Hirsch, The dissociation of dislocations in GaAs, Phil. Mag. A 38:733 (1978)

8. H. Gottschalk, G. Patzer and H. Alexander, Stacking fault energy and ionicity of cubic III-V compounds, Phys. Stat. Sol. (a) 45:207 (1978)

9. J. W. Matthews and A. E. Blakeslee, Defects in epitaxial layers, J. Cryst. Growth 27:118 (1974)

10. W. Hagen and H. Strunk, A new type of source generating misfit dislocations, Appl. Phys. 17:85 (1978)

11. J. W. Matthews, Defects associated with the accommodation of misfit between crystals, J. Vac. Sci. Technol. 12:126 (1975)

12. C. A. Ball and J. H. Van der Merwe, The growth of dislocation-free layers, in: "Dislocations in Solids," F. R. N. Nabarro, ed., North Holland, Amsterdam (1983)

13. R. People and J. C. Bean, Calculation of critical layer thickness versus lattice mismatch for Ge_xSi_{1-x}/Si strained layer heterostructures, Appl. Phys. Lett. 47:322 (1985)

14. P. M. J. Maree, J. C. Barbour, J. F. van der Veen, K. L. Kavanagh, C. W. T. Bulle-Lieuwma and M. P. H. Viegers, Generation of misfit dislocations in semiconductors, J. Appl. Phys. 62:4413 (1987)

15. I. J. Fritz, P. L. Gourley and L. R. Dawson, Critical layer thickness in $In_{0.2}Ga_{0.8}As$/ GaAs single strained quantum well structures, Appl. Phys. Lett 51:1004 (1987)

16. P. L. Gourley, I. J. Fritz and L. R. Dawson, Controversy of critical layer thickness for InGaAs/GaAs strained-layer epitaxy, Appl. Phys. Lett. 52:377 (1988)

17. F. R. N. Nabarro, "Theory of Crystal Dislocations", Clarendon, Oxford (1967)

18. J. W. Matthews, S. Mader and T. B. Light, Accommodation of misfit across the interface between crystals of semiconducting elements or compounds, J. Appl. Phys. 41:3800 (1970)

19. G. R. Booker, J. M. Titchmarsh, J. Fletcher, D. B. Darby, M. Hockly and M. Al-Jassim, Nature, origin and effect of dislocations in epitaxial semiconductor layers, J. Cryst. Growth 45:407 (1978)

20. M. Gal, P. J. Orders, B. F. Usher, M. J. Joyce and J. Tann, Observation of compressive and tensile strains in InGaAs/GaAs by photoluminescence spectroscopy, Appl. Phys. Lett. 53:113 (1988)

21. S. A. Erofeeva and Y. A. Osip'yan, Mobility of dislocations in crystals with the sphalerite lattice, Sov. Phys. - Solid State 15:538 (1973)

22. H. Booyens, J. S. Vermaak and G. R. Proto, The asymmetric deformation of GaAs single crystals, J. Appl. Phys. 49:5435 (1978)

23. S. K. Choi, M. Mihara and T. Ninomiya, Dislocation Velocities in GaAs, Jap. J. Appl. Phys. 16:737 (1977)

24. G. A. Rozgonyi, P. M. Petroff and M. B. Panish, Control of lattice parameters and dislocations in the system $Ga_{1-x}Al_xAs_{1-y}P_y$/GaAs, J. Cryst. Growth 27:106 (1974)

25. H. Booyens, M. B. Small, R. M. Polemski and J. H. Basson, Misfit dislocations and the morphology of gallium aluminum arsenide epitaxial layers grown on gallium arsenide, J. Appl. Phys. 52:4328 (1981)

26. M. Hockly, TEM studies of defects in GaInAs and GaInP epitaxial layers, D. Phil thesis, Oxford (1983)

27. M. S. Abrahams, J. Blanc and C. J. Buiocchi, Like-sign asymmetric dislocations in zinc-blende structure, Appl. Phys. Lett. 21:185 (1972)

SUMMARY OF DISCUSSION ON INSTRUMENTAL REQUIREMENTS FOR THE EVALUATION OF ADVANCED SEMICONDUCTOR MATERIALS BY ELECTRON MICROSCOPY

J.M. Gibson

AT&T Bell Laboratories
Murray Hill, NJ 07974

The discussion was divided into three sections: 1) instruments for in-situ studies of surfaces; 2) funding of instruments in Europe and 3) general discussion of instrumentation and post-mortem on the workshop. Throughout the informal and animated discussions there were several common themes. There was enthusiastic response to the need for in-situ studies: that is the use of the electron microscope as other than a post-mortem method of characterizing structures and more as an experimental tool. This was viewed to be particularly important for semiconductors because of the need for complementary information and well-controlled conditions. The importance of complementary studies of the same sample, whether in-situ or ex-situ, was viewed as of paramount importance for progress with semiconductor science, particularly in understanding the relationship between electrical properties and structure. The semiconductor field, despite its "high-tech" image, still relies heavily on empiricism and reproducibility of electrical data is not of the highest level, even in the same lab. As a result, individual microscopists working only on the structural aspects of an otherwise uncharacterized material, will have less of value to contribute than the concerted collaborative effort involving complementary techniques. A final theme arose strongly during funding discussions and that was the need to present a coherent front as a community in stimulating grants.

1. Instruments for Surface Science

Following a lively day on electron microscopy of surfaces, some future ideas for surface instruments were discussed. Prof. Bauer had shown superb results from low energy electron microscopy which enables the identification of the microscopic features giving rise to details in a Low-Energy-Electron Diffraction (LEED) pattern. Furthermore any electron emission mechanism such as photo or thermionic emission can be imaged with angular information.

It was clear that such an instrument was of great value in surface studies but that there remained a role for high energy electron diffraction and imaging as has been exploited by Takayanagi (Tokyo U.) and Gibson (AT&T Bell Laboratories), and in new instruments coming on line at Arizona State University (A.S.U.) and elsewhere. The penetration and kinematical diffraction capabilities of transmission diffraction were seen as unique, and the surface sensitivity and spectroscopic capabilities of reflection electron diffraction also make it unique.

Spence (ASU) described the recently installed UHV HREM based on a Phillips 300kV EM 430 modified by GATAN Inc. The design maintains the $\sim 2\text{Å}$ spatial resolution of the EM430 with an ambient specimen vacuum $\sim 4 \times 10^{-9} \tau$ and extensive in-situ specimen thinning, cleaning and deposition capabilities. Dr. Bauer commented on the rather poor vacuum, a problem shared to a degree by Gibson's and Takayanagi's machines. The reason for such problems could be partly laid at the door of the design requirement for maintenance of high resolution. Because of this, the specimen is held between the polepieces of an immersion objective lens with very limited vacuum conductance, and facing large surface area of materials chosen for their magnetic and not their vacuum properties. It may become clear that some sacrifice in resolution is desirable in future in return for improved vacuum and alternative surface characterization.

Venables (Sussex/ASU) pointed out that until 1985 no company made ultra-high vacuum microscopes, as a preamble to his description of the new "MIDAS" machine at ASU made by Vacuum Generators. This field-emission Scanning Transmission Electron Microscope (STEM) is fully equipped with preparation facilities in a special chamber, with no facilities for *in-situ* studies directly. It has a special lens design permitting the extraction of Auger electrons when the specimen is in the high-resolution imaging position: an exciting feature for simultaneous structural and chemical studies of surfaces at high resolution. Both the A.S.U. instruments are available as user facilities, although it is anticipated that most research will be done collaboratively with an inside expert. Note that A.S.U. has money for visiting specialists to spend extended periods of time working on collaborative projects.

John Spence described some initial results of a combined Scanning Tunneling Microscope (STM) and Reflection Electron Microscope (REM). This instrument promises important insight into the STM imaging process and the ability to improve the field of view from the conventional STM limit. Operating at the moment in a poor vacuum, Spence found the STM attracted contamination.

With regard to more ready access to clean surface studies, Mike Treacy (Exxon) stated that some catalytic specimens can be transferred in an inert atmosphere, using a glove bag, into a microscope and severe oxidation etc., can be inhibited. This direction could be proved useful for those without sophisticated UHV instruments and may be adequate for many purposes. One such purpose that came out in discussion of high resolution imaging is the poor signal to noise ratio of images arising from damage and contamination/oxidation films on specimen surfaces. If this can be removed chemically and air exposure avoided, significant improvement in quantitive accuracy may result.

Peter Dobson (Phillips) described an idea to improve time resolution in electron-beam studies of surfaces using photoelectron sources (Elsayd-Ali & Maurou, Appl. Phys. Lett. $\underline{52}$, 103 (1988)). Dobson also discussed combined optical photocurrent spectroscopy and diffraction using the RHEED beam as a "wire" contact to the specimen.

2. Funding of Instruments

Early one morning we convened to discuss the harsh reality of advanced instruments: the funding situation. B. Jouffrey (Toulouse) summarized the findings of last year's European meeting in Toulouse[1] on this subject. Taking the new JEOL 4000EX and Phillips EM430 instruments as an example, he noted that the European total (in 1987 = 16) is less than half the US total of 34 (Japan has 15). This discrepancy in investment is not uniform across all the sciences, for example in Raman laser labs the USA and France are equally well equipped.

Jouffrey stated that the existence of local industry helps to stimulate instrument sales e.g. with Vacuum Generators in England. However, it was noted that there are no transmission electron microscope manufacturers in the USA! Another point raised was the large number of young scientists leaving Europe to do postdoctoral studies in the USA, despite the fact that it is easy (in France) to get postdoctoral funding.

Dr. Jouffrey showed an impressive viewgraph of the future desires for electron microscopy, at the center of which lay, surprisingly, the Toulouse high-voltage microscope! The Toulouse meeting had decided that intermediate voltages $\sim$ 300 kV were ideally suited for materials studies but that field-emission guns (as yet unavailable at this voltage) were desirable for analytical work. Electron and X-ray spectroscopy, convergent beam diffraction, holography, surface studies, low temperature cryostages and luminescence were among the top future priorities of the Toulouse report.

In discussing ways to improve the funding situation in Europe, Jouffrey suggested more use of the European Economic Community (EEC). He noted that the French government funding through CNRS (Centre National pour Researches Scientifique) was very poor. The total annual equipment budget for scientific instruments last year through CNRS was 13,000,000 F.F. ($\sim$ $2,000,000) in basic research and about twice this for engineering sciences.

The European Committee for the Development of Science and Technology (CODEST) is an alternative source through the EEC which could be exploited by any member countries, particularly on co-operative ventures involving more than one country. There was considerable discussion about the success of lobbying for the synchrotron which will be funded through EEC. It was widely accepted that one serious political fault of the electron microscopy community is its lack of ability to create a united front in political matters affecting its future. This was recognized to be a world-wide problem.

This theme arose again in a presentation by Colin Humphreys on the funding siluation within the United Kingdom aptly entitled "Microscopic Funding Levels in the U.K.". He showed that matters had in fact improved considerably this year from the very low funding levels of £ 0.2M in 1981/82 for electron microscopes to £ 1.6M from from the Science & Engineering Research Council (SERC).

After the dreadful situation in 1981/82 in which £ 4M of applications competed for only £ 0.2M of awards, an SERC working party was set up to investigate "proper" levels of funding. This concluded an outlay of £ 1.44M per annum at 1983 prices was an absolute minimum annual investment, in addition a 30% contribution from universities was expected. It is hoped that funding levels can be maintained at recent levels in the future. The moral of the story is that "materials people got their act together and said that funding was dreadful", again stressing the need for coherent policy with regard to funding bodies.

Dr. Humphreys finally noted that the one remaining blight on the University funding landscape was the lack of direct involvement by the semiconductor industry, in contrast to the behavior of other materials industries.

3. Discussion of Future Instrumentation

On the last evening of the conference, in the midst of clearly flagging interest from the participants, it was ingeniously decided to convene the final discussion session in the bar: bringing the mountain to Mohammed as it were. A viewgraph projector was installed and a well lubricated and enjoyable discussion of future instrumental directions occurred. In addition a "post-mortem" was held on the conference itself.

One area which was well covered in the meeting and was seen as a frontier was "Atomistic Mechanisms of Thin Film Growth" (Spence, ASU). Obviously, in-situ studies will play a major role in this area. Amongst important areas which were missing from the meeting were holography and image processing. Particularly the field ion atom probe was seen as a very valuable instrument for studying chemical composition in semiconductors.

A major theme of the discussion became the reproducibility, or lack of it, which is involved in semiconductor characterization. Those directly involved in crystal growth (e.g. Dobson, Phillips) recognized the difficulty of achieving reproducible electrical results even from the same growth chamber in successive runs. Since it was widely accepted that the primary goal of semiconductor characterization was to understand the electrical properties, it was realized that isolated studies on structural aspects alone were of less and less value. The importance of close collaborations with crystal growers and electrical engineers was accepted. This has been easier in industrial laboratories but should be striven for in university studies also. The use of complementary techniques in characterizing semiconductor material was also stressed, even from a structural point-of-view. For example, electron microscopy suffers from the obviously small sample volume so that x-ray diffraction could be very useful in completing the overall picture. Rutherford ion backscattering and secondary ion mass spectroscopy also possess far better chemical sensitivity than analytical electron microscopy for uniform systems. On the other hand, P. Augustus (Plessey) had demonstrated an *inverse* correlation between X-ray double-crystal rocking curve half width and dislocation density in epitaxial GaAs on Si, stressing the importance of microscopic measurements.

Another frontier of semiconductor characterization in which electron microscopy was seen to have a major role was in the understanding of the electrical properties of defects. Individual defects can be studied by catholuminescence (Steeds, Bristol) and by low energy loss electron spectorscopy (Batson, IBM). In such studies it is not necessary to combine all the techniques in one instrument as specimen transfer through air between instruments is usually acceptable.

The provocative question was raised "Is Silicon an Advanced Electronic Material?" and the answer appears to be yes, there's still life in the old man yet. This was well illustrated in the conference program, where Si based studies equalled those in III-V's, although Dobson (Phillips) suggested that proprietary reasons may limit publication of III-V studies more than Si. Nonetheless, the use of heteroepitaxy clearly opens Si-based materials to new scientific and technological horizons and studies can be more scientifically fruitful since Si itself is a better understood and characterized material.

High resolution electron microscopy was discussed and it was accepted that although image processing is useful, improvement of a poor signal-to-noise ratio by obtaining cleaner and flatter samples is desired. Quantification of HREM is seen as the next frontier to allow estimation of validity for models. Clearly inelastic scattering must be included in calculations (even if excluded from images by spectroscopy (Stobbs, Cambridge), due to its effect on elastic multiple scattering). Several people raised questions about potential errors in image simulation programs and proposed a "round-robin" error-checking exercise on these complex pieces of code in routine use.

The participants expressed overall satisfaction, indeed pleasure, with the content of the workshop. It was widely agreed that David Cherns' idea of well-focussed sessions covering specific topics, although prone to missing some areas, was very successful in elucidating sensible discussion and illuminating the common problems and successes of microscopy in the characterization of advanced semiconducting materials. For his pivotal role in running a very successful and timely workshop, David Cherns should be widely applauded.

4. References

1. European Workshop on the "Future of Electron Microscopy-Prospects and Instrumentation," Toulouse, Jan. 1987, Final Report ed., B. Jouffrey.